Handbook of
Child Behavior Therapy

Issues in Clinical Child Psychology

Series Editors: **Michael C. Roberts,** *University of Kansas–Lawrence, Kansas*
Lizette Peterson, *University of Missouri–Columbia, Missouri*

A Continuation Order Plan is available for this series. A continuation order will bring delivery of each new volume immediately upon publication. Volumes are billed only upon actual shipment. For further information please contact the publisher.

Handbook of
Child Behavior Therapy

Edited by

T. Steuart Watson
Mississippi State University
Starkville, Mississippi

and

Frank M. Gresham
University of California, Riverside
Riverside, California

Plenum Press • New York and London

Library of Congress Cataloging-in-Publication Data

Handbook of child behavior therapy / edited by T. Steuart Watson and
  Frank M. Gresham.
        p.   cm. -- (Issues in clinical child psychology)
    Includes bibliographical references and index.
    ISBN 0-306-45548-X
    1. Behavior therapy for children.   I. Watson, T. Steuart.
  II. Gresham, Frank M.   III. Series.
  RJ505.B4H346 1997
  618:92'89142--dc21   97-40442
                                                                 CIP

ISBN 0-306-45548-X   6/21/99

© 1998 Plenum Press, New York
A Division of Plenum Publishing Corporation
233 Spring Street, New York, N.Y. 10013

http://www.plenum.com

10 9 8 7 6 5 4 3 2 1

Printed in the United States of America

To Dorothy, for her unwavering strength and support, and to Mackenzie, Tucker, and Addison, who put life events into proper perspective and who make it all worthwhile

—T. S. W.

To my son Matt, whose attitude toward life and will to survive stands as a model of inspiration to me and his mother, Laura

—F. M. G.

Contributors

Keith D. Allen • Division of Pediatric Psychology, Munroe-Meyer Institute for Genetics and Rehabilitation, and University of Nebraska Medical Center, Omaha, Nebraska 68198-5450

Robert T. Ammerman • Allegheny General Hospital, Department of Psychiatry, MCP♦ Hahnemann School of Medicine, Allegheny University of the Health Sciences, Pittsburgh, Pennsylvania 15212

Phillip J. Belfiore • Education Division, Mercyhurst College, Erie, Pennsylvania 16546

Brad Donohue • Center for Psychological Studies, Nova Southeastern University, Fort Lauderdale, Florida 33314

George J. DuPaul • School Psychology Program, Lehigh University, Bethlehem, Pennsylvania 18015-4793

V. Mark Durand • Department of Psychology, University at Albany, State University of New York, Albany, New York 12222

Patrick C. Friman • Father Flanagan's Boys' Home, Boys Town, Nebraska 68010; and Creighton University School of Medicine, Omaha, Nebraska 68178-0001

Peter Gernert-Dott • Department of Psychology, University at Albany, State University of New York, Albany, New York 12222

Frank M. Gresham • School of Education, University of California–Riverside, Riverside, California 92521-0102

Kathryn E. Hoff • School Psychology Program, Lehigh University, Bethlehem, Pennsylvania 18015-4793

Jeffrey M. Hutchinson • Education Division, Mercyhurst College, Erie, Pennsylvania 16546

Kevin M. Jones • Father Flanagan's Boys' Home, Boys Town, Nebraska 68010

Christopher A. Kearney • Department of Psychology, University of Nevada–Las Vegas, Las Vegas, Nevada 89154-5030

Katina M. Lambros • School of Education, University of California–Riverside, Riverside, California 92521-0102

Jeff Laurent • Department of Psychology, Illinois State University, Normal, Illinois 61790-4620

Thomas R. Linscheid • Division of Psychology/Pediatrics, Children's Hospital/The Ohio State University, Columbus, Ohio 43205

Amy B. Mace • School Psychology Program, Lehigh University, Bethlehem, Pennsylvania 18015-3094

F. Charles Mace • The University of Pennsylvania and Children's Seashore House, Philadelphia, Pennsylvania 19104

Eileen Mapstone • Department of Psychology, University at Albany, State University of New York, Albany, New York 12222

Judith R. Matthews • Division of Pediatric Psychology, Munroe-Meyer Institute for Genetics and Rehabilitation, and University of Nebraska Medical Center, Omaha, Nebraska 68198-5450

Joan Mayfield • Division of Pediatric Psychology, Munroe-Meyer Institute for Genetics and Rehabilitation, and University of Nebraska Medical Center, Omaha, Nebraska 68198-5450

Janice McAllister • Division of Pediatric Neurology, University of Nebraska Medical Center, Omaha, Nebraska 68198-2165

Colleen M. McMahon • School of Education, University of California–Riverside, Riverside, California 92521-0102

Raymond G. Miltenberger • Department of Psychology, North Dakota State University, Fargo, North Dakota 58105

Jodi Mindell • Department of Psychology, St. Joseph's University, Philadelphia, Pennsylvania 19131-1395

George H. Noell • Department of Psychology, Louisiana State University, Baton Rouge, Louisiana 70803-5501

Lizette Peterson • Department of Psychology, University of Missouri–Columbia, Columbia, Missouri 65211

Kirsten I. Potter • Department of Psychology, Illinois State University, Normal, Illinois 61790-4620

Patrick R. Progar • The University of Pennsylvania and Children's Seashore House, Philadelphia, Pennsylvania 19104

Sheri L. Robinson • School Psychology Program, Mississippi State University, Mississippi State, Mississippi 39762

Lisa Saldana • Department of Psychology, University of Missouri–Columbia, Columbia, Missouri 65211

Mark D. Shriver • Division of Pediatric Psychology, Munroe-Meyer Institute for Genetics and Rehabilitation, and University of Nebraska Medical Center, Omaha, Nebraska 68198-5450

Christopher H. Skinner • School Psychology Program, Mississippi State University, Mississippi State, Mississippi 39762

Jeffrey Sprague • College of Education, University of Oregon, Eugene, Oregon 97403

Heather Elise Sterling • School Psychology Program, Mississippi State University, Mississippi State, Mississippi 39762

George Sugai • College of Education, University of Oregon, Eugene, Oregon 97403

Judith A. Sylva • School of Education, University of California–Riverside, Riverside, California 92521-0102

Cheryl A. Tillotson • Department of Psychology, University of Nevada–Las Vegas, Las Vegas, Nevada 89154-5030

Timothy R. Vollmer • The University of Pennsylvania and Children's Seashore House, Philadelphia, Pennsylvania 19104

Hill Walker • College of Education, University of Oregon, Eugene, Oregon 97403

William J. Warzak • Department of Psychology, Munroe-Meyer Institute for Genetics and Rehabilitation, and University of Nebraska Medical Center, Omaha, Nebraska 68198-5450

T. Steuart Watson • School Psychology Program, Mississippi State University, Mississippi State, Mississippi 39762

Donald A. Williamson • Department of Psychology, Louisiana State University, Baton Rouge, Louisiana 70803-3103

Joseph C. Witt • Department of Psychology, Louisiana State University, Baton Rouge, Louisiana 70803-5501

Leslie G. Womble • Department of Psychology, Louisiana State University, Baton Rouge, Louisiana 70803-3103

Douglas W. Woods • Department of Psychology, Western Michigan University, Kalamazoo, Michigan 49008

Kathleen Zelis • Center for Psychological Studies, Nova Southeastern University, Fort Lauderdale, Florida 33314

Nancy L. Zucker • Department of Psychology, Louisiana State University, Baton Rouge, Louisiana 70803-3103

Preface

The genesis of this book occurred several years ago in Seattle on the veranda of a Chilean cafe overlooking Pikes Place Market during a National Association of School Psychologists conference. We were discussing, along with several other behavioral school psychologists, how the field of child behavior analysis and therapy has experienced rapid growth over the past forty years, but lamenting that books in the area did not reflect the advancements made in the assessment and treatment of a wide variety of problem behaviors evidenced by children. That is not to say that there are no good books available to the child behavior therapist. In fact, most readers of this book undoubtedly have bookshelves lined with noteworthy volumes on this very topic. What was missing, in our opinion, was a book reflecting the relationship between assessment and treatment, more specifically functional assessment/analysis, and describing the process a clinician uses when treating a particular behavior problem.

Without diminishing the contributions of the many excellent books on child behavior therapy currently available, it seems that most have followed a formula or "cookbook" approach. That is, the authors give a brief introduction to the topic, discuss possible etiologies and contributing factors, and then review the assessment and treatment literature on that topic. Although there is nothing patently wrong with this approach, it seems to communicate the wrong message to the reader; namely that the function of a behavior is less important than knowing what treatment to implement. We believe that effective treatment arises from a process: identifying the problem behavior, discerning the function of a behavior, formulating an intervention, and evaluating that intervention. In essence, effective intervention is more than just knowing what has worked in the past. Thus, the aim of this book is to provide readers with not only the "what to do" of child behavior therapy, but the "how to do it" as well. Each of the chapters guides the reader through the clinical decision-making process, from identifying a problem to evaluating the effectiveness of a chosen intervention.

One of the difficulties in assembling an edited book is ensuring a high degree of continuity and similarity between chapters, without infringing on the individual writing style of the authors. This book is certainly no exception. To help with continuity, we provided the authors with an outline to use as a guide as they prepared their manuscripts. The operative word here is "guide." Authors were free to alter the outline but not so dramatically as to violate the basic premise of the book. For example, prevention of injuries is an extremely important social concern for anyone involved in the care and treatment of children. It is not, however, a traditional area where a behavior therapist would intervene in a clinical setting. Therefore, the outline we provided did not readily accommodate the information on this topic. It was then up to the chapter authors (Saldana and Peterson, in this case) to modify the headings as necessary while maintaining as much integrity as possible with the original intent of the book. Thus, in comparing the structure of the chapters, the reader will notice that authors have taken a degree of liberty in describing the assessment and treatment process and in deciding what information goes under each major heading.

Many radical behaviorists or applied behavior analysts who read a couple of the chapters in this book will undoubtedly be offended by the occasional use of the "c" word: cognitive. Those who will be offended are reminded to say "intraverbal behavior" every time they read "cognitive" to reduce the unpleasantness associated with this word.

At first, we were tempted to inform authors to either avoid "cognitive" or recast the information in behavioral terms. We resisted this impulse for several reasons: (1) as long as the information is empirical, it should not be summarily discarded; (2) it does not harm behavior analysts to read chapters from a less than radical behavioral perspective so that they may learn what is happening outside their field; and (3) it allows the behavior analyst to reinterpret what the authors have written, thus strengthening their verbal repertoire regarding behavior analysis.

The organization of a book is important for many reasons, the primary reason being that it provides a conceptual context that communicates to the reader what the authors/editors deem important. The organization of this book attempts to communicate the notion of the importance of ecological considerations in the identification, assessment, treatment, and evaluation of child behavior problems. Thus, we grouped problem behaviors into the settings where the problem is usually manifested/identified, assessed, treated, and evaluated, all the while realizing that such clear distinctions do not often exist. We also included a "Foundations" section that provides basic information in important adjunctive areas of child behavior therapy: behavioral assessment, single subject research designs, and behavioral consultation. Without a working knowledge of the information within each of these adjunctive areas, the behavior therapist is little more than a technician implementing a prescribed treatment protocol.

The two overriding themes of this book are functional assessment/analysis and behavioral consultation. We stress functional assessment in addition to experimental functional analysis with the acknowledgment that practitioners will use the former most of the time as opposed to the latter. Functional assessment/analysis provides a *methodology* by which to identify the variables that are related to a specific problem so that the likelihood of treatment effectiveness is greatly enhanced. Behavioral consultation is a *process* that one uses when working with parents, teachers, or other behavior change agents to deliver psychological services, including functional analysis. We hope that by presenting assessment and treatment from a behavioral consultation perspective, where functional analysis is the primary methodology for designing interventions, both experienced and novice behavior therapists will learn new skills and approaches for a wide array of child problems.

Completing a book requires inordinate amounts of time, energy, and assistance and credit to many individuals. Our foremost appreciation is extended to the chapter authors who delivered manuscripts that exceeded our expectations in terms of quality and innovativeness. Our editor, Mariclaire Cloutier, first approved the prospectus and saw the potential in a book espousing a different method and approach for treating child behavior problems. Mariclaire dispensed valuable advice to a relative novice (TSW) and was also extremely patient and considerate when intervening circumstances made completion of this book difficult. Lizette Peterson and Michael Roberts, co-editors of Plenum's Issues in Clinical Child Psychology series, helped to organize and shape the content into a meaningful and coherent text for the reader. We sincerely thank our behavioral colleagues in school psychology, pediatric psychology, and child-clinical psychology for their support of this idea and for their many suggestions. Finally, we thank our families for their enduring support and encouragement, not only for completing the project, but for making it easier for us to produce a quality book.

T. Steuart Watson
Frank M. Gresham

Contents

Handbook of
Child Behavior Therapy

I

Foundations of Child Behavior Therapy

The chapters in this section present some of the basic elements necessary for the practice of effective child behavior therapy. Although the more experienced behavior analyst/therapist will be conversant with the content of these chapters, the novice or less seasoned behavior therapist must have a conceptual basis for applying the knowledge detailed in subsequent chapters. These three chapters are intended to provide that conceptual basis. Although there are many topics that may be considered essential for the practice of child behavior therapy, we have chosen three that permeate both the science and practice of the field and that are integral for reading this book. These chapters are not meant to be comprehensive treatments of the literature, but rather descriptions of how to utilize the knowledge already available to approach treatment, assess behavior, and evaluate behavior change.

Accurate assessment of behavior is a hallmark of behavioral psychology. Chapter 1, "Behavioral and Functional Assessment," is intended as a conceptual organizer or setting event for functional assessment information that follows in each of the chapters. Gresham does not evaluate specific behavioral assessment methods, rather he reviews the philosophy, assumptions, principles, and issues in behavioral and functional assessment.

One only has to look at the major journals that publish behavior change articles to see that single-subject designs are the preferred method for evaluating the effects of a chosen intervention. Many people mistakenly believe that single-subject designs are synonomous with case studies, in which and treatments are described without any emphasis on measuring behavior change. Knowing how to evaluate behavioral change using single-subject methodology is an absolute requirement for anyone working in an applied setting or conducting treatment-related research. Gresham, in Chapter 2, describes the most common designs used in applied settings, the advantages and disadvantages associated with each design, and the conceptual principles that govern the evaluation process.

John Bergan (1977) presented what has become one of the most widely used problem-solving models in psychology. Since that time, many articles have been written attesting to the effectiveness of Bergan's Behavioral Consultation model for providing a methodology for delivering behavioral services to clients. As with any model of service delivery, questions emerge that challenge some of the assumptions and practices inherent in the model. Behavioral consultation is certainly no different. Noell and Witt (Chapter 3) present some of the recent challenges and questions surrounding the practice of behavioral consultation and provide directions for more fully integrating behavioral technology within the consultation paradigm.

Reference

Bergan, J.R. (1977). *Behavioral consultation*. Columbus, OH: Charles E. Merrill.

1

Behavioral and Functional Assessment

FRANK M. GRESHAM AND KATINA M. LAMBROS

Introduction

As a specialty, behavioral assessment is relatively new in the broad field of psychological assessment. In 1979, two new journals devoted exclusively to behavioral assessment were published: *Behavioral Assessment* (by the Association for Advancement of Behavior Therapy), edited by Rosemary Nelson, and *Journal of Behavioral Assessment* (now *Journal of Behavioral Assessment and Psychopathology*), edited by Henry Adams. Although behavioral assessment procedures certainly predated the publication of these journals, the creation of these outlets gave formal recognition to the behavioral approach to assessment. In the inaugural editorial statement for *Behavioral Assessment,* R. Nelson (1979) described behavioral assessment as follows:

> Behavioral assessment is broadly conceived to include assessment, design, methodology, statistics, dependent variables, and program evaluation, regardless of population or setting. Behavioral assessment is distinguished from other types of assessment in its emphasis on meaningful response units and on their controlling variables (both environmental and organismic) and to its responsiveness to intervention strategies. . . . Behavioral assessment excludes trait assumptions and sign-oriented approaches to measurement. While psychometric procedures may be applied to behavioral techniques, traditional conceptualization is generally incompatible with a behavioral approach. (p. i)

Although behavioral assessment shares many of the same methods with "traditional" assessment,

these two broad approaches differ dramatically in the assumptions they make about behavior, its "causes" or controlling variables, and the use of assessment information for treatment planning and evaluation. Generally speaking, behavioral assessment is based on a situational analysis of discrete, observable behaviors; judges behavioral performances relative to the individual (idiographic) rather than to others (nomothetic); uses low levels of inference in interpreting these behavioral performances; and looks to current environmental events as maintaining behavior (A.R. Ciminero, 1986; Shapiro & Kratochwill, 1988). In short, behavioral assessment involves the measurement of meaningful response units and their controlling variables for the purposes of understanding and altering human behavior (R.O. Nelson & Hayes, 1979).

More recently, experts within the applied behavior analysis camp have distinguished between functional *assessment* and functional *analysis.* Functional *assessment* refers to a full range of procedures used to identify potential controlling variables (antecedents and consequences) on behavior (Horner, 1994). Functional *analysis,* on the other hand, refers to the experimental manipulation of environmental events under tight experimental conditions to identify the environmental determinants of specific behaviors in an individual's repertoire (Iwata, Dorsey, Slifer, Bauman, & Richman, 1982; Neef & Iwata, 1994). Not all functional assessment procedures (e.g., interviews, ratings) yield functional analytic information. Functional analysis is but one type of functional assessment, and perhaps is the most important aspect of assessment, because it verifies that a given environmental event (e.g., escape, social attention, self-stimulation) controls problem behavior (Carr, 1994).

FRANK M. GRESHAM AND KATINA M. LAMBROS • School of Education, University of California–Riverside, Riverside, California 92521-0102.

Handbook of Child Behavior Therapy, edited by Watson and Gresham. Plenum Press, New York, 1998.

The purpose of this chapter is to provide an overview of the philosophy, assumptions, and issues in behavioral and functional assessment. We distinguish between behavioral and functional assessment because not all behavioral assessment yields information about the function(s) of behavior. We do not review specific behavioral assessment methods except for illustrative purposes. Each of the chapters in this book describes its own set of behavioral and/or functional assessment procedures that are used in problem identification, problem analysis, and treatment evaluation. This chapter is intended to provide a conceptual organizer or setting event for the chapters that follow. It will become clear after reading this book that some behavior problems and response classes are more amenable to certain behavioral assessment or functional assessment procedures than others. We will highlight this in our discussion of specific procedures and classes of behavior.

Epistemologies in Traditional and Behavioral Assessment

In order to provide a context for discussing behavioral assessment, it is instructive to consider differing epistemologies of behavioral and traditional assessment models. Differential interpretations of assessment information in traditional and behavioral assessment are based on fundamental assumptions each model makes about the nature of human behavior. These assumptions represent extremes of each position and, as such, focus on virtually opposite interpretations of the meaning of assessment data. We realize that these assumptions fall on a continuum rather than into a strict dichotomy. For example, within the behavioral assessment camp, there are factions closer to what might be considered a traditional assessment viewpoint than to a purely *behavioral* assessment viewpoint. This is particularly true of behavior problems that reside primarily in the cognitive response mode (e.g., depression, anxiety, and obsessions). On the other hand, those persons operating out of a strict applied behavior analytic framework would more closely parallel what we will present as assumptions within behavioral assessment.

Kurt Lewin (1931) detailed fundamental differences between two approaches in psychology in his paper entitled "The Conflict Between Aris-

totelian and Galilean Modes of Thought in Contemporary Psychology." Lewin suggested that an Aristotelian approach to psychology views behavior as being caused by person variables, much as Aristotle believed that properties of physical objects caused them to "behave" in certain ways. There is a direct parallel between an Aristotelian mode of thought and personality trait theories, in that both view behavior as being manifestations of (i.e., "caused" by) within-person variables. Moreover, an Aristotelian philosophy of psychology views the frequent as scientifically lawful and utilizes group statistical methods to determine "truth." Thus, members of a particular group whose measured behavior is different from the average of the group are considered to have "error" in their measured behavior. Also, an individual whose score changes its relative position in a distribution of scores from Time 1 to Time 2 (in the absence of treatment or maturation) is considered to have error in measured behavior. Error in both cases is defined as deviations from an average score of a group or change in the relative ordinal position in a group.

In contrast, Lewin's interpretation of a Galilean approach to psychology views behavior as being caused by a person-X–environment interaction and considers all behavior lawful. An individual's measured behavior in a group is not considered to have error and is considered just as lawful as the group's measured behavior. An individual following a Galilean approach would seek to identify the conditions under which a person's behavior occurs. If identified, these conditions obviously cannot contribute to errors of measurement. Data analysis in a Galilean world employs single-subject (idiographic) designs using subjects as their own controls. A good example of a Galilean approach to assessment is curriculum-based assessment in which academic deficits are viewed as being functionally related to classroom environmental variables occurring contiguously to academic behavior (Fuchs & Fuchs, 1986; Lentz & Shapiro, 1986).

To summarize, traditional and behavioral assessment evolved, in part, from two distinct philosophies of science. Traditional assessment and measurement follows an Aristotelian approach based on nomothetic comparisons. Behavioral assessment and measurement typically takes more of a Galilean path based on idiographic comparisons. Skinner (1953) made a similar distinction in his discussion of *conceptual inner causes* of behavior. Traits or characteristics, for many psychologists working from an Aristotelian epistemology, are believed to cause behavior. We believe that this is the most popular viewpoint of psychologists and lay persons alike. In this approach, the trait of aggression causes aggressive behavior, a person drinks because he has a drinking habit, or a person plays the flute well because of her musical ability. Those psychologists operating out of a Galilean epistemology do not accept these conceptual inner causes of behavior, but rather rely on functional assessment/analysis information to explain the occurrence of behavior.

Core Assumptions

As previously mentioned, there are several camps within behavioral psychology in general and behavioral assessment in particular, (e.g., applied behavior analysis, social learning theory, cognitive–behavioral psychology) and these camps fall somewhere on a continuum regarding core assumptions each makes about the meaning of assessment data. All camps could probably the generally agree on some core assumptions governing behavioral assessment. The following assumptions represent a distillation of views from each camp within behavioral assessment. These assumptions are based, in part, on the writings of pioneers in the field of behavioral assessment (e.g., Cone, 1978, 1979; Goldfried & Kent, 1972; Hartmann, Roper, & Bradford, 1979; R.O. Nelson & Hayes, 1979).

Causes of Behavior

A fundamental assumption of behavioral assessment is that the causes or maintaining conditions of behavior exist in the current environment. This stands in direct contrast to traditional assessment which looks to either intrapsychic factors or traits as causative of human behavior. Some behavioral assessors acknowledge that temporally and situationally remote environmental events can occasion and maintain behavior. This can be either setting events (R. Wahler & Fox, 1981) or establishing operations (Michael, 1993).

Other behavioral assessors view unobservable behaviors such as cognitive behavior as being causative of some behavior problems (Meichenbaum,

1977; Mahoney, 1974; Kendall & Cummings, 1988). Depression is a classic example of this type of problem (see Laurent, this volume). S.C. Hayes and Hayes (1992) suggested that cognitive-behavior therapists view thoughts as being causative of overt behavior (e.g., Frank's negative self thoughts cause him to engage in a depressed behavior pattern). More traditional behavior therapists, however, would take an opposite view in that overt behavior is seen as influencing thoughts (Frank's depressed behavior pattern causes him to think negatively about himself). A contextualistic behaviorism would view thought–behavior as well as behavior–behavior relationships as being reciprocally or bidirectionally causative (e.g., Frank's depressed behavior pattern causes negative thoughts and negative thoughts contribute to Frank's depressed behavior pattern) (S.C. Hayes & Hayes, 1992).

Still other behaviorists, such as applied behavior analysts, distinguish between *causes* and *correlates* of behavior (Iwata et al., 1982; Horner, 1994). Functional analysis, an experimental demonstration of the function of behavior, is viewed as causative, whereas functional assessment, which looks at the temporal relationships between antecedents and consequences and the occurrence of behavior, is viewed as correlational. A fundamental difference between cognitive–behavioral and applied behavior analytic views of causation is the *observability,* and hence the *accessibility,* of the covert behavior that is considered causative in the occurrence of overt behavior.

Situational Specificity

Another core assumption of behavioral assessment is that behavior is considered a sample of behavior in a specific situation. This assumption views behavior as being maintained primarily by the environmental events present at that time in a given situation or setting. Although setting events and establishing operations can be functionally related to behavior in other settings and situations, the emphasis of behavioral assessment is clearly on temporally and situationally contiguous environmental events and behavior.

A major implication of the situational specificity assumption is that behavior that is assessed under a restricted range of assessment conditions might be generalizable only to those restricted sets of environmental conditions. For example, the behavior of a child assessed in the psychologist's office may not be generalizable to behavior of that child in the classroom the next day. R.G. Wahler (1975) showed that clusters of behavior in the home setting were not generalizable to those same behavioral clusters in the school setting.

The situational specificity assumption dictates that behavioral assessors obtain a representative sample of behavior in a representative sample of situations. In other words, this assumption implies that the results of a behavioral assessment should not be generalized beyond the settings and/or situations in which the behavior samples were obtained. This assumption creates difficulties for psychologists who restrict their assessments only to clinic or other restricted settings.

Treatment Validity

Treatment validity, sometimes referred to as treatment utility, refers to the degree to which assessment information contributes to beneficial treatment outcome(s) (S. Hayes, Nelson, & Jarrett, 1987). A key distinguishing feature of behavior therapy is the clear relationship between assessment data collected and treatment planning. This holds true not only for applied behavior analysts, but also for social learning and cognitive–behavioral theorists. For example, an applied behavior analyst conducting a brief functional analysis documenting that a problem behavior is maintained by social attention might select a treatment utilizing extinction for problem behavior and differential reinforcement of other behavior (DRO). A therapist operating out of a social learning framework might assess social self-efficacy to design a treatment using a combination of performance accomplishments and modeling to increase the frequency and enhance the quality of social skills performances. A cognitive–behavior therapist treating a child's social anxiety might teach the child progressive relaxation exercises coupled with positive self-talk regarding social interactions with peers. In each case, there is a direct link between assessment information and intervention strategies. What differs in each of the above cases is what is assessed and its relationship to the design of treatment (e.g., social attention, self-efficacy, or self-statements).

Although the concept of treatment validity evolved from the behavioral assessment field, it shares several characteristics and concepts with the traditional psychometric validity literature. One, treatment validity is based, in part, on Sechrest's (1963) notion of incremental validity, in that it requires that an assessment procedure improve prediction above and beyond existing assessment procedures. Two, treatment validity contains the idea of utility and cost-benefit analysis, which is common in the personnel selection literature (Mischel, 1968; Wiggins, 1973). Three, treatment validity is related to Messick's (1995) evidential basis for test interpretation and use, particularly as it relates to construct validity, relevance/utility, and social consequences. It is entirely possible for an assessment procedure to have construct validity, but to have little relevance or utility for a particular use of that assessment for treatment planning (i.e., treatment validity) (S. Hayes et al., 1987). Treatment validity is a fundamental assumption of behavioral assessment. For any assessment procedure to have treatment validity it must lead to identification of target behaviors, result in more effective treatments, and be helpful in evaluating treatment outcomes.

Level of Inference

Level of inference refers to the relationship between behavior actually observed and the interpretation, meaning, and/or generalizability of that observation to other situations, settings, or times. The level of inference can range on a continuum from simple, straightforward, precise descriptions of what was seen or observed (no inference) to quite abstract and remote interpretations of the meaning of behavior (high inference). Behavioral assessment relies on relatively low levels of inference to interpret assessment data.

Standards for Educational and Psychological Testing (American Psychological Association, 1985) defines validity as the degree to which empirical evidence supports the inferences made from test scores. That is, what is validated in assessment are the *inferences* drawn from assessment and not assessment instruments per se. In behavioral assessment, the meaning of "test scores" is relatively straightforward because low levels of inference are used to interpret rather straightforward assessment data. For example, frequencies, durations, and rates of behavior require little or no inference for accurate interpretation. Behavioral assessment uses a *sample* interpretation rather than a *sign* interpretation of assessment data. That is, behavior is interpreted as a sample of some behavior or response class of interest in a specific situation rather than as a sign of some underlying personality trait or characteristic (Goldfried & Kent, 1972).

It should be noted that some behavioral assessors rely on more inferences than do others in their assessments. For example, behavioral assessors utilizing analogue behavioral role-play tests to assess social skills *infer* that these performances can be generalized to social skill performances in naturalistic settings. Similarly, behavioral assessors conducting a problem identification interview with a teacher about a student's disruptive behavior rely on the inference that this information represents the student's typical classroom disruption. In both cases, inferences are being made that this *indirect* assessment information represents direct behavioral performances.

In contrast, applied behavior analysts collecting durations of negative social interactions on the playground or observational data on rates of classroom disruption do not have to make such cross-setting inferences. What is inferred, however, is that these observations represent *typical* behavioral performances that can be generalized to other observation sessions. This point will be discussed in more detail in the section on the quality of behavioral assessment data.

Idiographic Bias

Two contrasting approaches to behavioral assessment have been described by Cone (1986, 1988): the *nomothetic-trait approach* and the *idiographic-behavior approach.* In the nomothetic-trait approach, the focus is on assessing syndromes or characteristics such as depression, conduct disorder, or hyperactivity, using norm-referenced instruments (e.g., ratings scales, structured or semistructured interviews, self-reports). An individual is classified as atypical or having the syndrome based on his or her relative position in a distribution of scores. For example, T-scores of 70 and above (>98th percentile) on a teacher and parent behavior rating scale might be used as indicators of hyperactivity. An individual's status as having or not having a syndrome is based on how far his or her scores deviate from the average or

typical score of some group of individuals. Cone (1986, 1988) argues that while assessment based on norm-referenced instruments may be useful for describing differences among individuals, they are not sensitive enough to be used to evaluate the effects or outcomes of interventions.

The idiographic-behavior approach focuses on the assessment of specific behaviors of individuals and measuring these behaviors repeatedly over time. This is clearly the emphasis in an applied behavior analytic approach to behavioral assessment and is the primary approach advocated in this book. An idiographic-behavior approach to assessment rests on the intensive study of individual cases using assessment procedures that are sensitive to intervention effects and which can be administered repeatedly over time without being reactive. An idiographic-behavior approach develops its assessment procedures *inductively* in collecting a large amount of data on relatively few individuals. In contrast, the nomothetic-trait approach develops its assessment procedures *deductively* in gathering a relatively small amount of data on a large number of individuals. Although both approaches are used in behavioral assessment, the idiographic-behavior approach is more useful for target behavior selection, customizing interventions, and evaluating treatment outcomes.

Repeated Measurement

A hallmark of applied behavior analysis and behavior therapy is the repeated measurement of behavior over time. Unlike traditional group experimental designs using repeated measures (e.g., pretest–posttest designs), behavioral approaches use much more frequent measurements of behavior both during baseline and intervention phases. The individual's baseline levels of performance are used as the criterion against which treatment effects are compared or evaluated.

This repeated measurement yields *intrasubject variability,* which in and of itself can be used as a basis for functional analysis. That is, intrasubject variability may be functionally related to specifiable environmental and/or physiological stimulus or setting events. In short, variability in the repeated measurement of a single individual is viewed as data that can be identified, isolated, functionally analyzed, and controlled. Readers will note, in the chapters to follow, that authors advocate the repeated measurement of behavior over time to establish baseline levels of behavior, to evaluate responsiveness to treatment, and to evaluate treatment outcomes.

Conceptual Principles for Behavioral Assessment

Table 1 presents a behavioral assessment model that is a useful heuristic for guiding practitioners through the assessment of any given behavior problem. The assessment model presented in Table 1 is an extension of the Behavioral Assessment Grid (BAG) first proposed by Cone (1978). Note that this model is based on the concurrent consideration of six major aspects of behavioral assessment: (1) the direction or nature of the behavior problem(s) (excesses, deficits, and situational inappropriateness), (2) the dimensions of behavior assessed (e.g., frequency, intensity,

duration), (3) the repertoire or system through which behaviors are expressed (i.e., cognitive–verbal, overt–motoric, or physiological–emotional), (4) the methods used to assess behavior (e.g., functional interviews, ratings by others, direct observations), (5) the quality of assessment data, and (6) social validity.

Many of the components and concepts presented in Table 1 have been discussed extensively elsewhere in the behavioral assessment literature (see Bellack & Hersen, 1988; A. Ciminero, Calhoun, & Adams, 1986; Shapiro & Kratochwill, 1988). We present several "rules," or guiding principles, for translating the behavioral assessment model in Table 1 into assessment practice. The following five principles are presented as a useful means of guiding the behavioral assessment process.

Principle of Problem Solving

The assessment model presented in Table 1 can be viewed as a problem-solving process similar to

TABLE 1. Behavioral Assessment Model

I. Type of behavior problem	2. Stability
A. Excess	3. Interobserver agreement
B. Deficit	B. Validity
C. Situationally inappropriate	1. Content
II. Dimensions of behavior	2. Criterion-related
A. Frequency	3. Convergent
B. Temporality	4. Discriminant
1. Duration	5. Treatment
2. Latency	C. Generalizability
3. Interresponse time	1. Observer
C. Intensity/magnitude	2. Behavior
D. Permanent products	3. Method
III. Behavioral repertoire	4. Time
A. Cognitive/verbal	5. Setting
B. Overt/motoric	6. Dimension
C. Physiological/emotional	D. Accuracy
IV. Methods of assessment	VI. Social validation
A. Direct methods	A. Social significance of goals
1. Naturalistic observations	1. Consumer opinions
2. Self-monitoring	2. Habilitative validity
3. Physiological monitoring	B. Social acceptability of procedures
B. Indirect methods	1. Pretreatment acceptability
1. Interviews	2. Posttreatment acceptability
2. Ratings by others	3. Use and integrity
3. Self-reports	C. Social importance of effects
4. Analogue role-play	1. Subjective judgments
5. Permanent products	2. Social comparisons
V. Quality of data	3. Combined social validation procedures
A. Reliability	4. Reliable change index
1. Internal consistency	5. Functional effects

the model of behavioral consultation provided by Bergan and Kratochwill (1990). In this model, consultation is divided into four stages: problem identification, problem analysis, plan implementation, and treatment evaluation. Indeed, these stages represent the conceptual outline for the chapters to follow in this text. Behavioral assessment can be conceptualized as consisting of these same four stages, in which the purposes of assessment are to identify behavioral excesses or deficits, analyze antecedent and consequent events maintaining behavioral excesses, differentiate acquisition from performance deficits, implement an intervention plan, and evaluate the effectiveness of the intervention plan.

Viewing behavioral assessment as a process of identifying and analyzing behavioral excesses and deficits as well as implementing and evaluating interventions for problem behaviors is a significant departure from the traditional process of classifying children using a system such as the *Diagnostic and Statistical Manual of Mental Disorders* (*DSM-IV*) (American Psychiatric Association, 1994), which is based on the topography rather than the function of behavior, and thereby has little or no treatment validity (see Gresham & Gansle, 1992). The problem-solving approach to behavioral assessment puts the behavioral assessor in the role of problem solver rather than that of an accountant who merely collects numbers and assigns sometimes questionable diagnoses based on this information.

Principle of Functional Assessment

Most assessment information collected using a traditional assessment model is not useful for designing interventions. For instance, intelligence tests, projective techniques, and standardized tests of academic achievement are virtually worthless for intervention purposes because, among other things, they do not identify the function(s) of behavior. Behavioral assessment, on the other hand, seeks to determine the relationship between environmental events and behavior such that these environmental events can be changed or manipulated to effect changes in behavior. This process is called the functional assessment of behavior.

Functional assessment describes the full range of procedures that can be used to identify the antecedents and consequences associated with the occurrence of behavior. *Functional analysis* refers to

the experimental manipulation of environmental events to assess their impact on the occurrence of behavior. Horner (1994) suggested that functional analysis is one approach to functional assessment. Mace (1994) indicated that treatment matched to the operant function of behavior follows two strategies: (a) weakening the maintaining response-reinforcer relationship (e.g., punishment or extinction) and (b) establishing or strengthening a response-reinforcer relationship for adaptive behavior that replaces the function of the inappropriate or maladaptive behavior (e.g., DRO, differential reinforcement of communicative behavior [DRC], or differential reinforcement of incompatible behavior [DRI]).

Functional assessment methods have been categorized as: (a) indirect, composed of interviews and rating scales, (b) direct or descriptive methods, consisting of systematic behavioral observations in naturalistic settings, and (c) experimental methods involving standardized experimental manipulations intended to isolate contingencies controlling problem behavior (see Mace, 1994). Both indirect and direct methods can be used to identify variables controlling behavior in naturalistic settings. However, only functional analysis can rule out other variables that are not functional in controlling behavior. A chief disadvantage of functional analysis methodologies is that they usually are conducted in analogue rather than naturalistic settings, thereby limiting their generalizability. A notable exception to this was the functional analyses reported by Lewis and Sugai (1996) in general education classroom settings.

Functional assessment and functional analysis methodologies have found that problem behaviors sometimes serve multiple functions. Carr (1994) suggested that problem behavior may be controlled by four categories: (a) social attention, (b) escape/avoidance of tasks, (c) sensory reinforcement, and (d) access to tangible items or events. Within each of these categories, there may be subcategories of controlling environmental events. For example, social attention may be peer-related or teacher-related; escape/avoidance may be task-related or socially related. The goal in functional assessment is to precisely identify the function of behavior so that interventions based on this assessment can be designed and implemented.

Carr (1993) provided an insightful critique of the goals and philosophy of behavior analysis which suggested that behavior analysts are primarily, if not exclusively, concerned with the *functions* of behavior. In this critique, Carr suggested:

> true behavior analysts have, paradoxically, very little interest in behavior. Thus, knowing that a young boy diagnosed as autistic exhibits self-injury is, by itself, not very interesting. What is interesting is why the self-injury occurs (i.e., of what variables is it a function). . . . Topography (behavior) does not matter much; function (purpose) does. . . . behavior is not the thing of interest to behavior analysts. (p. 48)

We believe that the logic just discussed applies to the behavior problems described in the following chapters. That is, the primary purpose of what is called "problem analysis" is to identify the function(s) of behavior. Once these functions are identified, interventions can be designed to change target behaviors.

Principle of Multiple Operationalism

A comprehensive model of behavioral assessment is based on the premise that behavior should be assessed from a variety of perspectives using a number of assessment methods and information sources. Table 1 lists a number of direct and indirect behavioral assessment methods that are used to assess children's behavior problems. It should be noted that for some behavioral difficulties, only one or two behavioral assessment methods are used. For example, assessment of self-injurious behavior and stereotypy (see Vollmer and Mace, this volume) relies almost exclusively on direct observations of behavior. In contrast, the assessment of social skills (see Gresham, this volume) uses multiple methods of assessment, including direct observations, ratings by teachers and parents, peer ratings and nominations, and self-reports.

The principle of multiple operationalism is based on the multimethod-multitrait (MTMM) approach to construct validation using the concepts of convergent and discriminant validity. Campbell and Fiske (1959) argued that validity evidence could be established by demonstrating relatively higher correlations among several different methods of measuring the same trait (*convergent validity*) and showing relatively lower correlations among different traits measured by the same method (*discriminant validity*). Campbell and Fiske defined validity as "the agreement between two attempts to measure the same trait through maximally different methods" (p. 83). Any given assessment method may reflect as much the method used in the assessment as it does the behaviors being assessed. The MTMM approach attempts to separate *method* from *trait* variance such that the convergent validity of a particular construct can be evaluated.

Cone (1979) reinterpreted the MTMM model from a behavioral assessment standpoint by calling for *multimethod-multibehavior-multicontent matrices*. In this reformulation, "traits" are reinterpreted as response classes or behaviors that can occur across different content areas or behavioral repertoires (e.g., cognitive–verbal, overt–motoric, or physiological–emotional) using different assessment methods. A person may be observed to breathe rapidly and perspire in response to anxiety-provoking situations or stimuli (direct observation of physiological–emotional content). The same person may self-report that she breathes rapidly and perspires in anxiety-provoking situations (self-report of overt–motoric behavior). The correlations between direct observation and self-report of these two behaviors between and within these behavioral repertoires allows for the separation of method, behavior, and content variance, thereby providing convergent validity for the response class or behaviors being assessed.

In practice, the principle of multiple operationalism would require the assessment of behavior using most of the assessment methods listed in Table 1. By multiply operationalizing behavior in this way, behavior therapists can evaluate the convergence or agreement of data from multiple sources and methods. The lack of convergence or agreement among different sources does not necessarily invalidate the assessment data. Disagreement between methods of assessment (e.g., teacher and parent ratings of behavior) may reflect the situational specificity of behavior (Achenbach, McConaughy, & Howell, 1987; Kazdin, 1979), rather than the invalidity of the measures used. The primary reason for multiply operationalizing behavior is that the lack of agreement among assessment methods should prompt behavior therapists to conduct more in-depth assessments of those setting and/or situational variables that may be functionally related to these behavioral differences.

Principle of Quality Assessment

Although the primary purpose of behavioral assessment is to identify target behaviors and to specify the environmental variables of which these behaviors are a function, one must also ensure the quality of the data obtained (i.e., reliability and validity). Some writers in the area of behavioral assessment argue that traditional concepts of reliability and validity are irrelevant in a behavioral assessment framework, because they are based on assumptions that stand in direct contradiction to behavior theory (Cone, 1988; R. Nelson, 1983; R. Nelson, Hayes, & Jarrett, 1986). Others, however, argue that psychometric standards for reliability and validity are appropriate for evaluating the quality of behavioral assessment data (Barrios & Hartmann, 1986; Haynes & Wilson, 1979; Linehan, 1980; Silva, 1993; Strosahl & Linehan, 1986). Given the importance of these two perspectives for evaluating the quality of behavioral assessment data, it is instructive to discuss these opposing viewpoints. Table 2 presents comparisons and contrast of psychometric concepts in traditional and behavioral assessment.

Reliability

Reliability is defined in classical test theory as the correlation between true and fallible scores (Nunnally & Bernstein, 1994). An individual's test score on a particular measurement occasion is viewed as a

TABLE 2. Psychometric Concepts in Traditional Behavioral Assessment

	Traditional	Behavioral
I. Reliability	Based on the correlation between true and fallible scores	Based on agreement between observers viewing the same behavior at the same time
II. A. Homogeneity	Reflects the average interitem correlation in a domain	Reflects the agreement among observers viewing the same behavior at the same time
B. Stability	Degree to which observed scores fluctuate around true scores over time	Degree to which measurement is due to systematic factors operating in measurement situations over time
C. Errors of measurement	Imperfect correlation between parallel tests and/or the degree of random error in obtained scores over time	Disagreements among observers or lack of correspondence between observed value and true value of behavior
III. Validity	Quality inferences drawn from test data in terms of forecasting behavior, meaning of hypothetical constructs, and the content	Degree to which behavior is a true reflection of behavior in natural settings
A. Content validity	Degree to which text items representatively sample a content domain of interest	Degree to which the conditions under which behavior is observed represent all sets of conditions to which one is interested in generalizing (settings, situations, observers, and times)
B. Criterion-related validity	Degree to which test scores predict a criterion	Degree to which behavior can be predicted across situations
C. Construct validity	Meanings of underlying constructs as they occur in a nomological network, agreement between two or more methods of measuring the same trait, and the degree to which constructs can be differentiated	Sample of behavior or response class in a specific situation and differentiation of behaviors in a response class using multiple assessment methods
IV. Accuracy	Degree to which test scores are free from systematic and random errors measurement	Correspondence between measured behavior and the true value of behavior
V. Treatment validity	Not formally addressed, except in terms, of aptitude × treatment interactions (ATIs)	Degree to which assessment data contributes to positive or beneficial treatment outcomes

random sample of one of many possible test scores that the individual could have earned on repeated measurement occasions or test administrations or, more accurately, on a set of strictly parallel forms of that test. Classical psychometric theory assumes that individuals possess stable characteristics or traits (true scores) that persist through time, that error scores are completely random, and that fallible scores (obtained scores) result from the addition of true scores and error scores (Ghiselli, Campbell, & Zedeck, 1981).

Reliability in behavioral assessment, specifically in applied behavior analysis, refers to agreement among observers (or some measuring instrument) viewing the same behavior at the same time (Baer, 1977b; Johnston & Pennypacker, 1980). Unlike classical test theory, behavioral assessment is primarily interested in the degree of homogeneity among observers of behavior rather than the homogeneity of test items in a content domain. Strosahl and Linehan (1986) suggested that reliability in behavioral assessment uses the principle of equivalent forms in that it reflects the degree to which two observers are behaving as equivalent measuring instruments. In short, reliability in behavioral assessment refers to the consistency with which repeated observations of the same behavioral event yield equivalent information (Cone, 1981).

Classical test theory typically discusses two types of reliability: homogeneity and stability. *Homogeneity* is the degree to which items in a content domain are correlated and is reflected in the average interitem correlation (*coefficient alpha*). Homogeneity in behavioral assessment may reflect the relationships among behaviors in a response class much as classical test theory conceptualizes item homogeneity. Baer (1977b), however, suggested that homogeneity of behaviors, at least measured by time sampling, should not be expected because the occurrence of a behavior in one time-sampled interval should not necessarily be predictive of the occurrence of that same behavior in another time-sampled interval. Baer (1977b) also defines homogeneity in terms of observer homogeneity rather than behavior homogeneity. That is, any given number of observers using the same definition of a behavior should be able to look at that behavior and agree on its occurrence or nonoccurrence, duration of occurrence, and so forth.

Stability in classical test theory reflects the degree to which a person's observed score fluctuates around the true score over time (Crocker & Algina, 1986). Interpretations of stability coefficients are not as straightforward as interpretations of internal consistency estimates. For example, a low stability coefficient may indicate that the phenomenon being measured is unstable, yet this instability may have nothing to do with the theoretical reliability coefficient. State anxiety and stress are examples of response classes that are greatly affected by environmental events. This creates a situation in which an individual's true score may change as a function of changes in environmental circumstances or states of the individual.

This instability issue in classical test theory forms the basis for the behavioral assessment interpretation of stability or instability. Behaviorally, instability reflects the changeability of behavior over time as a function of situational factors. Given the identification of these situational factors through either functional assessment or functional analysis, the instability of behavior cannot be due to unreliability and therefore cannot contribute to error. In fact, behavioral assessment makes no assumptions about "true" scores or "errors of measurement" in the sense of classical test theory. So-called errors of measurement in behavioral assessment stem from two sources: (a) disagreements among observers recording the same behavior at the same time and (b) lack of correspondence between the true value of behavior and the observed value of behavior. This latter concept has been termed the *accuracy* of measurement (Cone, 1986, 1988; Johnston & Pennypacker, 1980).

Validity

Validity is traditionally defined as the quality of inferences drawn from test scores (L.J. Cronbach, 1988; Messick, 1988). These inferences are of three basic types: (1) the content domain of interest (content validity), (2) forecasting behavior (criterion-related validity), and (3) the meaning of hypothetical constructs (construct validity). According to *Standards for Educational and Psychological Testing* (American Psychological Association, 1985): "Validity . . . refers to appropriateness, meaningfulness, and usefulness of the specific inferences made from test scores" (p. 9). We limit our discussion here to content validity, given its importance to behavioral assessment.

Validity in behavioral assessment is the degree to which test behavior is a true reflection of behavior in naturalistic settings (Cone, 1986, 1988). Behavioral assessment validity is defined as the correspondence between behavior measured in the testing situation and behavior as it occurs in nontest situations. For example, the extent to which behavior assessed by analogue role-play measures represents that same behavior on the playground is an indicator of the validity of the role-play measure.

Linehan (1980) suggested that content validation represents the most important and relevant type of validity for behavioral assessment data. In describing content validity in behavioral assessment, Linehan (1980) indicated as follows:

> the absence of generalizability can be attributed to a failure to represent adequately in the assessment sample the behavioral universe to be predicted. . . . It is precisely this lack of assumed generalizability across diverse settings, response classes, etc., which necessitates attention to content validity (i.e., representative sampling from all settings, responses, etc. of interest) in the development of behavioral assessment procedures. (p. 152)

The fundamental question in behavioral assessment is as follows: How well does the measurement of behavior in a particular situation at a given point in time by a particular observer represent that same behavior measured in other situations, at other times, and by different observers? That is, behavioral assessment invariably takes samples of behavior in baseline and makes inferences about the operant rate of behavior (Linehan, 1980). Similarly, behavioral assessors take samples of behavior during treatment and assume that these samples are representative of that individual's actual behavior during treatment. Both scenarios require some degree of inference by behavioral assessors.

Generalizability

One alternative to traditional distinctions between reliability and validity, as well as a potential means of resolving some conceptual disagreements between traditional and behavioral assessment, can be found in *generalizability theory* (L. Cronbach, Gleser, Nanda, & Rajaratnam, 1972). Generalizability theory conforms to many, but not all, assumptions of behavioral assessment, particularly as these assumptions relate to the generalizability of

results of data collected at different times, by different observers, in different settings, and by different methods. It should be noted, however, that the empirical basis for generalizability theory rests on nomothetic or group rather than idiographic data. Cone (1977) identified six "universes" of generalizability that are relevant to behavioral assessment: (1) scorer, (2) behavior, (3) time, (4) setting, (5) method, and (6) dimension.

Scorer generalizability is similar to inter-observer agreement in behavioral assessment. Time generalizability is roughly equivalent to stability or test–retest reliability in classical test theory. Method generalizability is similar to convergent validity in the Campbell and Fiske (1959) sense. Item generalizability is like internal consistency reliability. Setting generalizability is similar to criterion-related validity in classical test theory and response generalization in operant learning theory. Dimension generalizability is somewhat like discriminant validity in the MTMM model. A more detailed discussion of generalizability theory can be found in several sources (Cone, 1977; Crocker & Algina, 1986; L. Cronbach et al., 1972; Gresham & Carey, 1988).

Practically speaking, data collected by a behavior therapist at a given point in time, in a specific setting, and by a given method may or may not be generalizable to data collected by other behavior therapists, at other times, and by different methods. Generalizability theory dictates that there should be relative levels of agreement among these various universes of generalizability. This constitutes not only good assessment practice, but also increases the probability that assessment data will be generalizable to other situations or conditions.

Conclusions

The assessment of assessment quality is made difficult by the core assumptions of behavioral assessment. On the one hand, if one adopts an idiographic approach to assessment, then psychometric standards based on group (nomothetic) data would appear to contradict this assumption. When one obtains data having low reliability and validity, the question becomes, Is variability in behavior creating the illusion of low reliability and validity, or is it the poor quality of the assessment instrument?

Johnston and Pennypacker (1980) argued that measurement in psychology is based predominantly on relative measurement ("vaganotic") in which the attributes being measured are based on the variation in a set of observations. The variability is then used as one basis for evaluating assessment quality. Measurement scales (e.g., ordinal or interval) define attributes on the basis of relative variability rather than absolute values of the attributes under consideration. For example, a student's level of reading achievement might be indexed by an ordinal scale (e.g., 16th percentile) or an interval scale (T score = 40). These scores, however, are based on the distance the student's score is from the mean of some standardization sample. The student's performance on this reading test is interpreted relative to the performances of others rather than the student's absolute level of academic proficiency (i.e., an interindividual comparison.

Another approach to measurement in psychology described by Johnston and Pennypacker (1980) is based on absolute measurement, which utilizes absolute and standard units and whose existence is established independent of the phenomenon being measured ("idemnotic"). Physical and natural sciences such as physics, chemistry, and biology utilize this absolute approach to measurement, basing their measurement systems on natural phenomena (e.g., distance, mass, time). Early psychologists such as Pavlov, Thorndike, and Ebbinghaus used an absolute approach to measurement, using measures of secreted saliva volume, elapsed time to solve puzzles, and frequency of remembered words, respectively, as outcome measures in their experiments. Present-day behavioral assessors, primarily applied behavior analysts, use absolute, unit-based measurement in their assessments. Measures of frequency, rate, duration, latency, and permanent products are typically used in this approach to behavioral assessment.

The foregoing discussion of relative and absolute measurement strategies highlights the differences between traditional psychometric and behavioral assessment approaches to assessment. We believe that it would be inappropriate to choose one measurement approach to the exclusion of the other and that behavior therapists should retain both models, depending on the purpose of assessment.

Relative measurement approaches are indispensable when one wishes to sample the same behavior or response classes of a group of individuals and to determine deviant (different) responses of an individual in a group. Thus, a relative approach to measurement is appropriate for screening, selection, and classification purposes. For instance, the Systematic Screening for Behavioral Disorders (Walker & Severson, 1992) uses a combination of teacher nominations, teacher ratings, and direct observations with a normative database to identify children at risk for externalizing and internalizing behavior disorders. In addition, the Child Behavior Checklist, Teacher Rating Form and Youth Self-Report (Achenbach, 1991) use relative or norm-based comparisons to identify and classify children as having externalizing, internalizing, or mixed (comorbid) profiles of psychopathology. Psychometric standards of reliability (test–retest, interrater) and validity (criterion-related, discriminant, construct) are appropriate for evaluating the quality of these approaches.

Absolute measurement approaches are indispensable when one is interested in conducting a functional assessment of behavior, collecting baseline data, monitoring responsiveness to intervention, and evaluating treatment outcome. Measures of frequency, temporality (duration, latency, interresponse time), intensity, and permanent products are sensitive to the effects of intervention, are typically nonreactive, and are amenable to repeated measurement over time (Cone & Foster, 1986; Hawkins, 1986; R. Hayes et al., 1986). The quality of these measures should be evaluated using idiographic approaches such as interrater agreement, accuracy, treatment validity, and social validity (to be discussed in the following section).

Curriculum-based measurement probes (e.g., number of words read correctly), for example, are more sensitive to the effects of reading interventions than are standardized tests of reading achievement (Shinn, 1989). Permanent products of written expression (e.g., spelling errors or grammatical errors in written language) are more accurate and content valid than are standardized tests of spelling and written expression (see Skinner, this volume). Similarly, durations of negative social interactions and time spent alone on the playground are more sensitive to the effects of social skills interventions than are teacher rating scales and sociometrics (Gresham, 1981, 1997; Walker, Colvin, & Ramsey, 1995).

Principle of Social Validity

Social validity deals with three fundamental questions faced by behavior therapists: What should we change? How should we change it? How will we know it was effective? There are sometimes disagreements among professionals as well as between professionals and consumers on these three fundamental questions. Wolf (1978) is credited with originating the notion of social validity, and it has become common parlance among many researchers and practitioners, particularly those operating from an applied behavior analytic perspective. Social validity refers to the assessment of the *social significance* of the goals of an intervention, the *social acceptability* of intervention procedures to attain those goals, and the *social importance* of the effects produced by the intervention.

For all intents and purposes, social validation is a means of assessing and analyzing consumer behavior. Schwartz (1991) indicated that the most important element in studying consumer behavior is the decision-making process. In the study of consumer behavior, this decision-making process consists of four steps: (1) recognizing the problem, (2) evaluating alternative solutions, (3) buying the product or service, and (4) evaluating the decision. This decision-making sequence parallels the problem-solving model of behavioral consultation (Bergan & Kratochwill, 1990), which involves problem identification, problem analysis, plan implementation, and treatment evaluation. Each of these levels of social validation will be discussed briefly in the following sections.

Social Significance of Goals

Deciding the goals to be accomplished in behavior therapy is perhaps the most vital aspect of the entire intervention process. One of the most important aspects of the behavioral consultation process is the adequacy of problem identification (Bergan & Kratochwill, 1990). An adequate definition of behavior, however, does not necessarily establish its social significance. It may be even easier to identify and define simplistic, trivial behaviors than complex, socially significant behaviors. The social significance of behavior can be established in relation to how consumers value certain behaviors. In other words, do consumers consider the behavior to be a socially significant behavior rather than a trivial or insignificant behavior? For instance, reading at grade level or completing math skill sheets with 100% accuracy may be more socially signifi-

cant than being on-task 100% of the time. This would be particularly important, given the fact that there is often little or no relationship between time on-task and academic production or accuracy (Shapiro, 1989).

Social validity is typically assessed using questionnaires that sample consumer opinions. These assessments are designed to measure the opinions of relevant communities of consumers and to use this information to select or change program goals or consumer opinions (Schwartz & Baer, 1991). Baer (1987) suggested that social invalidity is not necessarily the inverse of social validity. Instead, social invalidity is represented by consumers who disapprove of or complain about some aspect of an intervention program and who do something about that disapproval. For example, some conservative groups might express their disagreement with the goals of a program designed to increase knowledge and prevent sexually transmitted diseases by writing letters, placing telephone calls to school board members, and writing newspaper editorials.

Schwartz and Baer (1991) argue that social validity and invalidity should be assessed early and the reasons for consumer likes and dislikes should be detailed so that they can be accurately predicted in future intervention programs, rather than become an "early warning sign" of program rejection. Cataloging the positive and negative aspects of intervention programs, as well as the reasons for these evaluations, could allow behavior therapists to tailor specific interventions for their consumers. Although constructing a catalog of reasons for positive and negative evaluations of program goals, procedures, and outcomes may seem valuable at first glance, there are some potential drawbacks in this methodology. Should our major goal be to change behaviors that consumers dislike or wish to be changed? Should our goal be to "please" all consumers even though our empirically based opinions would suggest otherwise? Is the reduction or absence of complaints indicative of successful behavior therapy practice?

Hawkins (1991) argued that the term *social validity* is misleading because what is really being measured in social validation is consumer satisfaction. Basically, consumer satisfaction is obtained by asking for a second opinion from another source. If the second opinion agrees with the behavior therapist's opinion, the goals of an intervention are considered "socially validated." If the second opinion disagrees with that of the behavior therapist, the goals are viewed as social invalid or insignificant. It may well be the case, however, that second opinions obtained from consumers are less informed than are those of the behavior therapist. Disagreement between behavior therapists and consumers merely reflect the absence of interobserver agreement and not necessarily the invalidity of goals, procedures, or outcomes. For example, most cardiac patients would probably consider medication to be preferable to a triple bypass operation, although the former treatment may not solve the patient's problem in terms of a medically important outcome (the prevention of death).

Hawkins (1991) makes a strong case for using the concept of *habilitative validity* instead of social validity. Goals, procedures, and outcomes in behavior therapy should teach or promote behaviors that allow for successful functioning or adaptation to school, home, and community settings. Habilitative validity can be defined as the degree to which the goals, procedures, and/or outcomes of an intervention maximize the overall benefits and minimize overall costs to that individual and to others (Hawkins, 1991). Noell and Gresham (1993) used a similar heuristic in their model of consultation based on the notion of functional outcome analysis. In this model, the goals of interventions are considered socially valid if the benefits of an intervention (both objective and subjective) outweigh the costs.

Establishing the social significance of target behaviors is an exercise in the identification of functional behaviors. The questions asked in the process are these: Is this a functional target behavior to change? Will changing it result in short-term and long-term benefits? Is the cost of changing this behavior less than the benefits produced by the change (a positive cost–benefit ratio)? Consumers may not always be in the best position to judge the habilitative or functional validity of target behaviors: As Hawkins (1991) observed, "The validity of such consumer judgments has yet to be established; they should not be viewed as a validity criterion but rather as a second opinion from a lay person which may or may not be better informed and less biased than the professional is" (p. 26).

Social Acceptability of Procedures

Not all interventions developed in behavior therapy and behavior analysis are necessarily acceptable to consumers. Kazdin (1981) defined treatment acceptability as a judgment as to whether a given treatment is fair in relation to a given problem, is reasonable and nonintrusive, and is consistent with what a treatment should be. Witt and Elliott (1985) developed a model of treatment acceptability that specified reciprocal interrelationships among four elements: treatment acceptability, treatment use, treatment integrity, and treatment effectiveness. Elliott (1988) suggested that *acceptability* is the initial issue in treatment selection and use. If a treatment is considered acceptable, then the probability of using that treatment is high relative to treatments judged less acceptable. Use and effectiveness of treatments are linked by the integrity with which treatments are implemented. Gresham (1989) suggested that the lack of integrity is a major reason for the ineffectiveness of many treatments developed in behavioral consultation. Finally, treatment effectiveness is based on whether the outcomes of the treatment meet or exceed the expectations of treatment consumers.

Virtually all of what we know about the acceptability of treatments has been from research conducted with behavioral treatments in analogue situations. The typical paradigm involves presentation of a written problem and treatment followed by evaluative ratings of the treatment (Elliott, 1988). Most of what we know about the acceptability of behavioral treatments is based on hypothetical rather than consumers' actual experiences with using various treatments (i.e., pretreatment acceptability). What we do know about pretreatment acceptability is that complex treatments are less acceptable than simpler treatments, positive treatments are more acceptable than negative (punishment-based) treatments, all treatments become more acceptable as behavior problem severity increases, and that consumers more knowledgeable of behavioral principles rate all treatments as more acceptable than do their less knowledgeable peers (see Elliott, 1988, for a review).

This literature, while informative with respect to pretreatment acceptability, may not correspond to what consumers might tell us about the acceptability of treatments after they have tried them. The pretreatment acceptability paradigm is similar to judging the sales and consumption of products based on verbal descriptions and ratings in relation to similar products rather than on actual sales or consumption. A more direct measure of acceptability would use the concepts of *integrity* and *use* as direct behavioral indices of acceptability. If a treatment is not implemented as planned, then some aspect(s) of that treatment might be considered unacceptable. Similarly, if a treatment is not used, for whatever reason, it can be considered unacceptable. In this revised conceptualization, integrity and use are behavioral markers for treatment acceptability (see Gresham & Lopez, 1996, for a comprehensive discussion).

Consumer satisfaction with intervention procedures may not reflect the most effective treatment procedures or what is in the best interests of children. Walker and colleagues (1995) suggested that surgeons' choice of a procedure having a 20% mortality rate over one having a 10% mortality rate because (a) they like it better, (b) it is easier to do, and (c) they are trained in it, might be considered unethical. Some consumers (e.g., parents and teachers) may reject legitimate interventions simply because they lack the skills for their implementation, because they are philosophically opposed to them, or because they may have motives other than the implementation of interventions. The net effect of any of these reasons is that children may not receive the best practices of behavioral intervention, because of consumer dissatisfaction with treatment procedures.

Social Importance of Effects

The social importance of the effects produced by an intervention establishes the clinical or practical significance of behavior change. That is, does the quality or quantity of behavior change make a difference in an individual's functioning? Does the change in behavior have habilitative validity (Hawkins, 1991)? Is the behavior now in a "functional" range? All of these questions capture the essence of what is meant by establishing the social importance of intervention effects.

Fawcett (1991) suggested that the social importance of effects could be evaluated at several levels: the level of proximal effects, that of intermediate effects, and that of distal effects. Proximal effects represent changes in target behaviors as a function of an intervention (e.g., increased sight word vocabulary, increased social skills, increased math work completion). Intermediate effects represent concomitant, positive changes in collateral behaviors and outcomes as a function of changes in target behaviors (e.g., reading fluency, peer acceptance, higher math grades). Distal effects represent long-term changes in behavior or outcomes as a function of proximal and intermediate effects (e.g., increased recreational reading, increased friendships, successful completion of advanced math coursework).

One reason that many practitioners may fail to utilize the research literature in guiding their practice is that this literature is not presented in a readily "consumable" form. Conventional methods for reporting research outcomes have relied primarily on parametric statistics. Although parametric statistics have contributed to our understanding of intervention, these methods do not present research outcomes in a readily understandable and usable form.

There is often no relationship between statistical significance and practical significance, particularly when statistical significance is a function of large sample sizes rather than strong effects of intervention (Baer, 1977a; Gresham, 1991; Gresham & Noell, 1993; Jacobson, Follette, & Revenstorf, 1984). Traditional statistical analyses were not designed for and therefore cannot address the issue of what constitutes beneficial outcomes. Establishing the practical significance of interventions involves the determination of whether or not intervention effects are *socially important*. Jacobson et al. (1984) suggested that most behavior problems vary on a continuum of functioning involving a range of scores on any given dependent variable. Some approaches to social validation (e.g., Kazdin & Wilson, 1978) contend that a result is socially validated if the problem is successfully resolved. This approach, however, leads to thinking about outcomes in terms of false dichotomies (problem present versus problem absent) (Jacobson et al., 1984).

One means of establishing the social importance of intervention effects is to conceptualize behavioral functioning as belonging to either a *functional* or *dysfunctional* distribution. Hawkins (1991) would consider this as an exercise in determining whether or not a behavior change had habilitative validity. For example, we could socially validate a reading intervention by demonstrating that a child moved from a dysfunctional to a functional range of reading performance. This could be established by calculating the probability that the child's reading score belonged to a functional rather than a dysfunctional distribution. Jacobson and colleagues (1984) emphasized that this approach to social validation is problematic because it requires a normative database for both functional and dysfunctional populations. Many of the behaviors targeted for intervention do not have a normative database and fewer still have separate norms for functional and dysfunctional populations.

More practical approaches to establishing the social importance of intervention effects were first proposed by Kazdin (1977) and were extended by others (Fawcett, 1991; Hawkins, 1991; Schwartz & Baer, 1991; Van Houten, 1979). Kazdin (1977) recommended three general approaches to social validation: social comparison, subjective evaluations, and combined social validation procedures. Social comparison involves comparing an individual's behavior after intervention with the behavior of relevant peers. Social comparisons, however may not necessarily reflect changes in behavior that have habilitative validity. It is entirely possible to produce changes in a child's behavior so that it is comparable to his or her peers, yet the behavior may not be in a functional range of performance. For example, if an entire classroom is functioning two to three grade levels below grade placement in mathematics, moving the child into the a comparable range of mathematical performance would have little, if any, habilitative validity. Fawcett (1991) suggested that in evaluating the social importance of effects, we should specify various levels of performance. For example, one could specify *ideal* (the best performance available), *normative* (typical or commonly occurring performance), or *deficient* (the worst performance available). Interventions moving a child from a deficient level of performance to normative or ideal levels of performance could be considered socially important.

Subjective evaluations represent another approach to establishing the social importance of effects. These evaluations consist of having treatment consumers rate the qualitative aspects of the child's behavior. These global evaluations of behavior assess how well the child is functioning and provide an overall assessment of performance (Kazdin, 1977). Subjective evaluations can be used not only for assessing the quality of behavior change, but also to assess consumer satisfaction with treatment procedures, teaching methods, and therapist behavior. Recent studies have used this type of assessment in homework completion studies to supplement more objective indices of treatment outcome (see Miller & Kelley, 1994; Olympia, Sheridan, Jenson, & Andrews, 1994).

Combined social validation procedures take advantage of social comparisons and subjective evaluations in assessing the social importance of effects. The practical significance of behavioral interventions could be bolstered if we could demonstrate that (a) the child's behavior moved into the same normative range (or higher) than nonreferred peers, and (b) treatment consumers felt that the intervention had produced socially important changes in behavior. The combined approach captures not only how much a behavior changed (a quantitative criterion), but also how consumers of intervention view that change (a qualitative criterion).

Another approach to establishing the social importance of intervention effects is to calculate a reliable change index. First proposed by Nunnally and Kotsche (1983), later expanded by Jacobson and colleagues (1984), and revised by Christensen and Mendoza (1986), a reliable change index (RC) has been recommended for quantifying the social importance of effects. RC is defined as the difference between a posttest score and a pretest score divided by the standard error of difference between posttest and pretest scores: RC = Posttest–pretest/ standard error of difference. The standard error of difference describes the spread of the distribution of change scores that would be expected if no actual change had occurred. An RC of +1.96 ($p < .05$) would be statistically significant, and, given this value, one could conclude that an intervention produced reliable changes in behavior. This formula for establishing the social importance of intervention outcomes has the following advantages: (a) data are reported for individuals rather than groups, (b) reliable changes from pretest to posttest for individuals are indexed by the standard error of difference, and (c) confidence intervals can be constructed around change scores to avoid overinterpretation of a particular result.

It should be noted that RC is strongly affected by the reliability of the dependent measure used. For instance, if a measure is highly reliable (e.g.,

.90 or higher), then small changes in behavior could be considered statistically reliable, but not socially important. Conversely, if a measure has low reliability, then large changes in behavior might not be statistically reliable, but could be socially important. For these reasons, both social validation (social comparisons and subjective judgments) and RC should provide a means of documenting clinically and statistically significant changes in behavior.

Summary and Conclusions

Behavioral assessment is an approach to assessment that, at least conceptually, differs from what is typically called traditional psychological assessment. We noted that behavioral assessment eschews *sign* or trait interpretations of assessment data and instead focuses on the assessment of *samples* of behavior and controlling variables. We noted, however, that behavioral assessment shares many of the same assessment methods with traditional assessment (e.g., interviews, self-reports, ratings by others). The primary difference in the two approaches lies in the interpretation of assessment data based on philosophical epistemologies and core assumptions that each model makes about human behavior.

We indicated that traditional and behavioral assessment evolved from two distinct philosophies of science, Aristotelian and Galilean, respectively. The Aristotelian approach to assessment emphasizes a trait-oriented approach and uses nomothetic comparisons to interpret assessment information. This approach is similar to Skinner's (1953) depiction of traditional personality interpretations as conceptual inner causes of behavior. A Galilean path to assessment assumes that behavior results from person-X–environment interactions and uses an idiographic approach to interpret assessment information.

The Galilean epistemology dictates several core assumptions on which most behavioral assessors would probably agree. These core assumptions include (a) causes of behavior (primarily environmental), (b) situational specificity of behavior, (c) treatment validity of assessment data, (d) low levels of inference, (e) an idiographic bias toward assessment interpretation, and (f) repeated and frequent measurement of behavior over time. These core assumptions distinguish behavioral assessment from most approaches to traditional assessment and are clearly more oriented toward treatment than is traditional assessment, which emphasizes diagnosis or classification.

Some would argue that traditional and behavioral assessment approaches are more alike than different (see McReynolds, 1986; Mischel, 1988; Silva, 1993). According to these views, behavioral assessment, like traditional assessment, is both idiographic and nomothetic, is both criterion-referenced and norm-referenced, and is governed by psychometric standards of reliability and validity. We believe that this statement is somewhat broad and ignores not only the purposes of assessment (screening versus classification versus treatment), but also the nature of the response class being assessed; for example, narrow, discrete behaviors (selective mutism or self-injurious behavior) versus larger, interrelated response classes (social competence or depression). As we mentioned earlier in this chapter, behavioral assessors fall on a continuum regarding their stance in relation to epistemology and the core assumptions regarding human behavior that emanate from their epistemology. We hope that this chapter provides a framework for the chapters to come and serves as a useful conceptual organizer for the diverse problems presented to child behavior therapists.

References

Achenbach, T. (1991). *Integrative guide for the 1991 CBCL/4-18, YSR, and TRF profiles*. Burlington, VT: University of Vermont, Department of Psychiatry.

Achenbach, T., McConaughy, S., & Howell, C. (1987). Child/adolescent behavioral and emotional problems: Implications of cross-informant correlations for situational specificity. *Psychological Bulletin, 101*, 213–232.

American Psychiatric Association. (1994). *Diagnostic and statistical manual of mental disorders* (4th ed.). Washington, DC: Author.

American Psychological Association. (1985). *Standards for educational and psychological testing*. Washington, DC: Author.

Baer, D. (1977a). "Perhaps it would be better not to know everything." *Journal of Applied Behavior Analysis, 10*, 1676–172.

Baer, D. (1977b). Reviewer's comment: Just because it's reliable doesn't mean that you can use it. *Journal of Applied Behavior Analysis, 10*, 117–120.

Baer, D. (1987, March). *A behavior-analytic inquiry into early intervention*. Paper presented at the Banff International Conference on Behavioral Science, Banff, Alberta, Canada.

Barrios, B., & Hartmann, D. (1986). The contributions of traditional assessment: Concepts, issues, and methodologies. In

R. Nelson & S. Hayes (Eds.), *Conceptual foundations of behavioral assessment* (pp. 81–110). New York: Guilford.

Bellack, A., & Hersen, M. (Eds.). (1988). *Behavioral assessment: A practical handbook.* New York: Pergamon.

Bergan, J., & Kratochwill, T. (1990). *Behavioral consultation and therapy.* New York: Plenum.

Campbell, D., & Fiske, D. (1959). Convergent and discriminant validation by the multitrait-multimethod matrix. *Psychological Bulletin, 56,* 81–105.

Carr, E.G. (1993). Behavior analysis is not ultimately about behavior. *The Behavior Analyst, 16,* 47–49.

Carr, E.G. (1994). Emerging themes in the functional analysis of problem behavior. *Journal of Applied Behavior Analysis, 27,* 393–399.

Christensen, L., & Mendoza, J. (1986). A method of assessing change in a single subject: An alteration of the RC index. *Behavior Therapy, 17,* 305–308.

Ciminero, A., Calhoun, K., & Adams, H. (Eds.). (1986). *Handbook of behavioral assessment* (2nd ed.). New York: Wiley Interscience.

Ciminero, A.R. (1986). Behavioral assessment: An overview. In A.R. Ciminero, K. Calhoun, & H. Adams (Eds.), *Handbook of behavioral assessment* (2nd ed., pp. 3–11). New York: Wiley.

Cone, J.D. (1977). The relevance of reliability and validity for behavioral assessment. *Behavior Therapy, 8,* 411–426.

Cone, J.D. (1978). The Behavioral Assessment Grid (BAG): A conceptual framework and a taxonomy. *Behavior Therapy, 9,* 882–888.

Cone, J.D. (1979). Confounded comparisons in triple response mode assessment research. *Behavioral Assessment, 1,* 85–95.

Cone, J.D. (1981). Psychometric considerations. In M. Hersen & A. Bellack (Eds.), *Behavioral assessment: A practical handbook* (pp. 38–70). New York: Pergamon.

Cone, J.D. (1986). Idiographic, nomothetic, and related perspectives in behavioral assessment. In R.O. Nelson & S.C. Hayes (Eds.), *Conceptual foundations of behavioral assessment* (pp. 111–128). New York: Guilford.

Cone, J.D. (1988). Psychometric considerations and the multiple models of behavioral assessment. In A. Bellack & M. Hersen (Eds.), *Behavioral assessment: A practical handbook* (pp. 42–66). New York: Pergamon.

Cone, J.D., & Foster, S. (1986). Direct observation in clinical psychology. In P. Kendall & J. Butcher (Eds.), *Handbook of research methods in clinical psychology* (pp. 311–354). New York: Wiley Interscience.

Crocker, L., & Algina, J. (1986). *Introduction to classical and modern test theory.* New York: Holt, Rinehart, & Winston.

Cronbach, L., Gleser, G., Nanda, H., & Rajaratnam, N. (1972). *The dependability of behavioral measures.* New York: Wiley.

Cronbach, L.J. (1988). Five perspectives on validity argument. In H. Wainer & H. Braun (Eds.), *Test validity* (pp. 3–18). Hillsdale, NJ: Erlbaum.

Elliott, S.N. (1988). Acceptability of behavioral treatments in educational settings. In J. Witt, S. Elliott, & F. Gresham (Eds.), *Handbook of behavior therapy in education* (pp. 121–150). New York: Plenum.

Fawcett, S. (1991). Social validity: A note on methodology. *Journal of Applied Behavior Analysis, 24,* 235–239.

Fuchs, L.S., & Fuchs, D. (1986). Curriculum-based assessment of progress toward long-term and short-term goals. *The Journal of Special Education, 20,* 69–82.

Ghiselli, E., Campbell, J., & Zedeck, S. (1981). *Measurement theory for the behavioral sciences.* San Francisco: Freeman.

Goldfried, M.R., & Kent, R. (1972). Traditional versus behavioral personality assessment: A comparison of methodological and theoretical assumptions. *Psychological Bulletin, 77,* 409–420.

Gresham, F.M. (1981). Assessment of children's social skills. *Journal of School Psychology, 17,* 120–133.

Gresham, F.M. (1989). Assessment of treatment integrity in school consultation and prereferral intervention. *School Psychology Review, 18,* 37–50.

Gresham, F.M. (1991). Moving beyond statistical significance in reporting consultation outcome research. *Journal of Educational and Psychological Consultation, 2,* 1–14.

Gresham, F.M. (1997). Social skills. In G. Bear, K. Minke, & A. Thomas (Eds.), *Children's needs II: Development, problems, and alternatives* (pp. 39–50). Bethesda, MD: National Association of School Psychologists.

Gresham, F.M., & Carey, M. (1988). Research methodology and measurement. In J. Witt, S. Elliott, & F. Gresham (Eds.), *Handbook of behavior therapy in education* (pp. 37–66). New York: Plenum.

Gresham, F.M., & Gansle, K.A. (1992). Misguided assumptions of the DSM-III–R: Implications for school psychological practice. *School Psychology Quarterly, 7,* 79–95.

Gresham, F.M., & Lopez, M.F. (1996). Social validation: A unifying concept for school-based consultation research and practice. *School Psychology Quarterly.*

Gresham, F.M., & Noell, G.H. (1993). Documenting the effectiveness of consultation outcomes. In J. Zins, T. Kratochwill, & S. Elliott (Eds.), *Handbook of consultation services for children* (pp. 249–273). San Francisco: Jossey-Bass.

Hartmann, D., Roper, B., & Bradford, D. (1979). Some relationships between behavioral and traditional assessment. *Journal of Behavioral Assessment, 1,* 3–21.

Hawkins, R. (1986). Selection of target behaviors. In R. Nelson & S. Hayes (Eds.), *Conceptual foundations of behavioral assessment* (pp. 331–385). New York: Guilford.

Hawkins, R. (1991). Is social validity what we are interested in? Argument for a functional approach. *Journal of Applied Behavior Analysis, 24,* 205–213.

Hayes, S., Nelson, R., & Jarrett. R. (1987). The treatment utility of assessment: A functional approach to evaluating assessment quality. *American Psychologist, 42,* 963–974.

Hayes, S.C., & Hayes, L.J. (1992). Some clinical implications of contextualistic behaviorism: The example of cognition. *Behavior Therapy, 23,* 225–249.

Haynes, S., & Wilson, C. (1979). *Behavioral assessment.* San Francisco: Jossey-Bass.

Horner, R.H. (1994). Functional assessment contributions and future directions. *Journal of Applied Behavior Analysis, 27,* 401–404.

Iwata, B., Dorsey, M., Slifer, K., Bauman, K., & Richman, G. (1982). Toward a functional analysis of self-injury. *Analysis and Intervention in Developmental Disabilities, 2,* 3–20.

Jacobson, N., Follette, W., & Revenstorf, D. (1984). Psychotherapy outcome research: Methods for reporting variability and evaluating clinical significance. *Behavior Therapy, 15,* 336–352.

Johnston, J., & Pennypacker, H. (1980). *Strategies for human behavioral research.* Hillsdale, NJ: Erlbaum.

Kazdin, A. (1977). Assessing the clinical or applied significance of behavior change through social validation. *Behavior Modification, 1,* 427–452.

Kazdin, A. (1979). Situational-specificity: The two-edged sword of behavioral assessment. *Behavioral Assessment, 1,* 57–75.

Kazdin, A. (1981). Acceptability of child treatment techniques: The influence of treatment efficacy and adverse side effects. *Behavior Therapy, 12,* 493–506.

Kazdin, A., & Wilson, T. (1978). *Evaluation of behavior therapy: Issues, evidence, and research strategies.* Cambridge, MA: Ballinger.

Kendall, P., & Cummings, L. (1988). Thought and action in educational interventions: Cognitive–behavioral approaches. In J. Witt, S. Elliott, & F. Gresham (Eds.), *Handbook of behavior therapy in education* (pp. 403–418). New York: Plenum.

Lentz, F.E., & Shapiro, E.S. (1986). Functional assessment of the academic environment. *School Psychology Review, 15,* 346–357.

Lewin, K. (1931). The conflict between Aristotelian and Galilean modes of thought in contemporary psychology. In D. Adams & K. Zener (Eds.), *A dynamic theory of personality: Selected papers of Kurt Lewin.* New York: McGraw-Hill.

Lewis, T.J., & Sugai, G. (1996). Functional assessment of problem behavior: A pilot investigation of the comparative and interactive effects of teacher and peer social attention on students in general education settings. *School Psychology Quarterly, 11,* 1–19.

Linehan, M. (1980). Content validity: Its relevance to behavioral assessment. *Behavioral Assessment, 2,* 147–159.

Mace, F.C. (1994). The significance and future of functional analysis methodologies. *Journal of Applied Behavior Analysis, 27,* 385–392.

Mahoney, M.J. (1974). *Cognition and behavior modification.* Cambridge, MA: Ballinger.

McReynolds, P. (1986). History of assessment in clinical and educational settings. In R. Nelson & S. Hayes (Eds.), *Conceptual foundations of behavioral assessment* (pp. 42–80). New York: Guilford.

Meichenbaum, D. (1977). *Cognitive–behavior modification: An integrative approach.* New York: Plenum.

Messick, S. (1988). The once and future issues of validity: Assessing the meaning and consequences of measurement. In H. Wainer & H. Braun (Eds.), *Test validity* (pp. 33–46). Hillsdale, NJ: Erlbaum.

Messick, S. (1995). Validity of psychological assessment: Validation of inferences from persons' responses and performances as scientific inquiry into score meaning. *American Psychologist, 50,* 741–749.

Michael, J. (1993). Establishing operations. *The Behavior Analyst, 16,* 191–206.

Miller, D., & Kelley, M.L. (1994). The use of goal-setting and contingency contracting for improving children's homework performance. *Journal of Applied Behavior Analysis, 27,* 73–84.

Mischel, W. (1988). [Review of Nelson, R.O., & Hayes, S.C. (Eds.), *Conceptual foundations of behavioral assessment*]. *Behavioral Assessment, 10,* 125–128.

Neef, N., & Iwata, B. (1994). Current research on functional analysis methodologies: An introduction. *Journal of Applied Behavior Analysis, 27,* 211–214.

Nelson, R. (1983). Behavioral assessment: Past, present, and future. *Behavioral Assessment, 5,* 195–206.

Nelson, R., Hayes, S., & Jarrett, R. (1986). Evaluating the quality of behavioral assessment. In R. Nelson & S. Hayes (Eds.), *Conceptual foundations of behavioral assessment* (pp. 461–503). New York: Guilford.

Nelson, R.O. (1979). Note from the editor: [Editorial statement]. *Behavioral Assessment, 1,* i–ii.

Nelson, R.O., & Hayes, S.C. (1979). Some current dimensions of behavioral assessment. *Behavioral Assessment, 1,* 1–16.

Noell, G.H., & Gresham, F.M. (1993). Functional outcome analysis: Do the benefits of consultation and prereferral intervention justify the costs? *School Psychology Quarterly, 8,* 200–226.

Nunnally, J., & Bernstein, I. (1994). *Psychometric theory* (3rd ed.). New York: McGraw-Hill.

Nunnally, J., & Kotsche, W. (1983). Studies of individual subjects: Logic and methods of analysis. *British Journal of Clinical Psychology, 22,* 83–93.

Olympia, D., Sheridan, S., Jenson, W., & Andrews, D. (1994). Using student-managed interventions to increase homework performance. *Journal of Applied Behavior Analysis, 27,* 85–100.

Schwartz, I. (1991). The study of consumer behavior and social validity: An essential partnership for applied behavior analysis. *Journal of Applied Behavior Analysis, 24,* 241–244.

Schwartz, I., & Baer, D. (1991). Social validity assessment: Is current practice state of the art? *Journal of Applied Behavior Analysis, 24,* 189–204.

Sechrest, L. (1963). Incremental validity: A recommendation. *Educational and Psychological Measurement, 23,* 153–158.

Shapiro, E.S. (1989). *Academic skills problems: Direct assessment and intervention.* New York: Guilford.

Shapiro, E.S., & Kratochwill, T.R. (Eds.). (1988). *Behavioral assessment in schools: Conceptual foundations and practical applications.* New York: Guilford.

Shinn, M. (Ed.) (1989). *Curriculum-based measurement: Assessing special children.* New York: Guilford.

Silva, F. (1993). *Psychometric foundations and behavioral assessment.* Newbury Park, CA: Sage.

Skinner, B.F. (1953). *Science and human behavior.* New York: Free Press.

Strosahl, K., & Linehan, M. (1986). Basic issues in behavioral assessment. In A. Ciminero, K. Calhoun, & H. Adams (Eds.), *Handbook of behavioral assessment* (2nd ed., pp. 12–46). New York: Wiley Interscience.

Van Houten, R. (1979). Social validation: The evolution of standards of competency for targets. *Journal of Applied Behavior Analysis, 12,* 581–591.

Wahler, R., & Fox, J. (1981). Setting events in applied behavior analysis: Toward a conceptual and methodological expansion. *Journal of Applied Behavior Analysis, 14,* 327–338.

Wahler, R.G. (1975). Some structural aspects of deviant child behavior. *Journal of Applied Behavior Analysis, 8,* 27–42.

Walker, H.M., Colvin, G., & Ramsey, E. (1995). *Antisocial behavior in school: Strategies and best practices.* Pacific Grove, CA: Brooks/Cole.

Walker, H.M., & Severson, H. (1992). *Systematic screening for behavioral disorders.* Longmont, CO: Sopris West.

Wiggins, J. (1973). *Personality and prediction: Principles of personality assessment.* Reading, MA: Addison-Wesley.

Witt, J.C., & Elliott, S.N. (1985). Acceptability of classroom intervention strategies. In T. Kratochwill (Ed.), *Advances in school psychology* (Vol. 4, pp. 251–288). Hillsdale, NJ: Erlbaum.

Wolf, M.M. (1978). Social validity: The case for subjective measurement or how applied behavior analysis is finding its heart. *Journal of Applied Behavior Analysis, 11,* 203–214.

2

Designs for Evaluating Behavior Change

Conceptual Principles of Single Case Methodology

FRANK M. GRESHAM

Introduction

Documenting and evaluating the efficacy of procedures to change behavior is a hallmark of behavior therapy and applied behavior analysis. Psychologists trained in behaviorally oriented programs are taught to empirically evaluate their treatments and make treatment decisions based on empirical data. This is not to say that all behavior therapists function as researchers. Malott (1992) suggested that there are two categories of behavior analysts based on the goals and requirements of one's job: researchers and practitioners. Researchers are primarily interested in manipulating independent variables and observing their unique effects on dependent variables using tight experimental control. Practitioners are more interested in implementing a treatment program and bringing the dependent variable into acceptable ranges very quickly rather than isolating the unique effects of an independent variable. These two goals, while differing in detail and methodological rigor, are based on the same principle: data based, empirical evaluation of treatment effects or outcomes. Some may allude to the former as "applied research" and to the latter as "program evaluation." Most behavior therapists/analysts would probably agree that collecting data on treatment outcomes is one of the most important aspects of the entire behavior change process.

This view, however, is not held by most practicing psychotherapists. A survey of clinical practitioners in the American Psychological Association by Morrow-Bradley and Elliott (1986) concerning the use of psychotherapy research by practicing psychotherapists indicated that questions addressed in research often are not clinically relevant; the variables studied are not representative of typical clinical practice; the forms in which results are reported (e.g., mean differences, F ratios) do not represent clinically important changes or differences; single case research is infrequent; and practical or relevant measures of psychological change often are not used. In short, practicing psychotherapists are relatively unaffected by psychotherapy research and do not find it useful in their daily practice.

Why would these practitioners hold such a low opinion of behavior change research? One explanation may be that practicing psychotherapists, unlike behavior therapists/analysts, are not trained in a research tradition that values empirically based evaluation of treatment outcomes. In fact, many of the issues addressed in conventional psychotherapy are often not amenable to measurement and empirical evaluation. Another explanation is that the way research is presented, packaged, and marketed is often alien, incomprehensible, and irrelevant, speaking little to the practical significance of research findings. D. Barlow (1981) suggests in his criticisms of psychotherapy research that perhaps the literature

FRANK M. GRESHAM • School of Education, University of California–Riverside, Riverside, California 92521-0102.

Handbook of Child Behavior Therapy, edited by Watson and Gresham. Plenum Press, New York, 1998.

itself, rather than the practitioner, is to blame for the underutilization of clinical research.

The purpose of the present chapter is to present readers with fundamental conceptual principles governing the planning, design, and evaluation of behavioral intervention procedures. This chapter focuses exclusively on single case methodologies used in documenting the efficacy of intervention procedures. Not all child behavior therapists or researchers adhere exclusively to a single case approach; however, this approach is the preferred, if not exclusive, experimental design methodology of modern-day applied behavior analysts. Given our emphasis in this book on behavior analysis, we will focus on the use of within-subject, single case experimental designs.

Overview of Research Paradigms

Two general paradigms of experimental research exist in psychology. The first approach, which is by far the most common, uses group or nomothetic data to make statements about average differences between two groups or among several groups. The second approach uses repeated measures of behavior on a single individual or on a small number of individuals to make statements about differences between control and experimental phases or conditions of an experiment. These two research paradigms differ in their goals and strategies and in the inferences made about the effects of independent variables on dependent variables.

Baer (1977) perhaps most clearly differentiated these two approaches in his classic article "Perhaps it would be better not to know everything":

> If behavior might be different under a condition known as "A" than it is under a condition known as "B", and if it were important to find out whether that possibility was an actuality, then two basic paradigms would be available for its examination. A number of subjects might be recruited and divided at random into two equal groups. One of these groups would be exposed to the "A" condition, and its behavior noted; the other would be exposed to the "B" condition, and its behavior similarly noted. The mean behavior of those exposed to "A" could be compared to the mean behavior of those exposed to "B." A difference in those means might be interesting. Alternatively, a single subject might be recruited and exposed to the "A" condition for some time to behavior repeatedly under its influence. Then the "A" condition would be replaced by the "B" condition, and the ongoing behavior would con-

tinue to be monitored as before. An alteration of "A" and "B" conditions would continue, and the repeated patterns of behavior seen under the repeated "A's" would be compared to the repeated patterns of behavior seen under the repeated "B's". A consistent difference in those arrays might be interesting. (p. 167)

Baer (1977) argues that the group design paradigm defends itself against spurious findings or "chance" by using samples to estimate whether or not there are population mean differences. This is accomplished by randomly sampling from a population or randomly assigning subjects to groups; these procedures, however, are not the same. What is typically done in this paradigm is to ignore this problem and assume that the difference between "A" and "B" conditions is zero.

In single case designs, defense against chance is accomplished by observing repeated patterns of behavior under repeated and alternated "A" and "B" conditions. If behavior under the repeated "A" conditions is repeatedly different under the repeated "B" conditions, then it is concluded that these differences were not due to chance. These differences, however, are typically not subjected to statistical analyses to determine what degree of confidence researchers have in their findings (e.g., $p < .05$ or .01).

Researchers operating out of the group paradigm guard against errors in statistical decisions by controlling Type I errors (false rejection of a true null hypothesis). This error rate traditionally has been set at .05, thereby indicating that if a researcher concludes that the null hypothesis is false, then there is a 5% chance that this conclusion would be erroneous. Cohen (1994), a well-respected group design methodologist and statistician, argued convincingly against the use of traditional null hypothesis significance testing (NHST). He suggested that this approach has failed in advancing psychological knowledge and has actually impeded it. Cohen indicates that the chief problem in NHST is that it does not tell us what we want to know. What we want to know is, "Based on these data, what is the probability the null hypothesis is true?" In terms of a treatment outcome study involving two groups (experimental and control), what is the probability that there are not differences in the groups' mean scores. Unfortunately, what NHST tells us is, "If the null hypothesis is true, what is the probability that these data occurred by chance?" (a Type I error). These two questions, however, are not the same.

In contrast, Baer (1977) indicates that Type I errors in single case methodology are not precisely computable, but the error rate is less than .05. Instead, the single case researcher uses visual inspection of repeated "A" and "B" differences to guard against Type I errors. Consequently, single-subject researchers make very few Type I errors and a large number of Type II errors (i.e., retaining a false null hypothesis), whereas group researchers make more Type I errors but relatively few Type II errors. In summing up his arguments regarding single case and group paradigms of research, Baer (1977) stated:

> Individual-subject-design practitioners, operating without calculation of the pertinent probabilities necessarily fall into very low probabilities of Type 1 errors and very high probabilities of Type 2 errors, relative to their group-paradigm colleagues. As a result, they learn about fewer variables, but these variables are typically more powerful, general, dependable, and—very important—sometimes actionable. These are exactly the variables on which a technology of behavior might be built. (pp. 170–171)

In short, Baer indicates that applied behavior analysts are interested in discovering strong treatments and are willing to conclude that a treatment was not a functional one in changing behavior when, in fact, it might have been (a Type II error). In contrast, group design researchers often discover weak effects through statistical analysis and NHST which may not be meaningful in a powerful science of behavior change.

Cohen (1994) and Baer (1977) agree that there are rather substantial problems with traditional group experimental design logic, particularly as it relates to null hypothesis testing. Cohen (1994), a group methodologist by training and philosophy, comes down on the side of the behavioral philosophy of science by stating:

> We appeal to inductive logic to move from the particular results in hand to a theoretically useful generalization. . . . we have a body of statistical techniques, that used intelligently, can facilitate our efforts. But given the problems of statistical induction, we must finally rely, as have the older sciences on replication. (p. 1002)

Problems with the Group Design Paradigm

The group comparison or nomothetic approach has a long history in psychology and dominates research endeavors in both experimental and applied psychological research. One only has to glance at any recent journals such as *Journal of Educational Psychology, Journal of Consulting and Clinical Psychology,* or *Journal of Experimental Psychology: Human Perception and Performance,* to confirm this. Given psychology's obvious acceptance of this research paradigm, what, then, could be wrong or problematic with this way of studying behavior? We saw in the preceding section that Baer (1977) outlined substantial differences between the group and single case paradigms. We also saw that Cohen (1994) totally rejects the tradition of NHST because not only does it not tell us what we want to know, it does not contribute to an inductive understanding of psychological phenomena. These differences emanate, in part, from the two differing epistemologies, Aristotelian and Galilean, discussed in Chapter 1 (see Gresham & Lambros, this volume).

Perhaps the most forthright criticisms of the group experimental design paradigm can be found in Johnston and Pennypacker (1993). These authors argue that behavior is an individual phenomenon resulting from the interaction between an organism and its environment. Therefore, behavior change agents should be interested only in an individual's behavior under various environmental conditions. Johnston and Pennypacker suggest that behavior analysis should be considered a natural science (e.g., biology) rather than a social science. Unlike the social sciences, there are relatively little group comparison research and inferential statistics in either the physical or natural sciences (with the exception of, perhaps, medicine).

D.H. Barlow and Hersen (1984) noted five limitations of the group comparison approach in behavior therapy. First, there are some *ethical concerns* regarding the use of the group comparison paradigm. This is particularly problematic when the design calls for a no-treatment or delayed-treatment control group. As D.H. Barlow and Hersen correctly point out, these concerns are based on the assumption that we know the intervention is effective a priori, which would obviate the need for running the experiment in the first place. In the single case paradigm, control groups are not needed because each subject serves as his or her own control.

A second concern relates to the *practical difficulties* in collecting large numbers of subjects homogenous for particular behavior problems or diagnoses. Many of the problems child behavior therapists and behavior analysts see are low-incidence conditions such as autism, selective mutism, and chronic illnesses of childhood. Trying to select a representative sample large enough for adequate statistical power for these problems would be difficult and expensive.

A third issue that strikes at the heart of group comparison research is the *averaging of results,* which masks the outcome of intervention for any given individual in a group. Common wisdom in psychotherapy research suggests that some clients improve, some stay the same, and some deteriorate as a function of therapeutic intervention. Thus, the mean or average score will not necessarily represent any person in that group. Also, the measurement of attributes in much of psychology uses what Johnston and Pennypacker (1993) call *vaganotic,* or relative, measurement strategies. Vaganotic measurement systems are based on the variation in a set of underlying observations rather than on absolute values. Therefore, for example, the meaning of a child's score on any of the subscales of the Child Behavior Checklist or Teacher Rating form (Achenbach, 1991) is based on how far his or her score deviates from the T-score mean of 50 ($SD = 10$). Johnston and Pennypacker (1993) argue that this approach to measurement is unique to the social sciences and is not unlike measuring the weight of objects by weighing all available objects, computing a mean and standard deviation, and then assigning values to these objects based on the deviation of each object from the mean value of all objects.

A fourth concern of the group comparison approach voiced by D.H. Barlow and Hersen (1984) deals with the *generality of findings.* Results from group studies do not inform or reflect changes in individuals and thus are not particularly useful for practicing behavior therapists. This was described earlier in this chapter in regard to practicing psychotherapists' low opinions of the value of published research for guiding their practice. Johnston and Pennypacker (1993) aptly point out that Sir Ronald Fisher (1956), the father of modern statistics, clearly indicated that inferences can be made only from samples to populations and not from samples to individuals. Based on this logic, any results of group comparison research can inform us only about the performance of a group as a whole rather than about that of any individual child within that group.

D.H. Barlow and Hersen (1984) mention a final problem with the group paradigm: the degree of *intersubject variability.* One way in which researchers have dealt with variability in performances of subjects is to consider it to be intrinsic to the individual and not due to environmental or experimental factors (see Johnston & Pennypacker, 1993; Sidman, 1960). Therefore, the significance of Group A's mean score and Group B's mean score is determined by the amount of intersubject variability within each group. Any deviation of an individual's score from the mean in a given group is considered "error," whereas the differences between groups are considered to result from the effects of the independent variable. In contrast, most behavior therapists and behavior analysts view variability in behavior to be extrinsic. Extrinsic behavior is behavior that is describable and predictable, and in which variation in performance can be explained by reference to other organismic and/or environmental phenomena (Johnston & Pennypacker, 1993).

Single Case Experimental Design

Background

Single case experimental designs are not new, but are often underutilized in clinical practice (Hayes, 1981). Gresham and Kendell (1987) made a similar observation regarding research and practice of school-based consultation. Hayes (1981) specified several reasons for the infrequent use of single case methodology in clinical practice: (a) Single case methodology is either untaught or undertaught in most training programs, most typically by statisticians or experimental psychologists having little or no interest in or familiarity with clinical problems; (b) single case methodology has not been directed toward the practicing clinician and therefore is perceived as impractical; (c) the methodology is associated with behavioral approaches, although it, like the group comparison approach, is theoretically neutral; (d) many clinicians may think of research only in terms of group comparison research, thereby ignoring the single case paradigm as a viable research alternative; (e) there are few publication outlets for "on-line" clinical research (most journals require a methodological rigor that exceeds the practicalities of doing clinical research); and (f) many institutions (e.g., clinical agencies, schools) provide little or no support or incentive for doing research.

The reasons specified by Hayes (1981) some 15 years ago still hold true. Only a relatively small number of researchers are trained in the single case approach; most of these are applied behavior analysts. In fact, the author is aware of several cases at major universities in which prospective faculty job applicants were severely criticized and were rejected because they had presented a single case design colloquium. This is unfortunate, given the contributions single case methodology has made in our understanding of human behavior. The fact is that the hypothectico-deductive, theory-building approach to research continues to dominate American psychology.

Fundamental Principles of Single Case Methodology

Experimental designs, whether they be group or single case, have the same basic purpose: to assess the unique effects of an independent variable on a dependent variable while controlling threats to experimental validity. Group experimental designs do this by randomly assigning subjects to experimental or control conditions and comparing their average scores on some dependent measure. Single case experimental designs, on the other hand, compare the same subject's performance or that of several subjects, under baseline and treatment conditions, using subjects as their own controls. Besides this fundamental difference, there are some core elements that distinguish single case methodology from traditional group experimental designs. These core elements have been described by others in the literature and have consental agreement from most experts in the field of behavior therapy and behavior analysis (see D. Barlow, Hayes, & Nelson, 1984; D.H. Barlow & Hersen, 1984; Hayes, 1981; Kazdin, 1992; Johnston & Pennypacker, 1993; Tawney & Gast, 1984). These core elements or essential principles are: (a) repeated measurement, (b) analysis of behavioral variability, (c) dynamic experimental design, (d) specification of conditions, and (e) replication. Each of these core elements will be discussed briefly in the following sections.

Repeated Measurement

The most fundamental principle of single case methodology is the repeated measurement of behavior under standard (baseline) and experimental conditions. These repeated measurements of behavior are based on precise, operational definitions of behavior which remain the same throughout the entire experiment. A central concern in single case design is obtaining a sufficient number of measurements of the target behavior under baseline and treatment conditions, because these measurements are the basis of determining the effects of the treatment.

Another consideration in the repeated measurement of behavior is establishing and analyzing stable or *steady state responding*. Johnston and Pennypacker (1993) define steady state responding as a pattern of responding that varies little in its measured qualities over time. Obviously, stable or steady state responding can only be assessed through the repeated measurement of behavior over time. Johnston and Pennypacker (1993) discuss several reasons for the importance of establishing steady state responding. First, stable responding provides information about behavior and its influences. For example, behavior might show a great deal of variability when measured by *duration,* and show steady state responding when measured by *frequency.* Alternatively, behavior might show considerable variability when observed in the afternoon, but may reflect steady state responding when observed in the morning. In either case, stability or variability in repeated measurements of behavior informs researchers and practitioners about particular environmental or organismic influences on behavior.

Second, repeated measurement of behavior assists in evaluating the degree of experimental control over a dependent variable. For example, a high level of behavioral variability during baseline makes conclusions regarding the effects of the independent variable difficult, if not impossible. Similarly, if a great degree of behavioral variability occurs during treatment conditions, then assessing the unique effects of the independent variable is compromised.

Third, repeated measurement of behavior allows for comparisons between baseline and experimental conditions for individuals. Each individual's behavior is assessed under baseline and experimental conditions, thereby allowing for within-subject rather than between-subject comparisons. If stable responding is established under baseline and treatment conditions, then the effects of treatment on behavior can be more clearly established. In contrast, if highly variable performances are seen under baseline and/or treatment conditions, researchers are better able to identify extraneous variables that may be causing this variability.

Finally, repeated measures of behavior can be used to assess *trends* in behavior over time. Steady state responding shows an absence of trends or no consistent changes in direction over time. Increasing or decreasing trends in behavior under baseline conditions make it virtually impossible to conclude that an independent variable was responsible for the behavior change. Thus, steady state or stable responding during baseline conditions is essential for drawing valid experimental conclusions.

Analysis of Behavioral Variability

Analysis of intrasubject variability is another cardinal feature of single case research and is the context in which levels and trends in repeatedly measured behavior are evaluated (Hayes, 1981). Behavioral variability is the window through which the single case researcher views what is going on in an experiment, and it serves as the basis for evaluating the effects of treatment. Johnston and Pennypacker (1993) suggest that behavioral variability takes at least three forms: (a) it can refer to differences in features of behaviors that may be part of the same response class (e.g., frequency of disruptive behavior versus duration of academic engaged time); (b) it can refer to variations in different dimensions of the same behavior (e.g., frequency vs. duration vs. interresponse times of aggressive episodes); and (c) it can refer to variations in measures of behavior across sessions or phases of an experiment.

As mentioned earlier, variability can also be masked by averaging individual responding across sessions or days. D.H. Barlow and Hersen (1984) provide several examples of how highly variable data can be made to look quite stable by this averaging. Averaging is problematic because decisions regarding phase changes and responsiveness to treatment may be inaccurate if they are based on averaged data. Intrasubject variability is common in repeated measurement of behavior, and how much variability an experimenter or practitioner is willing to tolerate is based on a judgment call, rather than on some formal decision rule (D.H. Barlow & Hersen, 1984).

Johnston and Pennypacker (1993) suggest that behavioral variability serves three functions. First, variability in behavior prompts and guides researchers to ask questions about their data. For example, why do some children respond to response cost procedures, whereas others may respond better to overcorrection? Second, variability in behavior assists in designing and modifying experiments as well as determining length of baseline and experimental phases. As Johnston and Pennypacker (1993) state: "[V]ariability serves the same navigational role in leading the researcher through the many decisions involved in designing experiments and conducting comparisons that will clarify the influence of experimental variables" (p. 179). Third, behavioral variability serves as the basis for interpreting one's experiments. Graphic displays of this variability during different phases of the experiment allow for certain conclusions to be drawn from the data.

Unlike group experimental designs which treat intrasubject variability as error, behavioral variability in the single case paradigm is an extremely valuable source of information. Intrasubject variability is the context in which important decisions regarding experimental arrangements and conclusions are drawn about the effects of an intervention. Johnston and Pennypacker (1993) argue that two experimental strategies are used concurrently to deal with behavioral variability. The first strategy seeks to isolate and control extraneous sources of environmental influences responsible for variability. For example, the effects of using DRO for reducing aggressive and disruptive behavior could not be evaluated if the client was placed on psychotropic medication midway through the experiment. A second strategy is the primary purpose of the experiment: the deliberate manipulation of an independent variable and observation of its effects on the dependent variable. The purpose of this manipulation is to observe how this changes steady state responding observed from a baseline condition to the variability created by introduction of a treatment condition.

Dynamic Experimental Design

Another fundamental characteristic of single case design is the dynamic, interactive nature of the design, or what Hayes (1981) calls an attitude of investigative play. In group experimental designs, the design, numbers of subjects, sampling, and the like are planned before the experiment is conducted. Once an experiment is decided and begun, the design is unchanging and static and does not use data collected at any time during the experiment as a basis for changing the design. Single case designs, on the other hand, are always tentative and subject to change based on how subjects respond to various experimental arrangements.

An example illustrates this dynamic nature of single case designs. A researcher may take baseline data on frequency of disruptive behavior in a classroom and establish steady state responding. An interdependent group contingency is implemented and disruptive behavior may not be significantly decreased. In looking at the individual data, the researcher may discover that two students are responsible for 95% of disruptive behavior. Having determined this, the researcher changes the intervention from an interdependent to a dependent group contingency, in which the two most disruptive students earn reinforcement for the rest of the group. This change results in dramatic decreases in disruptive behavior rates for the class. The researcher returns to baseline and then replicates this effect in a subsequent phase, thereby demonstrating a reliable effect. Clearly, this procedure probably would not have been attempted in a group experimental design, the study would have been deemed a failure, and it certainly would not have been published in a reputable journal.

Replication

Replication is at the heart of all scientific investigation, because results of any experimental manipulation should be repeated by the same researcher and by other researchers to have scientific credibility. In single case experimental designs, replications often occur within phases of the experiment (within baseline and treatment conditions), as well as across two or more baseline and treatment conditions, as in ABAB or withdrawal designs. Replications can also be demonstrated across baseline and treatment conditions for subjects, settings, or behaviors, as in multiple baseline designs, or between two or more treatments that are rapidly changed, as in alternating treatments designs.

Replications also must be demonstrated across different experiments studying the same phenomena. The replications are the basis of the external validity or generality of findings in single case experimental designs. D.H. Barlow and Hersen (1984) mention that replication is relevant to three types of generality that are important for external validity of results: (a) It is important to demonstrate that behavior changes for one client can be replicated with other clients; (b) it is important that behavior change produced by one therapist, teacher, or change agent can be reproduced by other therapists or change agents; and (c) replication requires that changes produced in one setting can be generalized to other settings.

Johnston and Pennypacker (1993) suggest that replication serves two functions: (a) it provides information on the reliability of original findings, and (b) it provides information regarding the generality of findings. Sidman (1960) perhaps summed up the nature of generality of single case designs best:

> It is unrealistic to expect that a given variable will have the same effects upon all subjects under all conditions. As we identify and control a greater number of the conditions that determine the effects of a given experimental operation, in effect we decrease the variability that may be expected as a consequence of the operation. It then becomes possible to produce the same results in a greater number of subjects. Such generality could never be achieved if we simply accepted intersubject variability and gave equal status to all deviant subjects in an investigation. (p. 190)

Specification of Conditions

Without clear and unambiguous specification of the independent variable, there can be no definitive conclusions regarding a functional analysis of behavior (Johnson & Pennypacker, 1993; Sidman, 1960). This specification requires the representation of the treatment procedures (the independent variable) by known physical parameters of an environmental event. Treatment specification is important for two extremely important aspects of experimental research: (a) *treatment integrity* and (b) *replication*.

Treatment integrity refers to the extent to which a treatment is implemented as planned and is concerned with the accuracy and consistency with which treatments are implemented (Gresham, 1997; Gresham, Gansle, & Noell, 1993). Treatments that are not well specified cannot be subjected to integrity assessments, and, thus, conclusions regarding the effects of treatments are compromised. Treatments that are not well specified also cannot be replicated by other researchers. Unless an independent researcher or practitioner knows precisely what was done, how it was done, and how long it was done, then replication is impossible. If replication means to duplicate, copy, or repeat what was done, then this replication depends entirely upon a complete and unambiguous specification of experimental procedures *and* an assessment of whether or not they were implemented as planned (treatment integrity).

Experimental Design Models

All experimental designs, whether they are traditional group experimental designs or single case designs, are built from a relatively few core or essential elements. Kirk's (1995) classic text, *Experimental Design,* indicates that although there are a "bewildering array" of designs available to researchers, all of these group designs can be reduced to three simple building-block designs (completely randomized designs, randomized block designs, and Latin square designs). All experimental designs represent variations and/or combinations of these core experimental designs. Others have variously classified experimental designs into between subjects designs, within subjects designs, and combined or mixed designs (Linquist, 1953; Winer, 1971). In between subjects designs, subjects are randomly assigned to two or more experimental conditions and their scores on some dependent variable are compared. Within subjects designs expose each subject to all experimental conditions in a counterbalanced fashion and thereby use each subject as its own control. Mixed or combined designs represent some combination of the first two.

Hayes (1981) similarly has reduced the large number of single case experimental designs into three core elements organized by the logic of their data comparisons. These strategies are within series strategies, between series strategies, and combined series strategies. These strategies parallel the within,

between and mixed (combined) classifications of group experimental designs; however, the sampling units are different. In group designs, the sampling units typically are persons exposed to two or more conditions. In single case designs, the sampling units are samples of repeatedly measured behavior of the same subject(s) over time within and across baseline and experimental conditions. Theoretically, there are an infinite number of experimental designs that could be constructed to answer research questions from these three core strategies. Table 1 lists some examples of frequently used experimental designs characteristic of each of these strategies, and intervention questions. The logic and examples of each approach are described in the following sections.

Within-Series Strategies

The most common experimental arrangements in single case designs have traditionally been based on comparing changes within a series of data points under two baseline and two treatment conditions. Baer, Wolf, and Risley (1968) described the logic of this design as follows:

> There are at least two designs commonly used to demonstrate reliable control of an important behavioral change. The first can be referred to as the "reversal" technique. Here a behavior is measured, and the measure is examined over time until its stability is clear. Then, the experimental variable is applied. The behavior continues to be measured, to see if the variable will produce a behavioral change. If it does, the experimental variable is discontinued or altered, to see if the behavioral change just brought about depends on it. If so, the behavioral change should be lost or diminished (thus, the term "reversal"). The experimental variable then is applied again, to see if the behavioral change can be recovered. . . . It may be reversed briefly again, and yet again, if the setting in which the behavior takes place allows further reversals. (p. 94)

It is also possible to compare two or more treatments using simple phase changes such as ABAC, BCBC, or any of a number of combinations or sequences of experimental arrangements. For example, one might be interested in knowing if response cost (B) is more or less effective in reducing classroom disruptive behavior than is time-out (C). This question might lead to an ABAC design; however, there may be better ways of answering this experimental question that would control for the obvious sequence effects (e.g., a multielement design described later).

TABLE 1. Intervention Questions and Single-Case Design Arrangements to Answer Them

Intervention question	Within series	Between series	Combined series
Does an intervention work?	(a) Withdrawal design ABAB and its variations (b) Changing criterion design	Multielement designs (alternating treatments design)	(a) Multiple baseline designs (across subjects, settings, and behaviors); (b) Replicated crossover designs
Does one intervention work better than another?	Simple phase changes (e.g., BCBC)	Multielement designs comparing B & C treatments (alternating treatments designs)	(a) Multiple baselines comparing B & C Controlling for order (b) Replicated crossover design comparing B & C
Do different intervention elements interact to produce behavior change?	Complex phase changes (e.g., B/B + C/B or C/B + C/C, etc.)	Multielement designs (alternating treatments) (e.g., comparing B with B + C)	(a) Mutiple baseline designs comparing B with B + C and C with B + C (b) Replicated crossovers comparing B with B + C and C with B + C
Do treatment effects maintain after treatment is withdrawn?	(a) Sequential withdrawal design (b) Partial-withdrawl design (c) Partial sequential withdrawal design	Complex phase changes with withdrawals (e.g., B/B + C/B/A)	(a) Mutiple baseline designs with withdrawal of treatment (b) Replicated crossovers with withdrawal of treatments
Does the child have the behavior in his or her repertoire?			Multiple probe technique in multiple baseline designs

Note: Adapted from S.C. Hayes. Single case experimental design and empirical clinical practice. *Journal of Consulting and Clinical Psychology, 49,*
     193–211.

Experimental designs using *complex phase changes* seek to uncover the combined or interactive effects of two or more treatments on behavior. The purpose of these designs is to evaluate and analyze the effects of two or more treatments separately and in combination and replicate these findings across experimental phases (D.H. Barlow & Hersen, 1984). These designs use the same logic as the simple phase change, but add and subtract treatment components in various sequences to determine experimental effects. For example, a behavior analyst might be interested in the unique and combined effects of overcorrection and response cost on inappropriate verbalizations in a classroom setting. This experimental design might take the following sequence: A/B/B+C/B/A/C/B+C, where A is baseline, B is overcorrection, and C is response cost. R.H. Barlow and Hersen (1984) present numerous examples of these types of experimental designs.

Rusch and Kazdin (1981) described variations of the withdrawal design that are useful for assessing response maintenance after experimental control has been established. In addressing the importance of response maintenance and its assessment, Rusch and Kazdin suggested:

> In acquisition studies investigators are interested in demonstrating, unequivocally, that a functional relationship exists between treatment and behavioral change. In maintenance studies, on the other hand, investigators attempt to conclude that behavior is maintained after the intervention is withdrawn. . . . If the investigator is evaluating acquisition or maintenance, he or she should be able to conclude which variables are responsible for behavior change or maintenance. (pp. 131-132)

There are three variations of the withdrawal design: (a) sequential-withdrawal, (b) partial-withdrawal, and (c) partial-sequential withdrawal. In the sequential-withdrawal design, one component of a multicomponent treatment is withdrawn at a time until all components have been withdrawn. Thus, each component is withdrawn *sequentially* in consecutive experimental phases. For example, a multicomponent treatment might involve a combination of token reinforcement, DRI, and praise to increase academic engaged time. After experimental control is established, the researcher removes the token reinforcement component and assesses response maintenance. Next, the researcher removes the DRI component and similarly notes maintenance. Finally, the praise component is removed and the effect observed. In this hypothetical example, it may be that withdrawal of the token reinforcement and DRI components did not result in loss of maintenance, but when praise was withdrawn, behavior deteriorated. This would indicate that praise alone was sufficient in maintaining responding.

In a partial-withdrawal design, one component of a multicomponent treatment, or the entire treatment, is withdrawn from one or several baselines in a multiple baseline design (across, subjects, settings, or behaviors). For example, response cost and overcorrection might be used to decrease rates of disruptive behavior, inappropriate verbalizations, and out-of-seat behavior in a multiple baseline across-behaviors design. The response cost component might be removed for disruptive behavior and the effects observed. If rates of disruptive behavior increased, it might be predicted that the same effects would happen if response cost were removed for inappropriate verbalizations and out-of-seat behavior. However, as Rusch and Kazdin (1981) point out, withdrawing a treatment or a component may not represent the data pattern for all behaviors, subjects, or settings/situations.

The partial-sequential-withdrawal design involves withdrawing an entire multicomponent treatment or a component of that treatment from one of the baselines in a multiple baseline design across subjects, settings, or behaviors. Rusch and Kazdin (1981) suggest that this design seeks to determine whether maintenance of treatment effects occur when various components of the intervention are removed. It involves sampling of subjects or behaviors to obtain a preview of what might happen with other subjects and behaviors. As an example, a researcher might use a combination of verbal prompts, positive practice, and praise to increase rates of positive social interactions across three subjects. For Subject 1,

the researcher removes the entire treatment and rates of social interaction return to baseline levels. The researcher concludes the same effect would occur with Subject 2 and removes only the prompt component. This manipulation produces no significant decrease in responding. For Subject 3, both prompts and positive practice components are removed with no significant decrements in performance. The researcher concludes that praise alone is necessary to maintain behavior and should be continued.

One caveat that Rusch and Kazdin (1981) present is that the *order* in which treatment components are withdrawn may have differential effects and this may interact with individual subjects and multiple behaviors. Thus, because partial-sequential-withdrawal designs involve sampling, it is impossible to conclude that the same effects would be observed when treatment components are removed in different orders with other subjects, behaviors, and settings.

Another within series strategy is known as the *changing criterion design* (Hartmann & Hall, 1976), in which changes in a given criterion level for reinforcement are implemented in a stepwise fashion across several experimental phases. If the target behavior changes in relation to these criteria, then experimental control is demonstrated and the experimenter can be confident in concluding that the treatment (criteria for reinforcement) was responsible for behavior change. Changing criterion designs are especially useful for evaluating the effects of academic interventions in which the criteria might be increasing levels of work completion or accuracy. This is known as an *accelerating changing criterion* design. For example, a child's baseline levels of performance in math computation might range between 25% and 30%. The behavior therapist might set the first criterion for reinforcement for the next five days at 50%, for the next five days at 70%, for the next five days at 80%, and for the final five days at 90%. Each day the child meets the criterion, he or she receives reinforcement. If math accuracy tracks the various criteria, experimental control is established.

Changing criterion designs can also be *decelerating;* here the goal is to reduce a target behavior from baseline levels. For instance, the goal of an intervention might be to reduce the number of classroom rule infractions from baseline levels. The behavior analyst would systematically change the criterion for reinforcement in a decelerating fashion until the target behavior reaches acceptable levels.

Between Series Strategies

Between series strategies make comparisons between a series of two or more data points across time. Between series strategies compare rapid and repeated alterations of treatment conditions. Unlike within series strategies, there is no need (or possibility) to establish stability, level, and trend within phases because a given data point may be preceded or followed by measurements of other conditions (Hayes, 1981). Between series strategies are especially useful for comparing the effects of two or more treatments, although there are some difficulties with multiple treatment interference, sequential confounding, carryover effects, and contrast effects (see D. Barlow et al., 1984, for a complete discussion).

The most common between series strategy is the *alternating treatments design* (ATD) described by D.H. Barlow and Hayes (1979), but referred to by Sidman (1960) as a multielement design and as a multiple schedule design by others (D.H. Barlow & Hersen, 1973; Hersen & Barlow, 1976). The basic logic of this design is rapid alteration of two or more treatment conditions (e.g., discriminative stimuli, schedules of reinforcement) so that responding under these differential conditions can be compared.

Hains and Baer (1989) prefer the term *multielement* design and indicate that these designs are best suited for studying effects of stimulus control rather than for comparing different methods for teaching new skills, which may require a more slow-paced series of within series comparisons (e.g., withdrawal designs). An excellent example of a multielement design is the classic study by Iwata and colleagues on the functional analysis of self-injurious behavior (SIB) (Iwata, Dorsey, Slifer, Bauman, & Richman, 1982). In this investigation, subjects were exposed to each of four different conditions (social disapproval, academic demand, unstructured play, and alone) to assess the functional relationships among these conditions and rates of SIB. This investigation showed that rates of SIB were consistently associated with specific stimulus conditions and were not due to within subject "random" variability. Multielement designs of this sort have essentially become the "gold standard" design used in functional analytic work with SIB (Vollmer, Marcus, Ringdahl, & Roane, 1995) as well as brief functional analyses of aberrant behavior (Derby et al., 1992).

Multielement or ATD designs possess several advantages over within series strategies. First, these designs typically produce effects much more rapidly than withdrawal or reversal designs. Second, there is no need to establish a stable baseline or to be concerned with increasing or decreasing trends within phases, because a data point is associated with a given condition and is not part of a consecutive series of data points. Third, these designs are especially useful in functional analytic work in which specific stimulus conditions can be rapidly alternated. As mentioned previously, a major threat to these designs, however, is multiple treatment interference and its variations (e.g., contrast effects, sequential confounding, order effects).

Combined Series Strategies

Combined series strategies make comparisons both within and between a series of data points to determine experimental control. The most common of these strategies is the *multiple baseline design,* which allows for sequential comparisons between baseline and treatment conditions for persons, settings, or behaviors. D. Barlow and colleagues (1984) argue that the term "multiple baseline" might be a misnomer, because what is actually being done in the design are *multiple phase changes* and multiple baselines are not really required by the design's logic. In any event, multiple baselines control for the weaknesses in simple phase change designs by reducing the likelihood that extraneous events could be responsible for experimental effects. This is accomplished by replicating the effects of a treatment at different points in time over a series of data points across persons, settings, or behaviors.

There are several variations of the multiple baseline design that are worth noting. For example, R.D. Horner and Baer (1978) described a variation of the multiple baseline for studying acquisition behavior called the *multiple probe technique,* which does not require continuous baseline measurement and instead "probes" responding. R.D. Horner and Baer suggest that multiple probes are appropriate when (a) extended baselines may be reactive, (b) it is impractical, and/or (c) there are strong a priori assumptions of stability of responding. Multiple probe designs are particularly useful for investigating chains or successive approximations of behavior (e.g., tooth brushing, toileting, language). In summarizing the multiple probe technique, R.D. Horner and Baer (1978) state as follows:

> the multiple-probe technique provides a procedure for collecting data that will permit a thorough functional analysis of the variables related to the acquisition of behavior across the components of a chain or successive approximation sequence. In addition, intermittent probes provide an alternative method for establishing stable baselines when continuous measurement during multiple baselines proves impractical, unnecessary, or reactive. (p. 196)

Another variation of the multiple baseline design was described by Wacker and colleagues as the *sequential alternating treatments* design (Wacker et al., 1990). This design combines the logic of the ATD with that of a multiple baseline and is useful when a baseline is either not practical or does not provide an adequate contrast for the experimental conditions and can be used across subjects, behaviors, and settings/tasks. Wacker and colleagues detail the advantages and disadvantages of the sequential ATD with and without baseline conditions.

Another combined series approach is known as the *crossover design,* in which two concurrent phase changes are implemented in reverse order of one another (Hayes, 1981; Kazdin, 1992). In this design, subjects are first exposed to one treatment condition and, midway through the study, the subjects "cross over" and receive the second treatment. A good example of the crossover design can be found in the study by Gettinger (1993) in which pairs of subjects (one below-average student and one above-average student) were assigned to either an invented spelling condition or to a direct instruction condition for five consecutive weeks. After five weeks, the conditions were reversed for another five weeks. After the second five weeks, each spelling condition was replicated for each pair of children for another three consecutive weeks. As Gettinger pointed out, one drawback of this design is the possibility of carryover effects of each treatment, in spite of attempts to control for sequence effects by counterbalancing replications.

Issues and Considerations in Single Case Designs

The use of single case experimental designs is an efficient way of dealing with issues of experimental control and randomization required in large-scale group experimental designs. As we have seen, single case designs using within-series, between-series, and combined-series strategies can be used to establish relationships (correlational or functional) between independent and dependent variables. In spite of the versatility of these designs, there are several issues which should be considered in interpreting interventions based on this methodology. These issues include: (a) quantification of effects, (b) social validation, and (c) experimental validity.

Quantification of Effects

One issue that is somewhat controversial in single case design concerns the most appropriate way of quantifying the effects of intervention. In group designs, conventional statistical methods test the significance of between-group or between-treatment differences by using within-group variability as "error." If between-group differences are large relative to within-group differences, then statistical significance is achieved (e.g., $p < .05$).

Visual Inspection

Visual inspection of graphed data is the most common way of analyzing data from single case designs (D.H. Barlow & Hersen, 1984; Johnston & Pennypacker, 1993). Effects of intervention are determined by comparing baseline levels of performance to postintervention levels, to detect treatment effects. Unlike complex statistical analyses, this method uses the "interocular" test of significance. Visual inspection of graphed data has been criticized on the grounds that it is an insensitive method of determining treatment effects (Kazdin, 1984). That is, the procedure identifies only large effects and fails to detect subtle (and perhaps cumulative) changes in the dependent variable, and would thus create a Type II error.

There is a considerable body of research, however, suggesting that even highly trained behavior analysts cannot obtain consensus in evaluating single case data using visual inspection (Center, Skiba, & Casey, 1985–1986; DeProspero & Cohen, 1979; Knapp, 1983; Matyas & Greenwood, 1990, 1991; Ottenbacher, 1990). It would therefore appear that visual inspection of graphed data often results in erroneous conclusions regarding the presence or absence of experimental effects. Baer's (1977) position regarding Type I and Type II error rates in single case and group experimental designs was discussed earlier in this chapter. Recall that Baer suggested that visual inspection produces low Type I error rates and relatively higher Type II error rates than do group experimental designs. A study by Matyas and Greenwood (1990) showed that Type I error rate ranged from 16% to 84% with autocorrelated data. A subsequent study by Matyas and Greenwood (1991) of data published in the *Journal of Applied Behavior Analysis* showed that the Type I error rate was approximately 10%. The results from this study do not support Baer's (1977) position that visual inspection of single case data produces few Type I errors.

Given the problems with parametric statistical analyses in determining treatment effects for individual clients, and given the often unacceptably high Type I error rate using visual inspection, what procedures are available to the single case researcher to quantify treatment effects? At least three alternatives have been proposed for quantifying the effects of intervention in single case experimental designs: (a) reliable changes in behavior, (b) time-series analyses, and (c) effect size estimates.

Reliable Changes in Behavior

A major problem with group design statistics (e.g., F ratios or t tests) is the reliance on mean differences between groups of subjects to determine a treatment effect. This averaging masks the effects for individuals and ignores potentially valuable information (e.g., characteristics of responders and nonresponders to treatment). Although one could calculate the percentage of clients who "improved" in a group design, this improvement may not represent statistically reliable improvement.

Nunnally and Kotsche (1983) first proposed a *reliable change index* (RCI) to determine the effectiveness of an intervention for individuals. This RCI was later expanded by Jacobson, Follette, and Revenstorf (1984) and revised by Christensen and Mendoza (1986). The RCI is defined as the difference between a posttest score and a pretest score divided by the standard error of difference between posttest and pretest scores. The standard error of difference is the spread or variation of the distribution of change scores that would be expected if no actual change had occurred. An RCI of +1.96 ($p < .05$) would be considered to be a reliable change in behavior.

With single case design data, RCIs must be computed for baseline (pretest) and intervention (posttest) phases of the design. For instance, in an ABAB withdrawal design, pretest scores would be calculated from the initial baseline (A) and posttest scores from the mean of the two intervention, or B, phases. Similarly, in a multiple baseline design, pretest scores would be calculated from the baselines of each subject, setting, or behavior, and posttest scores from the means of the respective intervention phases. The standard error of difference would be based on the autocorrelation and variation of baseline and intervention phases. The advantage of RCIs are that changes are reported for individuals rather than groups, reliable changes can be quantified from pretest to posttest (baseline to intervention) and confidence intervals can be placed around change scores to avoid overinterpretation of results.

Time Series Analysis

Time series analysis is an analytical technique that estimates changes in *level* and *trend* in a series of repeated observations collected over time. A change in level reflects a change in behavior at the point intervention is introduced, and changes in slope reflect changes in trend both within and between phases of an intervention. Kazdin (1984) and Center and colleagues (1985–1986) describe some fundamental considerations in using time series analyses with single case data. Although potentially valuable, time series analyses have several limitations, particularly in clinical practice. First, these analyses are fairly complex, and therefore are not particularly user-friendly. Second, fitting regression models to data with relatively few data points often yields inaccurate results, because it is impossible to meet the statistical assumptions of regression-based analyses. Third, effect sizes, particularly in the piecewise regression approach recommended by Center and colleagues (1985–1986) are awkwardly expressed as standard errors of estimate (prediction errors from the regression model).

Several alternatives to time series analyses have been proposed over the years, none of which is entirely satisfactory. *Randomization tests* in which treatments are randomly assigned to days or sessions have been recommended (Edgington, 1980; Levin, Marascuilo, & Hubert, 1978). However, this technique is applicable only to experimental designs in which baseline and treatment phases are rapidly alternated, as in multielement (alternating treatments) designs. *Rank tests* have been recommended for use in multiple baseline designs in which ranks of scores before and after the introduction of the intervention are compared across settings, subjects, and behaviors (see Wolery & Billingsley, 1982). Finally the *split-middle technique,* which makes use of a celeration line reflecting *rate of responding* to predict future performances, is employed (White, 1974). This is the method used to predict and plot expected performances in curriculum-based assessment (see Skinner, this volume). Kazdin (1984) suggests that this technique is used to *describe* change within and between phases, rather than an inferential statistical technique.

Effect Sizes

Another way of quantifying single case data is through the use of effect sizes. Effect sizes are used in meta-analytic research, which integrates bodies of literature by converting results of independent studies to a common metric. This metric, the effect size, is computed by subtracting the mean of an experimental group from the mean of a control group and dividing this difference by the standard deviation of the control group (see Rosenthal & Rosnow, 1991). The effect size is expressed as a z score having a mean of 0 and a standard deviation of 1.

Busk and Serlin (1992) have proposed two approaches for calculating effect sizes in single case studies. The first approach makes no distributional assumptions, and calculates the effect size by subtracting the treatment mean from the baseline mean and dividing by the standard deviation of the baseline mean. The second approach, based on the homogeneity of variance assumption, is the same, except that it uses the pooled within-phase variances as the error term (i.e., the denominator). Effect sizes calculated in this way are interpreted the same way as traditional effect size estimates. They can be used to estimate effect sizes for a treatment in a single study, for comparing two or more treatments in a single study, or for synthesizing numerous independent single case studies (i.e., meta-analysis).

Effect sizes can also be calculated by computing the percentage of *nonoverlapping data points* (PNOL) between baseline and treatment phases (Mastropieri & Scruggs, 1985–1986). PNOL is computed by indicating the number of *treatment data points* that exceed the *highest baseline data point* in an expected direction and dividing by the total number of data points in the *treatment phase.*

For example, if 10 of 15 treatment data points exceed the highest baseline data point, then PNOL is 67%. The method provides for quantitative synthesis of single case data that is relatively easy to compute. Although there are situations in which this method would not be appropriate (e.g., inappropriate baseline trends, nonorthogonal slope changes, floor and ceiling effects), overall, it is a reasonable estimate of treatment effectiveness.

Functional Outcome Analysis

A final method that could be used to quantify effects in single case designs is known as *functional outcome analysis* or FOA (Gresham & Noell, 1993; Noell & Gresham, 1993). FOA derives from cost-effectiveness or cost–benefit analyses (Yates, 1985) and principles of ecological behavior analysis (Martens & Witt, 1988). Within this framework, the functional relationship between resources invested in treatment and outcomes is examined. FOA is designed to permit efficient, ecologically valid interventions.

Intervention costs can be conceptualized along two dimensions: objective and subjective. Objective costs consist of time and money. Within an FOA framework, time would be employed as the primary objective cost metric to enhance the utility of results. Time data would permit evaluation of feasibility of interventions in settings with differing personnel costs. Time data would also permit evaluation of feasibility of interventions in settings in which personnel costs represent not new personnel, but, rather, new time demands on existing personnel. Material costs would be reported in monetary terms.

Subjective costs are the phenomenological costs (e.g., hassle, discomfort, inconvenience) of implementing an intervention. Subjective costs could also be conceptualized as response cost to the intervention provider for carrying out the intervention. Subjective cost data may be collected through rating scales or by interview.

Benefits can also be conceptualized as objective and subjective. Objective benefits can be either increases in available resources, or desired behavior change. In cases of child behavior problems, the most probable resource increase is in available time. The time a teacher or parent no longer spends in dealing with inappropriate behavior represents an objective benefit (i.e., increased available resources). Behavioral change benefits might include increased academic engaged time, decreased aggression, and improved grades.

Subjective benefits are also phenomenological in nature. These benefits might include reduced stress, decreased depression, increased happiness, and improved self-esteem. Both the child and treatment implementors may be beneficiaries of subjective benefits. Subjective benefits, like costs, could be assessed through rating scales, observations, and interviews. Subjective benefits and costs should be assessed using the same method with similar scaling properties to permit comparisons of results.

One way of empirically indexing the objective and subjective costs and benefits of interventions is the *efficiency ratio* (ER). Similar to an interest rate, the ER describes the amount of return per unit of investment. An ER above 1 indicates that the intervention was profitable (benefits exceeded costs) whereas an ER less than 1 means the intervention was unprofitable (costs exceeded benefits). In most cases, behavioral interventions have multiple ERs because objective and subjective costs represent conceptually different domains, thereby requiring computation of separate ERs for each domain.

The *objective efficiency ratio* (OER) reflects the ratio of objective benefits to objective costs and is ordinarily computed by comparing time savings to time costs. For example, an intervention saving 600 minutes of a teacher's time with an investment of 100 minutes has an OER of 6, a highly cost beneficial intervention. Where necessary, time data may be converted to money data (based on salary or wages) to permit computation. As a result, the OER normally has no units because time and money appear in both the numerator and the denominator. In this sense, the OER is like an interest rate.

An OER may also be computed by comparing time invested to degree or level of behavior change. OERs computed in this way may be useful in comparing interventions, but they do not represent absolute efficiency. For instance, OERs could be computed by comparing gains in oral reading performances using direct instruction, versus whole-language methods per $100 expended per student. Subjective Efficiency Ratios (SERs) can be computed in the same way.

The OER and SER are intended to help guide the evaluation of interventions during their course and at their termination. The ERs relevant to an intervention should be computed and graphed on an ongoing basis. Interventions showing negative trends may need to be changed or modified. Interventions that are objectively efficient (OER > 1), but noxious to the consumer (SER < 1) may need to be modified to identify a more acceptable treatment with roughly equal objective benefits.

Social Validation

Social validation was discussed extensively in Chapter 1 as a means of determining the *social importance of effects* in behavioral interventions (see Gresham & Lambros, this volume). The social importance of effects produced by an intervention establishes the clinical or practical significance of behavior change rather than its statistical significance. In other words, did the change produced by the intervention represent a socially important change that has habilitative validity for an individual?

Social importance can be determined by subjective judgments obtained from treatment consumers, by social comparisons between treated and untreated clients, or by a combination of these two procedures (Kazdin, 1977; Van Houten, 1979; Wolf, 1978). Fawcett (1991) suggested that one could socially validate a treatment on three levels: by specifying a priori *ideal* (best performance), *normative* (typical performance), and *deficient* (worst performance) performance levels. Thus, interventions moving a child from deficient to normative or ideal performance levels would be considered to have produced socially important changes in behavior. Readers are encouraged to refer to Chapter 1 and other sources (Hawkins, 1991; Schwartz, 1991; Schwartz & Baer, 1991) for more details on social validation.

Experimental Validity

Experimental validity of research design refers to how confident one can be in the results of a given experiment. Cook and Campbell (1979) described four types of experimental validity: (a) internal validity, (b) external validity, (c) construct validity, and (d) statistical conclusion validity. Two of these, internal and external validity, are most germane to single case designs. Internal validity refers to the extent to which changes in the dependent variable can be attributed to systematic changes in the independent variable and not to other factors extraneous to the experiment. External validity refers to the extent to which findings from an investigation can be generalized to other settings, other subjects, and other intervention agents.

With respect to internal validity, several threats may compromise the conclusions drawn from an intervention (e.g., history, maturation, instrumentation, statistical regression). For the most part, single case experimental designs (e.g., withdrawal, multiple baseline, multielement) control for most threats to internal validity.

Perhaps the biggest concern in single case experimental designs falls under the rubric of external validity. Threats to external validity (e.g., sample characteristics, reactivity, novelty effects) may hinder efforts to generalize from a given investigation to other subjects, settings, and treatment agents. Multiple treatment interference, drawing conclusions about a given treatment in the context of other treatments, is particularly problematic in multielement and within series, complex phase change (interaction) designs. Johnston and Pennypacker (1993) argue that findings produced by single case methodology can be generalized (i.e., establish external validity) by replications of experiments by the same and other researchers. An excellent example of this type of replication can be found in functional analysis of behavior for self-injurious behavior (see reviews by Carr, 1994; R.H. Horner, 1994; Mace, 1994).

Treatment Integrity

Internal and external validity of experiments can also be compromised by the poor integrity with which treatments are implemented. Treatment integrity refers to the degree to which treatments are implemented as intended (Gresham et al., 1993; Moncher & Prinz, 1991; Peterson, Homer, & Wonderlich, 1982). Treatment integrity is concerned with the *accuracy* and *consistency* with which independent variables are implemented. Treatment integrity is necessary, but not sufficient, for the demonstration of functional relationships between experimenter-manipulated independent variables (treatments) and dependent variables (target behaviors). Some independent variables may be implemented with perfect integrity yet show no functional relationship with a dependent variable (a weak treatment). Other independent variables may be functionally related to a dependent variable; however, this functional relationship may be unknown or weak because of the poor integrity with which it was applied.

Failure to ensure the integrity of treatments poses numerous threats to valid inference making in behavioral research (Moncher & Prinz, 1991). If significant behavior change occurs and if there are no data concerning the implementation of the independent variable, then the internal validity of the experiment may be compromised. Similarly, if significant behavior change does not occur and if the integrity of the treatment is not monitored, then one has difficulty in distinguishing between an ineffective treatment and an effective treatment implemented with poor integrity (Gresham, 1989; Wodarski, Feldman, & Pedi, 1974).

In terms of external validity, poorly defined, inadequately described, and idiosyncratically implemented treatments make replication and evaluation of treatments difficult (Johnston & Pennypacker, 1980; Moncher & Prinz, 1991). The absence of information concerning treatment definition and integrity limits the generalizability of treatments across settings, situations, subjects, and treatment implementors (Kazdin, 1992).

Johnston and Pennypacker (1980) define a replication as the degree to which *equivalent environmental manipulations* (i.e., independent variables) associated with earlier observations are duplicated. Replications provide information regarding the generality of a functional relationship over a range of conditions (e.g., subjects, settings, experimenters). Failure to assess the degree to which treatments are implemented as planned compromises the science of building a replicative history.

Two reviews of the applied behavior analysis literature suggest that researchers do not frequently monitor the integrity of their treatments. Peterson et al. (1982) reviewed all empirical studies published in *Journal of Applied Behavior Analysis* between 1968 and 1980 (539 studies). This review showed that only 20% of the 539 studies reported data on the integrity of treatments. In addition, more than 16% of studies did not provide an operational definition of the independent variable. In a subsequent review, Gresham and colleagues (1993) reviewed all studies (158 studies) published in the *Journal of Applied Behavior Analysis* between 1980 and 1990 that were child studies (i.e., subjects under 19 years of age). Of the 158 child studies, only 32.4% (54 studies) provided an operational definition of the independent variable. Only 15.8% of the 158 studies systematically measured and reported levels of treatment integrity.

Failure to gather data on the integrity of treatments, no matter how inconvenient this procedure may be, compromises the science of behavioral intervention efforts. This lack of treatment integrity assessment or monitoring prevents our learning about functional relationships between independent and dependent variables. If there is no reliable measurement of *both* the independent and dependent variable, then the experimental validity of an intervention must certainly be questioned.

References

Achenbach, T. (1991). *Integrative guide for the 1991 CBCL/4-18, YSR, and TRF profiles.* Burlington, VT: University of Vermont, Department of Psychiatry.

Baer, D. (1977). "Perhaps it would be better not to know everything." *Journal of Applied Behavior Analysis, 10,* 167–172.

Baer, D., Wolf, M., & Risley, T. (1968). Some current dimensions of applied behavior analysis. *Journal of Applied Behavior Analysis, 1,* 91–97.

Barlow, D. (1981). On the relation between clinical research and clinical practice: Current issues, new directions. *Journal of Consulting and Clinical Psychology, 49,* 147–155.

Barlow, D., Hayes, S., & Nelson, R. (1984). *The scientist practitioner.* New York: Pergamon Press.

Barlow, D.H., & Hayes, S.C. (1979). Alternating treatments design: One strategy for comparing the effects of two treatments in a single subject. *Journal of Applied Behavior Analysis, 12,* 199–210.

Barlow, D.H., & Hersen, M. (1973). Single case experimental designs: Uses in applied clinical research. *Archives of General Psychiatry, 29,* 319–325.

Barlow, D.H., & Hersen, M. (1984). *Single case experimental designs: Strategies for studying behavior change* (2nd ed.). New York: Pergamon.

Busk, P.L., & Serlin, R.C. (1992). Meta-analysis for single-case research. In T. Kratochwill & J. Levin (Eds.), *Single-case research design and analysis* (pp. 187–212). Hillsdale, NJ: Erlbaum.

Carr, E.G. (1994). Emerging themes in the functional analysis of problem behavior. *Journal of Applied Behavior Analysis, 27,* 393–399.

Center, B.A., Skiba, R.J., & Casey, A. (1985–1986). A methodology for the quantitative synthesis of intra-subject design research. *The Journal of Special Education, 19,* 387–400.

Christensen, L., & Mendoza, J. (1986). A method of assessing change in a single subject: An alteration of the RC index. *Behavior Therapy, 17,* 305–308.

Cohen, J. (1994). The earth is round p<.05). *American Psychologist, 49,* 997–1003.

Cook, T., & Campbell, D. (1979). *Quasi-experimentation: Design and analysis for field settings.* Chicago: Rand McNally.

DeProspero, A., & Cohen, S. (1979). Inconsistent visual analyses of intrasubject data. *Journal of Applied Behavior Analysis, 12,* 573–579.

Derby, K.M., Wacker, D., Sasso, G., Steege, M., Northrup, J., Cigrand, K., & Asmus, J. (1992). Brief functional assessment techniques to evaluate aberrant behavior in an outpatient clinic: A summary of 79 cases. *Journal of Applied Behavior Analysis, 25,* 713–721.

Edgington, E.S. (1980). Validity of randomization tests for one-subject experiments. *Journal of Educational Statistics, 5,* 235–251.

Fawcett, S. (1991). Social validity: A note on methodology. *Journal of Applied Behavior Analysis, 24,* 235–239.

Fisher, R. (1956). *Statistical methods and scientific inference.* London: Oliver & Boyd, Ltd.

Gettinger, M. (1993). Effects of invented spelling and direct instruction on spelling performance of second-grade boys. *Journal of Applied Behavior Analysis, 26,* 281–292.

Gresham, F.M. (1989). Assessment of treatment integrity in consultation and prereferral intervention. *School Psychology Review, 18,* 37–50.

Gresham, F.M. (1997). Treatment integrity in single subject research. In R.D. Franklin, D.B. Allison, & B.S. Gorman (Eds.), *Design and analysis of single case research* (pp. 93–117). Hillsdale, NJ: Erlbaum.

Gresham, F.M., Gansle, K., & Noell, G. (1993). Treatment integrity in applied behavior analysis with children. *Journal of Applied Behavior Analysis, 26,* 257–263.

Gresham, F.M., & Kendell, G. (1987). School consultation research: Methodological critique and future research directions. *School Psychology Review, 16,* 306–316.

Gresham, F.M., & Noell, G.H. (1993). Documenting the effectiveness of consultation outcomes. In J. Zins, T. Kratochwill, & S. Elliott (Eds.), *Handbook of consultation services for children* (pp. 249–276). San Francisco: Jossey-Bass.

Hains, A.H., & Baer, D.M. (1989). Interaction effects in multielement designs: Inevitable, desirable, and ignoble. *Journal of Applied Behavior Analysis, 22,* 57–69.

Hartmann, D.P., & Hall, R.V. (1976). The changing criterion design. *Journal of Applied Behavior Analysis, 9,* 333–339.

Hawkins, R. (1991). Is social validity what we are interested in? Argument for a functional approach. *Journal of Applied Behavior Analysis, 24,* 205–213.

Hayes, S.C. (1981). Single case experimental design and empirical clinical practice. *Journal of Consulting and Clinical Psychology, 49,* 193–211.

Hersen, M., & Barlow, D.H. (1976). *Single case experimental designs: Strategies for studying behavior change.* New York: Pergamon.

Horner, R.D., & Baer, D.M. (1978). Multiple-probe technique: A variation of the multiple baseline. *Journal of Applied Behavior Analysis, 11,* 189–196.

Horner, R.H. (1994). Functional assessment contributions and future directions. *Journal of Applied Behavior Analysis, 27,* 401–404.

Iwata, B., Dorsey, M., Slifer, K., Bauman, K., & Richman, G. (1982). Toward a functional analysis of self-injury. *Analysis and Intervention in Developmental Disabilities, 2,* 3–20.

Jacobson, N., Follette, W., & Revenstorf, D. (1984). Psychotherapy outcome research: Methods for reporting variability and evaluating clinical significance. *Behavior Therapy, 15,* 336–352.

Johnston, J.M., & Pennypacker, H.S. (1980). *Strategies and tactics of human behavioral research.* Hillsdale, NJ: Erlbaum.

Johnston, J.M., & Pennypacker, H.S. (1993). *Strategies and tactics of behavioral research* (2nd ed.). Hillsdale, NJ: Erlbaum.

Kazdin, A.E. (1977). Assessing the clinical or applied significance of behavior change through social validation. *Behavior Modification, 1,* 427–452.

Kazdin, A.E. (1984). Statistical analyses for single-case experimental designs. In D. Barlow & M. Hersen. *Single case experimental designs: Strategies for studying behavior change* (pp. 285–324). New York: Pergamon.

Kazdin, A.E. (1992). *Research design in clinical psychology* (2nd ed.). New York: Macmillan.

Kirk, R.E. (1995). *Experimental design: Procedures for the behavioral sciences* (3rd ed.). Pacific Grove, CA: Brooks/Cole.

Knapp, T.J. (1983). Behavior analysts' visual appraisal of behavior change in graphic display. *Behavioral Assessment, 5,* 155–164.

Levin, J., Marascuilo, L., & Hubert, L. (1978). N=1: Nonparametric randomization tests. In T. Kratochwill (Ed.), *Single-subject research: Strategies for evaluation change* (pp. 167–197). New York: Academic.

Linquist, E.F. (1953). *Design and analysis of experiments in psychology and education.* Boston: Houghton Mifflin.

Mace, F.C. (1994). The significance and future functional analysis methodologies. *Journal of Applied Behavior Analysis, 27,* 385–392.

Malott, R.W. (1992). Should we train applied behavior analysts to be researchers? *Journal of Applied Behavior Analysis, 25,* 83–88.

Martens, B.K., & Witt, J.C. (1988). Expanding the scope of behavioral consultation: A systems approach to classroom behavior change. *Professional School Psychology, 3,* 271–281.

Mastropieri, M., & Scruggs, T. (1985–1986). Early intervention for socially withdrawn children. *The Journal of Special Education, 19,* 429–441.

Matyas, T.A., & Greenwood, K.M. (1990). Visual analysis of single-case time series: Effects of variability, serial dependence, and magnitude of intervention effects. *Journal of Applied Behavior Analysis, 23,* 341–351.

Matyas, T.A., & Greenwood, K.M. (1991). Problems in the estimation of autocorrelation in brief time series and some implications for behavioral data. *Behavioral Assessment, 13,* 137–157.

Moncher, F., & Prinz, R. (1991). Treatment fidelity in outcome studies. *Clinical Psychology Review, 11,* 247–266.

Morrow-Bradley, C., & Elliott, R. (1986). Utilization of psychotherapy outcome research by practicing psychotherapists. *American Psychologist, 41,* 188–197.

Noell, G.H., & Gresham, F.M. (1993). Functional outcome analysis: Do the benefits of consultation and prereferral interventions justify the costs? *School Psychology Quarterly, 8,* 200–226.

Nunnally, J., & Kotsche, W. (1983). Studies of individual subjects: Logic and methods of analysis. *British Journal of Clinical Psychology, 22,* 83–93.

Ottenbacher, K.J. (1990). When is a picture worth a thousand p values? A comparison of visual and quantitative methods to analyze single case data. *The Journal of Special Education, 23,* 436–449.

Peterson, L., Homer, A., & Wonderlich, S. (1982). The integrity of independent variables in behavior analysis. *Journal of Applied Behavior Analysis, 15,* 477–492.

Rosenthal, R., & Rosnow, R. (1991). *Essentials of behavioral research: Methods and data analysis* (2nd ed.). New York: McGraw-Hill.

Rusch, F.R., & Kazdin, A.E. (1981). Toward a methodology of withdrawal designs for the assessment of response maintenance. *Journal of Applied Behavior Analysis, 14,* 131–140.

Schwartz, I. (1991). The study of consumer behavior and social validity: An essential partnership for applied behavior analysis. *Journal of Applied Behavior Analysis, 24,* 241–244.

Schwartz, I., & Baer, D. (1991). Social validity assessment: Is current practice state of the art? *Journal of Applied Behavior Analysis, 24,* 189–204.

Sidman, M. (1960). *Tactics of scientific research.* New York: Basic Books.

Tawney, J.W., & Gast, D.L. (1984). *Single subject research in special education.* Columbus, OH: Merrill.

Van Houten, R. (1979). Social validation: The evolution of standards of competency for targets. *Journal of Applied Behavior Analysis, 12,* 581–591.

Vollmer, T.R., Marcus, B., Ringdahl, J., & Roane, H. (1995). Progressing from brief assessments to extended experimental analyses in the evaluation of aberrant behavior. *Journal of Applied Behavior Analysis, 28,* 561–576.

Wacker, D., McMahon, C., Steege, M., Berg, W., Sasso, G., & Melloy, K. (1990). Applications of a sequential alternating treatments design. *Journal of Applied Behavior Analysis, 23,* 333–339.

White, O.R. (1974). *The "split middle": A "quickie" method of trend estimation.* Seattle, WA: University of Washington, Experimental Education Unit, Child Development and Mental Retardation Center.

Winer, B.J. (1971). *Statistical principles in experimental design* (2nd ed.). New York: McGraw-Hill.

Wodarski, J., Feldman, R., & Pedi, S. (1974). Objective measurement of the independent variable: A neglected methodological aspect in community based behavioral research. *Journal of Abnormal Child Psychology, 2,* 239–244.

Wolery, M., & Billingsley, F. (1982). The application of Revusky's R test to slope and level changes. *Behavioral Assessment, 4,* 93–103.

Wolf, M.M. (1978). Social validity: The case for subjective measurement or how applied behavior analysis is finding its heart. *Journal of Applied Behavior Analysis, 11,* 203–14.

Yates, B.T. (1985). Cost-effectiveness analysis and cost–benefit analysis: An introduction. *Behavioral Assessment, 7,* 207–234.

3

Toward a Behavior Analytic Approach to Consultation

GEORGE H. NOELL AND JOSEPH C. WITT

Introduction

Of the developments in psychology and education over the last 50 years, those in behavioral psychology have been among the most important. Behavioral psychology has amassed an impressive technology for responding effectively to many problems with important social and pragmatic implications. Many volumes such as this one and entire scholarly journals have been devoted exclusively to descriptions of the effectiveness of behavioral technology for a wide array of problems. The application of behavioral technologies through a problem-solving process serves as the foundation for this volume. The efficacy of the application of behavioral technologies in a wide range of settings, targeting an array of problems, and incorporating a diversity of treatment agents is evident in the continuing stream of publications in this area. Unquestionably, the technology has been invented and validated.

The purpose of this chapter is not to add to the important literature on *what* to do for specific problems; rather, our focus is the *use* of existing technology. The solution of problems in applied settings requires three important elements:

1. An accurate analysis of the problem.
2. An intervention that will address the controlling variables identified by the analysis.

3. Implementation of the intervention with fidelity to the intervention protocol.

The focus on this chapter will be on elements 1 and 3 as they are conducted *in combination with* a parent or teacher. A central premise here will be that these elements are as important to successful problem resolution as the intervention. An intervention that addresses the wrong problem or that is not implemented properly is not likely to have its intended effect. An intervention as seemingly simple in application as time-out can frequently exacerbate problem behaviors (Shriver & Allen, 1996). Obviously, the necessity for a behavior analyst to collaborate with another person further complicates the situation. Obtaining a valid behavioral analysis and accurate implementation are more difficult when these tasks are being completed by an individual who is probably untrained and possibly unmotivated than it is when the behavior analyst is providing the service directly. In addition to having to measure, monitor, and produce effects in the behavior of the client (i.e., child), the behavior analyst may be required to measure, monitor, and produce effects in the person who provides the direct service to the client.

The primary goal of this chapter is to describe a behavioral approach to what is called consultation. The practices to be discussed will be referred to as consultation because they involve a consultant and consultee working together for the benefit of a client (see Bergan and Kratochwill, 1990 for a more complete discussion of the defining characteristics of consultation). The chapter will begin

GEORGE H. NOELL AND JOSEPH C. WITT • Department of Psychology, Louisiana State University, Baton Rouge, Louisiana 70803-5501.

Handbook of Child Behavior Therapy, edited by Watson and Gresham. Plenum Press, New York, 1998.

with a review of some fundamental assumptions of behavior analysis. These assumptions will be briefly compared with the tenet underlying behavioral consultation (Bergan & Kratochwill, 1990), which is the dominant model of consultation for those who practice from a behavioral perspective. We will conclude by describing a structured process for building and then implementing an intervention.

What Makes Behavioral Consultation Behavioral

Behavioral consultation emerged to give professionals with expertise in behavior analysis and behavior modification a general case methodology for providing behavioral technology in service delivery to meet the needs of clients and consultees (Bergan & Kratochwill, 1990). Empirical interest in this method of disseminating behavioral technology is evidenced by a disproportionate number of studies of behavioral consultation in the consultation literature (Gresham & Kendell, 1987), combined with the rapid increase in consultation research over the past decade. The publication of the seminal works in the area (Bergan, 1977; Bergan & Kratochwill, 1990) has led to a modal model for this form of service delivery simply called behavioral consultation (BC). The interviews and procedures that constitute BC have become the basis for most if not all of the work in this area.

Although it is the standard model for behavioral consultation, it is not equivalent to all of the possible methods of providing behavioral technologies and behavior analysis in service delivery (Bergan & Kratochwill, 1990; Noell, 1996). BC is a particular model for accomplishing a task that might be achieved in a number of ways. Rather than reviewing the status of BC and presenting the BC model, this chapter will focus on the broader range of practices and possibilities in the response class of behavioral consultation. Readers interested in a review of BC are referred to excellent sources already available on that subject (see Bergan & Kratochwill, 1990; Kratochwill, Elliott, & Rotto, 1995; Martens, 1993). Throughout the balance of this chapter, "BC" will be used to refer to the model of consultation described by Bergan and Kratochwill (1990), while "behavioral consultation" will be

used to refer to the broader range of possibilities examined in this chapter.

The impetus to examine modifications of BC and alternative practices originated in several concerns regarding the current modal model of behavioral consultation. Perhaps the most important concern is that, in the attempt to make BC efficient, some of the fundamental principles of behavior analysis were given slight consideration or rejected outright (Witt, Gresham, & Noell, 1996). This has raised the further concern that in the attempt to achieve efficiency, the efficacy of behavior analytic procedures may have been eroded. The authors' concerns regarding the assumptions underlying BC, procedures comprising BC, and the data supporting BC have been described elsewhere (see Noell & Witt, 1996; Witt et al., 1996). Rather than reviewing these concerns again here, this chapter will examine the challenges inherent in incorporating some of the fundamental principles of behavior analysis into behavioral consultation.

Fundamental Assumptions

Assumption 1: Measurement at each step must be conducted with direct, low-inference methods that are both valid and reliable. The direct measurement of behavior has been one of the defining characteristics of behavioral research (Johnston & Pennypacker, 1993) and applied behavior analysis (Baer, Wolf, & Risley, 1968). Baer and colleagues stated this principle as, "Accordingly a subject's verbal description of his own non-verbal behavior usually would not be accepted as a measure of his actual behavior unless it were independently substantiated" (p. 93). While the use of direct measures of behavior has been fundamental to the development of applied behavior analysis, obtaining them can present a considerable challenge to behavioral consultants.

In most practice environments, the consultant is not able to be in the containing environment on a daily basis and will not have trained observers readily available. The consultee may have difficulty incorporating data collection into his or her schedule and is unlikely to be trained in behavioral data collection procedures in any case. Simply shifting to indirect measures of behavior such as interview of the consultee may appear to be a simple and logical solution to this problem. Unfortunately, this raises the question of the treatment validity (Cone, 1988) of relying primarily on data obtained through interviews. Is the type of data obtained appropriate for the purposes for which it will be used? Are interviews an empirically validated technique for determining the function of the client's behavior and the skills the client possesses? Many functional assessment reports describe using interviews as a beginning point for assessment (e.g., Umbreit, 1995), but none of the studies located by the current authors limited assessment to interview.

However, determining that direct measures of behavior are an epistemological and empirical requirement of a behavior analytic approach to consultation does not resolve the question of how to obtain direct evidence of behavior. One obvious solution is to devote the time to train the consultee in an appropriate data collection procedure (Watson & Robinson, 1996). However, exclusive reliance on the consultee as the observer raises new problems. Observer drift and experimental expectancy (Foster & Cone, 1986) may result in changes in the measure that are unrelated to the phenomenon of interest. The use of a hybrid data collection strategy has previously been recommended as a solution for this particular problem (Noell & Gresham, 1993). A hybrid strategy in this instance requires that the consultant collect intermittent data, while the consultee collects data frequently. The consultant could then use his or her direct data either to provide feedback to the consultee on data collection procedures or to adjust his or her interpretation of the data obtained by the consultee.

Applied behavior analysis has developed a wide range of assessment techniques that complement data collecting in the containing environment (see Ciminero, Calhoun, & Adams, 1986; Gresham, this volume; Shapiro & Skinner, 1993). These techniques may permit a more efficient assessment of some dimensions or functions of behavior than are possible in the containing environment. The creation of direct tests of important hypotheses regarding client functioning may mean that assessment can be completed more quickly with more definitive data than would be possible if the only assessment technique is observation of the behavior in the containing environment. Many forms of direct tests such as behavioral role-plays or skills inventories can be completed in a timely manner through the cooperative efforts of consultants and consultees.

Assumption 2: Assessment and intervention activities must be conducted on an ongoing basis in the containing environment. If the behavior measured as described in the preceding section is analogous to the dependent variable contained in a research report, then the intervention developed during consultation would be equivalent to the independent variable. Attributing change in the dependent variable to changes in the independent variable requires specification and measurement of the independent variable (Johnston & Pennypacker, 1993). Obtaining adequate assessment data may be a necessary condition for targeting and changing important behaviors, but it will not be sufficient. The intervention must be implemented properly in order for it to have any benefit to the client or consultee (Bergan & Kratochwill, 1990; Gresham, 1989). The fact that the consultee, rather than the consultant, is likely to be in frequent contact with the client in the targeted environment logically dictates that the consultee will be the one who implements the intervention.

Implementation of the intervention by the consultee in the containing environment is consistent with much of applied behavioral research. The bulk of behavioral intervention reports, particularly those employing operant procedures, are implemented in the containing environment. This apparent synergy between behavioral consultation and the treatment research that informs it obscures some important challenges. One of the most crucial challenges is discovering how to develop an intervention that is compatible with the demands made by the consultee's other responsibilities.

No empirically validated procedure currently exists for ensuring that an intervention is compatible with the other demands on the consultee's attention and time. The majority of the attempts to deal with this question might be characterized as discussion and consideration of issues that may affect the practicality of intervention implementation. One method for attempting to ensure that an intervention is practical is to examine how the intervention will fit into the behavioral ecology (Martens & Witt, 1988). Consideration of the behavioral ecology requires that the intervention be compatible with important behavioral regularities that already exist in the environment; modification or reallocation of existing consultee behaviors, therefore, would generally be preferred over the introduction of completely novel intervention procedures. Functional assessment may contribute to this type of intervention development by identifying the factors in the environment that are maintaining the problematic behaviors (Mace, 1994). However, the present state of the art in assuring the practicality of interventions is likely to consist of a discussion between the consultee and the consultant that examines intervention costs and anticipated benefits (Noell & Gresham, 1993).

From a behavioral perspective, this problem can also be conceptualized as a concurrent reinforcement schedule for the teacher. The teacher will choose to engage in activities which evolve out of consultation if those responses pay off at a higher rate than other responses. For example, the teacher can choose to intervene or the teacher can do nothing and allow the child's behavior to worsen. The consultant may presume that seeing improvement in the child would reinforce the teacher. The teacher, however, may have a reinforcement history that has indicated that the interventions recommended by this particular consultant are effective only 25% of the time. On the other hand, the teacher has learned that doing nothing will result in the child being identified as in need of additional services about 80% of the time.

Assumption 3: Preparation of the consultee to use the intervention is accomplished through careful training followed by supervised implementation and follow-up in the containing environment. At each step of the process, the behavior analyst takes no chances and makes no inferences. The approach at this step is a relatively simple one: Seeing is believing. That is, the behavioral consultant assumes that a verbal explanation of the intervention to the consultee is a necessary but not sufficient condition for enabling the consultee to implement the intervention. Acceptable proof that the consultee can implement the intervention is direct observation of implementation in the containing environment.

Providing consultant-directed training and monitoring of implementation appears to contradict the collaborative and co-equal descriptions that have typically been incorporated into consultation (Bergan & Kratochwill, 1990; Conoley & Conoley, 1982; J.E. Zins & Erchul, 1995). In contrast to these traditional assumptions regarding consultation, Watson and Robinson (1996) describe an approach to consultation that includes direct teaching of the consultee. The purpose of providing the consultee with

direct instruction in intervention implementation, where necessary, is not to establish a hierarchical relationship. Rather, the purpose is to provide needed technical support so that the consultee can implement the intervention accurately and confidently.

Assumption 4: Continued implementation of an intervention by the consultee will occur only when controlling variables support consultee implementation behaviors. The entire intervention implementation process appears to be primarily a problem of generalization that is subject to the same principles as other behaviors. Generalization, according to Johnston and Pennypacker (1993) is not a magical process, but instead relies on understanding the controlling variables. For example, if a teacher implements the intervention with 100% integrity with the consultant present but does not implement the intervention when the consultant is not present, then something to do with the consultant's presence is related to implementation. The generalization task would be to discover an intermediate step in which the consultant could monitor implementation intermittently or in which permanent product evidence of implementation could be subject to consultant review at any time. If the intermediate step fails, then it was either too large a step or there was an incomplete understanding of the controlling variables.

How can the consultant help the consultee generalize intervention behaviors from the consultation meeting to the relevant setting and occasions? If obtaining treatment integrity is conceptualized from this perspective, the full range of procedures for establishing behavior and for generalizing behavior are potentially applicable. Generalization procedures such as programming contingencies for implementation, programming discriminative stimuli, or training sufficient exemplars (Stokes & Osnes, 1989) are potential candidates for incorporation within consultation. However, experimental examinations of generalization procedures targeting the treatment implementation by consultees have not been conducted to date. In the absence of research examining procedures targeting generalization of consultee behavior, any recommendations for use of specific procedures can only be regarded as hunches or guesses. Extensive consideration of generalization strategies may be premature, given that initial descriptions of consultation efficacy are arguably lacking in measurement of consultee implementation of treatment (Witt et al., 1996).

Obtaining treatment integrity (Peterson, Homer & Wonderlich, 1982; Yeaton & Sechrest, 1981), might be characterized as an emerging area of inquiry. The importance of treatment integrity is indicated by a meta-analysis that found moderate correlations ($r = .51$ to .58) between measures of treatment integrity and treatment outcome (Gresham, Gansle, Noell, Cohen, & Rosenblum, 1993). Despite the intuitive appeal of and empirical support for the importance of treatment integrity in treatment outcome, relatively little is currently known about how to obtain adequate integrity for interventions implemented through consultation (Noell & Witt, 1996).

Assumption 5: Consultation must be cost-effective and reinforcing or it will decrease in frequency. A final element linking behavioral consultation and applied behavior analysis is practical rather than empirical or epistemological: time. An essential element of BC's raison d'être is that, through the use of indirect services and extensive use of interviews as measures, a small professional staff will be able to serve a large number of clients (Erchul & Schulte, 1996). Examination of the issues discussed previously and the procedures described in the following sections should give the impression that incorporating a greater range of the procedures and core epistemological elements of behavior analysis into behavioral consultation would run counter to BC's reason for being. Stated more simply, increasing the technical assistance provided in consultation to include more direct assessment and teaching will decrease the number of clients a consultant can serve.

Acknowledging that time is a finite quantity, if more time is devoted to some consultation activities it will take time away from other activities or cases. One possible partial solution would be to decrease time devoted to meetings and reallocate that time to direct assessment or teaching. The intent of this chapter is not to create a new standard for the practice of consultation. Although the tools of behavior analysis are well documented, a sufficient database examining their implementation in consultation in a manner inconsistent with BC does not exist. The intent of the discussion to this point and the sections that follow is to explore how the breadth of applied behavior analysis can be brought to bear in consultation.

It appears intuitively obvious that the nature and intensity of consultant involvement necessary to assist consultees resolve referral concerns will cover a wide range. Some referrals may be resolvable through simple advice offered during an informal conversation. Other client-consultee pairs may have sufficiently intense needs that the referral may be successfully resolved only through an extensive direct assessment conducted by the consultant, followed by intensive direct instruction in how to implement the intervention. A crucial concern here is not just efficiency, but also efficacy. Incorporating the conservative core epistemological elements, the range of available procedures, and varying intensities of consultant technical support of applied behavior analysis allows a more flexible behavioral consultation to be developed. Although consultation with more direct service elements may not be necessary in all cases, failing to find a method to incorporate behavior analysis into behavioral consultation unnecessarily reduces the available tools and potential efficacy of consultation. Reduced strength of behavioral consultation may significantly reduce the number of clients for whom behavioral consultation is an effective and viable form of service delivery.

Procedures, Processes, and Tactics for Implementation of a Behavior Analytic Approach to Consultation

The remaining sections of this chapter describe an approach to solving problems and consultation that incorporates a range of behavior analytic procedures and technologies. The procedures described herein diverge from current behavioral consultation models (Bergan & Kratochwill, 1990; Zins & Erchul, 1995) by placing greater emphasis on differentiated complementary roles for the consultant and consultee, on direct assessment of the referral concern, and on analysis of intervention plan implementation. The implementation sections are predicated on the assumption that consultees are seeking knowledgeable assistance regarding problematic behaviors and environments that they have been unable to resolve independently. Stated differently, consultees are assumed to want assistance from consultants who have knowledge different from theirs regarding the factors controlling human behavior. The consultant's role as an expert in human behavior and the consultee's primary responsibility for caring for the client are assumed to create complementary roles in consultation. The consultant is responsible for providing technical assistance, guiding assessment, and providing a limited amount of direct assistance, while the bulk of intervention activities and progress monitoring activities are the responsibility of the consultee. These complementary roles may be more consistent with previous findings that teachers prefer consultation interviews in which the consultant is more directive (Erchul & Chewning, 1990).

Behavioral principles and procedures were developed based on direct evidence regarding the behavior of individuals; this indicates the importance of direct assessment, if a behavior analytic approach is to be employed in consultation. In addition, the consultee's request for assistance suggests that he or she may not understand the client's behavior, even though the consultee may understand and respond effectively to other children and/or adults. In the absence of direct assessment, the development of the intervention is based on the recollections of a person who is sufficiently upset or discouraged about the situation to seek professional assistance. In addition, a consultant's failure to perform any form of direct assessment may undermine the consultant's credibility with the consultee.

Two important limitations of the behavior analytic description of consultation presented in this chapter should be noted. First, the great quantity of material available on behavior change and applied behavior analysis precludes a comprehensive presentation of that material in this chapter. The following description will focus on how applied behavior analytic technologies can be incorporated into consultation, with particular attention to novel issues related to consultation. Second, not all referrals to a psychologist are driven by a desire to change client behavior, nor is change in client behavior always an appropriate goal for consultation. Consultees may seek out consultants with goals such as the removal of the client to another environment (e.g., special education) or reassurance that a child's development is within expected limits. In addition, some referrals may arise from developmentally inappropriate expectations. The procedures outlined below are intended to assist consultants and consultees in changing client behavior, and will not be the most appropriate strategies when this is not the goal of consultation.

Pretreatment Assessment

Conceptually, all of the activities related to solving referral concerns can be described as assessment. Implementation of a treatment is an assessment of the impact and function of a particular environmental manipulation (Martens, 1993). This section will focus on assessment activities that take place prior to implementation of an intervention in the environment. The pretreatment assessment section examines assessment issues primarily from the perspective of important questions to be answered. Specific procedures for obtaining data, such as interview, frequency recording, or behavioral role-play tests, are not given extensive consideration.

However, choosing the person or persons who will collect the data and determining what data will be collected to make decisions within consultation are important considerations. As the following sections reveal, the authors recommend an increased reliance on direct measures of client behavior rather than on recollections obtained from interviews. The reliance on direct measures of behavior is a fundamental element of applied behavior analysis (Baer et al., 1968). Although relying primarily on verbal exchanges to make decisions about what behavioral treatment to adopt is consistent with BC, it is inconsistent with the methods that were used to develop and evaluate behavioral treatments. BC (Bergan & Kratochwill, 1990) has developed elaborate methods for obtaining verbal recollections (e.g., behavior specification elicitor), but these elaborate methods do not change the nature of the underlying data. No matter how precisely an interview is conducted, information from the interview is still subject to the range of limitations inherent in human memory (Weingardt, Loftus, & Lindsay, 1995).

If direct behavioral data are preferred over recollections about behavior, assignment of responsibility for collecting those data assumes increased importance. The following sections assume that data collection and analysis would be a responsibility shared between the consultant and consultee. The consultant must possess sufficient technical knowledge to design an appropriate assessment and intervention for this process to be appropriate. An understanding of applied behavior analytic procedures is a prerequisite for the consultant to design an assessment that can be completed cooperatively with the consultee. It will often be necessary for the consultant to assist the consultee in data collection, either directly or by providing appropriate materials and training for data collection. For example, the consultant may need to provide the scatter plot and explain how it is completed. Alternatively, the consultant and consultee might together complete a role-play assessment of client skills. A number of reports appear in the experimental literature in which persons in the targeted individual's environment have collaborated with researchers in the collection of pretreatment assessment data (e.g., Lalli, Browder, Mace, & Brown, 1993; Umbreit, 1995).

Problem Identification

Specification and definition of the target concern is a crucial initial step in consultation. Teachers are likely to report concerns in a vague and global manner (Lambert, 1976) that may be incompatible with assessment of the target concern or development of an intervention. Specifying the concern is necessary to the development of an assessment plan and has been found to be related to intervention implementation (Bergan & Tombari, 1976). Although problem definition is an important assessment activity within consultation, a modal method for identifying problems has not emerged. In practice, initial problem identification is likely to be an informal process that occurs in an interpersonal interaction or interview. While a single method for identifying problems has not emerged, a number of authors have examined issues related to problem identification.

Hawkins (1991) has argued for the evaluation of intervention targets and effects based on habilitative criteria. An intervention outcome that had habilitative validity would increase the individual's ability to successfully adapt to his or her environment. Hawkins (1991) distinguishes habilitative validity from social validity (Schwartz & Baer, 1991). A socially valid target concern would be one that would be valued by important consumers of consultation services such as parents or teachers. Social validity typically would be assessed by asking consumers if they valued intervention goals or outcomes (Schwartz & Baer, 1991). In contrast, habilitative validity would be established when it can be demonstrated that changes in the target behavior produced greater adaptive success in the target environment. While social and habilitative validity

may often converge, they will not necessarily do so. A teacher may be most immediately concerned that a student remain quiet and seated (a socially valid target), while the student's learning to complete assignments accurately may permit greater success in school (a target with habilitative validity).

The concept of keystone behaviors (Barnett, Bauer, Ehrhardt, Lentz, & Stollar, 1996) has been described as important to target selection in consultation, and it is related to habilitative validity. Barnett and colleagues (1996) describe keystone behaviors as pivotal behaviors whose modification can have diverse collateral benefits and serve as a foundation for adaptation in the present and future environments. The concept of keystone behaviors extends the concept of habilitative validity by specifically acknowledging that changes in some response classes can have diverse benefits. Increasing compliance can serve to collaterally decrease a variety of maladaptive behaviors (Parrish, Cataldo, Kolko, Neef, & Engel, 1986) without actually targeting the individual maladaptive responses. Reading skills have the potential for being keystone academic behaviors, because they should facilitate success in a variety of activities beyond reading.

The burgeoning functional analysis literature has contributed an empirical method for identifying habilitative behaviors that may be keystone behaviors. A hallmark of some of this research is the identification of adaptive behaviors that can serve as functional replacements for maladaptive behaviors. Functional communication training (Carr & Durand, 1985) provides an excellent example of this methodology. During the analysis stage of Carr and Durand's (1985) study, the function of maladaptive behaviors was identified; during the treatment phase, appropriate communicative behaviors were developed to replace the maladaptive responses. The functional analytic approach to assessment and target selection may also benefit the client by preventing an overly negative treatment focus. Using this type of methodology, the focus of treatment would be on increasing adaptive communicative behavior, rather than exclusively on decreasing maladaptive behavior. This positive (behavior increasing) treatment focus is consistent with previous recommendations for target selection (Evans, 1993).

Drawing from the work described above, an ideal target behavior for increase would be a behavior that would have a broad adaptive benefit to the client. Increases in this keystone target behavior might also benefit other consultation consumers, such as peers, parents, or teachers. The identification of keystone targets may require an assessment process that includes interviews, examination of response classes, task analyses, template matching, or functional assessment (see Barnett et al., 1996). If the initial target behavior is a behavioral excess, an alternative adaptive response that can replace the maladaptive behavior should be identified. This will help prevent a negative treatment focus and would prevent the problems associated with having goals specifying only the absence of behavior (Johnston & Pennypacker, 1993). If identification of keystone targets is a goal of the problem definition, the assessment will be ideographic in nature and is likely to extend beyond a single interview.

Because the completion of classroom work is so central to what schools are about, an obvious choice for an initial intervention in schools is to establish an intervention directed toward getting the student engaged in his or her primary job, that is, academic performance. The default option for an initial intervention for relatively common problems, such as academic performance deficits or mild to moderate behavior problems, is the establishment of systematic procedures for increasing academic performance. The logic here is that if the teacher's classroom routine does not support appropriate behavior, then many students will choose inappropriate behavior to gain peer attention or other sources of reinforcement. Academic performance is an appropriate intervention outcome goal even if the problem is behavioral. Batsche and Knoff (1995) have noted that the identification of replacement behaviors (i.e., behaviors that will replace problem behaviors) is the first step in intervention planning for two reasons:

> First, interventions that focus on the reduction of a behavior assume that the negative behavior will be replaced, automatically, by a prosocial behavior. . . . Unless the reductive intervention is continued, the negative behavior will return as soon as conditions warrant. . . . Second, interventions designed to reduce behaviors are not educative and do not draw on the teaching skills of school personnel. Interventions that *teach* use the same teaching processes of modeling, role play, performance feedback and transfer of training that teachers use every day to teach academics. Therefore the "behavioral regularity" of the

teacher remains intact and the number of new skills required to implement interventions are minimized. (p. 571 emphasis in original)

The development of an intervention designed to increase academic performance will provide information to the consultant about several important questions. First, given that the child is given work which is appropriately difficult and that this work is monitored and consequenced, is the child able to perform in the classroom? Second, is there a collateral decrease in disruptive behavior, or are there behaviors which will require some specific attention? Third, can the teacher implement this academic intervention, which represents only a minimal departure from normal classroom routines, or does the teacher have skill and/or performance deficits in the area of intervention implementation? This information can be used later to develop alternative interventions for the child or to intensify consultant behaviors which will result in increased treatment integrity (i.e., reteaching the intervention or providing performance feedback).

Problem Analysis and Assessment

A clear and absolute boundary between definition of the target concern and assessment of the target concern will not be established in all cases. This may be particularly true if a functional assessment is undertaken. The functional assessment may lead to a broadening of the target concern to include adaptive alternative behaviors. The assessment procedures described in the following sections focus on determining the client's skills and identifying environmental variables that have functional control over the emission of adaptive and problematic behaviors.

An important part of the assessment phase will be collection of baseline data. Ideally the ongoing baseline data collection procedure will not be burdensome to implement and will not interfere with the consultee's other responsibilities (J.E. Zins & Erchul, 1995). Recording the products of behavior, such as scores on in-class work assignments or slips from referrals to the principal's office, may provide simple, meaningful data with low time pressure for data recording. It is also worth noting that the procedures for data collection may need to be modified if assessment results lead to additional or alternative target behaviors.

Functional Assessment

One of the essential purposes of behavioral assessment is the identification of variables that control the emission of targeted behaviors (Nelson & Hayes, 1979). The understanding gained through the identification of controlling variables should subsequently facilitate the modification of the target response. The identification of functional relationships can also be described as functional assessment. A functional assessment examines the relationship of antecedent and consequent variables to the behavior of interest (Bijou, Peterson, & Ault, 1968; Iwata, Dorsey, Slifer, Bauman, & Richman, 1982). The assessment attempts to determine what antecedents set the occasion for the behavior and what consequences maintain the behavior.

Before examining functional assessment techniques, it is important to acknowledge that it is not always necessary to understand the function of behavior to change it. Using powerful reinforcers may be sufficient to change behavior in the absence of any knowledge of function. A limitation of this approach is that it assumes that powerful reinforcers will be readily available and acceptable. In addition, it may create a matching situation (Herrnstein, 1990) in which the target behavior continues to occur at low rates as the schedules of reinforcement compete. Finally, designing interventions in the absence of knowledge of function can lead to counterintuitive and counterproductive results. For example, if the function of the behavior is escape, time-out would serve to increase the rate of problematic behavior (e.g., Plummer, Baer, & LeBlanc, 1977; Solnick, Rincover, & Peterson, 1977). Functional assessment can allow the consultant and consultee to avoid the risks that are associated with intervention in the absence of assessment, and may permit interventions to be developed that do not require reinforcers that are incompatible with the behavioral ecology.

A wide variety of assessment techniques can potentially contribute to a functional assessment: they can be categorized as either descriptive or experimental.

Descriptive Functional Assessments. Descriptive functional assessment techniques examine the sequences of events associated with the target behavior and use these sequences to generate hypotheses about the function the behavior may serve (Lerman & Iwata, 1993). Direct observation in the containing environment and interviews can contribute to a descriptive assessment.

The Problem Analysis Interview (PAI) component of BC (Bergan & Kratochwill, 1990) is one form of functional assessment. This assessment follows the pattern of the antecedent, behavior, and consequent (ABC) analysis described by Bijou and colleagues (1968). This form of descriptive analysis attempts to discover function by looking for patterns in the occurrence of environmental events and behavior. For example, a student may consistently exhibit tantrums when seat work is assigned, and these tantrums may be followed by removal from class. This descriptive analysis could lead to the hypothesis that tantrums served to obtain escape from seat work. The same hypothesis might be developed based on direct observation in the containing environment or the use of a scatter plot (Touchette, MacDonald, & Langer, 1985) combined with interview data.

Descriptive assessment has some limitations, despite its long history of use and its intuitive appeal. Functional relationships may not be readily apparent through direct observation (Barnett et al., 1996). The consequence of the behavior that is salient to the observer may be a coincidental effect of the behavior that has no functional relationship to the behavior. In addition, a single behavior may produce several consequences. In the instance of tantruming behavior described above, the tantrums may produce escape, teacher attention, and peer attention. The behavior may be functionally related to one, some, or none of these consequences. A descriptive analysis provides a basis for developing initial hypotheses, but is not useful in selecting between plausible rival hypotheses. Testing rival functional hypotheses requires manipulation of environmental variables.

In addition to the limitations of functional assessments in general, assessment that is driven primarily or exclusively by interview data is subject to the limitations inherent in memory and perception (Weingardt et al., 1995). Informants may be reluctant to report events that they believe will be regarded negatively. Functionally important variables that are not salient to the informant may not be reported. Memory biases may cause the informant to remember highly salient or upsetting behaviors as occurring more frequently than they actually do. These limitations of functional assessment based on interview data do not negate the utility of interview as an assessment tool. All referrals and assessments are likely to begin with an interview. The utility of interviews in functional assessment might better be summarized as developing hypotheses that guide the initial direct assessment and identifying important targets for assessment.

Functional Analysis. The alternative to a descriptive analysis of the target concern is the experimental assessment, which has been described as a functional analysis. A functional analysis is an experimental manipulation of environmental events to identify variables that suppress or maintain a targeted behavior (Iwata et al., 1982, Vollmer & Northup, 1996). During a functional analysis, the impact of differing antecedents and contingencies is tested during a series of experimental sessions. The impact of these contingencies on behavior then is typically determined by comparisons of graphed data from varying conditions. Experimental conditions have included free play, alone, reprimands (attention), removal of task demands, and access to material reinforcers, among others. Functional analyses have been conducted in both the target environment (e.g., Lalli et al., 1993) and analog settings (e.g, Iwata et al., 1982). Researchers have found interpretable differences between conditions using very few sessions per condition (Northup et al., 1991; Umbreit, 1995).

A functional analysis permits determination of the function of a behavior. This determination of function permits the development of an intervention that is relevant to the function of the behavior. Using functionally relevant interventions can lead to more powerful interventions that potentially can be more compatible with the behavioral ecology (Vollmer & Northup, 1996). If the function of tantrums was experimentally determined to be escape from the task, the escape function of the behavior could be blocked. The assignment could be sent with the student to the principal's office, where the student would be required to complete the assignment before returning to class. If a student's disruptive interruptions were determined to be functionally controlled by teacher attention, an intervention in which attention was provided when the student complied with the classroom routine and disruptive

statements were ignored might be developed (differential reinforcement). In addition, if the function of a problematic behavior can be determined, an alternative adaptive response that can serve as a functional replacement for the problematic behavior may be identified and targeted for increase.

While functional analyses provide powerful assessment data, they have a number of limitations. First, the resources required to conduct the analysis may exceed those available to the consultant and consultee (Lerman & Iwata, 1993). Second, results obtained in analog situations may not generalize to the environment of interest. Third, it may not be possible to obtain useful functional analysis data if conditions cannot be identified in which the behavior will occur at moderate rates. If the target concern is an explosive outburst that occurs once per week, a functional analysis may not be possible. In addition, if the focus of the assessment is the absence of important social or academic behaviors, a functional analysis may not return the most informative data. This would be especially true if the client lacked the skill to perform the behavior.

Assessment of Skill and Performance Deficits

The last limitation of functional analysis described above, determination of skills, logically leads to consideration of assessment by different means for differing purposes. At some point in the assessment or problem definition phase, an adaptive behavior should be targeted for increase. A referral resulting from poor reading or poor social skills may lead to an adaptive behavior target during the problem identification phase. Alternatively, the adaptive behavior may be identified during the assessment phase. This might arise if a goal of intervention was to teach a child to solicit parental attention in a socially acceptable manner rather than through aggressive behavior. However, identification of the adaptive target behavior raises a new question. Is the skill necessary to complete the target response present in the client's repertoire?

Gresham (1986) described the conceptual basis for this type of assessment as it relates to social skills. Gresham (1986) identified skill deficits, performance deficits, and self-control deficits as useful categories of social skill problems. An individual with a skill deficit would not exhibit the target behavior because he or she lacks the skill, while an individual with a performance deficit possesses the skill, but does not perform the skill frequently enough. In the case of performance deficits, the absence or infrequence of socially skilled behavior results from inadequate stimulus control or reinforcement contingencies. Gresham (1986) described individuals who exhibit self-control deficits as failing to exhibit socially skilled behavior due to responses deriving from some type of emotional arousal (e.g., anxiety or anger). In addition to the self-control deficit, the individual either possesses the skill (self-control performance deficit) or does not possess the social skill (self-control skill deficit).

Although this categorization of reasons for poor performance was developed to describe social skills, the same conceptual framework can be extended to other adaptive behaviors. The basis for a client's poor mathematics performance could be found to be either a skill or a performance deficit. In addition, a competing behavior, such as socializing with peers, may interfere with mathematics performance. The term *competing behavior* may have a greater general case utility in understanding and treating behaviors that block emission of adaptive responses than the term *self-control deficit*. A student's socializing with peers during class may result from competing schedules of reinforcement, rather than a cross-situational trait. The use of the term competing behaviors, rather than self-control deficit, is not intended to indicate that some children do not exhibit self-control deficits that would be an important target for intervention. Rather, the concept of competing behaviors permits extension of Gresham's (1986) conceptualization to the broad array of behaviors that can block the performance of adaptive responses.

The categories of skill deficits, performance deficits, and competing behaviors can provide conceptual anchors when the goal of assessment is to determine why the client does not exhibit the targeted adaptive response. Any alternative behavior that occurs on the occasions when the targeted adaptive behavior should occur constitutes a competing behavior. Determining the environmental variables that have functional control over the occurrence of the competing behavior is a question that can best be addressed through some form of functional assessment (see the preceding section). However, the absence of the target response in the containing environment will not provide definitive information about the client's skills (Gresham, 1986, 1989).

A crucial first step in assessing client skills is to identify meaningful standards for evaluating performance. For example, instructional placement standards (e.g., Fuchs & Deno, 1982) can be used to evaluate the adequacy of academic skills. Alternatively, evaluation of social skills could be based on performance of steps in a task analysis of a skill such as social entry, or on outcomes such as successfully entering a play group (Gresham, 1986). Once standards for acceptable performance have been established, information can be gathered through a wide range of assessment techniques. Interview, observational data, or review of permanent products can be used to determine whether the client exhibits competent performance on some occasions. If the client exhibits the skill on some occasions or in some settings, the lack of competent performance on targeted occasions is likely to be the result of a performance deficit.

The absence of the targeted response does not preclude the possibility of a performance deficit. A history of punishment may have suppressed the behavior, environmental cues may not be sufficient to elicit the behavior, or available reinforcement may not be sufficient to control the response. The basic technique for determining client skills requires assessing them under conditions which are relatively ideal for eliciting the behavior for that individual. These conditions will be idiographic in nature. For a client motivated by positive social attention, the simple request to demonstrate his or her best example of the targeted skill in a role-play test may yield valuable assessment data. For a client who exhibits high rates of oppositional behaviors, an assessment based on a request may not be informative regarding skills.

Another assessment alternative is to provide a contingency for adequate performance. A recent investigation found that implementing curriculum-based assessment (CBA), with and without contingencies for reading performance, yielded data indicating differing appropriate instructional placement for some of the students assessed (Noell, Witt, & Gansle, 1996, unpublished raw data). In this study, some students read above an instructional goal when reading fluently led to access to a preferred stimulus, while access to a preferred stimulus did not affect the CBA reading fluency of other students. The former students could be described as exhibiting a performance deficit, while the latter might be described as exhibiting a skill deficit.

An important limitation should be noted regarding the attempt to demonstrate a skill deficit. It is not possible within behavioral assessment or the scientific method to conclusively demonstrate the absence of a skill. If 25 assessment techniques failed to elicit the skill, that does not exclude the possibility that assessment technique number 26 would elicit competent performance. For practical purposes, however, an assessment that examines plausible conditions that may elicit the behavior from the client should be adequate for treatment planning. If competent behavior does not occur in the environment or under relatively ideal assessment conditions, a skill deficit hypothesis appears to be tenable.

Plan Implementation

Developing the Intervention Plan

At the conclusion of the assessment phase, the consultant and consultee should be able to state hypotheses regarding the function of problematic behaviors and identify the skills the client possesses relevant to the targeted concern. Identification of intervention options should derive directly from the assessment data. If the client exhibits a skill deficit for the targeted adaptive behavior, skill training should be an important component of the intervention plan. Intervention elements might include coaching, behavioral rehearsal, systematic prompting, shaping (Sulzer-Azaroff & Mayer, 1991), or direct instruction (Engelmann & Carnine, 1982). Alternatively, if the behavioral deficit is determined to be a performance deficit, the intervention would logically focus on generalization strategies for increasing performance of that skill. Intervention elements are likely to attempt to bring performance of the target behavior under stimulus control in the containing environment through manipulation of antecedents and/or consequences.

Many referral concerns will include the reduction of problematic behaviors as an important treatment focus. The functional assessment described previously should lead to hypotheses regarding the function of the problematic behavior. These func-

tion hypotheses should in turn lead to treatment options with a high probability of success. For example, a functional assessment reported by Lalli and colleagues (1993) demonstrated that one of the participant's targeted aggressions accelerated when it was followed by attention. During a subsequent treatment phase, the aggressive behavior was reduced by withholding attention subsequent to aggression. In a final treatment phase, the aggression was eliminated and an adaptive alternative response developed through a combination of skill training and differential reinforcement of alternative behaviors.

At the end of the assessment phase, a number of intervention options are likely to be available. A problematic behavior might be reduced by time-out or differential reinforcement. Performance of a social skill might be increased through peer initiations or contingent reinforcement. A primary consultant role at this stage is to discuss and interpret the assessment data with the consultee. This review of assessment data should lead naturally to a discussion of intervention options. The selection and development of an intervention plan is a critical stage in the consultation process, and the complementary nature of the relationship between consultant and consultee is crucial. Because the consultee is likely to have primary or exclusive responsibility for implementing the intervention plan, it has been regarded as important that she or he find the intervention plan acceptable (Elliott, 1988; J. Zins & Ponti, 1990). However, recent research has suggested that treatment integrity is related to consultee training, not to the consultee's positive appraisal of treatment prior to its use (Sterling, Watson, Wildman, Watkins, & Little, in press).

Several factors have been found to be related to treatment acceptability. Treatments which are behavior-increasing, target severe misbehavior, are not time-consuming to implement, and are reported to be effective have been found to be more acceptable than treatments having the reverse characteristics across a number of studies (Elliott, 1988). In addition, teachers who are knowledgeable about behavioral principles have been found to rate a variety of treatments as more acceptable (Elliott, 1988). These findings have particular importance for the development of interventions within consultation. If the consultant can adequately explain why the intervention should be effective for this specific client based on the assessment data (effectiveness information), and can explain how it will work (knowledge), the consultee may perceive the intervention as more acceptable. Despite the numerous parametric findings regarding acceptability, within the context of any consultation case the particular consultee's acceptability evaluations will be the variable of interest.

Once an acceptable intervention option has been identified, planning for implementation should begin. All of the elements of the plan should be discussed and written. The responsibilities of each participating individual should be identified and recorded to reduce the risk of misunderstanding and to facilitate accountability (J. Zins & Ponti, 1990). Implementation may be enhanced if the consultant contributes some resources to either intervention preparation or implementation (Noell & Gresham, 1993). In addition, the specific skills needed to implement the intervention should be identified and discussed. It may be necessary for the consultant to teach the consultee how to implement some or all of the intervention elements (Watson & Robinson, 1996; Witt, Noell, LaFleur, & Mortenson, in press). Taking the time to ensure that the consultee knows how to implement the intervention accurately and understands the rationale for each of the steps of the intervention may contribute to obtaining adequate treatment integrity. Frequently it will be necessary to observe the consultee's implementation of the intervention in the containing environment while prompting behaviors as needed.

A final element of the plan development stage is to decide on a treatment monitoring or data collection procedure. The importance of a progress monitoring plan is highlighted by the meta-analysis finding that systematically monitoring and graphing student achievement produced a 0.80 effect size (Fuchs & Fuchs, 1986). The issues in devising a data collection procedure closely parallel those of intervention development with regard to acceptability, assisting with preparation, and implementing training as needed. Ideally, the discussion of the data collection procedures will be a review of procedures that were established for baseline data during the assessment phase.

Treatment Integrity

The intervention implementation phase is arguably the most important phase of consultation. A consultation process that does not result in an intervention that is implemented is unlikely to benefit either the client or the consultee. Although the implementation phase may be the most crucial stage of consultation, relatively little research has been conducted using direct measures of treatment integrity to identify variables that contribute to adequate integrity (Witt et al., 1996). An additional challenge of this phase of consultation is identifying an appropriate method for assessing treatment integrity (see Gresham, 1989). Although simply asking the consultee about implementation seems to be an obvious choice, one empirical investigation of teacher self-report of integrity found teacher report to yield much higher levels of integrity than were revealed by direct observation (Wickstrom, 1995). If the intervention produces permanent products, such as self-monitoring records, these products may be useful in examining both treatment integrity and treatment outcome.

Whether treatment integrity is assessed by consultee report or by a more direct measure, the remaining question is how to increase treatment integrity when it is low or maintain it when it is adequate. The issues related to ensuring adequate integrity are of increased importance when the intervention is part of a legal entitlement such as Section 504 accommodation or services under the Individuals with Disabilities Education Act. In some cases, implementing the intervention may produce effects that reinforce its use (Noell & Gresham, 1993). This appears to be most likely to occur when the intervention produces effects that benefit the consultee as well as the client. Implementing an intervention that increases order and decreases conflict in the classroom might directly reinforce continued use of the treatment by a teacher.

An additional possibility for enhancing treatment integrity is to increase the sense that the intervention is a shared responsibility in which several individuals are accountable to one another for implementation. Conjoint behavioral consultation (Sheridan, Kratochwill, & Elliott, 1990) may provide a method for increasing integrity by sharing responsibility between educators and parents. However, this is a logically derived potential benefit of this consultation procedure that has not yet been subjected to an empirical test.

Social support and feedback delivered by the consultant has been shown to increase treatment integrity in an experimental study (Witt et al., in press). In this study, consultants met with teachers to review treatment implementation data obtained from permanent products and to discuss implementation issues. Child outcome data were also reviewed in these brief meetings. The teachers demonstrated increased treatment integrity during the phase in which they received daily feedback and support. One of the four teachers did not demonstrate high levels of integrity until a case conference was implemented. It is also worth noting that the consultants in this study were doctoral students who did not have any administrative authority in the schools. This form of support and feedback was effective in the absence of a hierarchical relationship.

Plan Evaluation

The modal model for BC (Bergan & Kratochwill, 1990; Kratochwill, Elliott, & Rotto, 1995) calls for a formal Plan Evaluation Interview (PEI) at which the effectiveness of the intervention is reviewed. This evaluation would typically be accomplished by comparing graphed data from the treatment phase with data from the baseline phase and with the goal level set during problem identification or analysis (Martens, 1993). Based on a review of the data, decisions can be made regarding how to proceed. If the client demonstrates a trend toward the goal, but has not yet achieved the goal, the intervention might be continued. If performance has stabilized above goal levels, treatment might be shifted to a maintenance procedure. Finally, inadequate client progress or poor treatment integrity may indicate the need to modify the intervention or provide additional assistance to the consultee in implementing the plan.

While acknowledging that a formal PEI may have many benefits, the present authors would favor a greater emphasis on ongoing evaluation. This might be accomplished through frequent and brief contacts in which implementation and outcome data are reviewed. The meta-analysis summarized previously (Fuchs & Fuchs, 1986) indicates that frequent formative evaluation may produce large positive effects. Witt and colleagues' (in press) study included a modest form of daily program evaluation during feedback phases; this may have facilitated treatment integrity. Frequent formative evaluation in consultation can also permit small refinements in the intervention plan, to be implemented in a timely

manner that benefits both the consultee and the client. Finally, more frequent evaluation can prevent implementation problems or treatment side effects from becoming unmanageable before consultant support is provided.

Regardless of how often the consultant and consultee review the data, plan evaluation has two basic elements. The first is determining if the client's performance of the targeted behavior has attained the goal set during the problem identification or assessment phases. The second is deciding whether changes in the client's behavior can be attributed to the intervention. The first question should be readily answerable through review of the progress monitoring data. Through review of these data decisions regarding continuing the intervention, modifying the treatment, or shifting to a maintenance procedure can be made. To be able to attribute changes in client behavior to the intervention requires some form of experimental manipulation. Limiting evaluation to baseline and treatment data does not control several potential confounds (Barlow & Hersen, 1984). A variety of single case experimental designs are available that can be compatible with consultation and permit more conclusive determination of intervention effects (Chapter 2, this volume; Hayes, 1981; Kazdin, 1994).

Summary and Directions for Future Research

The behavior analytic approach to consultation described in this chapter placed a wide range of behavior analytic techniques within a consultation framework. This description examined some of the issues and possibilities as they related to including more of the epistemological bases and procedures of behavior analysis within consultation. The impetus for this description was the exclusion of many of the tools of behavior analysis from much of the writing relevant to consultation. The traditional dichotomous distinction between direct service and consultation was abandoned because it appears to be a barrier to the development of a broader range of options for the practice of behavioral consultation. Within the present context, direct consultation service might be more accurately described as a continuous variable. The amount of direct assessment, teaching, and technical assistance provided by the consultant is assumed to be driven by the needs of the consultee–client dyad.

The issues discussed in this chapter highlight the need for lines of research that are both new and old. For example, a continuing need exists for research examining methods of obtaining assessment data and progress monitoring data that are as time efficient as possible, are reliable, and have treatment validity. While the body of applied behavioral research continues to provide new possibilities for data collection, the need for time-efficient direct measures of behavior remains at least partially unfulfilled. If the implementation of more direct functional assessment is to be incorporated into behavioral consultation, new lines of inquiry may be needed. Research examining how direct behavioral assessment can be incorporated into the interpersonal process of consultation is needed. Additional investigations examining direct behavioral assessment implemented jointly by consultants and consultees are also needed.

The central challenge facing consultation researchers is the same now as it was when Bergan (1977) published his seminal book on behavioral consultation. What procedures can behavioral consultants employ to ensure adequate treatment integrity? Without implementation of the intervention, behavioral consultation degenerates into little more than social support for frustrated teachers, parents, and direct service providers. While social support has merits, there are less expensive and complex means of providing social support than behavioral consultation. Behavioral consultation's relevance to the problems faced by consultees and clients resides not in the consultation process, but in the implemented interventions the process produces. Some of the answers to the most important question facing behavioral consultation researchers, that of how to obtain treatment integrity, are likely to lie within behavioral consultation's roots: applied behavior analysis.

References

Baer, D.M., Wolf, M.M., & Risley, T.R. (1968). Some current dimensions of applied behavior analysis. *Journal of Applied Behavior Analysis, 1,* 91–97.

Barlow, D.H., & Hersen, M. (1984). *Single case experimental designs* (2nd ed.). New York: Pergamon.

Barnett, D.W., Bauer, A.M., Ehrhardt, K.E., Lentz, F.E., & Stollar, S.A. (1996). Keystone targets for change: Planning for widespread positive consequences. *School Psychology Quarterly, 11,* 95–117.

Batsche, G.M., & Knoff, H.M. (1995). Best practices in linking assessment to intervention. In A. Thomas & J. Grimes (Eds.), *Best practices in school psychology III* (pp. 569–585). Washington, DC: National Association of School Psychologists.

Bergan, J.R. (1977). *Behavioral Consultation.* Columbus, OH: Merrill.

Bergan, J.R., & Kratochwill, T.R. (1990). *Behavioral consultation and therapy.* New York: Plenum.

Bergan, J.R., & Tombari, M.L. (1976). Consultant skill and efficiency and the implementation and outcomes of consultation. *Journal of School Psychology, 14,* 3–14.

Bijou, S.W., Peterson, R.F., & Ault, M.H. (1968). A method to integrate descriptive and experimental field studies at the level of data and empirical concepts. *Journal of Applied Behavior Analysis, 1,* 175–191.

Carr, E.G., & Durand, V.M. (1985). Reducing behavior problems through functional communication training. *Journal of Applied Behavior Analysis, 18,* 111–126.

Ciminero, A.R., Calhoun, K.S., & Adams, H.E. (1986). *Handbook of behavioral assessment* (2nd ed.). New York: Wiley.

Cone, J.D. (1988). Psychometric considerations and the multiple models of behavioral consultation. In A.S. Bellack & M. Hersen (Eds.), *Behavioral assessment* (3rd ed., pp. 42–66). New York: Pergamon.

Conoley, J.C., & Conoley, C.W. (1982). *School consultation: A guide to practice and training.* New York: Pergamon.

Elliott, S.N. (1988). Acceptability of behavioral treatments in educational settings. In J.C. Witt, S.N. Elliott, & F.M. Gresham (Eds.), *Handbook of behavior therapy in education* (pp. 121–150). New York: Plenum.

Engelmann, S., & Carnine, D. (1982). *Theory of instruction: Principles and applications.* New York: Irvington.

Erchul, W.P., & Chewning, T.G. (1990). Behavioral consultation from a request centered relational communication perspective. *School Psychology Quarterly, 5,* 1–20.

Erchul, W.P., & Schulte, A.C. (1996). Behavioral consultation as a work in progress: A reply to Witt, Gresham, and Noell. *Journal of Educational and Psychological Consultation, 1,* 345–354.

Evans, I.M. (1993). Constructional perspectives in clinical assessment. *Psychological Assessment, 5,* 264–272.

Foster, S.L., & Cone, J.D. (1986). Design and use of direct observation. In A.R. Ciminero, K.S. Calhoun, & H.E. Adams (Eds.), *Handbook of behavioral assessment* (2nd ed., pp. 253–324). New York: Wiley.

Fuchs, L.S., & Deno, S.L. (1982). *Developing goals and objectives for educational programs.* Washington, DC: American Association of Colleges for Teacher Education.

Fuchs, L.S., & Fuchs, D. (1986). Effects of systematic formative evaluation on student achievement: A meta-analysis. *Exceptional Children, 53,* 199–208.

Gresham, F.M. (1986). Conceptual and definitional issues in the assessment of children's social skills: Implications for classification and training. *Journal of Clinical Child Psychology, 15,* 3–15.

Gresham, F.M. (1989). Assessment of treatment integrity in school consultation and prereferral intervention. *School Psychology Quarterly, 18,* 37–50.

Gresham, F.M., Gansle, K.A., Noell, G.H., Cohen, S., & Rosenblum, S. (1993). Treatment integrity of school-based behavioral intervention studies: 1980–1990. *School Psychology Review, 22*, 254–272.

Gresham, F.M., & Kendell, G.K. (1987). School consultation research: Methodological critique and future research directions. *School Psychology Review, 16*, 306–316.

Hawkins, R.P. (1991). Is social validity what we are interested in? Argument for a functional approach. *Journal of Applied Behavior Analysis, 24*, 205–213.

Hayes, S.C. (1981). Single case experimental design and empirical clinical practice. *Journal of Consulting and Clinical Psychology, 49*, 193–211.

Herrnstein, R.J. (1990). Rational choice theory: Necessary but not sufficient. *American Psychologist, 45*, 356–367.

Iwata, B.A., Dorsey, M., Slifer, K., Bauman, K., & Richman, G. (1982). Toward a functional analysis of self-injury. *Analysis and intervention in developmental disabilities, 2*, 3–20.

Johnston, J.M., & Pennypacker, H.S. (1993). *Strategies and tactics of behavioral research*. Hillsdale, NJ: Erlbaum.

Kazdin, A.E. (1994). *Behavior modification in applied settings* (5th ed.). Pacific Grove, CA: Brooks/Cole.

Kratochwill, T.R., Elliott, S.N., & Rotto, P.C. (1995). School-based behavioral consultation. In A. Thomas & J. Grimes (Eds.), *Best practices in school psychology III* (pp. 519–538). Washington, DC: National Association of School Psychologists.

Lalli, J.S., Browder, D.M., Mace, F.C., & Brown, D.K. (1993). Teacher use of descriptive analysis to implement interventions to decrease students' problem behaviors. *Journal of Applied Behavior Analysis, 26*, 227–238.

Lambert, N.M. (1976). Children's problems and classroom interventions from the perspective of classroom teachers. *Professional Psychology, 1*, 507–517.

Lerman, D.C., & Iwata, B.A. (1993). Descriptive and experimental analyses of variables maintaining self-injurious behavior. *Journal of Applied Behavior Analysis, 26*, 293–319.

Mace, C.F. (1994). The significance and future of functional analysis methodologies. *Journal of Applied Behavior Analysis, 27*, 385–393.

Martens, B.K. (1993). A behavioral approach to consultation. In J.E. Zins, T.R. Kratochwill, & S.N. Elliott (Eds.), *Handbook of consultation services for children* (pp. 65–86). San Francisco: Jossey-Bass.

Martens, B.K., & Witt, J.C. (1988). On the ecological validity of behavior modification. In J.C. Witt, S.N. Elliott, & F.M. Gresham (Eds.), *Handbook of behavior therapy in education* (pp. 325–342). New York: Plenum.

Nelson, R.O., & Hayes, S.C. (1979). Some current dimensions of behavioral assessment. *Behavioral Assessment, 1*, 1–16.

Noell, G.H. (1996). New directions in behavioral consultation. *School Psychology Quarterly, 11*, 187–188.

Noell, G.H., & Gresham, F.M. (1993). Functional outcome analysis: Do the benefits of consultation and prereferral intervention justify the costs? *School Psychology Quarterly, 8*, 200–226.

Noell, G.H., & Witt, J.C. (1996). A critical re-evaluation of five fundamental assumptions underlying behavioral consultation. *School Psychology Quarterly, 11*, 189–203.

Noell, G.H., Witt, J.C., & Gansle, K.A. (1996). [Identification of skill and performance deficits in oral reading]. Unpublished raw data.

Northup, J., Wacker, D.P., Sasso, G., Steege, M., Cigrand, C., Cook, J., & DeRaad, A. (1991). A brief functional analysis of aggressive and alternative behavior in an outclinic setting. *Journal of Applied Behavior Analysis, 24*, 509–521.

Parrish, J.M., Cataldo, M.F., Kolko, D.J., Neef, N.A., & Engel, A.L. (1986). Experimental analysis of response covariation among compliant and inappropriate behaviors. *Journal of Applied Behavior Analysis, 19*, 241–254.

Peterson, L., Homer, A., & Wonderlich, S. (1982). The integrity of independent variables in behavior analysis. *Journal of Applied Behavior Analysis, 15*, 477–492.

Plummer, S., Baer, D.M., & LeBlanc, J.M. (1977). Functional considerations in the use of procedural timeout and an effective alternative. *Journal of Applied Behavior Analysis, 10*, 689–706.

Schwartz, I., & Baer, D. (1991). Social validity assessment: Is current practice the state of the art? *Journal of Applied Behavior Analysis, 24*, 189–204.

Shapiro, E.S., & Skinner, C.H. (1993). Childhood behavioral assessment and diagnosis. In T.R. Kratochwill & R.J. Morris (Eds.), *Handbook of psychotherapy with children and adolescents* (pp. 75–107). Boston: Allyn and Bacon.

Sheridan, S.M., Kratochwill, T.R., & Elliott, S.N. (1990). Behavioral consultation with parents and teachers: Delivering treatment for socially withdrawn children at home and school. *School Psychology Review, 19*, 33–52.

Shriver, M.D., & Allen, K.D. (1996). The time-out grid: A guide to effective discipline. *School Psychology Quarterly, 11*, 67–75.

Solnick, J.V., Rincover, A., & Peterson, C.R. (1977). Some determinants of the reinforcing and punishing effects of time out. *Journal of Applied Behavior Analysis, 10*, 415–424.

Sterling, H.E., Watson, T.S., Wildman, M., Watkins, C., & Little, E. (in press). Treatment acceptability, direct training, and treatment integrity: Applications to consultation. *School Psychology Quarterly*.

Stokes, T.F., & Osnes, P.G. (1989). An operant pursuit of generalization. *Behavior Therapy, 20*, 337–355.

Sulzer-Azaroff, B., & Mayer, G.R. (1991). *Behavior analysis for lasting change*. Chicago: Holt, Rinehart, & Winston.

Touchette, P.E., MacDonald, R.F., & Langer, S.N. (1985). A scatter plot for identifying stimulus control of problem behavior. *Journal of Applied Behavior Analysis, 18*, 343–351.

Umbreit, J. (1995). Functional assessment and intervention in a regular classroom setting for the disruptive behavior of a student with attention deficit hyperactivity disorder. *Behavioral Disorders, 20*, 267–278.

Vollmer, T.R., & Northup, J. (1996). Some implications of functional analysis for school psychology. *School Psychology Quarterly, 11*, 76–92.

Watson, T.S., & Robinson, S.L. (1996). Direct behavioral consultation: An alternative to traditional behavioral consultation. *School Psychology Quarterly, 11*, 267–278.

Weingardt, K.R., Loftus, E.F., & Lindsay, D.S. (1995). Misinformation revisited: New evidence on the suggestibility of memory. *Memory and Cognition, 23*, 72–82.

Wickstrom, K. (1995). *A study of the relationship among teacher, process and outcome variables with school-based consultation.* Unpublished doctoral dissertation, Louisiana State University, Baton Rouge.

Witt, J.C., Gresham, F.M., & Noell, G.H. (1996). What's behavioral about behavioral consultation? *Journal of Educational and Psychological Consultation, 7,* 327–344.

Witt, J.C., Noell, G.N., LaFleur, L.H., & Mortenson, B.P. (in press). Teacher usage of interventions in general education settings: Measurement and analysis of the independent variable. *Journal of Applied Behavior Analysis.*

Yeaton, W., & Sechrest, L. (1981). Critical dimensions in the choice and maintenance of successful treatments: Strength, integrity, and effectiveness. *Journal of Consulting and Clinical Psychology, 49,* 156–167.

Zins, J., & Ponti, C. (1990). Best practices in school-based consultation. In A. Thomas & J. Grimes (Eds.), *Best practices in school psychology* (2nd ed., pp. 673–693). Washington, DC: National Association of School Psychologists.

Zins, J.E., & Erchul, W.P. (1995). School consultation. In A. Thomas & J. Grimes (Eds.), *Best practices in school psy-chology III* (pp. 609–624). Washington, DC: National Association of School Psychologists.

Bibliography

Bergan, J.R. (1977). *Behavioral Consultation.* Columbus, OH: Merrill.

Bergan, J.R., & Kratochwill, T.R. (1990). *Behavioral consultation and therapy.* New York: Plenum Press.

Fuchs, D., & Fuchs, L.S. (1989). Exploring effective and efficient prereferral interventions: A component analysis of behavioral consultation. *School Psychology Review, 18,* 260–279.

The number of seminal references in the area of behavioral consultation is limited by the fact that few studies have examined the relationship between a consultation process and a direct measure of treatment implementation.

II

School-Based Problems

Problems that occur in the school environment account for a large percentage of referrals to pediatricians, family physicians, school and clinical psychologists, and counselors. Certainly, reading skills, or the lack of reading skills, is especially problematic, particularly in the early grades. Skinner, in Chapter 4, covers some of the most recent developments related to improving accurate academic responding in students with academic difficulties, including reading, math, and spelling. He advocates a somewhat novel approach to remediating academic skills deficits by looking at the rate and efficiency of learning trials as opposed to simply strengthening learning trials. Chapter 5 (Belfiore & Hutchinson) presents a refreshing look at a topic that receives very little attention in the professional literature; namely, functional analysis and treatment of skills that are related to academic development. Included in this chapter are skills related to notetaking, study strategies, and homework.

One would be safe in saying that Attention-Deficit/Hyperactivity Disorder is the diagnosis of the decade. More children, at younger ages, are being diagnosed as having ADHD and are being prescribed some form of stimulant medication. Although ADHD symptoms may be displayed across settings, we included it in the school-based section because it is usually first recognized and diagnosed when children enter the more restrictive classroom environment. In addition, medication is often titrated according to a child's academic schedule. DuPaul and Hoff (Chapter 6) have written what we consider to be a prototype for functional analysis and intervention for a child with attention and concentration problems.

Speech disfluencies is a somewhat uncommon chapter for child behavior therapy books. Traditionally, treatment of speech problems, especially stuttering, was left to a speech pathologist. Miltenberger and Woods (Chapter 7), however, describe how behavior therapists can successfully treat stuttering. This chapter is a shining example of how operant principles can be applied to areas once considered outside the purview of behavior analysis.

Kearney and Tillotson (Chapter 8) illustrate how a behavior once considered to be maintained only by anxiety (i.e., school refusal) may actually be maintained by several different contingencies. Further, they thoroughly describe treatment based on the assessed function of the refusal behavior. Their chapter will be an invaluable guide to professionals working in the schools who have been referred cases of school refusal, regardless of the age of the child.

4

Preventing Academic Skills Deficits

CHRISTOPHER H. SKINNER

Introduction

A functional approach to remediating academic skills deficits differs from a functional approach designed to remediate inappropriate behavior. When addressing inappropriate behavior, often the goals are to reduce idiosyncratic behavior that may serve different functions across students and/or environments. Thus, individual behavior change programs may have to be implemented for each student. When addressing academic skill deficits there are similar goals across students, which include increasing or improving performance on academic skills. While some students may go through their education never requiring any psychoeducational services designed to remediate inappropriate social behavior, all students receive services designed to improve academic skills. Therefore, any discussion of approaches designed to remediate academic skills deficits should also address procedures designed to prevent academic skills deficits.

This chapter will not focus on procedures designed to increase specific academic skills such as reading, writing, and mathematics; rather, empirically validated procedures designed to increase target behavior associated with increases in specific academic skills will be described, discussed, and analyzed in order to highlight behavioral principles and procedures that can be used to increase skills across domains. This focus will include an emphasis on increasing learning trial rates as opposed to theories and techniques designed to strengthen

learning trials. However, before this is done, traditional assessment and intervention procedures designed to prevent and remedy learning problems will be described and analyzed.

Classifying or Diagnosing Mild Learning Problems

The majority of students who are referred for psychoeducational services are experiencing mild learning or academic problems (Algozzine & Korinek, 1985; Bergan & Kratochwill, 1990; Ownby, Wallbrown, D'Atri, & Armstrong, 1985; Reschly, 1987). Under traditional models of service delivery, referred students are assessed (Shapiro, 1987). to determine if the child is eligible for special education services (diagnosis). Another function of psychoeducational assessment is to link assessment to intervention (Meyers, & Kundert, 1988; Reschly & Ysseldyke, 1995; Shapiro, 1989; Ysseldyke & Christenson, 1988).

A variety of problems and limitations with current diagnostic systems have been identified and described. Many of these problems stem from a system that is based on a traditional diagnostic-prescriptive medical model of linking assessment to interventions. A basic assumption of the traditional model is that current academic problems are a symptom of, or caused by, some underlying pathology within the student (Hartmann, Roper, & Bradford, 1979; Shapiro, 1996; Ysseldyke, & Christenson, 1988). Assessment is then undertaken to diagnose the student and identify the underlying pathology. Under a medical model of service delivery, a diagnosis is supposed to lead to treatment. When students with mild disabilities meet special

CHRISTOPHER H. SKINNER • School Psychology Program, Mississippi State University, Mississippi State, Mississippi 39762.

Handbook of Child Behavior Therapy, edited by Watson and Gresham. Plenum Press, New York, 1998.

education eligibility requirements, instructional intervention options may increase due to increased levels of parental involvement, increased funds allocated for teaching specific children, and individualized education plans developed by teams, including psychoeducational professionals and parents (Reschly, 1988).

Some students who are experiencing academic problems do not meet eligibility requirements. When students referred for academic problems do not meet eligibility requirements they are often labeled "at-risk" or "underachievers." These are not common diagnostic categories and typically lack any specified differential-diagnostic criteria. Furthermore, in most cases, these students are not eligible to receive special education services. However, the fact that students do not meet special education criteria does not mean that they are not having learning problems (Lentz & Shapiro, 1986; Smith, 1984). In the past, these students would not be eligible for service to help remediate their present learning problems and to prevent more severe future learning problems (Shapiro, 1987). Currently, some school systems are attempting to provided needed services to these children through student assistance teams, consultation, and building-based support teams (Graden, Zins, & Curtis, 1988).

The second major purpose of assessment is to determine methods and procedures that may help remediate current learning problems and prevent future learning problems. Many psychoeducational instruments used for diagnosis have been designed to more specifically identify within-student underlying pathologies and underlying strengths. Internal causal variables or pathologies most often associated with these mild learning problems are information processing problems or weaknesses (Wong, 1986). Assessment instruments have been designed to measure students' ability to process information when it is presented in different topographies, forms, or modalities (e.g., Illinois Test of Psycholinguistic Abilities; Kirk, McCarthy, & Kirk, 1968) and/or in different sequences (e.g., K-ABC; Kaufman & Kaufman, 1983). Scatter score or profile analysis (Kaufman, 1994; Keith, 1994) assessment and interpretation procedures have also been developed to allow for the assessment of within subject processing strengths and weaknesses.

Exceptionality-Treatment and Aptitude-Treatment Interactions

The most serious problem with traditional psychoeducational diagnostic practices is that they often do not lead to more effective academic interventions. Although receiving a special education diagnosis can result in increased instructional options (e.g., IEPs, special education teachers), these diagnostic categories do little to indicate which interventions or instructional strategies would be most effective for students with mild learning problems (Deno, 1985). Research suggests that the same academic interventions appear to be effective for students with learning disabilities, students with mild mental retardation, at-risk students, and low-achieving students (Heller, Holtzman, & Messick, 1982; Morsink, Thomas, & Smith-Davis, 1987).

Meeting, or failing to meet, diagnostic criteria, in and of itself, may provide little information for planing instructional procedures designed to remediate learning problems in students experiencing mild learning problems. The research on aptitude–treatment interactions has yielded similar results (Speece, 1990). Under a traditional method of service delivery, once information-processing strengths and weaknesses are identified, teachers can attempt to improve students' learning rates through accommodation or remediation (Anderson, 1980). Accommodation involves providing academic stimuli in a manner that allows students to process that academic information using their within subject information process strengths. This is often referred to as teaching to students' strengths. Remediation involves any attempt to improve information-processing weaknesses. Unfortunately, researchers have shown that teaching to strengths or attempting to remediate information-processing weaknesses typically does not improve students' learning rates (e.g., Arter & Jenkins, 1979; Ayers & Cooley, 1986; Deno, 1986; Fisher, Jenkins, Bancroft, & Kraft, 1988; Kavale & Forness, 1987; Macmann & Barnett, 1994; Speece, 1990).

Problem Identification

When the search for underlying pathology is abandoned, the identification of learning problems focuses on educationally valid goals. For the most part, educators have adopted a fairly narrow view of academic achievement, focusing primarily or solely on increasing the accuracy of academic responses (Haring & Eaton, 1978; Leper, 1985). However, if academic skills such as reading, writing, and arithmetic are to be functional, students must be able to respond accurately and fluently across different academic stimuli. Furthermore, students must maintain these improvements over time.

Can't Do

One of the first steps in the identification of any academic problem is to determine if the student can perform the task or skills (Bergan & Kratochwill, 1990). Various standardized norm-referenced tests have been developed which provide achievement scores for students across specific skill domains. However, these test are imprecise measures. The imprecision of these measures is caused by several factors. First, the test often measures material that is not included in the student curriculum and fails to measure material that is included in the students' curricula (Martens, Steele, Massie, & Diskin, 1995). Shriner and Salvia (1988) used the term "chronic non-correspondence" to describe the lack of overlap between commonly used curricula and commonly employed standardized tests. These "one-shot" assessments are designed to be brief, but also to assess many skills. Therefore, it is often impossible to obtain a large enough sample of specific skills to determine whether they have been mastered. Student responses during these assessments often take a form (e.g., multiple choice) that differs from the goal or target response. Finally, these instruments typically assess only accuracy. Therefore, these instruments may not provide very precise data on students' skill levels (Skinner, 1950).

Haring and Eaton (1978) developed a learning hierarchy in which the first stage is focused on increasing students' accuracy. Although instruction often focuses on accuracy and stops after students display some level of accuracy, subsequent stages (fluency and maintenance building, generalization programming, and adaptation programming) are very important if a skill is to be learned to the point at which it is functional or useful. Although "can't do" problems may be caused by the student never acquiring the desired behavior, they may be related to or caused by the failure of students to increase

academic performance beyond the accuracy or acquisition stage.

When a student cannot respond to an academic stimulus accurately, the problem may be a maintenance problem, not an acquisition problem. Often students acquire, but fail to maintain, specific behavior or skills. Maintenance building is one component of Haring and Eaton's (1978) second stage of learning. The other component, fluency building, will be discussed later.

"Can't do" problems may also be caused by stimulus generalization deficits. Sometimes students acquire a skill but cannot apply that skill to other similar stimulus conditions. One example of this would include a student who learned a phonetic unit (e.g., ch) and can read the word chair, church, and chain, but cannot read the word porch. This student may have acquired the ability to accurately read "ch" when it is presented in the beginning of words, but not when it is presented at the end of words. Other times students make accuracy errors because they have acquired several skills, but they cannot discriminate which skill is required when responding to specific stimuli.

When a student cannot perform a specific task accurately, one cannot assume that the problem is a failure to acquire a skill. In order to prevent and remediate learning problems, educators must go beyond procedures designed to increase accuracy, and include programming designed to improve maintenance, fluency, and generalization of those accurate responses.

Won't Do

"Won't do" problems most often evoke the concept of choice (e.g., the student chooses not to do the work). Some may call this a motivation problem. Recent research related to the matching law, concurrent schedules of reinforcement, and choice behavior has the potential to have a tremendous impact on "won't do" problems (Mace, McCurdy, & Quigley, 1990; McDowell, 1988; Neef, Mace, & Shade, 1993; Neef, Mace, Shea, & Shade, 1992; Neef, Shade, & Miller, 1994). "Won't do" problems may also be related to fluency building, the other goal of Haring and Eaton's (1978) second stage of learning. Although this relationship will be discussed later in this chapter, the importance of automaticity or fluency will be briefly discussed.

Behavioral and cognitive researchers have suggested that accuracy is a poor target behavior and have recommended using the latency between stimuli and accurate responses as both target behavior and measures of learning (Breznitz, 1987; Daneman & Carpenter, 1980; LaBerge & Samuels, 1976; Lesgold & Perfetti, 1978). Automaticity is a cognitive term that is measured by the latency between a stimulus and response (Gagne, 1982; Hasselbring & Goin, 1986; Pellegrino & Goldman, 1987). Hasselbring, Goin, and Bransford (1987) describe a procedure designed to assess automaticity to specific mathematics problems using flash cards. This procedure requires students to respond to the math facts (e.g., $6 \times 7 =$) within one or two seconds. Similar procedures could be used to assess automaticity when reading specific words or when spelling words.

Behavioral psychologists have taken a more molar view of automaticity, which they often refer to as fluency (Shapiro, 1996; Shinn, 1989). Curriculum-based measurement procedures have been designed for evaluating speed of accurate responding across many stimulus items. Deno and Mirkin (1977) described procedures designed to measure students' performance across reading, mathematics computation, writing, and spelling. For reading, students are instructed to read passages from different grade-level text, and evaluators time their reading and score errors. Their performance on the passage is then converted to words correct and errors per minute. Similar procedures are used for writing, where students are given a story starter and words written per minute are measured. In mathematics, students are given assessment sheets containing multiple problems, and, again, their performance is timed. These scores are then converted to digits correct per minute. For spelling, student performance is measured in letter sequences per minute.

These rate measures have been correlated with other measures of academic achievement (Marston, 1989). For example, Marston cites more than 12 studies which have shown that word-correct-per-minute correlates with a variety of reading skills, including literal and inferential comprehension.

From a behavioral perspective, fluency or automaticity has implications for "won't do" problems. When given a choice of two behaviors, organisms may choose the behavior that requires the least effort and/or results in higher rates of reinforcement (C.H. Skinner, Robinson, Johns, Logan, & Belfiore, 1996). Therefore, increasing students' response fluency may increase rates of reinforcement and decrease the effort required to earn those reinforcers. This relationship between fluency and student choice will be analyzed further in the plan implementation stage.

Problem Analysis: Student Responding and Learning Trials as Target Behaviors

The goal of academic prevention and remediation programs is to increase students' acquisition, fluency, maintenance, and generalization of academic skills. Educators and teachers often focus on what they must do to teach, rather than on what students must do to learn (Lindgren & Suter, 1985). When the primary focus is shifted from teacher behavior to student behavior, we arrive at one of the primary stages of behavioral problem solving: identifying target behaviors. One of the hallmarks of applied behavior analysis is the focus on direct identification of target behaviors (Hartmann et al., 1979; Shapiro, 1987). Once these behaviors are identified, then stimulus conditions (teaching and instruction) can be manipulated in order to bring about changes in target behaviors. While teachers control the antecedent and consequent stimuli, student behavior is the target. A strong research base exists that focuses on student behavior, and correlates with and/or causes high levels of student achievement across acquisition, fluency, maintenance, response generalization, and stimulus generalization. Next, characteristics of student responses (frequency, rate, accuracy, and topography) will be described and analyzed.

Frequent Responding across the Hierarchy

Although Haring and Eaton's (1978) learning hierarchy described different interventions for each stage of learning, at each stage there is a common focus on student responding. The importance of students' actively responding to academic stimuli has been known for some time. Colloquialisms like "practice makes perfect" and "learning by doing" are supported by a strong research base for targeting active responding to increase skill mastery.

Providing more response or practice opportunities can be traced back to Aristotle and what became known as the law of frequency (Malone, 1990). Increasing the number of opportunities a student has to learn can lead to improving students' academic performance across the learning hierarchy. Increasing learning opportunities has been shown to increase accuracy (Albers & Greer, 1991), fluency (e.g., C.H. Skinner, Ford, & Yunker, 1991), and maintenance of academic performance gains (e.g., Ivarie, 1986). Stimulus generalization and response adaptation, programming and training, both require that students be exposed to a variety of different stimuli conditions. Therefore, increasing opportunities to respond allows for more opportunities for stimulus and response discrimination and generalization programming (Skinner, Fletcher, & Henington, 1996).

An opportunity to respond is provided when an antecedent stimulus is followed by an academic response (Greenwood, Delquadri, & Hall, 1984). If a student does not actively respond to the antecedent stimulus, then an opportunity to respond has not occurred. Researchers have shown that increasing the number of opportunities to respond to academic stimuli often results in increased learning (Anderson, 1982; Berliner, 1984; Darch, Carnine, & Gersten, 1984; Greenwood et al., 1984; C.H. Skinner & Shapiro, 1989).

Greenwood and colleagues (1984) describe an experiment conducted by Whorton and Delquadri, where an A-B-A-B design was used to compare traditional teacher-led instruction with classwide peer tutoring in reading. The Code for Instructional Structure and Student Academic Responses (CISSAR) developed by Stanley and Greenwood (1981) was used to measure students' rates of academic responding under the two instructional conditions. Results indicated that students' mean rates of responding were 39% and 35% during the two teacher-led instructional phases, compared with 68% and 73% during the two classwide peer tutoring phases. Consistent with the law of frequency, these results indicated that improvements in reading performance were much stronger during the peer-tutoring intervention phases.

Because the two conditions in the previously described study (peer tutoring versus teacher-led instruction) differed across so many variables, it is impossible to determine which specific variables caused the increase in learning rates. However, C.H. Skinner and Shapiro (1989) conducted a study where the only variable manipulated across three of the four conditions was the number of opportunities to respond. During this study, students read word lists. Under the drill condition, they read a list two times per session. Under the continuous assessment condition, they read the list one time per session, and under the intermittent assessment condition, they read a list once every third session. Although no instruction or feedback was provided, students' accuracy and fluency levels increased on each list. Furthermore, the increases were greatest under the drill condition and least under the intermittent assessment condition. Because these three conditions in this study were so sterile, the study provides strong evidence that increasing opportunities to respond causes increases in the level of academic performance.

Temporal Definition of Target Behaviors

One way to increase the frequency of student responses is to provide more time to learn. Paine, Radicchi, Rosellini, Deutchman, and Darch (1983) divide time into three distinct levels; school time, class time, and instructional time. Procedures that increase the amount of time students spend in school are typically resource inefficient and require broad systems-level changes. Providing longer school days, extending the school year, or starting children in school when they are younger provide more time for students to interact with academic stimuli, and therefore may allow for greater academic achievement gains (C.H. Skinner, Belfiore, & Watson, 1995). Class time is defined as the amount of time students spend in the classroom. Class time can be increased by reducing the time spent for lunch breaks, recess time, and transition times to and from classrooms (Paine et al., 1983). These changes typically require altering the procedures within each school system. For example, a school could choose to shorten the time allowed for students to make the transition from one classroom to another.

The final time variable identified by Paine et al. (1983) is the amount of time students and teachers are engaged in actual classroom activities. Time can be saved here by reducing student and teacher time engaged in nonacademic activities (Gettinger,

1995). For example, a teacher has more time to provide instruction if the teacher spends less time counting lunch money or returning homework. Other researchers and educators have further narrowed the definition of time students spend interacting with academic stimuli by focusing on increasing students' levels of on-task, school-work, and/or academic engagement behavior (Lentz, 1988). These target behaviors require students to be oriented toward academic stimuli (teacher, textbook, worksheets, etc.). Because these targets tend to be continuous, rather than discrete behaviors with clear beginnings and ends, they are measured with momentary time sampling and are duration estimates (Lentz, 1988; Shapiro & Skinner, 1990). When educators or teachers target these behaviors, the goal becomes to increase students' time spent oriented toward academic stimuli.

Although increasing time spent in school, in classrooms, and/or oriented toward academic stimuli has been shown to correlate with academic achievement (e.g., Lentz, 1988), providing more time for academic behavior does not guarantee that students will engage in those behaviors. There are several reasons why increasing time spent oriented toward academic materials may not result in skill improvement.

Increasing time spent oriented toward academic stimuli may not maximize learning rates if students are not responding to academic stimuli. For example, a student can spend time oriented toward their reading text, but rather than being engaged in silent reading, the student is planning what to wear for the school dance. Even when students are oriented to academic stimuli and are responding to academic stimuli, if those responses are inaccurate, achievement is unlikely to increase. For example, a student could be engaged in covert reading of the text but fail to comprehend the material.

Perhaps the biggest limitations associated with focusing on increasing time available for learning is that time is limited and beyond educators' control. Students with learning problems could be defined as students who require more time to learn (Gettinger, 1984). Many students who experience learning problems across one set of skills or objectives also experience learning problems across other areas (e.g., Kulak, 1993; Lapadat, 1991). Therefore, even though providing more time to learn may increase learning levels, it is often difficult for educa-

tors to schedule more time for improving one skill without reducing time allotted for altering other behavior. This time press becomes even more severe as educators are given the responsibility of teaching students appropriate social behavior (e.g., abstinence). However, that does not mean that time is not an important contextual variable (C.H. Skinner et al., 1995). Research on rates of student responding and the relationship of this target behavior to student learning problems will be discussed next.

Rates of Student Responding

Students with learning problems can be viewed as students who require more time to learn (Carroll, 1963; Gettinger, 1984). Therefore, while increasing the frequency of accurate academic responses may increase learning levels, it may not necessarily increase learning rates if those additional opportunities to respond require more time. When the number of responses is combined with time engaged in these learning activities, the target behavior becomes rate-based rather than merely frequency-based. Because students with learning problems often require more time to learn (Gettinger, 1984) this temporal context of student target behaviors must be taken into account (C.H. Skinner et al., 1995).

Berliner (1984) defined Academic Learning Time (ALT) as time students spend engaged in high rates of correct responding. ALT differs from previous temporal definitions of student academic behavior because it focuses on time students spend engaged in a more specific type of behavior, time spent engaged in *high rates* of *accurate* responding. Therefore, it is not surprising that this measure of time correlates more strongly with learning rates than do other measures of time. Research from the Beginning Teachers Evaluation Study (Berliner, 1984) concluded that student ALT correlates more strongly with student achievement gains than do other temporal measures of student behavior (i.e., allotted time, engaged time, and so forth). Berliner (1987) reported that over 40% of the variance in student learning could be accounted for by ALT.

With ALT, Berliner (1984) accounted for a temporal and behavioral aspect of learning problems. Few students with mild learning problems are actually failing to learn. Rather, most mild learning problems are better characterized as learning rate problems; students are not learning rapidly enough

(C.H. Skinner et al., 1995). By focusing on high rates of student responding, Berliner suggests that learning rates can be increased by providing more opportunities to respond within the same period of time.

Accuracy of Responses

Increasing rates of academic responding is unlikely to increase learning rates if students are making inaccurate responses. Increases in accuracy are often equated with increases in achievement or skill mastery (Haring & Eaton, 1978; C.H. Skinner, Turco, Beatty, & Rasavage, 1989). Furthermore, manipulating antecedent and consequent stimuli to occasion increases in accuracy is often equated with teaching. Therefore, a large research base which demonstrates procedures for increasing accuracy has already been developed. Some of these procedures will be briefly described below.

Haring and Eaton (1978) described four procedures designed to increase accuracy, including demonstration, modeling, cuing, and routine drills. The first three procedures focus on antecedent stimuli which are used to prompt accurate student responding. Although some would suggest that students will learn better if they are not shown how to respond to academic stimuli (constructivist and discovery learning approaches), directly prompting accurate responses may be the most efficient way to teach students at the acquisition stage. Without any sort of prompting, students who have not mastered basic skills that allow them to construct or discover may not be able to respond and learn (Carnine, Jones, & Dixon, 1994). Because demonstration and modeling are efficient and effective, they may be the most common procedures used to increase accuracy (Hendrickson & Gable, 1981).

Learning Trials and Immediate Feedback Systems

A learning trial differs from an academic response in that an academic response requires an active response to an academic stimulus. A learning trial consists of an antecedent academic stimulus, an academic response, and a consequence delivered contingent upon some aspect of that academic response (Albers & Greer, 1991). When an academic response is followed by feedback contingent upon some aspect of that response, a learning trial has occurred. Although providing feedback requires time, and therefore may decrease rates of student responding, it also completes a learning trail, which may increase learning.

Belfiore, Skinner, and Ferkis (1995) conducted a study to compare the effects of trial repetition with response repetition on sight-word reading accuracy and maintenance. During trial repetition, students were given five learning trials per day with one response opportunity per trial. During response repetition, students made five repeated responses within the same learning trial. Both conditions increased sight-word reading performance. Although both conditions occasioned the same number of accurate responses, results indicated that the trial repetition condition resulted in greater increases in reading accuracy than did the response repetition condition. These results suggest that merely increasing students' rates of accurate responding may not be as important as increasing complete stimulus–response–consequence (i.e., A-B-C) learning trials.

Although immediate corrective feedback is rarely delivered in classrooms (Leper, 1985), immediate feedback is an essential component of learning trials in which the goal is to increase accuracy. Following antecedent instructional procedures (e.g., demonstration, cuing, or modeling), routine drills are often implemented at the acquisition stage in order to increase opportunities to respond. Many students can learn a skill such as an algorithm or steps involved in borrowing during subtraction, but the fact that the student performs the behavior accurately one time does not mean they will perform it accurately during subsequent times.

Because students often make errors during the initial acquisition stage of learning, it is essential that students receive immediate feedback with respect to accuracy during this stage. Without this feedback, students may make frequent incorrect responses; this essentially results in practicing inaccurate responses. Feedback may also serve as a discriminative stimulus that encourages students to engage in behaviors that will allow them to respond correctly in the future. These behaviors might be, for example, asking a teacher, peer, or parent for help, or reviewing their curricula material to determine how to respond (Hansen, 1978; C.H. Skinner & Smith, 1992). Immediate feedback may also serve as a punisher for incorrect responding or as a reinforcer for accurate responses (Van Houten, 1984). These functions of immediate feedback may increase the probability of students' making accurate responses during routine drills designed to increase learning at the acquisition stage.

Increasing learning trials or learning trial rates is also important when the goal is to program generalizability. In order to successfully generalize skills, students must be able to discriminate when that skill is required for accurate responding and when the same skill will not result in accurate responding. Discrimination training is an essential component of stimulus generalization programming, and requires exposure to different stimuli that require similar and different responses (e.g., subtraction problems which requiring borrowing and those that do not). Therefore, increasing learning trial rates should allow for more exposure to different stimulus conditions within the same period of time. This should increase learning rates at the generalization stage. Without these generalization/ discrimination trials and feedback regarding accuracy during these trials, it would be difficult to increase learning at this stage.

Immediate Feedback Procedures

The type of immediate feedback is linked to the topography of the student response. When student responses are overt, many different forms of immediate corrective feedback are available. Immediate corrective feedback can be provided by having teachers work one-to-one with each student. Obviously, the inefficiency of this procedure prevents it from being implemented on a large scale.

Peers can also be used to provide immediate feedback regarding the accuracy of overt academic responses. One of the best examples of peer feedback procedures is the classwide peer tutoring system developed by researchers at the Junipers Gardens Children's Project (Greenwood, et al., 1987). In using peer feedback, one student makes overt responses to academic stimuli while another student evaluates the accuracy of those responses. Computers can also be used to provide immediate feedback following overt academic responses.

During self-managed academic interventions such as cover, copy, and compare (C.H. Skinner et al., 1989) and programmed instruction (Vargus &

Vargus, 1991), students obtain immediate feedback regarding accuracy by comparing their responses to printed examples of correct responses. In many cases, the student's original response was also in written form. However, since the students are both responding and evaluating their responses, it is possible for these self-evaluation procedures to be used when academic responses are covert (C.H. Skinner et al., 1991). Similarly, the sample that students compare their responses to does not have to be provided in printed form. Lalli and Shapiro (1990) demonstrated how students could use tape-recordings of word lists to evaluate their own responses to written words.

Immediate feedback can also be provided when students make covert responses to teacher-led instruction. For example, a teacher may deliver an antecedent academic stimulus (e.g., "What is 6 × 7?). Then, after several seconds, the teacher may call on a student to answer the question. Classmates can use the student's answer and the teacher's subsequent evaluation of that answer to evaluate their own responses.

Response Topography

As previously mentioned, educators and researchers operating under the assumption that information-processing weakness cause learning disabilities have focused on the topography or modality of the response (e.g., visual and auditory responding). Behavioral researchers have also focused on the topography of academic responses and the role topography may play in student learning.

Greenwood and colleagues (1984) suggested that academic responses during learning time take the same topography as do goal responses. The rationale for this argument is based on response generalization. If frequent student responding during learning trials is in a topography that differs from goal responding, then improvements in one form of responding may not generalize when goal responding requires these responses to be made in a different form. For example, if your goal is to improve students' written spelling performance, then students should be required to write words.

Keeping students' academic responses the same as goal responses prevents one from having to train in one form and hope that the improvements in that form of responding generalize to other forms

(Stokes & Baer, 1977). However, some goal responses are in covert forms which do not lend themselves to immediate corrective feedback. For example, individuals typically read silently to obtain information from text. The problem with silent reading is that it is difficult to determine if students are reading and if they are reading accurately. Greenwood and colleagues (1984) violated their own recommendation of keeping responses in a form similar to goal responses (i.e., they required students to respond *aloud* during ALT when *silent* reading comprehension was the goal) when constructing their classwide peer-tutoring reading interventions. However, by requiring students to make covert aloud responses (reading aloud), classwide peer tutoring allows other students to evaluate the accuracy, reinforce accurate responses, correct inaccurate responses, and punish inaccurate responses. Even though the target behavior during the intervention is not silent reading comprehension, research on the peer-tutoring intervention shows that it has resulted in educationally significant increases in silent reading comprehension (Greenwood, et al., 1987). Because there are often advantages to altering responses to a different topography from goal responses, researchers should investigate the process of response generalization in order to allow educators to better predict when response generalization is likely to occur and when it may not occur.

Plan Implementation: Procedures for Increasing Responding and Rates of Accurate Responding

If the goal is to obtain greater learning trial rates or rates of active, accurate academic responding, then "won't do" problems are particularly troublesome. If educators are not able to occasion responding from students, it will be very difficult to increase learning rates (Daly, Lentz, & Boyer, 1996). Next, "won't do" problems will be discussed in terms of competing schedules of reinforcement, student preference, and skill fluency. A description and analysis of research and procedures which have been shown to be effective for increasing learning trial rates or rates of active academic responding will follow.

Won't Do

During time allotted for academic responding, students with the prerequisite skills can choose to engage in active academic responding or chose to engage in other, sometimes disruptive, nonacademic behavior. One approach to decreasing the probability of students' choosing to engage in alternative, incompatible behavior, is to put those behaviors on extinction. However, implementing extinction programs in educational settings can be procedurally difficult. It is easy for educators and peers to unintentionally reinforce a student's nonacademic behavior. For example, assume teacher attention has been reinforcing a student's inappropriate behavior. Educators can attempt to ignore inappropriate behaviors, thereby putting the behavior on extinction. Unfortunately, teachers often do not and cannot behave consistently. This can result in an intermittent schedule of reinforcement, which is likely to make the inappropriate behavior even more resistant to extinction.

During extinction, teachers use the topography of student behavior to cue their own behavior. However, extinction-induced variability may result in students' altering the topography, intensity, or duration of these inappropriate behaviors. When they alter the topography, teachers may respond to other behaviors that where not originally targeted. Even when teachers attempt to ignore all inappropriate behavior, students may intensify their inappropriate behavior, (e.g., scream rather than talk, punch rather than poke). When these behaviors are intensified, teachers may not be able to ignore the behaviors.

Even when teachers are successful at eliminating their delivery of reinforcement for inappropriate behavior, peers may provide the reinforcement. It is very difficult for teachers to control all other students' behavior to ensure that they are not providing positive reinforcement contingent upon a peer's nonacademic behavior.

Negative reinforcement also makes it difficult to eliminate inappropriate behavior through extinction. Aversive stimuli can occasion behaviors which allow students to escape and/or avoid those aversive situations. The most prominent stimuli in educational environments should be instructional or academic stimuli (Dunlap & Kern, 1996). Unfortunately, students often find these stimuli and the task associated with these stimuli (academic responding) aversive. While some students may escape from academic demands by misbehaving, other students escape by merely not responding. Escape can be very simple and hard to detect under some circumstances. For example, while a teacher is providing group instruction (e.g., showing students how to perform long division steps using the blackboard), students should be paying attention and/or responding covertly. These covert responses are unobservable. Therefore, teachers look for behaviors that are observable (e.g., head and eyes oriented toward the teacher and the blackboard). Unfortunately, students who appear to be on-task may in fact be escaping the lecture. Because these quiet, escape-avoidance behaviors are unobservable, teachers are likely to have difficulty reducing rates of negative reinforcement when students engage in these nondisruptive escape-avoidance behaviors.

Relative Rates of Reinforcement

Given the procedural and practical difficulties associated with extinction, it is fortunate that behaviors are chosen based on relative rates of reinforcement. Herrnstein (1961) developed a formula that allows one to predict and manipulate two incompatible behaviors based on the relative rates of reinforcement for each behavior. When given the choice of two incompatible behaviors, an organism is more likely to engage in the behavior that results in higher rates of reinforcement. When both behaviors are on interval schedules of reinforcement, the larger the discrepancy between the rates of reinforcement, the more likely it is that the organism will choose to engage in the behavior that results in the higher rate of reinforcement. When both behaviors are on ratio schedules of reinforcement, once the reinforcement for appropriate behaviors exceeds the rate of reinforcement for inappropriate behaviors, only appropriate behaviors should be emitted (Meyerson & Hale, 1984). Herrnstein's (1961) formula, which is known as the "matching law," has been validated across species, organisms, behaviors, settings, and experimenters (de Villiers, 1977).

Matching law research should have a significant impact on learning, because students' behaviors are under multiple concurrent schedules of reinforcement in educational settings (McDowell, 1988). Recently, researchers have begun investigating students' choice behaviors in educational settings. Collecting data in a special education classroom, Martens and Houk (1989) demonstrated that Herrnstein's (1961) formula predicted levels of on-task and disruptive behaviors in an adolescent with mental retardation. Martens, Lochner, and Kelly (1992) experimentally manipulated similar behaviors by altering the rates of reinforcement in a fourth-grade elementary school classroom. In both of these studies, the greater the discrepancy between rates of reinforcement, the more likely the students were to engage in the behavior(s) that resulted in the greater rate of reinforcement.

Martens and colleagues' (1992) research demonstrates how educators can increase the probability of students' engaging or choosing to engage in academic work, as opposed to other behaviors. Although it may be extremely difficulty to eliminate positive and/or negative reinforcement for inappropriate behaviors, matching law research shows that non-target behaviors do not have to be put on absolute extinction schedules. Rather, this research shows that one can increase appropriate target behaviors, in this case rates of accurate academic responding, and decrease incompatible target behaviors by making the schedule of reinforcement for those target behaviors richer than that for competing behaviors. Because choice behaviors are made based on relative rates of reinforcement, educators can increase the probability of students responding to academic stimuli by ensuring that reinforcement for target academic responding behaviors exceeds reinforcement for other behaviors.

Procedures for Increasing Rates of Reinforcement for Academic Behaviors

Hall (1991) suggested that behavior analysis procedures and techniques may be underutilized by general education teachers because the procedures require resources unavailable to teachers in general education ecologies (e.g., teacher and student time, materials, additional staff). Fortunately, many efficient procedures have been designed that allow rates of reinforcement to be increased for accurate academic responding. Neef et al. (1994) demonstrated how computer technology can be used to monitor student behaviors and deliver exchangeable reinforcers at high rates. Computers can be used to immediately evaluate student responses and deliver points for number of accurate responses. Computers can then keep a running tally of these points, which can function like tokens, with students exchanging these points at a later time for reinforcers.

Peers can also be used to monitor the accuracy of academic responses and deliver points for accurate responses. During classwide peer tutoring, students evaluate each others' responses, correct errors, and deliver points for accurate responses. This system has been shown to be effective for increasing student achievement in reading, mathematics, and spelling. Finally, students could use self-monitoring procedures to evaluate their own responses. For example, Lalli and Shapiro (1991) had students evaluate the accuracy of their sight-word reading using tape-recordings of word lists. Students then tracked the accuracy of these responses and delivered their own reinforcers based on their evaluations. When these self-monitoring and self-reinforcement procedures are used, educators must monitor students to ensure that they follow procedures and do not deliver reinforcers following inaccurate responses or when they fail to respond.

When structuring reinforcement systems, if responding time is held constant, students are not only reinforced for accurate responding, but also for rates of accurate responding. By holding time constant (e.g., 10 minutes), and giving students enough material so that they cannot complete all responses in the allotted time, students are reinforced for *high rates* of accurate responding rather than for just accurate responding. These rate-based reinforcement systems should increase learning rates and may also keep students on-task and responding persistently (C.H. Skinner, Belfiore, Mace, Williams-Wilson, & Johns, 1997).

Student Preference

If students are given academic assignments that they prefer, they may be more likely to choose to engage in those assignments. Dunlap and Kern (1996) reviewed procedures used to increase student preference for academic task. Several of these studies show that providing students with preferred assignments can increase on-task levels and decrease disruptive behavior.

One way to make academic assignments more preferable is to increase rates of reinforcement associated with the assignment. Researchers have experimentally manipulated rates of reinforcement

and demonstrated that Herrnstein's formula could be used to predict and control students' choice of academic behaviors (Mace et al., 1990; Neef et al., 1992, 1993, 1994). If students choose one assignment over another, then there is direct evidence that a particular assignment is preferable.

Another procedure used to increase assignment preference is to alter the task so that the outcomes are meaningful to individual students. For example, Dunlap, Foster-Johnson, Clarke, Kern, and Childs (1995) found that they were able to increase a student's on-task levels and learning rates by altering a multistep assembly task. Initially, the student was required to put together pens. When the task was changed to making cracker sandwiches, on-task levels increased and inappropriate behavior levels decreased. Researchers suggested that the change in these behaviors was related to the outcome of the task: a complete sandwich was more meaningful and valued by the student than was a complete pen (i.e., a reinforcer of higher quality).

Although altering tasks to make outcomes more meaningful may work in some instances, this procedure may actually hinder learning rates. In the example provided in the previous paragraph, if the goal was merely to train students to perform a multistep chained task, then this solution was acceptable. However, if the goal was to teach the student to put together pens so that they could earn money at a sheltered workshop, then this solution would not be effective. Students often must engage in behaviors that are not immediately meaningful (Dunlap & Kern, 1996). For example, learning the "ch" sound or the times tables may have little immediate value to students. In these instances, educators must make the outcomes more valuable by reinforcing improved problem solving or word decoding. Therefore, when tasks do not have immediate value, it may be necessary to give those tasks value by reinforcing those responses. By providing reinforcers, teachers provide a function to behaviors that may not have immediate or clear value to students.

In the cracker sandwich example, the focus was on the function of the behavior. Building a cracker sandwich was functional for the target student because the student ate the sandwiches later in the day. Unfortunately, students may engage in academic behaviors to avoid punishment, not to obtain positive reinforcement. Evidence for this negative reinforcement paradigm comes from research on assignment length and contingent skipping. Dunlap and Kern (1996) described examples of instances where they reduced academic assignment length and found increased rates of student academic responding and decreased rates of inappropriate behaviors. Contingent skipping, (i.e., students are not required to complete additional academic assignment if they complete other assignments at specific performance levels), has been used to increase students' academic performance (e.g., Lovitt & Hansen, 1976). Students may prefer briefer assignments or reductions in assignments because the assignments are aversive. Furthermore, students may misbehave to avoid having to complete assignments.

Students may also prefer easier assignments. Cooke, Guzaukas, Pressley, and Kerr (1993) conducted research on students' assignment preference and assignment difficulty. In these experiments, researchers exposed students to assignments in which 100% of the items were unknown or difficult, and other assignments where they replaced 30% of the unknown or difficult items with known or easy items. In three separate experiments, they required students to work on distinct academic assignments: spelling, mathematics facts, and word reading. Results showed that students consistently preferred the assignments with the easy items.

Unfortunately, research suggests that learning rates may also be suppressed when difficult or unknown tasks are replaced with known or easy tasks, or when assignment length is reduced. For example, Roberts and Shapiro (1996) found that student learning rates were lowest when unknown or instructional items were replaced with known items. Further, the greater the percentage of unknown items that were replaced with known items, the smaller the learning rates. These results are not surprising, given the previously discussed research, which shows that increasing learning trials increases learning rates. By replacing target words with mastered words, educators reduce the opportunity students have to learn new words. A similar problem occurs when assignment length or the number of assignments (e.g., contingent skipping) is reduced. These procedures reduce learning trial frequency, and this may jeopardize curricula integrity and hinder student improvements across acquisition, fluency, maintenance, and generalization, because learning trials are reduced.

Another way to increase reinforcement rates during academic assignments may be to intersperse additional, more time-efficient, tasks (i.e. tasks that take less time to complete than do target tasks). In a study examining self-evaluation of mathematics, Laird and Winton (1991) suggested that immediate evaluation and feedback following the accurate completion of an academic task served as a strong reinforcer for accurate responding. During independent seat work, students are often required to complete many distinct academic tasks (e.g., completing different mathematics problems) with no immediate accuracy feedback or reinforcers. Under these no-feedback conditions, academic task completion may be either positively or negatively reinforcing. If task completion is reinforcing, then students may prefer or choose assignments when additional brief tasks are added and interspersed with assignments containing longer tasks, because this would increase problem completion rates (C.H. Skinner, Robinson, et al., 1996).

C.H. Skinner, Belfiore and colleagues (1997) exposed college students to two different academic assignments. One assignment contained 16 three-digit by two-digit multiplication problems. The other assignment contained 16 similar problems with one-digit by one-digit problems added and interspersed every three problems. Problem completion rates were higher on the assignments with the additional problems. Furthermore, students preferred the assignments with the additional brief, easy problems even though they contained more problems. In subsequent experiments, C.H. Skinner and colleagues rule out novelty effects (C.H. Skinner, Robinson, et al., 1996) or problem ease (C.H. Skinner, Fletcher, Wildmon, & Belfiore, 1996) as causal variables. In another experiment, researchers found similar results when seventh-grade students were asked to complete mathematics worksheets containing problems that they had been taught but had not yet mastered (Logan, Robinson, Johns, & Skinner, 1996).

In previous research, difficult items were replaced with known or easy items (Cooke et al., 1993). As previously stated, this may hinder learning rates (Roberts & Shapiro, 1996). However, C.H. Skinner and colleagues (C.H. Skinner, Fletcher, et al., 1996; C.H. Skinner, Robinson, et al., 1996) added the brief problems, thereby improving student preference for the assignment without reducing learning trials or jeopardizing curricula integrity. While these researchers provide no direct evidence that proved that completing a problem or task was reinforcing, the choice data is consistent with previous matching law research. Because additional resources (e.g., staff, computers) were not required to monitor and reinforce student behaviors, interspersing tasks that take less time to complete may be an efficient procedure for increasing rates of reinforcement in general education ecologies. Researchers should continue to investigate the effects of this procedure on student preference, learning rates, and on-task levels.

Choice and Effort: Between "Can't Do" and "Won't Do" Is Fluency

Although acquisition, maintenance, and generalization programming failures may account for "can't do" problems, automaticity and fluency problems may be related to "won't do" problems. Any consideration of choice behavior must also take into account the effort required to perform behaviors (Horner & Day, 1991). Because researchers have shown that more complex or effortful behaviors often take more time (Fitts, 1954; Hay, 1981; Horner & Day, 1991; Sugden, 1980) it is often difficult to determine what effect each of these variables (response effort versus time required to respond) has on student choice behavior (Skinner, Fletcher, Wildmon, et al., in press). Nevertheless, fluency or automaticity may play a major role in what may best be described as "can't do" problems.

A student who has the ability to respond both accurately and rapidly may be much more likely to chose to engage in a task than a student who can also respond accurately but requires more time and effort to make those responses. Response effort can influence whether rewards are more likely to occasion a behavior. While many students may complete brief, simple, low-effort tasks such as 20 one-digit by one-digit problems in order to receive a gold star, fewer students are likely to choose to complete a task which requires much more effort, such as completing 20 three-digit by two-digit problems, for the same reinforcer (Neef et al., 1994). The reinforcement is not worth the effort.

Rates of reinforcement are also related to speed of responding (Skinner & Schock, 1995). For example, suppose two students are given a mathemat-

ics sheet containing 100 two-digit by two-digit problems. Both students can respond at 90%–100% accuracy levels. Both are told that they will be given the same reinforcers if they complete these problems at 100% accuracy levels. The student who is not fluent may require 5 hours to complete the mathematics assignment, while the student who is fluent may need only 20 minutes to complete the assignment. The student who can complete the task in 20 minutes is reinforced at a higher rate. Therefore, this student may be more likely to complete the assignment (Mace et al., 1990; Martens & Houk, 1989; Martens et al., 1992).

Perhaps the best example of response effort and response time can be seen in students who choose to read for leisure versus those who do not. Students may read to acquire information or for enjoyment. Further, suppose that each of two students could acquire the same 60 bits of information and/or 60 bits of enjoyment by reading the same text. However, one student can read the text in 1 hour and the other needs 10 hours. The more rapid or fluent reader would be obtaining 1 bit of information or bit of enjoyment for every minute the student read. The other would be obtaining a bit of information or enjoyment at a much lower rate, one bit for every ten minutes the individual read. For this student, reading requires much more effort and results in a thinner schedule of reinforcement. These variables suggest that the slower reader may choose to engage in other behaviors that result in a thicker schedule of reinforcement and/or require less effort, because reading is not worth the time or effort.

For these reasons, it is essential that students do more than just acquire basic skills. If educators increase students' ability to perform these behaviors accurately and rapidly, they may increase rates of reinforcement for performing these behaviors and decrease the effort required to perform these behaviors. Both of these variables may increase the probability of students choosing to engage in future academic responding, thereby avoiding lower future learning rates and preventing behavior problems.

Increasing Learning Trial Rates

Preventing "can't do" problems requires students to be actively engaged in high rates of academic responding. The focus in the previous section was on occasioning student responses. In this section, research on procedures designed to increase rates of accurate academic responding or learning trial rates will be described and analyzed.

Response Variables: Topography and Rates of Responding

Response topography has been discussed in relation to information-processing strengths and weakness, error correction and feedback systems, and response generalization. However, responses also have a temporal component. Response latency is the time required to make an academic response follow an academic stimulus. Response latency is related to response topography, as responding in one form requires more time than responding in another form. Researchers have shown that requiring students to respond in more efficient forms can increase academic performance, even when the more efficient responses are topographically dissimilar from goal or assessed responses (C.H. Skinner et al., 1991; C.H. Skinner, Belfiore, et al., 1997).

C.H. Skinner, Belfiore, and colleagues (1997) used a multiphase alternating treatments design to compare the effects of two cover, copy, and compare (CCC) interventions on multiplication performance in two students with behavior disorders. During written CCC, students were required to look at a problem and answer, cover the problems and answer, write the problem and answer, and then uncover the problem and answer and evaluate their written response by comparing it to the initial stimulus. Verbal CCC was similar except that students stated the problem and answer aloud and then evaluated that response from memory after uncovering the response. Following the interventions, students were assessed by requiring them to write answers to problems as quickly as possible. Percentage of problems correct (accuracy) and number of digits correct per minute (fluency) served as dependent variables.

During the first intervention phase, with trials held constant, students completed 24 CCC learning trials under both the written and verbal conditions. Results showed small and approximately equal increases in accuracy and fluency across conditions. Furthermore, because writing problems and answers took longer than stating them aloud, written CCC procedures took much longer than the verbal CCC condition. In the next intervention phase (i.e., the time held constant phase), students were given the

average amount of time required to complete the written CCC condition (204 s and 229 s) to complete as many CCC learning trials as they could under both conditions. During this phase, one student completed, on average, 26 written CCC learning trials, but completed 86 verbal CCC learning trials in the same amount of time. The other student completed, on average, 33 written CCC learning trials, but completed 83 verbal CCC learning trials in the same amount of time. Even though the assessment procedures required students to respond in writing, assessment results indicated that students made greater gains in written fluency and accuracy on problems assigned to the verbal CCC intervention. Similar results were found by C.H. Skinner et al., (1991) who did not include the first trials held constant phase.

C.H. Skinner, Belfiore, and colleagues' (1997) study is important because it highlights the difference between increasing learning trial strength and increasing learning trial rates. If two learning trials result in equal improvements in academic performance, then learning trial strength is equal. In the trials held constant phase, C.H. Skinner, Belfiore, and colleagues (1997) demonstrated that the learning trials were of equal strength. However, if one of these trials takes much less time, then it may be possible for students to receive many more opportunities to respond using these trials in the same period of time. By increasing learning trial rates or responding rates, educators can increase learning rates (the amount of performance change in a fixed period of time).

As previously mentioned, one concern with altering responses during learning trials, such that the response does not match the topography of the goal response, is that response generalization may not occur. For example, students who become more accurate and fluent working mathematics problems on a computer may not show the same increases when the goal response is written paper and pencil mathematics and fluency. Therefore, when educators alter response topography and make it different from goal responses, they should assess students' responding in the goal topography to ensure that the desired generalization has occurred (C.H. Skinner et al., 1991).

Another procedure involving altering the topography of a response to increase complete learning trials is the use of response cards. Response cards may not actually increase stimulus-feedback rates, but may increase rates of student active responding during group recitations (C.H. Skinner, Fletcher, & Henington, 1996). Typically during group recitation, teachers ask questions and call on students to answer those questions verbally. One problem with this procedure is that only one student may actually respond to the question. During these situations, teachers cannot monitor responses of students who are not called on. Therefore, many students who were not called on may make not active, but covert, responses. Furthermore, other students may make inaccurate academic responses that the teacher cannot correct because they cannot be observed.

When response cards are used, all students are instructed to write brief responses to teacher questions. Narayan, Heward, Gardner, Courson, and Omness (1990) compared response card recitation procedures with typical verbal responding recitation procedures. When response cards were employed, stimulus-feedback rates were lower (1.2 questions per minute versus 1.9) because students were given more time to write answers following questions. However, during response card recitations, students made 15.6 written responses per session versus 11.6 hand raises per session. Assuming that students who raised their hands had covertly responded, these results suggest that response cards evoked a greater rate of group responding than the verbal responding procedure. Since a learning trial has not occurred if students have not made an active academic response, learning trial rates were higher under the response card condition. As expected, results also indicated that student learning rates were higher under the condition that occasioned the greatest number of student responses, (i.e., the response card condition). In a subsequent study, Gardner, Heward, and Grossi (1994) replicated these results and found that maintenance levels were also higher under the response card condition. Because teachers can ask the entire class to display their cards after they have responded, response cards have a further benefit in that, by making the entire class's covert responses overt, teachers can evaluate those responses and provide corrective feedback when errors occur.

Pacing: Intertrial Intervals and Wait Times

Response cards increase the number of students responding by altering the topography of those responses. Increasing wait times can be used to increase the number of students responding, and, consequently, the number of complete learning trials, by ensuring that students have enough time to respond (Rowe, 1974). A wait time is the term used to describe the interval between an academic stimulus being delivered (teacher asks the class a question) and some other stimulus being delivered that effectively ends the learning trial (e.g., a correct answer being given). During recitation, teachers can control these wait times by delaying the time between asking the question and calling on students.

Riley (1986) compared the effects of 1-, 3-, and 5-second wait times on students' achievement as measured by a teacher-constructed science test. Results showed that elementary students who received the 1-second wait time scored lowest on the test. Students who received the 3-second wait time scored highest on knowledge questions, and students who received the 5-second wait time scored highest on comprehension questions. These results can easily be explained in terms of the number of learning trials. Because the 1-second wait times did not allow all students enough time to respond before the trial was effectively ended, it occasioned the lowest learning rates. The 5-second wait time was strongest for the comprehension questions because these question took longer to answer. However, the one finding that may appear to be inconsistent was that the 3-second wait time resulted in higher accuracy levels on the knowledge questions than did the 5-second wait times. The 5-second wait times should have allowed as many, if not more, students to respond than the 3-second wait times. Research on pacing and intertrial intervals may explain this inconsistent finding.

Learning trial rates can be increased by reducing intertrial intervals, or the time between learning trials (Carnine, 1976; Darch & Gersten, 1985). Carnine (1976) found that when teachers delivered the next academic stimulus immediately after the previous learning trial ended, two low-achieving elementary students displayed higher levels of on-task behavior and greater rates of responding. Furthermore, when intertrial intervals were reduced, the accuracy of student responses increased. This simple procedure was shown to increase academic learning time (i.e., time spent engaged in high rates of accurate academic responding. Darch and Gersten (1985) found similar results when they compared five-second intertrial intervals with immediate intertrial intervals. The elementary students' reading accuracy levels and on-task behavior levels where higher during the reduced intertrial interval condition.

These studies where instructional pace was altered may explain why Riley (1986) found that the 3-second wait time resulted in greater increases in knowledge accuracy than did the 5-second wait times (C.H. Skinner, Fletcher, & Henington, 1996). Although both wait times may have provided sufficient time for most or all of the students to respond, the 3-second wait time resulted in faster teacher-paced learning trials. This faster pace may have increased on-task levels and the probability that students were responding covertly. Consequently, the brief intertrial intervals may have occasioned greater learning trials because more students were responding to more items. Future researchers should investigate the interaction between wait times and pacing (C.H. Skinner, Fletcher, & Henington, 1996).

Antecedent Stimuli: Timings and Time Limits

Increasing students' rates of accurate academic responding suggests that educators should be concerned with time allotted for responding. One stimulus control procedure that may increase students' rates of responding is timing. Derr and Shapiro (1989) found that students read aloud more rapidly when the experimenter overtly, rather than covertly, timed their performance. Although this study was conducted to investigate curriculum-based measurement assessment procedures, it does indicate that the timing process can serve as a stimulus for students to work more rapidly. Other researchers have shown that the process of timing and setting time limits in itself can increase rates of responding. Van Houten and Thomas (1976) investigated the impact of timing on second-grade students mathematics performance. During the baseline phase, students were given 30 minutes to complete as many problems as possible. During the experimental phases, the experimenter signaled students when each minute had passed and students then drew a line under the last problem they completed. Results showed higher rates of responding under the experimental condition.

Setting time limits is another antecedent stimulus that may be used to increase student rates of re-

sponding. Van Houten, Hill, and Parsons (1975) found that when they reduced the time allotted for students to complete their writing composition assignment from 20 to 10 minutes, fourth-grade students completed as much of their assignment in 10 minutes as in 20 minutes. One concern with reducing time allotted may be that students would rush and not complete assignments as well or as accurately. Although it is difficult to judge the quality of writing assignments, Van Houten and Little (1982) found that setting briefer time limits on mathematics assignments increased students' rates of assignment completion and also their accuracy levels. This suggests that these antecedent control procedures increase not only rates of responding, but response accuracy as well.

Contingencies for More Rapid Responding

When teachers deliver antecedent and consequent stimuli, they can control the pace of instruction and deliver reinforcement contingent upon accurate and high rates of responding. During independent seat-work teachers may be able to increase rates of accurate academic responding with procedures such as timing and setting time limits. However, these antecedent control procedures may not be effective over repeated sessions if students are not reinforced for these higher rates of responding during independent seat-work.

Several procedures can be used to reinforce higher rates of accurate responding during independent seat-work. In order to do this, educators must measure learning trial rates, not just number of learning trials. C.H. Skinner and colleagues (1991) held independent seat-work time constant throughout instructional procedures and recorded the number of learning trials each student completed during each session. Prior to each session, students were told their best previous rate and encouraged to try to beat this rate. Van Houten and Thomas (1976) also found that students' composition writing rates further increased when they included in their program a public posting component and praise for high rates of responding.

When responses are written, it is relatively easy for teachers to determine students' learning trial rates because written responses leave a permanent product. However, when responses are not written, teachers may have difficulty in determining each student's rate of responding. If teachers cannot monitor student learning trial rates, they cannot reinforce them. Greenwood and colleagues (1984) described a clever way around the problems of monitoring and consequently reinforcing high rates of accurate academic responding for reading. During classwide peer tutoring, the class is divided into two teams. Students are then paired based on team membership. Students are given a fixed amount of time to read aloud to each other. Oral reading does not result in a permanent product. However, the student's peer from the other team is given the task of following along, reading silently, while evaluating and recording the accuracy of the oral reading. Points are awarded for the amount of accurate reading completed in a fixed period of time. Because time is held constant, students earn more points by reading accurately and rapidly. This encourages them to read both accurately and rapidly. Furthermore, teachers do not have to monitor each student's oral reading, as students perform this task. This allows half of the class to make active overt reading responses and to receive feedback on those responses. Because points are earned on an individual basis and for the team, students are also reinforced for covert responding while they are following along. This occurs because the more errors the peer detects, the lower the other team's score.

Summary

The procedures and techniques described in this section allow educators to increase rates of accurate responding. This in turn can make learning time more efficient, thus increasing learning rates. However, these procedures in and of themselves will not be effective without quality instruction (modeling, demonstration, cuing, etc.). Furthermore, student should not spend every moment of every school day engaged in high rates of accurate responding. Rather, these procedures should be used to increase student performance across the learning hierarchy in an efficient manner, so that more time is available to address other student needs. By employing efficient procedures design to improve and maintain academic skills, educators may find more time available to allow students to engage in other activities, such as discovery or constructive learning or social skills training.

Plan Evaluation

When responses are overt, educators can directly observe and evaluate those responses. Educators can then increase rates of accurate responding by monitoring these behaviors, setting accurate response rate goals, and reinforcing high rates or increases in rates of accurate responding during instructional time (Greenwood et al., 1984; C.H. Skinner et al., 1991; Van Houten, 1984).

Formal methods can be used to evaluate rates of accurate student responding. For example, several direct observation systems have been developed which allow observers to collect data on rates of student responding (e.g., Greenwood, Carta, Kamps, & Delquadri, 1993; Saudargus, 1992; Stanley and Greenwood, 1981). While these formal direct observation systems are useful, they are not very resource efficient. Furthermore, they are not very effective for assessing the accuracy of student responses or rates of responding, particularly when responses occur at rapid rates or are covert.

Educators can use informal procedures to assess students' rates of accurate responding. For example, during independent seat-work, teachers can circulate around the room, checking students' work for both accuracy and speed of accurate responding. As previously mentioned, peers and computers can also be used to assess or evaluate rates of accurate responding during academic learning time (Greenwood et al., 1984; Leper, 1985). Finally, teachers can have students observe, evaluate, and record their own rates of accurate responding during academic learning time (C.H. Skinner & Smith, 1992).

Students' progress and performance should be assessed frequently. Frequent assessments can serve many purposes. They provide students with additional opportunities to respond which may increase learning rates (C.H. Skinner & Shapiro, 1989). Frequent assessments can also be used indirectly to reinforce high rates of accurate covert responding. For example, educators cannot directly determine who is silently reading and who is not. However, by assessing or testing students on that reading material, educators can indirectly determine those students who were performing the desired behaviors and can reinforce those behaviors based on these indirect assessments.

Frequent assessments can provide students with feedback on their progress and performance.

This feedback is essential if academic responding is to be maintained at high rates. Because high-rate responding requires student effort, this feedback may make students aware that their efforts are resulting in improved performance. Progress graphs can be used to track students' progress through different curricula objectives (Deno & Mirkin, 1977). As students master objectives, the progress is recorded on a cumulative graph and new unmastered items or objectives are added to their curricula (e.g., Pratt-Struthers, Bartalamay, Bell, & McLaughlin, 1994. This cumulative form of assessment prevents students from reaching ceilings, because new items or objectives are constantly added.

Assessment procedures that measure rates of accurate responding also prevent ceiling effects. Students who are 100% accurate have reached a ceiling and cannot improve their accuracy levels. However, repeated learning trials may function to increase rates of accurate responding, maintenance, fluency, and generalization. Therefore, educators should assess fluency or rates of accurate responding to avoid these ceiling effects. By providing feedback on, and reinforcement for, increased rates of accurate responding, educators can keep students responding and attempting to improve their academic skills even when they have reached 100% accuracy levels (McLaughlin & Skinner, 1996). Finally, if educators periodically test skills that were mastered previously, they can assess maintenance (Fuchs, 1992; Pratt-Struthers et al., 1994).

Summary and Direction for Future Research

In the past, many researchers have focused on increasing the strength of learning trials. This chapter focused on increasing learning trial rates or response rates. By focusing on these target behaviors, educators can increase not just learning levels, but also learning rates. Although the theory behind increasing learning trial rates is old, some may say "musty," increasing learning trial rates is effective. Future researchers should not neglect the investigation of procedures designed to increase these target behaviors.

Skill mastery includes accuracy, fluency, maintenance, and response and stimulus generalization. However, educators continue to make accuracy their primary goal, while neglecting these other

skill domains that are essential if skills are to be functional. Research on student preference, student choice, and response effort can also have a tremendous impact on student learning rates. If educators can alter academic stimulus conditions and/or academic assignments to make them more preferable, they may be able to increase academic responding, improve students' attitudes regarding learning in general and school work specifically, decrease disruptive behaviors, and improve learning rates. Researchers should continue with this line of applied research and perhaps focus on the relationship between fluency and student preference.

In several sections of this chapter response topography was discussed. Response topography has been addressed by cognitive researchers concerned with intraindividual processing strengths and weakness (i.e., modality strengths and weakness). However, the response itself is an integral part of any learning trial and should be addressed by behavioral researchers. Researchers may want to focus on the prediction and control of response generalization, as altering responses to a form different from goal responding can be used to allow for immediate feedback (Greenwood, et al., 1984) and increased rates of responding (C.H. Skinner et al., 1991; C.H. Skinner, Belfiore, et al., 1997).

Barlow & Hersen (1984) described the history of research on attention as a positive reinforcer and the failure of these positive reinforcement procedures to affect self-injurious and disruptive behaviors in some children. This problem was later addressed from a functional perspective, and researchers found that many of these behaviors were actually being maintained by escape avoidance (e.g., Carr, Newsome, & Binkoff, 1980). A similar line of investigation of negative reinforcement paradigms in the classroom environments may also result in significant advances in the assessment, prevention, and remediation of academic problems (C.H. Skinner, Fletcher, Wildmon, et al., 1996).

Finally, researchers must continue to take current advances in basic research and develop procedures designed to apply those advances in educational settings. Much of the research reviewed in the current chapter included special education subjects who had already experienced psychoeducational problems. Therefore, this research may be better characterized as remedial, rather than preventative. Although the science of applied behavioral analysis has made valuable contributions to the field of special education, behavioral theory and techniques have not been widely used in general education settings (Axelrod, 1991). Although a variety of reasons may account for this failure to transfer (Cooke, 1984, Pumroy & McIntire, 1991, Watson, 1994), Hall (1991) suggested that the nature of behavior analysis procedures and techniques may be the reason that general educators underutilize behavior analysis in their classrooms. Many behavioral procedures require resources (e.g., teacher and student time, materials, additional staff) unavailable to teachers in general education ecologies. Therefore, applied behavioral researchers should make efforts to construct effective academic interventions that are ecologically valid and can be run in general classroom environments. This focus may result in the prevention of psychoeducational problems across many students who now experience mild learning problems.

References

Albers, A.E., & Greer, R.D. (1991). Is the three term contingency trial a predictor of effective instruction? *Journal of Behavioral Education, 1,* 337–354.

Algozzine, B., & Korinek, L. (1985). Where is special education for students with high prevalence handicaps going? *Exceptional Children, 51,* 388–397.

Anderson, J.R. (1980). *Cognitive psychology and its implications.* San Francisco: Freeman.

Anderson, J.R. (1982). Acquisition of cognitive skills. *Psychological Review, 89,* 369–406.

Arter, J.A., & Jenkins, J.R. (1979). Differential diagnosis-prescriptive teaching: A critical appraisal. *Review of Educational Research, 49,* 517–555.

Axelrod, S. (1991). The problem: American education. The solution: Use of behavior analytic technology. *Journal of Behavioral Education, 1,* 275–283.

Ayers, R.R., & Cooley, E.J. (1986). Sequential versus simultaneous processing on the K-ABC: Validity in predicting learning success. *Journal of Psychoeducational Assessment, 4,* 211–220.

Barlow, D.H., & Hersen, M. (1984). *Single case experimental designs: Strategies for studying behavior change.* New York: Pergamon.

Belfiore, P.J., Skinner, C.H., & Ferkis, M.A. (1995). Effects of response repetition in sight-word training for students with learning disabilities. *Journal of Applied Behavior Analysis, 28,* 347–348.

Bergan, J.R., & Kratochwill, T.R. (1990). *Behavioral consultation and therapy.* New York: Plenum.

Berliner, D.C. (1984). The half-full glass: A review of research on teaching. In P.L. Hosford (Ed.), *Using what we know about teaching* (pp. 51–85). Alexandria: Association for Supervision and Curriculum Development.

Berliner, D.C. (1987, August). *New knowledge for new roles: Research on teaching.* Paper presented at the meeting of the American Psychological Association, New York.

Breznitz, Z. (1987). Increasing first graders' reading accuracy and comprehension by accelerating their reading rates. *Journal of Educational Psychology, 79,* 236–242.

Carnine, D. (1976). Effects of two teacher presentation rates on off-task behavior, answering correctly, and participation. *Journal of Applied Behavior Analysis, 9,* 199–206.

Carnine, D., Jones, E.D., & Dixon, R. (1994). Mathematics: Education tools for diverse learners. *School Psychology Review, 23,* 406–427.

Carr, E.G., Newsome, C.D., & Binkoff, J.A. (1980). Escape as a factor in the aggressive behavior of two retarded children. *Journal of Applied Behavior Analysis, 13,* 101–117.

Carroll, J.B. (1963). A model of school learning. *Teachers College Record, 64,* 723–733.

Cooke, N.L. (1984). Misrepresentations of the behavioral model in preservice teacher education textbooks. In W.L. Heward, T.E. Heron, D.S. Hill, & J. Trap-Porter (Eds.), *Focus on Behavior Analysis in Education* (pp.197–217). Columbus OH: Merrill.

Cooke, N.L., Guzaukas, R., Pressley, J.S., Kerr, K. (1993). Effects of using a ratio of new items to review items during drill and practice: Three experiments. *Education and Treatment of Children, 16,* 213–234.

Daly, E.J., Lentz, F.E., & Boyer, J. (1996). Academic responding: An essential link between assessment and intervention in reading. *School Psychology Quarterly, 11,* 369–386.

Daneman, M., & Carpenter, P.A. (1980). Individual differences in working memory and reading. *Journal of Verbal Learning and Behavior, 19,* 450–466.

Darch, C., Carnine, D.W., & Gersten, R. (1984). Explicit instruction in mathematics problems solving. *Journal of Educational Research, 4,* 155–165.

Darch, C., & Gersten, R. (1985). The effects of teacher presentation rates and praise on LD students' oral reading performance. *British Journal of Educational Psychology, 55,* 295–303.

Deno, S.L. (1985). Curriculum-based measurement: The emerging alternative. *Exceptional Children, 52,* 219–232.

Deno, S.L. (1986). Formative evaluation of individual student programs: A new role for school psychologists. *School Psychology Review, 15,* 358–374.

Deno, S.L., & Mirkin, P.K. (1977). Data-based program modification: A manual. Reston, VA: Council for Exceptional Children.

Derr, T.F., & Shapiro, E.S. (1989). A behavioral evaluation of curriculum-based assessment of reading. *Journal of Psychoeducational Assessment, 7,* 148–160.

de Villiers, P.A. (1977). Choice in concurrent schedules and a quantitative formulation of the law of effect. In W.K. Honig & J.E.R. Staddon (Eds.), *Handbook of operant behavior* (pp. 233–287). Englewood Cliffs, NJ: Prentice-Hall.

Dunlap, G., Foster-Johnson, L., Clarke, S., Kern, L., & Childs, K.E. (1995). Modifying activities to produce functional outcomes: Effects on the disruptive behaviors of students with disabilities. *Journal of the Association for Persons with Severe Handicaps, 4,* 248–258.

Dunlap, G., & Kern, L. (1996). Modifying instructional activities to promote desirable behavior: A conceptual and practical framework. *School Psychology Quarterly, 11,* 297–312.

Fisher, G.L., Jenkins, S.J., Bancroft, M.J., & Kraft, L.M. (1988). The effects of K-ABC-based remedial teaching strategies on word recognition skills. *Journal of Learning Disabilities, 21,* 307–312.

Fitts, P.M. (1954). The information capacity of the human motor system in controlling the amplitude of movement. *Journal of Experimental Psychology, 47,* 381–391.

Fuchs, L.S. (1992). Classwide decision making with computerized curriculum-based measurement. *Preventing School Failure, 4,* 30–33.

Gagne, R.M. (1982). Some issues in psychology of mathematics instruction. *Journal of Research in Mathematics Education, 14,* 7–18.

Gardner, R., Heward, W.L., & Grossi, T.A. (1994). Effects of response cards on student participation and academic achievement: A systematic replication with inner-city students during whole-class science instruction. *Journal of Applied Behavior Analysis, 27,* 63–71.

Gettinger, M. (1984). Achievement as a function of time spent learning and time needed for learning. *American Educational Research Journal, 21,* 617–628.

Gettinger, M. (1995). Best practices for increasing academic learning time. In A. Thomas & J. Grimes (Eds.), *Best practices in school psychology-III* (pp. 943–954). Washington, DC: National Association of School Psychologists.

Graden, J.L., Zins, J.E., & Curtis, M.E. (1988). *Alternative educational delivery systems: Enhancing instructional opportunities for all students.* Washington, DC: National Association of School Psychologists.

Greenwood, C.R., Carta, J.J., Kamps, D., & Delquadri, J. (1993). *Ecobehavioral assessment system software (EBASS): Observational instrumentation for school psychologists.* Kansas City: University of Kansas, Juniper Gardens Children's Project.

Greenwood, C.R., Delquadri, J.C., & Hall, R.V. (1984). Opportunity to respond and student academic performance. In W.L. Heward, T.E. Heron, J. Trap-Porter, & D.S. Hill (Eds.), *Focus on behavior analysis in education* (pp. 58–88). Columbus, OH: Merrill.

Greenwood, C.R., Dinwiddie, G., Terry, B., Wade, L., Stanley, S.O., Thibadeau, S., & Delquadri, J.C. (1987). Teacher-versus peer-mediated instruction: An eco-behavioral analysis of achievement outcomes. *Journal of Applied Behavior Analysis, 17,* 521–538.

Hall, R.V. (1991). Behavior analysis and education: An unfulfilled dream. *Journal of Behavioral Education, 1,* 305–316.

Hansen, C.L. (1978). Writing skills. In N.G. Haring, T.C. Lovitt, M.D. Eaton, & C.L. Hansen (Eds.), *The fourth R: Research in the classroom* (pp. 93–126). Columbus, OH: Merrill.

Haring, N.G., & Eaton, M.D. (1978). Systematic instructional procedures: An instructional hierarchy. In N.G. Haring, T.C. Lovitt, M.D. Eaton, & C.L. Hansen (Eds.), *The fourth R: Research in the classroom* (pp. 23–40). Columbus, OH: Merrill.

Hartmann, D.P., Roper, B.L., & Bradford, D.C. (1979). Some relationships between behavioral and traditional assessment. *Journal of Behavioral Assessment, 1,* 3–21.

Hasselbring, T.S., & Goin, L.I. (1986). CAMS: Chronometric analysis math strategies. [Computer program]. Nashville, TN: Expert Software.

Hasselbring, T.S., Goin, L.I., & Bransford, J.D. (1987). Developing automaticity. *Teaching Exceptional Children, 1,* 30–33.

Hay, L. (1981). The effects of amplitude and accuracy requirements on movement time in children. *Journal of Motor Behavior, 13,* 77–86.

Heller, K., Holtzman, W., & Messick, S. (Eds.). (1982). *Placing children in special education: A strategy for equity.* Washington, DC: National Academy Press.

Hendrickson, J.M., & Gable, R.A. (1981). The use of modeling tactics to promote academic skills development of exceptional learners. *Journal of Special Education Technology, 4*(3), 20–29.

Herrnstein, R.J. (1961). Relative and absolute strength of response as a function of frequency of reinforcement. *Journal of the Experimental Analysis of Behavior, 4,* 267–272.

Horner R.H., & Day, H.M. (1991). The effects of response efficiency on functionally equivalent competing behaviors. *Journal of Applied Behavior Analysis, 24,* 719–732.

Ivarie, J.J. (1986). Effects of proficiency rates of later performance of recall and writing behavior. *Remedial and Special Education, 7,* 25–30.

Kaufman, A.S. (1994). *Intelligence testing with the WISC-III.* New York: Wiley.

Kaufman, A.S., & Kaufman, N.L. (1983). *K-ABC: Kaufman Assessment Battery for Children.* Circle Pines, MN: American Guidance Service.

Kavale, K.A., & Forness, S.R. (1987). Substance over style: Assessing the efficacy of modality testing and teaching. *Exceptional Children, 54,* 228–239.

Keith, T.Z. (1994). Intelligence is important, intelligence is complex. *School Psychology Quarterly, 9,* 209–221.

Kirk, S., McCarthy, & Kirk, W. (1968). *Illinois Test of Psycholinguistic Abilities.* Champaign: University of Illinois Press.

Kulak, A.G. (1993). Parallels between math and reading disabilities: Common issues and approaches. *Journal of Learning Disabilities, 26,* 666–673.

LaBerge, D., & Samuels, S.J. (1976). Toward a theory of automatic information processing in reading. In H. Singer & R.R. Rudell (Eds.), *Theoretical models and processes of reading* (pp. 548–579). Newark, DE: International Reading Association.

Laird, J., & Winton, A.S.W. (1991). A comparison of self-instructional checking procedures for remediating mathematical deficits. *Journal of Behavioral Education, 3,* 143–164.

Lalli, E.P., & Shapiro, E.S. (1990). The effects of self-monitoring and contingent reward on sight word application. *Education and Treatment of Children, 13,* 129–141.

Lapadat, J.C. (1991). Pragmatic language skills of students with language and/or learning disabilities: A quantitative synthesis. *Journal of Learning Disabilities, 24,* 147–158.

Lentz, F.E. (1988). On-task behavior, academic performance, and classroom disruptions: Untangling the target selection problem in classroom interventions. *School Psychology Review, 17,* 243–257.

Lentz, F.E., & Shapiro, E.S. (1986). Functional assessment of the academic environment. *School Psychology Review, 15,* 346–357.

Leper, M.R. (1985). Microcomputers in education. *American Psychologist, 40*(1), 1–18.

Lesgold, A.M., & Perfetti, C.A. (1978). Interactive processes in reading comprehension. *Discourse Processes, 1,* 323–336.

Lindgren, H.C. & Suter, W.N. (1985). *Educational psychology in the classroom* (2nd ed.). Monterey, CA: Brooks/Cole.

Logan, P., Robinson, S.L., Johns, G.A., & Skinner, C.H. (1996, March). *Improving elementary students' preference for assignments by interspersing additional tasks.* Paper presented at the annual convention of the Association for School Psychologists, Atlanta, Georgia.

Lovitt, T.C., & Hansen, C.L. (1976). The use of contingent skipping and drill to improve oral reading and comprehension. *Journal of Learning Disabilities, 9,* 20–26.

Mace, F.C., McCurdy, B., & Quigley, E.A. (1990). A collateral effect of reward predicted by matching theory. *Journal of Applied Behavior Analysis, 23,* 197–205.

Macmann, G.M., & Barnett, D.W. (1994). Structural analysis of correlated factors: Lessons from the verbal-performance dichotomy of the Wechsler scales. *School Psychology Quarterly, 9,* 161–197.

Malone, J.C. (1990). *Theories of learning: A historical approach.* Belmont, CA: Wadsworth.

Marston, D.B (1989). A curriculum-based measurement approach to assessing academic performance: What is it and what does it do? In M.R. Shinn (Ed.), *Curriculum-based measurement: Assessing special children* (pp. 18–78). New York: Guilford.

Martens, B.K., & Houk, J.L. (1989). The application of Herrnstein's law of effect to disruptive and on-task behavior of a retarded adolescent girl. *Journal of the Experimental Analysis of Behavior, 51,* 17–27.

Martens, B.K., Lochner, D.G., & Kelly, S.Q. (1992). The effects of variable-interval reinforcement on academic engagement: A demonstration of matching theory. *Journal of Applied Behavior Analysis, 25,* 143–151.

Martens, B.K., Steele, E.S., Massie, D.R., & Diskin, M.T. (1995). *Journal of School Psychology, 33,* 287–296.

McDowell, J.J. (1988). Matching theory in natural human environments. *Behavior Analyst, 11,* 95–109.

McLaughlin, T.F., & Skinner, C.H. (1996). Improving academic performance through self-management: Cover, copy and compare. *Intervention in School and Clinic,* 113–118.

Meyers, J., & Kundert, D. (1988). Implementing process assessment. In J.L. Graden, J.E. Zins, & M.J. Curtis (Eds.), *Alternative educational delivery systems: Enhancing instructional opportunities for all students* (pp. 173–198). Washington, DC: National Association of School Psychologists.

Meyerson, J., & Hale, S. (1984). Practical implications of the matching law. *Journal of Applied Behavior Analysis, 17,* 367–380.

Morsink, C.V., Thomas, C.C., & Smith-Davis, J. (1987). Noncatagorical special education programs: Processes and outcomes. In M.C. Wang, M.C. Reynolds, and H.J. Walberg (Eds.), *The handbook of special education: Research and practice* (Vol. 3, pp. 287–311). Oxford, England: Pergamon.

Narayan, J.S., Heward, W.L., Gardner, R., Courson, F.H., & Omness, C.K. (1990). Using response cards to increase student participation in an elementary classroom. *Journal of Applied Behavior Analysis, 23,* 483–490.

Neef, N.A., Mace, F.C., Shea, M.C., & Shade, D. (1992). Effects of reinforcer rate and reinforcer quality on time allocation: Extension of matching theory to educational settings. *Journal of Applied Behavior Analysis, 25,* 691–699.

Neef, N.A., Mace, F.C., & Shade, D. (1993). Impulsivity in students with serious emotional disturbance: The interactive effects of reinforcer rate, delay, and quality. *Journal of Applied Behavior Analysis, 26,* 37–52.

Neef, N.A., Shade, D., & Miller, M.S. (1994). Assessing the influential dimensions of reinforcers on choice in students with serious emotional disturbance. *Journal of Applied Behavior Analysis, 24,* 575–583.

Ownby, R.L., Wallbrown, F., D'Atri, A., & Armstrong, B. (1985). Patterns of referrals for school psychological services. *Special Services in the Schools, 1,* 53–66.

Paine, S.C., Radicchi, J., Rosellini, L.C., Deutchman, L., & Darch, C.B. (1983). *Structuring your classroom for academic success.* Champaign, IL: Research Press Company.

Pellegrino, J.W., & Goldman, S.R. (1987). Information processing and elementary mathematics. *Journal of Learning Disabilities, 20,* 23–32, 57.

Pratt-Struthers, J.P., Bartalamay, H.R., Bell, S., & McLaughlin, T.F. (1994). An analysis of the add-a-word spelling program and public posting across three categories of children with special needs. *Reading Improvement, 31,* 28–36.

Pumroy, D.K., & McIntire, R. (1991). Behavior analysis/modification for everyone. *Journal of Behavioral Education, 1,* 283–294.

Reschly, D.J. (1987). Learning characteristics of mildly handicapped students: Implications for classification, placement, and programming. In M.C. Wang, M.C. Reynolds, & H.J. Walberg (Eds.). *The handbook of special education: Research and practice,* (Vol. 1; pp. 35–88). Oxford, England: Pergamon.

Reschly, D.J. (1988). Alternative delivery systems: Legal and ethical impact. In J.L. Graden, J.E. Zins, & M.J. Curtis (Eds.), *Alternative educational delivery systems: Enhancing instructional opportunities for all students* (pp. 525–561). Washington, DC: National Association of School Psychologists.

Reschly, D.J., & Ysseldyke, J.E. (1995). School psychology paradigm shift. In A. Thomas & J. Grimes (Eds.), *Best Practices in School Psychology-III* (pp. 17–31). Washington, DC: National Association of School Psychologists.

Riley, J.P. (1986). The effects of teachers' wait-time and knowledge comprehension questioning on science achievement. *Journal of Research in Science Teaching, 23,* 335–342.

Roberts, M.L., & Shapiro, E.S. (1996). Effects of instructional ratios on students' reading performance in a regular education program. *Journal of School Psychology, 34,* 73–91.

Rowe, M. (1974). Wait-time and rewards as instructional variables, their influence on language, logic and fate control. Part one: Wait time. *Journal of Research in Science Teaching, 17,* 469–475.

Saudargus, R.A. (1992). *State–Event Classroom Observation System.* Knoxville: University of Tennessee, Department of Psychology.

Shapiro, E.S. (1987). *Behavioral assessment in school Psychology.* Hillsdale, NJ: Erlbaum.

Shapiro, E.S. (1989). *Academic skills problems: Direct assessment and interventions.* New York: Guilford.

Shapiro, E.S. (1996). *Academic skills problems: Direct assessment and intervention* (2nd ed.).New York: Guilford.

Shapiro, E.S. & Skinner, C.H. (1990). Principles of behavioral assessment. In C.R. Reynolds & R. Kamphaus (Eds.),

Handbook of educational and psychological assessment in children: Personality, behavior, and context (pp. 342–364). New York: Guilford.

Shinn, M.R. (1989). *Curriculum-based measurement: Assessing special children.* New York: Guilford.

Shriner, J., & Salvia, J. (1988). Chronic noncorrespondance between elementary math curricula and arithmetic texts. *Exceptional Children, 55,* 240–248.

Skinner, B.F. (1950). Are theories of learning necessary. *Psychological Review, 57,* 193–216.

Skinner, C.H., & Schock, H.H. (1995). Best practices in assessing mathematics skills. In A. Thomas & J. Grimes (Eds.), *Best Practices in School Psychology-III* (pp. 731–740). Washington, DC: National Association of School Psychologists.

Skinner, C.H., & Shapiro, E.S. (1989). A comparison of taped-words and drill interventions on reading fluency in adolescents with behavior disorders. *Education and Treatment of Children, 12,* 123–133.

Skinner, C.H., & Smith, E.S. (1992). Issues surrounding the use of self-management interventions for increasing academic performance. *School Psychology Review, 21,* 202–210.

Skinner, C.H., Turco, T.L., Beatty, K., & Rasavage, C. (1989). Cover, copy, and compare: A method for increasing multiplication fluency in behavior disordered children. *School Psychology Review, 18,* 412–420.

Skinner, C.H., Ford, J.M., & Yunker, B.D. (1991). An analysis of instructional response requirements on the multiplication performance of behavior disordered students. *Behavior Disorders, 17,* 56–65.

Skinner, C.H., Belfiore, P.J., & Watson, T.S. (1995). Assessing the relative effects of interventions in students with mild disabilities: Assessing instructional time. *Assessment in Rehabilitation and Exceptionality, 2,* 207–220.

Skinner, C. H., Fletcher, P.A., & Henington, C. (1996). Increasing learning rates by increasing student response rates: A summary of research. *School Psychology Quarterly, 11,* 313–325.

Skinner, C.H., Fletcher, P.A., Wildmon, M., & Belfiore, P.J. (1996). Improving assignment preference through interspersal: Problem completion rates versus easy problems. *Journal of Behavioral Education, 6,* 427–437.

Skinner, C.H., Robinson, S.L., Johns, G.A., Logan, P., & Belfiore, P.J. (1996). Applying Herrnstein's matching law to influence students' choice to complete difficult academic tasks. *The Journal of Experimental Education, 65,* 5–17.

Skinner, C.H., Belfiore, P.J., Mace, H.W., Williams-Wilson, S., & Johns, G.A. (1997). Altering response topography to increase learning rates. *School Psychology Quarterly, 12,* 54–64.

Smith, D.K. (1984). Practicing school psychologists: Their characteristics, activities, and populations served. *Professional Psychology: Research and Practice, 15,* 798–810.

Speece, D.L. (1990). Aptitude-treatment interactions: Bad rap or bad idea? *The Journal of Special Education, 24,* 139–149.

Stanley, S.O., & Greenwood, C.R. (1981). *CISSAR: Code for instructional structure and students academic responses: Observers'manual.* Kansas City: University of Kansas, Bureau of Educational Research, Juniper Gardens Children's Project.

Stokes, T.F., & Baer, D.M. (1977). An implicit technology of generalization. *Journal of Applied Behavior Analysis, 10,* 349–368.

Sugden, D.A. (1980). Movement speed in children. *Journal of Motor Behavior, 12,* 125–132.

Van Houten, R. (1984). Setting up performance feedback systems in the classroom. In W.L. Heward, T.E. Heron, J. Trap-Porter, & D.S. Hill (Eds.), *Focus on behavior analysis in education* (pp. 112–125). Columbus, OH: Merrill.

Van Houten, R., Hill, S., & Parsons, M. (1975). An analysis of a performance feedback system: The effects of timing and feedback, public posting, and praise upon academic performance and peer interaction. *Journal of Applied Behavior Analysis, 12,* 581–591.

Van Houten, R., & Little, G. (1982). Increased response rate in special education children following an abrupt reduction in time limit. *Education and Treatment of Children, 5,* 23–32.

Van Houten, R., & Thomas, C. (1976). The effects of explicit timing on math performance. *Journal of Applied Behavior Analysis, 9,* 227–230.

Vargus, E.A., & Vargus, J.S. (1991). Programmed instruction: What is it and how to do it. *Journal of Behavioral Education, 2,* 235–251.

Watson, T.S. (1994). The role of preservice education in training teachers to serve behaviorally disordered children. *Contemporary Education, 65,* 128–131.

Wong, B.Y.L. (1986). Problems and issues in definition of learning disabilities. In J.K. Torgesen & B.Y.L. Wong (Eds.), *Psychological and educational perspectives on learning disabilities* (pp. 3–26). New York: Academic.

Ysseldyke, J.E., & Christenson, S.L. (1988). Linking assessment to intervention. In J.L. Graden, J.E. Zins, & M.J. Curtis (Eds.), *Alternative educational delivery systems: Enhancing instructional opportunities for all students* (pp. 91–110). Washington, DC: National Association of School Psychologists.

Bibliography

Daly, E. (1996). *School Psychology Quarterly,* Special Issue. Daly has edited a mini-series issue of *School Psychology Quarterly.* This issue contains many strong articles that address behavioral issues associated with academic interventions, some of which were discussed in this chapter. Educators and researchers may want to pay particular attention to the Dunlap and Kern article on student preference.

Gardner, R., Sainato, D.M., Copper, J.O., Heron, T.E., Heward, T.E., Eshleman, J., & Grossi, T.A. (1994). *Behavior analysis in education: Focus on measurably superior instruction.* Pacific Grove, CA: Brooks/Cole. This edited text contains 25 chapters written by leaders in the field of behavioral analysis and education. Chapters are historical, philosophical, and applied.

Shapiro, E.S. (1996). *Academic skills problems: Direct assessment and intervention* (2nd ed.). New York: Guilford. This text integrates the theory and practice of direct assessment and direct intervention. Also included is a workbook with many useful forms and training activities. The comprehensive nature of this text makes it a very useful tool for practitioners and researchers who wish to address remediation of academic skills problems.

5

Enhancing Academic Achievement through Related Routines

A Functional Approach

PHILLIP J. BELFIORE AND JEFFREY M. HUTCHINSON

Introduction

Academic test scores and academic achievement have been, and continue to be, a focal point in our educational system (National Commission on Excellence in Education, 1983; National Education Goals Report, 1994). Given the continued emphasis on academic achievement as an item on the educational agenda, educators, researchers, school psychologists, parents, and administrators continually seek out methodologies to identify, delineate, isolate, and maximize variables associated with student achievement on academic indicators. By identifying variables, or combinations of variables, associated with academic achievement, educational programs can be developed that benefit each student.

Greer (1994) suggested that effective educational programming is predicated on the assumption that schools must shift from a group oriented model to an individualized education model. This educational shift, from group to individual, places emphasis on mastery and fluency within the constraints of an individual's history (Greer, 1994). By taking an individual perspective to education, we can begin to (a) assess relationships between school-related variables (i.e., academic context) and student academic behavior(s) (i.e., academic en-

gagement), and (b) develop cross-curricular strategies that enhance performance in specific academic curriculum areas.

One set of school-related variables receiving limited attention, but pervasive throughout all of schooling, is academic related routines. Related routines in academics may be defined as those chains of skills necessary for academic achievement, but skill chains not directly related to teaching strategies within a single academic curriculum content area. Academic related routines represent strategies for enhancing academic achievement during school (e.g., notetaking, test preparation, study strategies), as well as strategies designed for times other than that allotted during school hours (e.g., homework). In addition, academic related routines represent mechanisms from which students with learning difficulties can better meet the challenges of an academic curriculum through more effective management of academic time.

If student academic performance is to be enhanced, effective assessment, design, and inclusion of academic related routines into the school curriculum must be targeted. First, an assessment of academic context and academic behavior must initially be conducted. The result of such a descriptive (Bijou, Peterson, & Ault, 1968), or ecobehavioral (Greenwood, Carta, & Atwater, 1991) assessment is the relationships observed between academic contexts (e.g., instructional arrangement, instructional format) and student academic engagement (e.g.,

PHILLIP J. BELFIORE AND JEFFREY M. HUTCHINSON • Education Division, Mercyhurst College, Erie, Pennsylvania 16546.

Handbook of Child Behavior Therapy, edited by Watson and Gresham. Plenum Press, New York, 1998.

homework accuracy, homework completion, test results, notetaking accuracy, note writing) under natural, not contrived, circumstances. One advantage of this type of assessment over traditional behavioral assessment is that behaviors may be assessed in terms of major and/or minor sets of contextual variables (Greenwood, et al., 1991). Specifically, ecobehavioral or descriptive assessments allow for analysis of intervention variables, as well as contextual variables, that may affect intervention variables.

Second, the design of any academic related routine must be empirically validated. Relations observed in the initial descriptive assessment must be validated under more controlled situations. For example, during step one (descriptive assessment), homework accuracy (a dependent variable), has been shown to increase when small groups of students (two to three) work on homework assignments 10 min before going home (independent variable). This second step (functional assessment) must validate what was initially observed to occur in the first step.

In concert with step two, the academic related routine must be tailored to, and included in, the academic content area in question. For example, a generic notetaking strategy (e.g., notetaking routine) that requires the student to identify key points of a class lecture, and then rewrite them in an outline framework form (see Figure 1) can be taught and mastered, but the generic strategy must then be tailored to the specific academic assignment and curriculum area. Any academic related routine must (a) be functionally related through assessment, and (b) following routine mastery, be content related to the academic curriculum area.

The goal of this link between descriptive and functional assessments is twofold. From the functional component, the link between academic variables and academic performance is (a) initially assessed through direct and indirect means to observe relationships between academic variable and student academic performance and then (b) empirically validated through more controlled conditions. The result of the functional component is an academic related routine incorporating classroom variables that have been shown to maximize student academic engagement. From the content component, the link between related routines and specific curriculum areas is (a) developed through generic

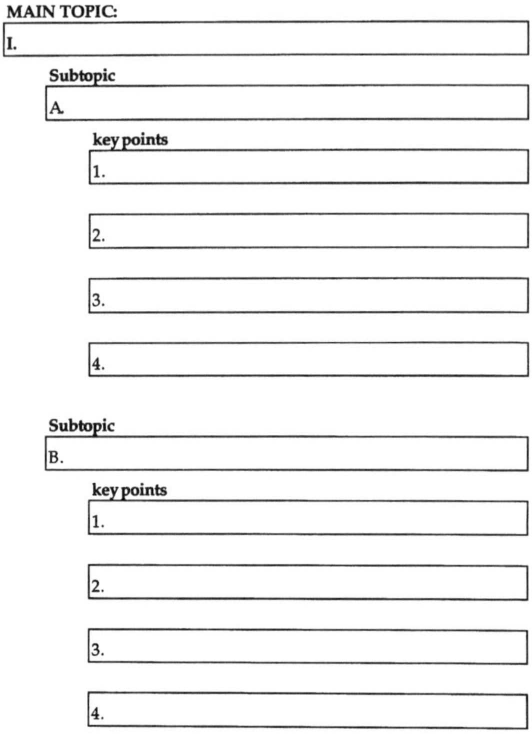

FIGURE 1. An example of a notetaking outline designed to provide cues to main topic, subtopics, and key points.

routines, and then (b) tailored to individual academic curriculum areas. The result of the content component is an academic related routine that can easily be included in academic curriculum areas requiring remediation.

The combination of functional and content components in understanding and utilizing academic related routines allows for content-specific routines that incorporate functionality between "school" variables and academic behavior. The result of this combination of approaches, content and functional, is the development of optimal educational strategies designed to enhance academic engagement by using related academic routines across content-specific curriculum areas. The purpose of this chapter is to examine the development of academic related routines on the academic achievement of students with learning difficulties. By taking a content *and* functional approach to developing effective related routines in academics, we can present to the reader a methodology that links instruction, home, and school variables with individual student academic performance.

Problem Identification: Descriptive Assessment

Academic achievement, or the ability to learn, depends on how the time available for academic engagement is utilized, not just the total amount of time available. More time does not necessarily produce more learning (Stallings, 1980). Academic achievement has been functionally related to the time actively engaged in academic contexts (Belfiore, Skinner, & Ferkis, 1955; Berliner, 1984; Greenwood, Delquardi, & Hall, 1984; Lentz, 1988; O'Melia & Rosenberg, 1994), rather than an inherent limit of aptitude. Greenwood (1991) has concluded that time actively engaged in academic situations was the single best indicator of achievement among students with learning difficulties. Therefore, instructional time becomes a critical variable when we attempt to understand and enhance academic achievement (Skinner, Belfiore, & Watson, 1995). If we consider instructional time a critical variable, then we can begin to look at students with learning difficulties as not failing to learn, but rather failing to learn at a rate commensurate with their fellow students. If we as educators can enhance learning rates through optimizing instructional time (i.e., better management of instructional time), then specific learning difficulties become a non-issue. From an applied behavioral perspective, a learning difficulty is a rate problem, not a level problem (Carroll, 1963; Gettinger, 1984).

Describing learning difficulties as problems in learning rate, rather than problems in learning levels or information processing, has led to a number of interventions related to such ideas as extended school year and longer school days. Although providing additional school time for academic instruction is problematic for students with learning difficulties (e.g., allocating more instructional time to mathematics may limit the time available for reading or language arts), developing more effective academic management and organizational skill competencies within a fixed amount of time is possible.

What needs to be determined is how instructional time can be enhanced through the use of academic related routines. The first step in enhancing instructional time through academic related routines is to conduct a descriptive assessment. In general, a descriptive assessment is designed to show naturally occurring relations between environmental variables and behavior (Bijou, et al., 1968; Mace, 1994). More specifically, an academic descriptive assessment examines the relations between academic context and academic performance. Following the descriptive assessment, generic academic related routines are developed and tested under more controlled conditions in a functional assessment. The functional assessment is conducted, incorporating generic routines into the academic curriculum content areas.

Initial Assessment: Home Inventory Checklist and Descriptive Assessment

One of the major strengths of incorporating a home inventory checklist and a descriptive assessment as the first step when determining academic related routines is the increased confidence that the results will generalize outside the controlled setting (Mace, 1994). For example, by observing in the descriptive assessment that a student's notetaking behavior is more accurate (higher percentage of keywords present in the outline) when a teacher verbalizes *and* writes the key words on the board, the behavioral interventionist can maximize the academic related routine by ensuring that both modes of teacher behavior are in place when notetaking is required. Furthermore, this information is enhanced if information can also be gleaned from the home environment. For example, we have determined that a student's notetaking behavior is more accurate when keywords are verbalized and written. In addition, from the home inventory, we found that the student goes to an after-school program directly from school, and there she can rewrite the notes taken in class with the help of a tutor. Using both direct and indirect information, we can better ensure that the student will have taken proper notes using the outline framework taught in the notetaking routine. Such a combination of information, home and school, results in the better management of instructional time.

The combination of indirect information gathered from the home and after-school setting, and direct information gathered from the classroom environment, will provide a more comprehensive picture of what variables may be incorporated into the development of academic related routines.

Home Variables—Indirect Assessment

One method for collecting descriptive information is through periodic checklists sent home with the student. The home, with the school, encompasses a majority of the student's environment and time. One assumption in a majority of published reports on academic related routines, and textbooks in special education, is that caregivers or parents are (a) available as home instructors, carrying out the continuing academic duties of the classroom teacher, and (b) willing to participate in after-school education (e.g., Jenson, Sheridan, Olympia, & Andrews, 1994; Miller & Kelly, 1994; Patton, 1994; Waldron, 1996) . In addition, it is often assumed that parents or caregivers are knowledgeable about the academic subject area(s) for which the assignment was made. Waldron (1996) suggested that the parents or caregivers create a home "environment for academic success" (p. 480). Waldron (1996) continues by suggesting that it is the job of the parent to provide a quiet place for homework completion, family interactions, reasonable bedtime schedules, and breakfast before leaving the house.

Unfortunately, this is not always the case. Single-head-of-household families, dual-parent working families, school-age student to care for younger siblings, and other realities of home life often limit the roles of parents/caregivers and available after-school time in the education of their children. The parent(s) or caregiver(s) may wish to assist in the educational activities of their children, but managing a household and/or providing primary financial income may take a priority. At times, the students who require the most academic assistance during nonschool times are the same students who do not get that assistance. Form 5.1 provides sample questions designed to obtain information from the home environment. This information can be used when determining whether academic related routines, such as homework, notetaking, and test preparation, can be carried out consistently in the home. If, for whatever reason, the home cannot be used as a consistent educational setting for after-school work, the teacher(s) must make sure test preparation, notetaking, and homework are carried out satisfactorily during school time, or in after-school programs, if available.

The inclusion of the home inventory checklist allows the teacher, guidance counselor, or school psychologist to determine the role post-school time can play in the enhancement of academic related routine. Too often it is assumed that post-school time is available, and frequently it is not. As educators, we must initially determine what role post-school time plays when academic related routines are involved.

FORM 5.1. Home Inventory Checklist

To be completed as best as possible by parent(s) or caregiver(s)
1. Does your son/daughter attend any after-school programs?
    if YES, what does does he or she attend, and for how long each day?
    if NO, are you aware of any after-school programs in the area?
2. Is there a time during the evening/morning for your son or daughter to do school work?
    if YES, for how long each day, and how many times a week?
    if NO, can a specific time each day be established?
3. Is there a specific location during the evening or morning for your son or daughter to do school work?
    if YES, where is that specific location?
    if NO, can a specific location be established?
4. Do you understand the homework assignments?
    if NO, please let me know how I can assist.
5. Would you be willing to attend a class with your child?
    if YES, when is best for you?
6. How best does your son or daughter do school work at the home?

alone?	YES ___	NO ___	NOT SURE ___
with others?	YES ___	NO ___	NOT SURE ___
in a quiet area?	YES ___	NO ___	NOT SURE ___
with music/TV?	YES ___	NO ___	NOT SURE ___

School Variables—Direct Assessment

A second method for obtaining descriptive data is through direct observation within the school environment. Again, the purpose of the descriptive assessment is to observe relationships between academic variables and academic engagement within a school context. Before any assessment can be conducted, variables and behaviors have to be identified. Teachers can identify classroom variables from random observations across the school day. Four general categories can be developed from observing the activities and interactions of the classroom: (a) contextual variables, (b) antecedent variables, (c) student behaviors, and (d) consequent variables. Table 1 provides several examples of variables within each of the four categories.

Once variables have been identified and defined, a data collection procedure must be determined. Momentary time sampling and partial interval recording systems provide a manageable system to incorporate. For example, using a momentary time sample (e.g., 15 s), allows the teacher to observe the context variables, antecedent variables, consequent variables, and target student at the end of a series of 15-s blocks (see Figure 2). As each 15-s block of time ends, the teacher observes the classroom variables in place at that moment,

TABLE 1. Examples of Variables to Be Included in a Descriptive Assessment

Context variables	Antecedent variables	Student behavior	Consequent variables
1. Instructional arrangement	1. Instructional format	1. Academic response	1. Feedback
—large lecture	—verbal instructions	—verbalization	—teacher
—small group	—written instructions	—writing	—support staff
—one-on-one	—discussion		—peers
—peer tutor			
—cooperative			
2. Physical arrangement	2. Teacher location	2. Academic engagement	2. Type
—at own desk	—front of room	—orienting towards	—positive
—on floor	—circulating	academic stimuli	—negative
—table	—out of view		—group
—quiet			—individual
—conversation			—general
			—specific

	:15	:30	:45	1	:15	:30	:45	2	:15	:30	:45	3	:15	:30	:45	4	:15	:30	:45	5
context var.																				
antecendent																				
behavior																				
consequent																				

FIGURE 2. An example of a 15-s interval data momentary time sampling collection sheet for descriptive and functional assessments. The total time for the sheet is 5 min.

and the behavior of the target student. At each 15-s interval, all variables and behaviors are checked off on the data sheet for that interval, and the teacher waits for the end of the next 15-s interval to record events. This procedure continues until the session (e.g., 40 min) or class period is over. Ideally, five to seven sessions can be run per student, over the course of several days, in situations that allow for as many variables identified to be observed. It would not be advantageous to observe the same class time, in the same class arrangement, during every observation. The purpose of the assessment is to observe, (i.e., "find") situations in which students are engaged in academic behavior.

Problem Analysis: Linking Descriptive and Functional Assessments

Once information is collected from both the home inventory checklist and the direct observation descriptive assessment, the results must be analyzed (e.g., "What relationships were observed to occur naturally?"). Information from the home inventory checklist can be summarized and used to augment results from the descriptive assessments. Data from a descriptive assessment can be summarized as the number of intervals scored as a specific response, given a specified antecedent condition, divided by the total number of intervals scored with that specified antecedent condition (Belfiore, Browder, & Lin, 1993). This type of descriptive analysis allows evaluation, given the power of the antecedent or context variable to occasion or evoke the target response. For example, if 40, 15-s intervals are scored as (a) peer tutoring, (b) verbal instruction, and 30 of those intervals are also scored with academic engagement, the percentage graphed is 75% (30/40). That is, seventy-five percent of the time the student was in peer tutoring with verbal instruction, that student was academically engaged. Given this information over repeated descriptive assessment sessions, the teacher may want to consider using peer tutoring and verbal instruction when assigning study groups for test preparation for that student.

A second method for analyzing descriptive assessment data is conditional probabilities. Kamps, Leonard, Dugan, Boland, and Greenwood (1991) have defined the conditional probability of a response as equal to the frequency of the response given a specified environmental condition, divided by the total response occurrence (total number of intervals scored as that response) of that response across all environmental conditions. Conditional probability gives the distribution of a given response across specified environmental conditions.

The combined results of the descriptive assessment and the home inventory checklist give a clearer picture as to the variables that can be included in effective academic related routines. The descriptive assessment yields those combinations of variables (context, antecedent, and consequent) that are observed to result in increased academic engagement. The home inventory checklist yields valuable information as to the time outside of school that can be included in the enhancement of academic related routines and academic engagement.

Although procedures such as the descriptive assessment, and similar systems (e.g., ecobehavioral assessments), help determine variables associated with academic engagement, these procedures do not provide empirical evidence as to the best environmental combination. Initially, data collected from the descriptive analysis show natural relationships among antecedent stimuli, subsequent stimuli, and the target response(s), without experimental manipulations. In addition, the home inventory checklist provides information as to the possible inclusion of home as an additional environment in which interventions can be incorporated. Data collected and analyzed from a descriptive assessment allow educators to form hypotheses as to which environmental variables may result in greater academic engagement (Skinner et al., 1995).

Direct assessments of the target behavior(s) under more controlled conditions can be used to test these hypotheses. These more controlled conditions, assessed using a functional analysis methodology (Iwata, Dorsey, Slifer, Bauman, & Richman, 1982), provide specific manipulations of the environment–behavior interactions initially observed in the descriptive assessment. For example, Kern, Childs, Dunlap, Clarke, and Falk (1994), following a descriptive assessment, developed a functional intervention strategy that included self-monitoring, short tasks, and nonwritten work to increase the time on task across spelling, English, and math for an elementary-age student with emotional challenges. Information from the initial descriptive assessment resulted in an intervention package designed to maximize on-task academic behavior across multiple curriculum areas.

The goal of the functional assessment is to isolate and manipulate variables occasioning and/or maintaining the target response(s) (Belfiore et al., 1993). Using both descriptive and functional assessment information provides firmer conclusions as to the relationships between academic variables and academic engagement.

Functional Assessment

Given information obtained from the descriptive assessment, a second step in developing effective academic related routines is a functional assessment. Cooper and colleagues (1992) have developed a brief procedure for conducting functional assessments. Brief multielement designs are established to manipulate and control variables identified in the descriptive assessment. For example, if the descriptive assessment showed that a student remained engaged in notetaking longer when teacher instruction was verbalized and written, the functional assessment would test this hypothesis. Using the same data-collection procedure as that discussed in the descriptive assessment (15 s momentary time sampling), and shorter sessions (10 min), data can be collected under one condition, in which the teacher gives both types of instruction throughout the entire 10-min session, and during a second condition, in which the teacher provides only verbal instruction throughout. Similarly, if we observed in the descriptive assessment that a student does better on a homework assignment when provided brief peer tutoring prior to leaving school, then we can set up two conditions to test this hypothesis: (a) a condition that allows for 10 min of peer tutoring, and (b) a second condition that allows for no peer tutoring following the homework assignment. Next day homework's are scored for accuracy. The conditions (written and verbal instruction versus verbal instruction only; 10 min of peer tutoring versus no peer tutoring) are alternated every other day over the course of two weeks in a multielement single subject design. If the functional assessment results support what was hypothesized from the descriptive assessment we can, with added confidence, begin to use this information in the development of academic related routines.

The data sheet in Figure 2 can also be used for the functional assessment. In the functional assessment only those context, antecedent, and/or consequent variables that are to be directly manipulated and tested are labeled. Once environment–behavior hypotheses are tested, the results of the functional assessment, along with information collected from the home inventory checklist, are included in the development of individualized academic related routines.

Academic Related Routine Development

Given the dilemma of fixed time for instruction, one set of academic variables that warrants discussion is academic related routines (i.e., notetaking, study strategies and test preparation, homework). As stated earlier in this chapter, related routines in academics are strategies that (a) are necessary for academic achievement, but not directly related to instruction within an academic curriculum area, (b) enhance academic achievement during school, as well as times other than time allotted during school hours (i.e., homework), (c) enhance the management of instructional time, and (d) represent mechanisms with which students with learning difficulties can better meet the challenges of an academic curriculum.

A routine can be defined as a chain, or sequence, of generalized, observable activities. Each activity that makes up the routine, or the routine itself, becomes the instructional objective when academic related areas are taught. For example, a routine designed to promote notetaking skills might include the following sequence: (a) obtain all necessary materials (e.g., book, pencils, outline framework [see Figure 1]), (b) find appropriate location, (c) engage in academic behavior (i.e., orient toward academic materials), (d) from teacher lecture, write main topic, subtopics, and key points in the outline spaces provided, and (e) compare main topic, subtopics, and key points from information reviewed. (In this example, remember that, from the functional assessment, it was demonstrated that notetaking accuracy was enhanced when the teacher verbalized and wrote lecture notes on the board.) This routine can be taught and assessed overtly at first, and later the student can self-monitor progress through the routine. Once mastered, this routine can be adapted to any curriculum area. Form 5.2 shows a data collection sheet that can be used initially by the teacher during instruction of the routine, and later by the student during self-monitoring.

FORM 5.2. Academic Related Routine: Notetaking

Student: _____   Date: _____

Subject area: _____   Time: _____

Steps to follow	Day 1	Day 2	Day 3	Day 4	Day 5	
1. Gather all materials	+					
2. Find appropriate location	+					
3. Academic engagement	+					
4. Write points on outline template	–					
5. Compare outline to notes delivered	–					
Notes:						

The academic related routine incorporates into it the information obtained from the descriptive assessment, the home inventory checklist, and the functional assessment. In the notetaking routine example above, the routine was developed from (a) observations made during the descriptive assessment, such as that academic engagement was greater when the teacher wrote and spoke lecture notes, (b) information from the home inventory checklist, such as that the student spends 30 min each Monday, Wednesday, and Thursday in an after-school program where notes can be reviewed, and (c) data collected from the functional assessment, such as that notetaking accuracy increased when the teacher verbalized and wrote lecture notes as compared to verbalizing alone. By incorporating the information gleaned from these assessments, we are more confident that the routine will better serve the student.

Implementation

Given the information compiled from the functional assessment and the development of generic academic routines, this section is designed to demonstrate how routines can be incorporated within specific academic content areas. This section will provide (a) a brief introduction to several academic related skill areas, (b) current related skill strategies designed to improve academic achievement, and (c) specific routines that can be developed and adapted, given information from the home inventory checklist, descriptive assessment, and functional assessment.

This section is not a "cookbook" of best practices for improving academic related skills. What is best for one student may not be best for another. For example, if after our descriptive and functional assessment we find that Emily completed more homework assignments when given written instructions and a 10-min practice with a peer the day before homework was due, we will design our routine with those tested components in place. If another student, Elisa, completed homework accurately with only verbal instructions the day before homework was due, we will not develop a routine that adds work for the teacher and provides less time for additional teaching. This section will provide techniques that have been shown to be effective, but those techniques must be paired with the results of the two-step assessment (descriptive and functional). The routines discussed for each academic related area will be generic enough for teachers to adapt following assessment, yet complete enough for teachers to see how the routine progresses.

Notetaking

Baker and Lombardi (1985) suggested that during lectures, in which main topics are presented, students miss at least one-half of those topics. Listening only while information is provided via lecture format does not provide the necessary structure for most students when testing on that information follows. Accuracy in test taking depends on more than just listening to lectures for information. Notetaking may involve information gathered while a teacher is lecturing on a specific topic, or information gathered from a media source (e.g., notes taken from a novel read, instructions taken from a computer program). Notetaking is not copying. Notetaking involves the transcribing of information gathered and writing the reorganized information into an outline framework.

Two elements appear key when developing notetaking routines: (a) a component of self-monitoring and (b) a specific outline format. Spires and Stone (1989) suggest that one reason notetaking does not necessarily result in information comprehension is that students do not always engage in self-monitoring during the notetaking. Laidlaw, Skok, and McLaughlin (1993) found that self-questioning, which involved asking questions to determine relationships between ideas, when explicitly instructed, enhanced the percentage correct on weekly science quizzes. Similarly, Spires and Stone (1989) developed a Directed Notetaking Activity (DNA), which included (a) a structured format for taking notes, (b) a self-questioning strategy, and (c) a direct and explicit teaching of notetaking. Self-monitoring during a notetaking routine may occur before taking notes (e.g., "What is the purpose of this assignment?"), while taking notes (e.g., "Am I discriminating between main topics and subtopics?"), and after taking notes (e.g., "Did I achieve my original goal?") (Spires & Stone, 1989). Self-monitoring during notetaking provides additional cues or prompts that result in a more comprehensive final product. Self-monitoring, after steps are overtly taught, also provides a mechanism with which students can work independently, allowing teachers more time for other instruction. In addition, self-monitoring before, during, and after notetaking also allows students to review materials in the home or in an after-school environment.

A second key element when developing a notetaking routine is the inclusion of an outline framework. Notetaking outlines are designed to introduce the student to main ideas, subtopics, and key words (Pieronek, 1994). Spires and Stone (1989) used a split-page method for notetaking which included (a) dividing the page into two columns, (b) placing main ideas in the left column, and (c) placing definitions, examples, and key words into the right column. Any outline framework requires the student to engage in more than just verbatim note recording. The outline provides discrimination for key parts of lectures to be written. Figure 1 provides an outline format designed to assist students in organizing topics from a lecture. This the outline also allows teachers to provide additional information to prompt students to complete the outline. For example, a teacher may provide the main topic and subtopics on the outline, requiring students to identify and fill in the key points.

The notetaking routine checklist in Form 5.2 provides a generic set of steps for teaching notetaking. Remember, information from the home inventory checklist and from the functional assessment will be used to supplement this routine, increasing its specificity, effectiveness, and efficiency. First, students must obtain all materials necessary for notetaking. For all students this should include an outline framework (see Figure 1), and for some students this should include a cassette recorder from which lecture notes can be replayed. Second, students must find a location where notetaking will take place. In school, this may be a table or desk, while at home the best location may be determined from home checklist information. Step three is academic engagement. The student must be engaged with the academic stimulus or stimuli. At home, this means reading notecards or listening to the recorded lesson. At school, this means observing the teacher and the board, reading notecards, or listening to the recorded lesson. Following academic engagement, the student must write notes. The last step involves a self-check between what has been written and what was lectured. As with all academic related routines, the steps are initially taught overtly, and, once mastered, they are self-monitored by the students.

Study Strategies and Test Preparation

Gearheart, Weishahn, and Gearheart (1996) have suggested that many, if not most, students with learning difficulties have not developed the necessary study skills for success in an academic curriculum. Decker, Spector, and Shaw (1992) defined study skills as encompassing a variety of skills, including notetaking, memory techniques, and test taking, that enhance the effectiveness and efficiency of learning. Study strategies are the link between notetaking and test taking. One feature of a study strategy is the preparation for tests and exams. If students are more accurate in the information they gather from lectures, class discussions, and written material, then study strategies are enhanced due to the organization of instructional materials. The best study strategy is of limited use if the material studies is not relevant to the final academic outcome (i.e., tests, exams, written reports, multimedia presentations). In essence, the first step of a study strategy routine is to develop an organized set of instructional materials from which to study (see Form 5.2 and Figure 1).

Archambeault (1992) suggested two variables important to maximizing study strategies: learner preference and environmental condition. Learner preference and environmental condition can best be determined through the combination of descriptive and functional assessments. The descriptive assessment shows relationships between academic variables and academic engagement. The functional assessment tests those relationships under more controlled conditions. Best study strategies related to context variables, antecedent variables, and consequent variables (see Table 1) are gleaned from the combined assessments. Information from the home inventory checklist is also instrumental in providing information as to best study strategies when outside of school. The questions in Form 5.1 give valuable information if teachers expect students to study in after-school programs or in the home. For example, one descriptive assessment showed that a student spent more time reviewing class notes while alone, with little feedback, and when the notes were rewritten in an outline framework (see Figure 1). The home inventory checklist showed that the student attended an after-school program 4 days a week from 3:00 to 3:30 p.m., and the student's mother required 30 min of study time prior to breakfast in the morning as a time for review. The functional assessment confirmed the relationships observed in the descriptive assessment by experimentally comparing conditions of (a) academic engagement—alone and (b) academic engagement—small group. Results of the functional assessment showed that the alone condition resulted in a greater number of intervals scored as academic engagement. An academic study routine was created to incorporate (a) developing an organizational time chart, (b) constructing an outline from lectures, and (c) selecting appropriate location (alone) (see Form 5.3). After the routine was taught and mastered, the student self-monitored accuracy in the routine, while the teacher monitored corresponding academic progress.

Although the preceding example shows that the study strategy selected was reorganizing lecture notes in outlines using a framework (step b, above), other strategies may be assessed and included into the routine. Archambeault (1992) suggested several

FORM 5.3. Academic Related Routine: Study Skills

Student: _____   Date: _____

Subject area: _____   Time: _____

Steps to follow	Day 1	Day 2	Day 3	Day 4	Day 5	
1. Develop organizational time chart	+					
2. Select study strategy from assessments	+					
3. Find appropriate location	−					
4. Academic engagement	+					
5. Review, if necessary	na					
Notes:						

strategies, including mnemonics, flash cards, and using a highlight marker. The purpose of selecting study strategies, (e.g., flashcards), is to determine how best to provide discriminable information to the student which in turn increases the probability of academic accuracy when that information is presented in a test or final project array.

Notetaking and study strategies co-exist in that accurate notes that capture the essence of the instructional materials is one fundamental requirement for efficient studying. If students do not follow a functional notetaking routine, the materials transcribed during the notetaking routine may be unorganized and irrelevant to the final product, hence making the studying inefficient. Effective study strategies may also influence the completion of homework assignments (Gajria & Salend, 1995). Without a specific study routine, homework may be difficult to complete, especially if new materials are included in the homework assignment. Decker and colleagues (1992) suggested that the integration of study strategies into the regular academic curriculum helps students do better because they are better organized and have a clearer idea of academic expectation.

Homework

Homework has been considered "the most common point of intersection among parent, child, and school activities related to formal learning" (Hoover-Dempsey, Bassler, & Burow, 1995, p. 435). Patton (1994) reported that homework has been identified as one of the most important strategies needing attention. Homework is also one of the primary strategies in which the majority of time is spent outside of school. Although, to be effective, homework must begin in the school with specific instructions (Waldron, 1996; O'Melia & Rosenberg, 1994), practice rehearsal (Waldron, 1996), and monitoring of completion and accuracy (Olympia, Sheridan, Jenson, & Andrews, 1994; Trammel, Schloss, & Alper, 1994), the bulk of the work is done without teacher supervision. This becomes problematic when the home environment is not conducive to homework completion (see outcome of home inventory checklist).

Any homework assignment must include detailed, explicit instructions as to the (a) outcome, (b) timetable, and (c) grading. If new materials are to be included in the homework assignment, the teacher should introduce and discuss that material, as well as provide guided and independent practice prior to the assignment (Waldron, 1996). In addition, Jenson and colleagues (1994) suggested that homework instructions be tailored to provide a clear connection between objectives in the classroom and what is expected from the homework assignment. Teachers must also remember that all homework assignments, like in-class work, must be functional and age-appropriate. If cooperative groups or peer dyads are working on homework in study halls, during free time before going home, or in after-school programs, detailed instructions and assignment of responsibilities must be provided.

Following the provision of instructions, Waldron (1996) suggested that teachers should encourage beginning the homework assignment in class. This will allow the teacher to determine whether instructions are clearly written and materials are not too novel for the students. In-class preparation of homework becomes critical for those students who do not have the time or assistance to complete homework at home. In this instance, class preparation may become the only situation in which homework can reliably be completed with assistance. Assistance in this instance can be given by peer tutors. Regardless of when or where homework is to be completed, a timeline must be established so that the student can manage the time available for completion. For example, a homework assignment given during a 45-min study hall may be due at the end of study hall, whereas a series of reading comprehension questions may be due the following morning.

Monitoring of homework completion and homework accuracy is a third area to target when developing a homework routine. Explicit instructions and available practice time are important, but without outcomes measures, the usefulness of homework routines is limited. The timely completion and grading of homework is critical to homework productivity (Jenson et al., 1994). O'Melia and Rosenberg (1994) created Cooperative Homework Teams (CHT) to examine the effect on rate of homework completion and homework accuracy in mathematics. Heterogeneous teams (three to four members) were set up, math assignments were assigned, and next-day team evaluations were conducted on the overnight assignment. Results showed that CHTs, in which teams evaluated, graded, reviewed, and re-graded homework during next-day team time, resulted in increased homework completion and increased homework accuracy. Trammel and colleagues (1994) showed how the introduction of homework assignment self-monitoring increased the number of assignments completed. Self-graphing and goal setting enhanced the self-monitoring results.

When developing the homework routine, teachers must remember to keep in mind (a) the necessity of clear instructions, (b) the usefulness of in-school practice time, and (c) the added benefits of teacher and student monitoring. The teacher must also remember that these three components can be evaluated as part of the descriptive assessment, the home inventory checklist, and the functional assessment. The format of instruction (i.e., instructional format, instructional arrangement, and physical arrangement) is observed and tested in the descriptive–functional assessment link. The inclusion of in-school support is a direct result from information obtained from the home checklist. Teacher monitoring is also determined by the descriptive–functional assessment link. The homework routine in Form 5.4 provides a sequence of steps necessary for homework completion. As with all the routines described

in this chapter, the sequences are only the required steps. Additional steps and strategies warranted are determined from the information collected and analyzed during the assessment phases.

Evaluation

As with any intervention, effectiveness can only be judged through evaluation. Earlier in this chapter it was explained how data collected from the descriptive assessment was analyzed using (a) the power of the antecedent to evoke the target response (Belfiore et al., 1993) and (b) the conditional probability (Kamps et al., 1991). From the descriptive assessment, relationships emerge and are graphed using single subject methodologies (for complete review, see Mace, Lalli, & Pinter-Lalli, 1991). Following the descriptive assessment, those relationships observed to occur naturally were tested under more controlled conditions in a single subject multielement design format. Once classroom variables were determined to occasion increases in academic responding and engagement (see Table 1), academic related routines were developed to include those variables.

FORM 5.4. Academic Related Routine: Homework

| Student: _____ | | Date: _____ |
| Subject area: _____ | | Time: _____ |

Steps to follow	Day 1	Day 2	Day 3	Day 4	Day 5	
1. Obtain requirements or outcome	+					
2. Obtain timeline for completion	+					
3. Gather all necessary materials	–					
4. Find appropriate location	+					
5. Complete assignment	+					
6. Turn in assignment, refer to timeline	–					
7. Monitor accuracy	+					
8. Monitor completion	+					
Notes:						

The evaluation of the effect of academic related routines on academic performance is determined using single subject methodologies looking at individual students' performance in a curriculum area. Graphs are established, and dependent variable data are collected and charted in repeated time-series format. Dependent measures to be evaluated may include, but are not limited to, (a) percentage of routine steps completed independently, (b) percentage of homework completed, (c) number of homework assignments turned in, (d) accuracy in homework assignment, (e) percentage of intervals engaged in notetaking, (f) number of key words written in outline framework, (g) percentage of intervals engaged in studying, (h) accuracy of self-monitoring, and (i) test performance. Daily session data are collected, scored, and graphed. Progress or maintenance is monitored, depending on the research question investigated. For example, teachers may be looking for progress on test performance or accuracy in homework assignments completed, or they may be looking for maintenance of routine independence or homework turned in on time. It is important to remember what the ultimate objective is when evaluating academic related routines. For example, developing a routine to increase homework completion is acceptable, but at some point homework accuracy must be addressed.

Procedural Integrity

Procedural integrity may be defined as the monitoring of intervention procedures to ensure that interventions are implemented as planned. Failure to monitor this poses threats to the validity of the project (Gresham, Gansle, & Noell, 1993; Peterson, Homer, & Wonderlich, 1982). In the case of academic related routines, teachers must be certain that interventions developed during the functional assessment and routine implementation are consistent over time. Periodically, a second observer (e.g., school psychologist, guidance counselor, another teacher, paraprofessional, parent) can collect and record integrity data in the classroom. For example, if the teacher is using the notetaking routine (Form 5.2), a second observer, following a checklist, makes sure the teacher delivers instructions according to the routine as defined in the checklist. Does the teacher verbalize the initiation of the routine? Does the teacher provide materials or directions for obtaining materials? Does the teacher provide written and/or verbal instructions during notetaking? All of these questions must be answered consistently if verbal initiation, directions for material gathering, and verbal directions are provided during the routine.

Generalization

Once a routine has been mastered by the student (as evaluated by the percentage of routine steps completed independently), the routine should be used across other academic curriculum areas and self-monitored by the student. Routine mastery does not mean that the routine is never assessed again; rather, the routine may be assessed for accuracy periodically, incidentally, or by the student through self-monitoring and self-graphing.

The notetaking, study/test preparation, and homework routines developed in this chapter can be generalized to other academic areas once mastery of the routine has been achieved. Once the routine has been individualized (from results of functional assessment and information from the home inventory checklist), the routine can be incorporated into other academic areas where notetaking, study and test preparation, and homework are required. For the student with learning difficulties, the academic related routines represent strategies that should be incorporated across *all* academic areas to maximize academic engagement.

Generalization over time (i.e., maintenance) is a critical and easily included component once routines have been mastered. Self-monitoring, self-graphing, and self-evaluation are all necessary elements if academic related routines are to be maintained following mastery. Trammel and colleagues (1994) used self-monitoring of daily homework assignments to increase homework completion by students ages 13 to 16 with learning disabilities. The self-monitoring consisted of requiring students to record homework assignments on an assignment sheet. After gaining self-monitoring proficiency, the students self-graphed daily homework completion. Later, self-initiated goals were set in an attempt to increase numbers of assignments completed (Trammel et al., 1994). Including generalization techniques will further enhance the instructional time of (a) teachers, because students will retain routine mastery with far less direct-instruction time, and (b) students, because they can now monitor their own performance on routines without waiting for teacher availability.

Summary and Future Directions

As educators attempt to meet the needs of every student, as well as mandates from local, state, and federal agencies, developing more effective approaches to utilizing instructional time is critical. Because instructional time cannot be increased, it must be managed more wisely. By identifying academic related routines, from direct observations in the school and from feedback from the home, educators can begin to create more efficient mechanisms for increasing or maintaining academic engagement.

The inclusion of functional, academic related routines not only enhances performance in curriculum areas in which notetaking, study and test preparation, and homework are required, but these routines provide an additional tool for students with learning difficulties to better meet the demands of time availability. Suggesting that students with learning difficulties spend more time on homework or extended school programs does not provide the answer. Providing tools to students with learning difficulties that assist them in managing the instructional time given is a more promising avenue to explore.

Once educators begin to look to the classroom context and the impact that context has on academic engagement, more functional and appropriate instructional strategies will emerge. When educators see that changes in the academic context can result in changes in student academic engagement, more time will be spent manipulating environmental variables when learning has stalled. Once educators realize that not all home environments (for whatever reason) allow for continued instructional time, they will begin to manage school time more efficiently, and after-school programs will be developed and staffed accordingly. When assessed and developed functionally, academic related routines in the areas of notetaking, study and test preparation, and homework provide cross-curricular options that will begin to meet the needs of students with academic learning difficulties.

ACKNOWLEDGMENTS

The authors would like to thank Tina King and the Program for Students with Learning Differences at Mercyhurst College for their assistance in this project. The authors would also like to thank Cynthia Johnson for her feedback on the development of the home inventory checklist.

References

Archambeault, B. (1992). Personalizing study skills in secondary students. *Journal of Reading, 35,* 468–472.

Baker, L., & Lombardi, B.R. (1985). Students' lecture notes and their relation to test performance. *Teaching of Psychology, 12,* 29–32.

Belfiore, P.J., Browder, D.M., & Lin, C.H. (1993). Using descriptive and experimental analyses in the treatment of self-injurious behavior. *Education and Training in Mental Retardation, 28,* 57–65.

Belfiore, P.J., Skinner, C.H., & Ferkis, M.A. (1995). Effects of response and trial repetition on sight-word training for students with learning disabilities. *Journal of Applied Behavior Analysis, 28,* 347–348.

Berliner, D.C. (1984). The half-full glass: A review of research on teaching. In P.L. Hosford (Ed.), *Using what we know about teaching* (pp. 51–85). Alexandria, VA: Association for Supervision and Curriculum Development.

Bijou, S.W., Peterson, R.F., & Ault, M.H. (1968). A method for integrating descriptive and experimental field studies at the level of data and empirical concepts. *Journal of Applied Behavior Analysis, 1,* 175–191.

Carroll, J.B. (1963). A model for school learning. *Teacher College Record, 64,* 723–733.

Cooper, L.J., Wacker, D.P., Thursby, D., Plagmann, L.A., Harding, J., Millard, T., & Derby, M. (1992). Analysis of the effects of task preferences, task demands, and adult attention on child behavior in outpatient and classroom settings. *Journal of Applied Behavior Analysis, 25,* 823–840.

Decker, K., Spector, S., & Shaw, S. (1992). Teaching study skills to students with mild handicaps: The role of the classroom teacher. *The Clearing House, 65,* 280–284.

Gajria, M., & Salend, S.J. (1995). Homework practices of students with and without learning disabilities. *Journal of Learning Disabilities, 28,* 291–296.

Gearheart, B.R., Weishahn, M.W., & Gearheart, C.J. (1996). *The exceptional student in the regular classroom.* Englewood Cliffs, NJ: Merrill.

Gettinger, M. (1984). Achievement as a function of time spent learning and time needed for learning. *American Education Research Journal, 21,* 617–628.

Greenwood, C.R. (1991). A longitudinal analysis of time to learn, engagement, and academic achievement in urban versus suburban schools. *Exceptional Children, 57,* 521–535.

Greenwood, C.R., Carta, J.J., & Atwater, J. (1991). Ecobehavioral analysis in the classroom: Review and implications. *Journal of Behavioral Education, 1,* 59–77.

Greenwood, C.R., Delquardi, J., & Hall, R.V. (1984). Opportunities to respond and student academic performance. In W. Heward, T. Heron, D. Hill, & J. Trap-Porter (Eds.), *Behavior analysis in education* (pp. 58–88). Columbus, OH: Merrill.

Greer, R.D. (1994). A systems analysis of the behaviors of schooling. *Journal of Behavioral Education, 4,* 255–263.

Gresham, F.M., Gansle, K.A., & Noell, G.H. (1993). Treatment integrity in applied behavior analysis with children. *Journal of Applied Behavior Analysis, 26,* 257–263.

Hoover-Dempsey, K.V., Bassler, O.C., & Burow, R. (1995). Parents' reported involvement in students' homework: Strategies and practices. *The Elementary School Journal, 95,* 435–450.

Iwata, B.A., Dorsey, M.F., Slifer, K.J., Bauman, K.E., & Richman, G.S. (1982). Towards a functional analysis of self-injury. *Journal of Applied Behavior Analysis, 27,* 3–20.

Jenson, W.R., Sheridan, S.M., Olympia, D., & Andrews, D. (1994). Homework and students with learning disabilities and behavior disorders: A practical, parent-based approach. *Journal of Learning Disabilities, 27,* 538–548.

Kamps, D.M., Leonard, B.R., Dugan, E.P., Boland, B., & Greenwood, C.R. (1991). The use of ecobehavioral assessment to identify naturally occurring effective procedures in classroom serving students with autism and other developmental disabilities. *Journal of Behavioral Education, 1,* 367–397.

Kern, L., Childs, K.E., Dunlap, G., Clarke, S., & Falk, G.D. (1994). Using assessment-based curricular intervention to improve the classroom behavior of a student with emotional and behavior challenges. *Journal of Applied Behavior Analysis, 27,* 7–20.

Laidlaw, E.N., Skok, R.L., & McLaughlin, T.F. (1993). The effects of notetaking and self-questioning on quiz performance. *Science Education, 77,* 75–82.

Lentz, F.E. (1988). On-task behavior, academic performance, and classroom disruptions: Untangling the target selection problem in classroom interventions. *School Psychology Review, 17,* 243–257.

Mace, F.C. (1994). The significance and future of functional analysis methodologies. *Journal of Applied Behavior Analysis, 27,* 385–392.

Mace, F.C., Lalli, J.S., & Pinter-Lalli, E. (1991). Functional analysis and the treatment of aberrant behavior. *Research in Development Disabilities, 12,* 155–180.

Miller, D.L., & Kelley, M.L. (1994). The use of goal setting and contingency contracts for improving children's homework performance. *Journal of Applied Behavior Analysis, 27,* 73–84.

National Commission on Excellence in Education. (1983) . *A nation at risk.* Washington, DC: U.S. Government Printing Office.

National Education Goals Report. (1994). *Building a nation of learners.* Washington, DC: U.S. Government Printing Office.

Olympia, D.E., Sheridan, S.M., Jenson, W.R., & Andrews, D. (1994). Using student-managed interventions to increase homework completion and accuracy. *Journal of Applied Behavior Analysis, 27,* 85–99.

O'Melia, M.C., & Rosenberg, M.S. (1994). Effects of cooperative homework teams on the acquisition of mathematics skills by secondary students with mild disabilities. *Exceptional Children, 60,* 538–548.

Patton, J.R. (1994). Practical recommendations for using homework with students with learning disabilities. *Journal of Learning Disabilities, 27,* 570–578.

Peterson, L., Homer, A.L., & Wonderlich, S.A. (1982). The integrity of independent variables in behavior analysis. *Journal of Applied Behavior Analysis, 15,* 477–492.

Pieronek, F. (1994, July/August). Using maps to teach note taking and outlining for report writing. *Social Studies, 48,* 165–169.

Skinner, C.H., Belfiore, P.J., & Watson, T.S., (1995). Assessing the relative effects of interventions in students with mild disabilities: Assessing instructional time. *Assessment in Rehabilitation and Exceptionality, 2,* 207–220.

Spires, H.A., & Stone, P.D. (1989). The directed notetaking activity: A self-questioning approach. *Journal of Reading, 33,* 36–39.

Stallings, J. (1980, December). Allocated academic learning time revisited, and beyond time on task. *Educational Researcher, 9,* 11–16.

Trammel D.L., Schloss, P.J., & Alper, S. (1994). Using self-recording, evaluation, and graphing to increase completion of homework assignments. *Journal of Learning Disabilities, 27,* 75–81.

Waldron, K.A. (1996). *Introduction to special education: The inclusive classroom.* Boston: Delmar.

Bibliography

Baer, D.M., Wolf, M.M., & Risley, T.R. (1987). Some still current dimensions of applied behavior analysis. *Journal of Applied Behavior Analysis, 20,* 313–327

Cooper, L.J., Wacker, D.P., Sasso, G.M., Reimers, T.M., & Donn, L.K. (1990). Using parents as therapists to evaluate the appropriate behavior of their children: Application to a tertiary diagnostic clinic. *Journal of Applied Behavior Analysis, 23,* 285–296.

DiVesta, F.J., & Gray, S.G. (1972). Listening and note taking. *Journal of Educational Psychology, 63,* 8–14.

Frederick, W.C., & Walberg, F. (1980). Learning as a function of time. *Journal of Educational Research, 73,* 183–204.

Kazdin, A.E. (1982). *Single-case research designs: Methods for clinical and applied settings.* New York: Oxford University Press.

Mastropieri, M.A., Scruggs, T.E., & Levin, J.R. (1985). Memory strategy instruction with learning disabled adolescents. *Journal of Learning Disabilities, 18,* 94–100.

Shapiro, E.S., & Lentz, F.E. (1986). Functional assessment of the academic environment. *School Psychology Review, 15,* 346–357.

Skinner, B.F. (1950). Are theories of learning necessary? *Psychology Review, 57,* 193–216.

Skinner, B.F. (1971). The shame of American education. *The American Psychologist, 39,* 947–954.

Sulzer-Azaroff, B., & Mayer, R.G. (1986). *Achieving educational excellence: Using behavioral strategies.* New York: Holt.

Wahler, R.G., & Fox J. (1981). Setting events in applied behavior analysis: Toward a conceptual and methodological expansion. *Journal of Applied Behavior Analysis, 14,* 327– 338.

Walberg, H.J. (1984). Improving the productivity of America's schools. *Educational Leadership, 41,* 19–30.

6

Attention/Concentration Problems

GEORGE J. DuPAUL AND KATHRYN E. HOFF

Introduction

Attention and concentration problems are among the most common behavior control difficulties exhibited by children and adolescents. Although attention problems typically are manifested across home, school, and community settings, these problems are most prominent in the classroom. Attention problems at school are represented by a variety of behaviors, including inconsistent completion of assigned seat-work, vision directed toward noninstructional activities (e.g., staring out the classroom window), and an inabililty to recall instruction and/or task directions. Among secondary school students, attention problems are manifested by poor organization skills such as not having appropriate materials for class, lack of homework completion, inconsistent and inefficient studying behavior, keeping an incomplete notebook, and failing test performance particularly on timed examinations. As a result, attention problems typically lead to impaired academic and social functioning (Barkley, 1990; DuPaul & Stoner, 1994).

Attention problems frequently are associated with high rates of impulsive behavior and physical activity (Achenbach, 1991). In the psychiatric nomenclature, the combination of significant inattention, impulsivity, and overactivity is referred to as Attention-Deficit/Hyperactivity Disorder, or ADHD (American Psychiatric Association, 1994). Impulsive behavior is characterized by the completion of work in a careless fashion, calling out without teacher permission, interrupting class activities and conversations, and engaging in physically dangerous acts without considering harmful consequences (e.g., running into the street to chase a ball). Overactivity is manifested by getting out of one's seat without permission, running about or climbing on furniture in the classroom, high rates of talking and noisemaking, and excessive movements of arms and legs while seated.

Research utilizing behavior rating scales completed by parents and teachers indicates that target behaviors in the inattention domain and behaviors in the impulsive-overactive domain are highly correlated (e.g., Achenbach, 1991; DuPaul, 1991). Although the behaviors comprising the category of ADHD are quite common in isolation, their combination at a high frequency is purported to occur in only 3% to 5% of the school-aged population, with boys outnumbering girls by approximately 5:1 (Barkley, 1990).

Most of the research examining the etiology of attention problems and ADHD has been conducted in the biomedical community. Therefore, investigations have been directed toward the roles of genetic factors, neuroanatomy, and neurotransmitters in the causation of behaviors comprising this syndrome (Hynd, Hern, Voeller, & Marshall, 1991). Although far from conclusive, the extant research literature indicates a strong association between neurological and familial-hereditary factors and the display of ADHD-related behaviors in both children and adults (Anastopoulos & Barkley, 1988). Nevertheless, it is important to point out that investigations in this area have been fraught with methodological difficulties that limit definitive conclusions. Further, there is no known

GEORGE J. DuPAUL AND KATHRYN E. HOFF • School Psychology Program, Lehigh University, Bethlehem, Pennsylvania 18015-4793.

Handbook of Child Behavior Therapy, edited by Watson and Gresham. Plenum Press, New York, 1998.

connection between the putative physiological cause of ADHD-related behaviors and treatment planning (Barkley, 1990).

Although physiological factors are associated with attention problems and ADHD, it is the interaction between these within-child variables and environmental stimuli that leads to the dysfunctional behaviors comprising this disorder (Barkley, 1990; DuPaul & Stoner, 1994). Both antecedent and consequent events are critical in determining the severity of attention problems, impulsive behavior, and high-rate physical activity. Important antecedent events that affect the probability of ADHD-related behaviors include the type of commands or instructions a child is given, the degree to which a child is supervised during independent work, and the number of children present during instruction (Barkley, 1990). A number of factors affect the degree to which consequences control behaviors related to attention and impulsivity, including the latency between behavior and consequent events, the frequency of reinforcement, how salient the consequences are to the child, and the manner in which verbal reprimands are delivered (Pfiffner & Barkley, 1990). Certainly the environmental factors just listed affect the behavior of all children; however, the behaviors of children with attention problems appear to be much more sensitive to these events.

Children who display high rates of ADHD-related behaviors also tend to exhibit problems in at least three key areas: academic achievement, aggression, and peer relationships (Barkley, 1990; DuPaul & Stoner, 1994). It is estimated that nearly 80% of children diagnosed with ADHD are underachieving academically (Cantwell & Baker, 1991). Presumably, this academic underachievement is due to the low rates of attention to instruction and to independent work that are associated with this disorder. Further, a significant minority (i.e., 20–30%) of children with ADHD are classified as "learning disabled" because of deficits in the acquisition of specific academic skills (DuPaul & Stoner, 1994).

The high correlation between overactivity and aggression is well documented in the research literature (Loney & Milich, 1982). The problems in the aggressive domain that are most frequently associated with ADHD include defiance or noncompliance with authority figure commands, display of angry verbal outbursts, and argumentativeness. In addition, more serious antisocial behaviors (e.g., stealing, lying, physical fighting) are displayed by approximately 25% of adolescents diagnosed with ADHD (Barkley, Fischer, Edelbrock, & Smallish, 1990). Thus, it should come as no surprise that youngsters with attention problems often encounter difficulties making and keeping friends. For instance, a number of studies have found uniformly high rates of peer rejection for children displaying ADHD-related behaviors (e.g., Milich & Landau, 1982; Pelham & Bender, 1982).

The behaviors comprising ADHD must be differentiated from similar behaviors that are due to other causes. First, it is not unusual to find concentration difficulties among children with academic skills deficits or learning disablities (DuPaul & Stoner, 1994). These attention and behavior control problems are presumably a manifestation of the frustration the student encounters during academic tasks. In a child with learning disabilities, attention problems are much less pervasive across time and settings than is the case for a student who is displaying inattention in the context of ADHD. A second possiblity is that the child is encountering emotional difficulties (e.g., depressive or anxiety-related behaviors) that have led to problems with concentration and behavior control. In such cases, the attention or concentration problems would be of recent onset and would be less pervasive over time and across settings relative to students diagnosable with ADHD. Finally, environmental factors such as poor or inconsistent academic instruction and/or ineffective behavior management can result in the display of attention and concentration problems. Whenever high rates of inattention and related behavior problems are occurring in only one or two classroom situations (e.g., math class), it is highly probable that such behaviors are primarily due to the quality of instruction and of behavior management in that situation.

Behaviors associated with ADHD typically begin during the preschool years and extend into adolescence (Weiss & Hechtman, 1993). In fact, 70% to 80% of elementary school students with ADHD will continue to exhibit significant deficits in attention, and greater impulsivity, relative to their classmates during adolescence (Barkley et al., 1990). Approximately 50% of these children will continue to display attention difficulties into adulthood (Barkley, 1990). In addition to continued ADHD-related behaviors, teenagers with this disorder are at higher than average risk for the display of anti-social behaviors, school suspensions, school drop-out, and, perhaps, substance abuse (Weiss & Hechtman, 1993). Unfortunately, it is quite clear that the prescription of psychostimulant medication (e.g., Ritalin) in isolation does little to affect the prognosis of individuals with this disorder (Barkley, 1990). Although longitudinal investigations of mul-timodal interventions (e.g., stimulant medication, behavior modification at home and school, aca-demic tutoring) have not been completed to date, it is presumed that nothing less than a long-term, multi-push treatment will be effective in altering the negative prognosis for children displaying ADHD-related behaviors.

The purpose of this chapter is to guide prac-titioners through several stages of assessment and intervention with the overriding goal being the amelioration of ADHD-related behaviors in class-room settings. These stages include problem identifi-cation, problem analysis, plan implementation, and plan evaluation. Activities at each stage will be delin-eated and illuminated through the use of case exam-ples. The chapter concludes with directions for future research and a bibliography of suggested readings.

Problem Identification

In the assessment of ADHD-related behaviors, a multimethod assessment approach is advocated (Barkley, 1990; DuPaul & Stoner, 1994). Multiple informant reports can yield a valuable sampling of behavior across situations, as well as help deter-mine environmental contingencies maintaining that behavior, thoughts related to the problem, areas of strengths and weaknesses, and settings in which attention/concentration problems may be exacer-bated. Based on the data yielded by these measures, an appropriate intervention can then be determined.

In the problem identification phase, the use of interviews, direct observation data, and standard-ized measures are all essential. They will be re-viewed in the following sections within the context of a behavioral consultation model. Further, devel-opmental considerations and factors for differential diagnosis will be discussed.

Interviews

Interviews are an invaluable tool for gaining information about the child and the nature of the problem behavior. In a comprehensive assessment, it is recommended that an interview be conducted with both the child's parents and the classroom teacher. Although past investigations have found low agreement between informants, this should not invalidate the use of a particular source (i.e., by assuming that they may be providing unreliable in-formation). Rather, the discrepancy between infor-mants may be a result of different behaviors being displayed across settings, as well as differing per-ceptions of the behavior across informants (e.g., Achenbach, McConaughy, & Howell, 1987).

Parent Interview

A parent interview provides valuable informa-tion regarding both the strengths and weaknesses of the child. An interview with the parents should be conducted to obtain relevant historical and develop-mental information about the child. Specifically, parents can provide information about the develop-mental and medical history of the child, such as the age of early milestones (e.g., walking, talking) or medical complications. Inquiring about the child's behavior at school can elicit information on the chronicity of school problems and can reveal any past assessments conducted on academic difficul-ties or inattentive behavior (Guevremont, DuPaul, & Barkley, 1990). Questioning parents on the child's behavior at home provides an indication of the chronicity and severity across home and school environments. For example, parents can be asked if attention/concentration problems are present when a child is doing homework or chores.

An example of a structured parent interview can be found in the appendix. This interview form was developed for use in conjoint behavioral consultation wherein teachers and parents systematically work to-gether with a consultant to address social, behavioral and/or academic concerns (Sheridan, 1993).

Teacher Interview

An interview with the child's classroom teacher is critical in determining the extent of the ADHD-related behaviors. A systematic problem-solving approach as described by Bergan and Kratochwill (1990) is a straightforward and effective method to use. Employing this semistructured interview technique (see the appendix) yields specific information regarding academic and behavior problems (e.g., magnitude, frequency), and typical classroom settings where problems may be exacerbated. Through this interview, the child's behavior is specified in concrete behavioral terms, rather than global statements. For example, rather than stating "Kelly does not pay attention," the interviewer would probe to eventually obtain a statement such as, "When Kelly is asked to do independent reading seat-work, she does not look at the work approximately 60% of the time, and only 40% of the work is completed." The teacher also is asked to identify antecedents and consequences of inattentive behavior, and to identify potential sequential conditions (e.g., time of day or day of week when behavior is most likely to occur). Typical antecedent events associated with inattentive behavior include the teacher instructing the class or asking the class to complete independent seat-work. Examples of consequent events that could be paired with inattentive behavior include incompletion of work (i.e., escape), laughter from peers, or verbal reprimands from the teacher.

When conducting a teacher interview, it also is crucial to ask about differences in attention and concentration across settings and as a function of varying situational demands. Inattentive behaviors typically do not manifest themselves in a consistent manner across settings. Rather, they fluctuate depending on environmental demands and expectancies within that environment. For example, an environment that provides more frequent reinforcement may elicit a greater frequency of attentive behaviors. In more restrictive settings, children with ADHD typically exhibit more disruptive behavior than do their normal counterparts, whereas in less structured settings (e.g., free play), differences in behavior across the two groups are much less apparent (Barkley, 1985). Further, inattentive behaviors may vary in frequency across different settings, academic subjects, or teachers. Teacher responses during the problem identification interview can serve as a guide to determine the settings in which to conduct direct observations of behavior.

Behavior Rating Scales

There are several advantages to using rating scales as part of a multimethod assessment for students exhibiting ADHD-related behaviors. Questionnaires can be used as reliable and valid indices of the general severity of the behavior difficulties in relation to a child's normative peers. Rating scales also provide information about general internalizing or externalizing problems that may be of concern. Finally, these measures are easy to obtain, and thus are very cost effective. Several well-standardized broad band, narrow band, and measures of associated difficulties are available for the assessment of ADHD-related behaviors. Some of the more common measures are mentioned briefly below; however, for a more in-depth review of these measures, the reader is referred to Barkley (1990).

Broad Band Scales

Broad band behavior rating scales provide information regarding parent and teacher perceptions of a wide range of possible behavior difficulties, including internalizing problems, aggression, and inattention. Measures in this category include the Child Behavior Checklist (CBCL; Achenbach, 1991), the Child Behavior Checklist—Teacher Report Form (Achenbach, 1991), the Behavior Assessment System for Children (Reynolds & Kamphaus, 1992), the Conners Parent and Teacher Rating Scales (Goyette, Conners, & Ulrich, 1978), and the Revised Problem Behavior Checklist (Quay & Peterson, 1983).

Narrow Band Scales

Narrow band rating scales provide specific information regarding parent and teacher perceptions of key ADHD-related behaviors. Examples of questionnaires in this category include the ADHD Rating Scale–IV (DuPaul, Anastopoulos, Power, Murphy, & Barkley, 1995), the Attention Deficit Disorder Evaluation Scales (McCarney, 1989), the ADD-H Comprehensive Teacher Rating Scale (Ullmann, Sleator, & Sprague, 1985), the Home and School Situations Questionnaires (Barkley, 1981) and the Revised Home and School Situations Questionnaires (DuPaul & Barkley, 1992).

Self-Report Questionnaires

Although children generally underreport externalizing behaviors (e.g., Landau, Milich & Widiger, 1991), they may provide information not easily obtained from parents or teachers. For example, children may provide important information regarding the presence and/or severity of internalizing problems (i.e., depression, anxiety) or covert antisocial behaviors (e.g., stealing, drug abuse). An example of a comprehensive self-report questionnaire is the Child Behavior Checklist-Youth Self-Report (CBCL-YSR; Achenbach, 1991) which can be completed by older children and by adolescents (i.e., those 11 years old or older).

Social Skills Assessment

Attention difficulties may be associated with significant social skills deficits and peer rejection (Landau & Moore, 1991). Unfortunately, few studies and interventions have examined peer relationships among students with attentional difficulties. Within a multmodal, multi-informant assessment protocol, however, it is important to gather information about this domain of functioning. Sociometric status can be assessed using a variety of peer-referenced assessment techniques, such as paired comparisons, peer assessment, peer nominations, peer ratings, and "mixed" assessments (for a discussion of the preceding techniques, see McConnell & Odom, 1986). All of these techniques involve collecting data from a group of individuals, and then converting these scores to measures of social functioning or sociometric status for each child (Gresham & Little, 1993). The decision about which peer assessment technique to use, however, depends on a variety of factors, such as the population being assessed and the length of time between assessments. Peer assessment measures also are associated with different psychometric characteristics. For example, the paired comparison test (McConnell & Odom, 1986) and peer rating techniques (Gresham & Little, 1993) appear to be the most reliable sociometric measures.

The use of peer nominations involves children answering questions, such as "Name three children you like to play with the most" and "Name three children you like to work with the most." Another type of sociometric measure is the use of peer ratings. For example, Asher and Dodge (1986) describe a procedure wherein every student rates his or her classroom peers on a 1–5 scale regarding how much she or he likes to play with and work with each child.

Although peer assessment data provide useful information, there are few empirical studies documenting their psychometric properties (McConnell & Odom, 1986). Further, they are time-consuming to obtain. A more efficient technique in targeting problem areas may be teacher ratings regarding the frequency and importance of specific social behaviors. A number of psychometrically sound instruments are available, including the Social Skills Rating System (Gresham & Elliott, 1990) and the Walker-McConnell Scale of Social Competence and School Adjustment (Walker & McConnell, 1988). Also, Demaray and colleagues (1995) have comprehensively reviewed available questionnaires. These instruments allow the teacher to identify a child's specific social skills deficits and/or suggest targets for intervention.

Direct Observation

Although informant reports are invaluable strategies in providing information about problem behaviors, these reports may be biased and do not provide information that is sufficient or specific enough for delineating targets for intervention. There are a variety of methods for coding direct observations of ADHD-related behaviors. These include the ADHD Behavior Coding System (Barkley, 1990), the Hyperactive Behavior Code (Jacob, O'Leary, & Rosenblad, 1978), and the Classroom Observation Code (Abikoff, Gittelman-Klein, & Klein, 1977). A review of the observation codes for ADHD found that children with ADHD could be distinguished from normal controls on measures of activity, inattention, and vocalizations, particularly when data were collected in school settings (Platzman et al., 1992).

Direct observations can focus on providing a quantitative measure of attentive behaviors, while also affording the opportunity to collect data on permanent products of behavior (e.g., rates of task completion and/or accuracy). It is important to observe the target behavior(s) in a variety of settings to provide a representative sampling of the behavior. For example, many students with ADHD perform inefficiently under less supervised conditions (e.g., independent seat-work) and behave more like their normal peers when being instructed on a one-to-one basis (Barkley, 1990). Observations should be conducted during both large- and small-group activities to gain an adequate sampling of behavior. Further, observations should be conducted at various time periods, as some children may be more attentive in the morning hours, while exhibiting more frequent off-task behavior after lunch (Porrino et al., 1983; Zagar & Bowers, 1983). Finally, it may be helpful to have the teacher identify a normative comparison peer (i.e., a typical student of the same gender) to determine the extent to which the target student deviates from his or her classmates.

Assessment of Academic Performance

Although many children with ADHD are referred for disruptive or inattentive behaviors, these children often also fall behind in their academic work. Children with attention problems have been found to employ inefficient and unorganized strategies for learning (Barkley, 1990). In addition, academic performance difficulties may be indicative of a learning problem. Thus, for many children exhibiting attention difficulties, an assessment of academic performance is necessary. Measures of academic functioning should help to determine whether the student is exhibiting a performance deficit, a skill deficit, or both (DuPaul & Stoner, 1994). Although direct observations may provide useful indirect data in this domain, often these data are not sufficient to pinpoint the nature of the child's academic difficulties. For example, a child may appear "on-task" to the observer, but may have a poor work completion rate or complete work inaccurately. Thus, it is helpful to obtain permanent product data regarding the amount of assigned work attempted during the observational session, as well as the percentage of items completed accurately. Contemporaneous data from the child's classmates can be collected to establish the deviance in academic productivity or accuracy difficulties. An observation of the academic environment should also be conducted across various academic periods (Shapiro, 1989). Curriculum-based measurement probes (Shinn, 1989) can be used to determine if the child

is being instructed at an appropriate place in the curriculum. Finally, teacher ratings on the Academic Competence subscale of the Social Skills Rating System or on the Academic Performance Rating Scale (DuPaul, Rapport, & Perriello, 1991) can be used to further pinpoint academic difficulties.

Developmental Considerations

When assessing attention/concentration problems, developmental factors should be taken into account. Specifically, there may be problems with potentially overidentifying attention and activity problems in preschoolers, due to the typically high activity levels exhibited by young children (Hinshaw, 1992). Alternatively, ADHD-related difficulties may be underidentified among adolescents, due to the covert nature of these problems in this age group (Barkley, 1990). As a general rule, developmental factors are addressed by using measures that have adequate norms broken down by age and gender. Further, assessment measures should have a high test–retest reliability in order to help determine whether the problem is merely a transient phenomenon, or is a more chronic concern. For example, levels of attention increase with age, and concerns regarding distractibility will obviously differ as a function of whether one is evaluating a preschooler or adolescent. To determine whether a problem exists, the practitioner needs to examine both the frequency and intensity of the problem behavior, and consider whether the problem is typical for a given age group and the problematic environment. Young children (i.e., preschool-aged) are especially prone to exhibiting variant behaviors across settings and adult caretakers. It is important to obtain the views of the older child or adolescent through an interview and administration of self-report questionnaires (DuPaul, Guevremont, & Barkley, 1991; Shelton & Barkley, 1990). Finally, interview and rating scale data should be obtained from several teachers when assessing a secondary-school student (DuPaul et al., 1991).

Differential Diagnosis of Inattentive Behavior

Problems with inattention may co-exist with a variety of other concerns, such as learning problems and anxious or depressive behaviors (DuPaul

& Stoner, 1994). In conducting a comprehensive assessment for problem identification, it is important to rule out competing hypotheses as to the origins of inattentive behavior. Attention problems may be a symptom of another disorder (e.g., depression), a manifestation of frustration due to a learning problem, or a reflection of an occurence within the child's environment (e.g., parental marital difficulties). For example, a child who is depressed may exhibit the same level of inattentive behaviors in the classroom as a child with ADHD. Therefore, in the problem identification stage, the teacher interview should elicit responses which may determine whether inattentive behaviors are a manifestation of another problem. Specifically, the teacher should be questioned as to whether inattentive behaviors occur more often during a specific subject, or whether there are significant stressors in the child's environment that have occurred during the past six months (e.g., divorce, move). This type of differentation can assist in guiding problem analysis and treatment planning, as different problems may require a specific mode of intervention (e.g., academic remediation) or a more comprehensive form of treatment (e.g., inclusion of pharmacotherapy).

Problem Analysis

The primary goal of the problem analysis stage is to ascertain the function(s) of a student's inattention and related behavior difficulties. Initially, a teacher interview is conducted to review data collected during the problem identification phase, to examine antecedent, sequential, and consequent conditions that may be associated with the behavior(s), and to brainstorm alternative treatment strategies to be implemented during the next stage (see Bergan & Kratochwill, 1990). Given that ADHD-related behaviors typically are exhibited across school and home settings, it may be fruitful to conduct a problem analysis interview jointly with the teacher and parent, using conjoint behavior consultation procedures as described by Sheridan (1993).

Through examination of antecedent and consequent events, hypotheses regarding the function(s) of ADHD-related behaviors can be developed. In our experience, we have found the following to be the most common hypothesized functions for inat-

tentive and disruptive behaviors displayed in classroom settings. The most likely function for inattentive behavior is to *escape effortful tasks*, particularly those that involve independent writing activity (e.g., seat-work). This is based on the assumption that presenting independent work is an antecedent for inattention which is followed by a lack of work completion. A second possible function is to *gain teacher and/or peer attention*. A frequent consequent event for inattention and disruption is a verbal reprimand from the teacher as well as nonverbal (e.g., smiles) and verbal reactions (e.g., laughter) from the student's classmates. An additional possible function of inattention is an increase in *sensory stimulation* that appears more reinforcing than do the stimuli that the student is expected to attend to. For example, when presented with a set of written math problems to complete, the student begins playing with a toy that he kept in his pocket. It is important to note that developing hypotheses as to behavioral functions is an idiographic process; thus, practitioners must form these hypotheses on an individual basis, using interview and observation procedures as described in the following discussion.

Descriptive Functional Analysis

Once initial hypotheses regarding the function of inattentive behavior are developed, additional data are gathered in the context of a descriptive functional analysis through semistructured interviews with the teacher (Dunlap et al., 1993) and student (Kern, Dunlap, Clarke, & Childs, 1995). In addition, observations are conducted regarding the student's classroom behavior in relation to antecedent and consequent events, using the observation form presented in Form 6.1. Data are used to confirm or disconfirm hypothesized functions of behavior, and alternative hypotheses are formulated for testing during the experimental functional analysis stage.

Ervin, DuPaul, Kern, and Friman (1996) conducted descriptive and experimental functional analyses with four boys diagnosed as ADHD and Oppositional Defiant Disorder (ODD). To provide an example of a descriptive functional analysis, we will examine the results of this analysis for one of the boys, Joey (age 13) who attended a middle school affiliated with a residential program for

FORM 6.1. Behavior Tracking Form

Youth's name: _____   Date: _____

Setting: <u>School</u>   Observer(s): _____

Behaviors & time of day			Situation/ antecedents			Get/ obtain			Escape/ avoid			Actual consequences		

a. not following instructions promptly | a. problems at home | a. teacher attention | a. avoids task | a. point loss

b. off-task looking looking | b. homework incomplete | b. peer attention | b. delays task | b. loss of free time

c. off-task motor | c. writing task | c. playing with object | c. escapes writing | c. accepting feedback

d. not on-time | d. verbal instruction | d. | d. delays consequence | d. office referral

e. homework incomplete | e. reading task | e. | e. | e. prompt

f. neatness (problem) | f. | f. | f. | f.

Comments/Concerns: _____

_____

_____

youth with family difficulties. Joey exhibited a variety of inattentive behaviors (e.g., looking out the window, playing with his pencil or other objects, sharpening his pencil excessively) that were hypothesized to be motivated by escape. Teacher interview and direct observation data indicated that these inattentive behaviors were reliably preceded by the teacher asking Joey to complete an independent writing task. During the student interview, Joey indicated that writing and English were his least favorite subjects and that he disliked writing intensely. Further, he stated that he would prefer to talk about things rather than write about them, and that he needed more time to think prior to beginning writing.

In Joey's case, a convergence among data gathered through direct observation, as well as teacher and student interviews, provided several important pieces of information. First, the function of his inattentive behavior was to escape assigned tasks. Second, a reliable antecedent of this behavior was the presentation of written tasks in the areas of reading and English. Finally, teacher and student interviews provided leads as to possible interventions that could reduce inattentiveness. More specifically, written tasks could be modified to be less aversive to Joey and he could be provided with a greater opportunity to think prior to writing. These ideas were used to formulate alternative hypotheses that were formally tested during the experimental functional analysis stage.

Experimental Functional Analysis

During this stage of problem analysis, one or more hypotheses are developed that are tested primarily through the collection of direct observation data. These hypotheses should delineate possible environmental conditions under which the inattentive behavior will change in a specified direction. Then these environmental conditions are systematically manipulated to determine whether reliable changes in off-task behavior are elicited.

Given the information obtained through the descriptive analysis, two hypotheses were formulated regarding Joey's inattentive behaviors. First, it was hypothesized that "Joey's off-task behavior will be reduced when he is given the opportunity to complete long (20 minutes or greater) writing tasks on the computer rather than by hand." An alternative writing method was posited to decrease the aversiveness of the task and thereby reduce the probability of escape behavior. The computer was chosen as the alternative writing method, given the availablity of a computer in the classroom and Joey's stated preference for this method. The direct observation data displayed in the top graph of Figure 1 are supportive of this hypothesis. The percentage of intervals in which Joey *did not* exhibit inattentive behaviors during long writing tasks was higher when he used the computer ($M = 96.8\%$) than when he was required to complete the task by hand ($M = 64.8\%$).

A second hypothesis was that "Joey's inattentive behaviors will be reduced when he is able to brainstorm with a peer prior to a short (i.e., 5 to 7 minutes) written task vs. when he is not allowed to brainstorm." Joey's teacher believed that he was more likely to be actively engaged in a short writing task if he participated in a discussion about the topic prior to writing. This was corroborated by Joey's belief that he needed more time to think prior to writing. The most feasible way for the teacher to ensure that Joey would think about what he was going to write was to have him spend a few minutes discussing his topic with a peer prior to beginning the assignment. Direct observation data confirmed this hypothesis (see bottom graph of Figure 1). The percentage of intervals in which Joey *did not* exhibit inattentive behaviors was higher when he discussed the topic with a peer prior to writing ($M = 91.4\%$) vs. when no discussion was allowed ($M = 63.2\%$).

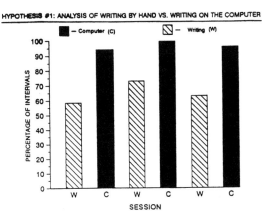

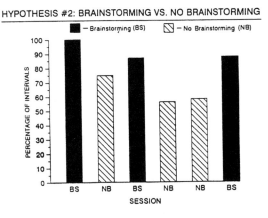

FIGURE 1. Results of an experimental functional analysis of two hypotheses for a 13-year-old boy diagnosed with ADHD. From Ervin et al., 1996.

Ideally, data gathered during the experimental analysis stage will be used to devise a plan that is formally evaluated at the next stage (see plan implementation). One of the primary concerns is how to determine when enough data have been gathered prior to the formal design and implementation of a treatment plan. Unfortunately, there are no empirically derived guidelines for use in making this decision in relation to ADHD-related behaviors. In lieu of empirically based guidelines, several considerations can guide clinical judgment in this area. First, one can determine how consistent the data are across sources of information. When agreement among teacher, student, and observational data is high (e.g., all agree that behavior is motivated by escape), then data collection at this stage may be relatively brief. Second, the stability of the observation data can be examined. The greater the stability across observation sessions, the fewer the data points that are necessary prior to plan implementation. In similar fashion, the greater the difference in behavior between the environmental conditions being manipulated, the fewer the observation sessions that are necessary. For example, in Joey's case, there were stark differences in his behavior under varying conditions, which were reliable across observation sessions. Thus, we did not need to conduct more than six observations for each hypothesis.

Plan Implementation

From a behavior analytic perspective, the primary functions of ADHD-related behavior are to (a) escape from effortful tasks, (b) gain attention from peers or adults, and/or (c) obtain sensory stimulation. Thus, to be effective, interventions must help the individual to exhibit functionally equivalent behaviors that are considered to be appropriate for the given circumstances. For example, in Joey's case he was able to escape the handwritten writing task by completing it under less aversive conditions. Based on the experimental analysis, an intervention that involved the combination of computer-completed tasks and peer discussion was implemented and found effective (see "Plan Evaluation").

In general, empirical investigations have documented the effectiveness of behaviorally based in-

terventions in the amelioration of ADHD-related behaviors (Barkley, 1990; DuPaul & Stoner, 1994). More specifically, contingent positive reinforcement and response cost techniques have been associated with clinically significant reductions in attention problems, with concomitant increases in academic productivity and accuracy (for review see Fiore, Becker, & Nero, 1993). Presumably these interventions increase the stimulation value of an assigned task (i.e., lower the probability of escape behavior) and/or teach the child that the display of appropriate behavior will result in access to attention from teachers or peers. Although fewer studies have addressed the manipulation of antecedent events in enhancing attentive behaviors, certain academic interventions (e.g., peer tutoring) also have been associated with positive results (e.g., DuPaul & Henningson, 1993). Antecedent-based interventions may increase the stimulation value of academic tasks and/or provide more opportunities to gain attention from others in the environment.

Most of the research on behavioral interventions for attention problems has been conducted in school settings or has involved clinic-based parent training. For the purposes of this chapter, we will focus on classroom-based interventions; however, similar techniques have been taught to parents for use in changing home behavior (see Anastopoulos & Barkley, 1990 for details). It should also be noted that school-based interventions have been primarily investigated in laboratory-school or special-education settings. In fact, DuPaul and Eckert (1995) found that approximately 60% of the extant studies have been conducted outside of general-education classrooms. Thus, when designing an intervention plan, the practitioner must be cognizant not only of the function of problematic behavior, but of the practicality and acceptability of the proposed intervention for the person(s) who are implementing the plan. Unfortunately, what has been found to be effective in controlled investigations is not always acceptable to our consumers (i.e., teachers and parents).

In this section, we discuss the most effective antecedent-based and consequent-based interventions for reducing attention problems. Further, we will provide specific details of what we believe to be the best options in each category. The importance of assessing treatment integrity will be delineated, along with some examples of how to assess integrity in a practical fashion. Finally, steps in planning for maintenance and generalization will be discussed. It is our contention that ADHD-related behaviors are optimally addressed through the manipulation of both antecedent and consequent events over a long time period. Given the chronicity and complexity of these problem behaviors, a less intensive intervention plan is likely to fail.

Antecedent-Based Interventions

Over the years, a number of task-related and instructional modifications have been suggested for the prevention of significant attentional difficulties (Barkley, 1990; DuPaul & Stoner, 1994). Suggested modifications have included (a) reducing the amount of seat-work or homework, (b) ensuring student understanding prior to beginning a task, (c) providing extra time for the completion of tests and/or long-term assignments, (d) posting rules with frequent reminders of expectations for rule-following behavior, and (e) teaching study skills and notetaking strategies. Unfortunately, most of these strategies have not been subjected to empirical scrutiny, at least not in the context of helping students with attentional problems.

Among the few antecedent-based interventions that have undergone empirical investigation are peer tutoring and allowing students to choose task activities. ClassWide Peer Tutoring (CWPT), as described by Greenwood, Delquadri, and Carta (1988), has been found to enhance the mathematics, reading, and spelling skills of students of all achievement levels (see for review, Greenwood, 1991). CWPT includes the following steps: (a) dividing the class into two teams; (b) within each team, classmates form tutoring pairs; (c) students take turns tutoring each other; (d) tutors are provided with academic scripts (e.g., math problems with answers); (e) praise and points are contingent on correct answers; (f) errors are corrected immediately with an opportunity for practicing the correct answer; (g) teacher monitors tutoring pairs and provides bonus points for pairs that are following prescribed procedures; and (h) points are tallied by individual student at the conclusion of each session. Tutoring sessions typically last 20 minutes with an additional 5 minutes for charting progress and

putting materials away. At the conclusion of each week, the team with the most points is applauded by the other team. Points are not usually exchanged for any back-up reinforcement.

Recently, the effects of CWPT on the attentional behavior and academic accuracy of students exhibiting significant ADHD-related behaviors have been investigated. DuPaul, Hook, Ervin, and Kyle (1995) found that the active engagement of 19 elementary-school-aged children (16 boys, 3 girls; M age = 7.5) with ADHD increased from an average of 21.6% during baseline to an average of 82.3% when CWPT was implemented by their general education teachers. Observational data were collected in a continuous fashion for each student in the context of an ABAB reversal design. In Figure 2, data for 3 children clearly demonstrate the effectiveness of this intervention. In addition, children's weekly posttest scores rose from an average of

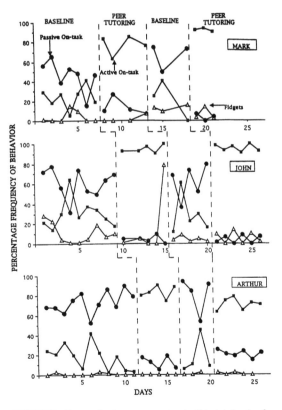

FIGURE 2. Rates of task engagement and off-task behavior for three children with ADHD as a function of baseline and Class-WidePeer Tutoring (CWPT) conditions. From DuPaul et al., 1995.

55.2% during baseline to 73% for CWPT conditions, thus indicating that this intervention affected both attentional behavior and academic performance. These results should not be surprising, given that peer tutoring incorporates strategies (e.g., provision of immediate, frequent feedback about performance, and the receipt of peer attention) known to optimize the performance of children with attention problems.

An advantage of some antecedent-based interventions is the ease with which they can be implemented in general education classrooms. For example, Dunlap and colleagues (1994) systematically varied whether independent tasks were teacher-assigned or were chosen by students from a menu. Rates of task engagement and disruptive behavior were functionally related to the manipulation of teacher vs. student choice, with the latter leading to higher levels of engagement and lower levels of disruptive behavior. Results for an 11-year-old boy with ADHD in the context of an ABAB reversal design are presented in Figure 3. It should be noted that this boy was being treated with desipramine 75 mg throughout this investigation, yet an environmental manipulation was necessary to elicit acceptable levels of task engagement.

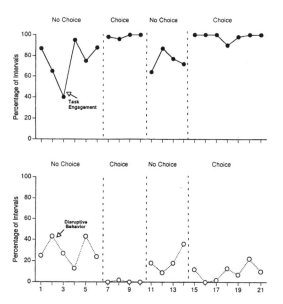

FIGURE 3. Percentage frequency of task engagement and disruptive behavior for a 12-year-old boy with ADHD as a function of teacher choice and student choice conditions. From G. Dunlap et al., (1994). Reprinted by permission.

Consequent-Based Interventions

There are two primary consequent-based approaches that are effective in addressing inattention and related behavior problems, including positive reinforcement contingent on the display of appropriate levels of attention and the use of response cost contingent upon off-task behavior. Typically, a combination of the two approaches will be optimal.

As is the case for most target behaviors, token reinforcement programs that target task-related attention and productivity typically lead to increases in these behaviors. The development of a token reinforcement program involves several steps. First, specific target behaviors must be delineated. It is best to follow the "dead man's" rule (Lindsley, 1991) in deciding which behaviors to target. This rule states that if a dead man can perform a behavior, then it is not a good target for intervention. Thus, the program will ultimately be more effective if it targets active, appropriate responding (e.g., completion of assigned work), rather than the lack of problematic behavior (e.g., stay in seat). The second step is to develop a menu of back-up reinforcers that can be earned. Our experience is that it is best to include a variety of preferred activities as reinforcers rather than concrete rewards, which many adults view as contrived attempts at "bribery." Also, the child should be involved in the selection of reinforcers. Finally, the specific time periods and/or situations for program implementation must be scheduled. To lessen the burdens on the teacher (and thereby increase the acceptability of intervention), it is best to initially implement the system for a short duration each day (e.g., during one academic period). As success is obtained, gradual implementation across settings and times could be accomplished. To achieve optimal treatment integrity, the practitioner must balance the comprehensiveness of treatment coverage with its acceptability by those who are implementing it.

Response cost, as it is typically implemented, involves providing an individual with a set number of token reinforcers at the outset of an activity and deducting tokens contingent on the display of inappropriate behavior (Kazdin, 1984). A variant of this procedure has been found effective for classroom use with students who are exhibiting attentional difficulties (e.g., Rapport, Murphy, & Bailey, 1982). The response cost tactic employed by Rapport et al. includes a number of steps. As is the case for a token reinforcement system, target behaviors and back-up reinforcers must be specified. Also, specific situations (e.g., independent seat-work) where the response cost system will be implemented are delineated. The student starts the work period with 0 points and is able to earn points periodically (e.g., once per minute) so long as she or he is exhibiting the target behavior (e.g., attending to seat-work). The teacher must award points on an interval schedule, thus necessitating periodic monitoring of the child's behavior. If the child exhibits significant off-task behavior, a point is deducted by the teacher. At the end of the specified work period, the student is able to exchange his or her final net points for a certain amount of time of a preferred activity.

This response cost procedure has been found to elicit on-task behavior equivalent to that associated with stimulant medication (Rapport et al., 1982). In addition, response cost plus positive reinforcement has been found superior to positive reinforcement alone in the maintenance of on-task behavior (Sullivan & O'Leary, 1990). Although under ideal circumstances practitioners would prefer to use positive reinforcement procedures in isolation, mild punishment strategies such as response cost appear necessary for many students with significant attentional problems. Further, response cost is acceptable to both students and teachers when it is delivered in the context of a management program weighted heavily in favor of positive reinforcement. In other words, the ratio of reinforcer delivery to response cost should be high (e.g., 3:1 or 4:1) and if a student consistently "zeroes out" in points, then the program components should be modified.

Treatment Integrity

In much of the behavioral intervention literature, the integrity of the independent variable (i.e., the degree to which the treatment was delivered as intended) has been sorely neglected (see Gresham, 1989; Peterson, Homer, & Wonderlich, 1982). Yet it is critical that adherence with intervention procedures not only be evaluated but also that procedures are used to increase the probability that treatment steps will be implemented correctly. Although treatment integrity is a universal issue, it is particularly important when designing interventions for children with attentional difficulties. ADHD-related behaviors tend to be chronic over time and are dis-

played across multiple settings. This necessitates the implementation of interventions by parents and teachers across multiple environments for a very long time. This is an enormously time-consuming enterprise that is all too easy to abandon, even if positive outcomes are achieved. Clearly, if integrity is not addressed in a proactive fashion, successful outcomes will be compromised.

Typically, treatment integrity is assessed through the completion of a checklist of intervention procedures during randomly selected treatment sessions (see Gresham, 1989, for details). An example of a treatment integrity checklist that we have used to monitor teacher implementation of CWPT procedures is displayed in Form 6.2. This checklist can be completed by an independent observer (e.g., school psychologist), the teacher, or even the identified student. Data can be compiled from completed checklists to determine: (a) the average percentage of steps adhered to across sessions and (b) the percentage of sessions where each specific step is implemented correctly. This provides valuable information on which steps, if any, need to be reviewed with the treatment implementer. For example, one might determine that an average of 90% of CWPT steps are completed with integrity, with most individual steps completed with 90% or greater accuracy. Further, it may be determined that one specific step (e.g., providing bonus points to tutoring pairs) is implemented at lower integrity levels, thus necessitating a reminder to the teacher to follow this step.

Beyond the ongoing assessment of treatment integrity, it is important to incorporate certain practices in the design of interventions to increase the probability of proper implementation (see Table 1). First, implementation planning should be a collaborative process between the consultant (e.g., school psychologist) and treatment implementer (e.g., teacher). For example, a brainstorming session could be utilized to generate as many intervention ideas as possible. Then the teacher selects the most acceptable, practical, and, it is hoped, effective intervention or combination of strategies. Second, acceptability of the intervention strategy should be assessed prior to beginning the treatment. Several checklists (e.g., Intervention Rating Profile-15; Witt & Elliott, 1985) are available for this purpose. Next, whenever possible, the emphasis should be on the manipulation of antecedent stimuli. Strategies such as task modifications, allowing task choices, and even peer tutoring

FORM 6.2. Teacher Monitoring Form

	Not at all	Somewhat	Very much	Not applicable
Target child _____ Date of observation _____				
Teacher _____ Tutor _____				
1. The teacher has instructional script(s) prepared.	0	1	2	NA
2. The teacher provided the appropriate amount of material to be tutored.	0	1	2	NA
3. The teacher periodically monitored the tutoring session.	0	1	2	NA
4. The teacher provided bonus points to tutors when appropriate.	0	1	2	NA
5. The teacher praised the efforts of the tutoring pair.	0	1	2	NA
6. The teacher provided assistance, when necessary.	0	1	2	NA
7. The teacher kept the tutoring pair on-task.	0	1	2	NA
8. The teacher signaled the students to switch roles.	0	1	2	NA
9. The teacher recorded points.	0	1	2	NA
10. The teacher charted progress.	0	1	2	NA

TABLE 1. Intervention Design Factors that Enhance Treatment Integrity

- Include treatment implementer (e.g., teacher, student) in intervention planning process
- Evaluate acceptability of intervention prior to implementation
- Emphasize manipulation of antecedent stimuli (e.g., task modifications)
- Initally implement interventions during a single academic period rather than entire school day
- Target behaviors that the teacher already monitors and that are considered important (e.g., permanent products like completed tasks)
- Design interventions that include the entire class rather than requiring an exclusive focus on a single student (e.g., ClassWide Peer Tutoring)
- Use available activities as reinforcers
- Provide feedback/reinforcement for accurate implementation
- Meet periodically to monitor progress and modify the intervention plan
- When working with a team, first take the path of least resistance

involve less time than typical consequent-based interventions. The less time involved, presumably the greater the integrity with which the intervention will be carried out. Further, it may be overwhelming to ask the teacher to implement the intervention for an entire school day. The teacher is more likely to follow through with the plan if she or he is doing so for only a segment of the day, at least initially.

Another factor that may enhance treatment integrity is the selection of target behaviors. Rather than asking a teacher to monitor how well as student pays attention (a cumbersome task, at best), the consultant should choose a behavior (e.g., task completion or percentage accuracy) that is already evaluated by the teacher. These targets typically have the additional advantages of not violating the "dead man's" rule, they reliably covary with attentive behavior, and they must be considered important by the teacher (otherwise, why would it be measured?).

Interventions that target a single student in a classroom of 25 to 35 children may be burdensome for the teacher to implement in the context of other duties. Thus, a teacher may be more likely to implement the strategy if she or he feels that it is benefiting the whole class (or small groups of students), so long as it is not too time-consuming. An example would be the use of CWPT, wherein students of all achievement levels participate.

Several other factors may enhance treatment integrity. Classroom activities (e.g., playing educational games, use of computer) are preferred as reinforcers over concrete rewards that may require teacher expense or may raise philosophical objections (e.g., reinforcement as bribery). Further, treatment strategies are more likely to be followed accurately when the implementer receives feedback about performance. Following treatment integrity checks, teachers should be provided with specific information about what they are doing well and the steps they need to improve upon. Periodic meetings should be held to monitor progress, modify the intervention plan, and provide feedback to the teacher about implementation. Feedback about treatment adherence is even more valuable when it is paired with reinforcement. Although this is not always feasible when working with adults, it is an important consideration when students are the primary intervention implementers. For example, bonus points provided to tutoring pairs can enhance student adherence with CWPT procedures.

Students, particularly at the secondary level, are taught by multiple teachers, all of whom may implement the intervention with varying levels of integrity. As a general rule, teachers who are most resistant to the intervention at the outset (i.e., find the plan to be unacceptable) are the least likely to follow procedures accurately. For this reason, it is generally a good idea to take the path of least resistance during the beginning stages of intervention. Initially, the plan would be implemented by the most flexible teacher, even if the student does not display his or her most significant behavioral difficulties in that class. As the plan is successful, it is gradually implemented by the more resistant faculty members. If generalization planning (discussed later) is carefully done, by the time the intervention is to be implemented by the most resistant teacher, the treatment has been modified to be less time- and resource-intensive than it was in the initial implementation.

Planning for Generalization

As is the case for the behavioral intervention literature in general, very few school-based intervention studies targeting students with attentional difficulties have assessed or explicitly programmed for generalization. In fact, DuPaul and Eckert (1995) found that fewer than 20% of studies in this area even included a follow-up assessment phase. Thus, beyond the recommendations offered in seminal articles by Stokes and Baer (1977), as well as Stokes and Osnes (1989), there is little in the published literature to guide practitioners in generalization programming. Beyond these general guidelines, it may be helpful to consider treatment methods that gradually transfer evaluation and reinforcement from an external agent (e.g., teacher) to the individual with attention problems.

Self-management interventions include strategies designed to teach individuals to monitor, evaluate, and reinforce their own behaviors. These strategies can be divided into two major groups: those that are cognition-based (e.g., self-instruction training) and those that are contingency-based (Shapiro & Cole, 1994). Although cognition-based approaches have been relatively unsuccessful in the treatment of ADHD (see Abikoff, 1985), a few empirical studies have supported the effectiveness of contingency-based, self-management approaches with this population (e.g., Barkley, Copeland, & Sivage, 1980; Hinshaw, Henker, & Whalen, 1984).

Hoff and DuPaul (1996) conducted a controlled case study of a contingency-based, self-management program for three children exhibiting significant ADHD-related behaviors in general-education classrooms. These children participated in several treat-

FORM 6.3. Self-Management Rating Criteria

5 = Followed classroom rules (see below) entire interval

4 = Minor infraction of rules (e.g., talked out of turn); followed rules remainder of interval

3 = Did not follow all rules for entire time, but no serious offenses

2 = Broke one or more rules to extent behavior was unacceptable (e.g., physically aggressive with classmate), but followed rules remainder of interval

1 = Broke one or more rules almost entire interval or engaged in higher degree of inappropriate behavior most of the time

0 = Broke one or more rules entire interval

Classroom rules:
1. Talking to classmates allowed only during group discussions.
2. Keep hands to self and own property unless you ask for teacher permission.
3. Follow teacher directives.

ment phases, beginning with a teacher-managed token reinforcement program and proceeding through successive stages of self-evaluation and self-reinforcement (a modification of procedures first reported by Rhode, Morgan, & Young, 1983). Prior to the first stage of self-management, each student was trained by the teacher to recognize target behaviors associated with ratings from 0 to 5 (see Form 6.3). These behaviors were modeled for the child, and the latter also role-played target behaviors while stating the rating associated with the behavior. During the first stage of self-management, the student and teacher independently rated the student's performance during one academic period. Ratings were compared wherein (a) if student rating was within one point of teacher's, the student kept the points he gave himself; (b) if student rating matched teacher's exactly, he received the points he gave himself plus one bonus point; and (c) if student and teacher ratings deviated by more than one point, then no points were awarded. As in the token reinforcement phase, points were exchanged on a daily basis for preferred activities.

During successive stages of the treatment, the frequency of teacher-student matches was gradually reduced to 0%. For example, during the 50% match stage, a coin was flipped following each rating period wherein the student was required to match the teacher an average of 50% of the time. Given that the outcome was random and unpredictable, the student could not assume prior to the coin flip that he didn't have to match the teacher's rating. On the occasions where he didn't have to match, the student automatically kept the points he gave himself. Figure 4 displays data for one of the students from Hoff

and DuPaul (1996) across self-management phases. Generalization across settings was programmed for and systematically evaluated. The data show that this student was able to maintain behavioral improvements initially elicited under token reinforcement, despite the fading of teacher feedback. It is important to note that by the end of the study, the student continued to provide written ratings of his performance and continued to receive back-up contingencies. The ideal outcome would be for written

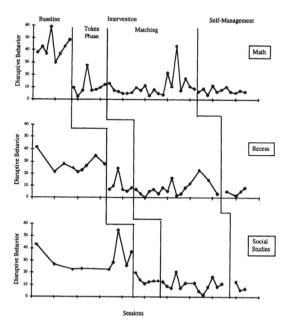

FIGURE 4. Percentage of disruptive behavior during a self-management intervention for an 8-year-old boy with ADHD across math, recess, and social studies periods. From Hoff & DuPaul, 1996.

ratings to be faded to oral ratings while back-up contingencies are phased out.

For some students exhibiting ADHD-related behaviors, the process of teaching self-management (i.e., achieving generalization across time and settings) will take several months, whereas for others this will take several school years. Unfortunately, for some youngsters with more severe attentional problems, this process may be a lifelong affair. Nevertheless, a contingency-based, self-management protocol may be a viable option for promoting the generalization of behavior change obtained under teacher-directed procedures.

Summary of Plan Implementation

ADHD-related behaviors typically are exhibited over long time periods and across multiple settings. Thus, intervention plans must be designed for long-term implementation and must include multiple components. Clearly, from a behavioral perspective, the most effective components will be contingent reinforcement and response cost as well as the manipulation of antecedent events (e.g., through the provision of academic instruction that takes the student's attention problems into account). In fact, school-based interventions that are contingency-based and/or include modifications of academic instruction are associated with large effect sizes (i.e., .69 to .94) that are significantly greater than effect sizes associated with cognitive–behavioral techniques (DuPaul & Eckert, 1995).

It should be acknowledged that psychostimulant medication (e.g., Ritalin or methylphenidate) is frequently administered to individuals exhibiting ADHD-related behaviors. Approximately 70% to 80% of children treated with methylphenidate demonstrate significantly greater levels of task-related attention and are much less impulsive and overactive (Barkley, DuPaul, & Costello, 1993). Research studies that have investigated the combination of behavioral interventions and stimulant medication have consistently documented that the combination of treatments is superior to either treatment in isolation (see, for review, Pelham & Murphy, 1986).

If one accepts the hypothesis that some children diagnosed with ADHD are "stimulation seekers" for biological reasons (Zentall & Meyer, 1987), then one of the purported functions of ADHD-

related behavior (i.e., to seek sensory stimulation) may be, in part, due to brain physiology. That is, brain physiology may affect the likelihood that stimulation-seeking behavior will occur, particularly in situations where the individual is faced with boring stimuli (e.g., independent seat-work). Stimulant medication may alter this behavior by temporarily changing the individual's brain functioning. Based on these assumptions as well as the extant literature, it our contention that the manipulation of environmental stimuli will be a necessary and sufficient treatment for some children with ADHD. Alternatively, other children (i.e., those who exhibit a greater number and/or frequency of ADHD-related behaviors) will require manipulation of both environmental and physiological events through the combination of behavioral interventions and medication. Finally, it is *never* appropriate to treat inattention and related behavior problems solely through the temporary alteration of physiological functioning (i.e., by using medication in isolation).

Plan Evaluation

Treatment Effectiveness

Evaluation of treatment effectiveness is essential to determine both the success of the intervention and to establish experimental control. Specifically, it must be determined that behavioral changes were caused by the employed intervention. Ideally, one should establish that no factors other than the intervention accounted for the behavior change (i.e., establish internal validity). Single subject design methodologies should be employed to establish whether treatment gains can be attributable to the intervention, rather than to chance or other environmental variables (see Kazdin, 1992). The most effective way to do this is by briefly returning to baseline conditions by either withdrawing or withholding treatment (i.e., ABA or reversal design). In some cases, the withdrawal of treatment will not be acceptable to the teacher and/or may not be considered ethical. In such cases, multiple baseline or changing criterion designs can be used. Unfortunately, in many instances the practitioner must use an AB or case study design that does not control for potential threats to internal validity. Nevertheless, there are several ways (e.g., collection of continuous data, phase changes planned in advance) to enhance the validity of the case study design (see Bergan & Kratochwill, 1990).

Direct observations of behavior typically provide the primary outcome data. These data are used to answer the question, "Did the intervention produce the desired changes within the classroom?" Statistics typically employed in single subject design research should be calculated for the baseline, treatment, and generalization/maintenance phases to assess quantitative changes in behavior as a result of the intervention. Specifically, the changes in mean performance and intercept across baseline and intervention phases should be calculated. Further, the trend of the data should also be graphed to determine if there are changes in the slope or rate of behavior change. For example, similar means may be obtained across the intervention and withdrawal phases, but there may be an increasing trend in the behavior during baseline, with a decreasing trend in the behavior associated with treatment. In addition to changes in the mean, intercept, and trend, it also is important to evaluate the variability of performance. For example, a student may be on-task an average of 70% of the time, but this behavior may range from 20% to 90%. This would indicate the need to continue the intervention, to stabilize behavior at a higher rate. Finally, the investigator should look at the percentage of nonoverlapping data points (Scruggs, Mastopieri, & Casto, 1987). This is the percentage of data points across the baseline and intervention phases that did not overlap (i.e., that were different).

An example of outcome data for a classroom intervention plan implemented for Joey is presented in Figure 5. Based on the data obtained during the problem analysis stage, an intervention was designed for writing class that involved the combination of brainstorming ideas with a peer and completing written assignments on a computer. An ABAB reversal design was employed wherein baseline phases were alternated with intervention phases. During the initial baseline phase, the percentage of intervals *without* off-task behaviors was variable and trending downward, with a mean of 67.7% (range: 54.2% to 83.3%). When the intervention was implemented, there was an immediate and stable increase in the percentage of intervals in which Joey did not engage in off-task behavior (*M*

= 96%; range: 93.7% to 98.3%). When the intervention was withdrawn for one day, the percentage of intervals without off-task behavior decreased to 62.7%. Once the intervention was reimplemented, Joey's behavior improved to a mean level of 95.4% (range: 90.7% to 98.7%). The percentage of nonoverlapping data points between baseline and intervention phases was 100%.

In addition to direct observations of behavior, narrow-band standardized assessment measures (e.g., behavior rating scales) can be used to evaluate treatment effects. Narrow-band measures can be used to document perceived treatment change and may be more sensitive to treatment effects than are broad-band rating scales or psychological tests. Behavior ratings are administered during both the baseline and intervention phase of the intervention to document treatment-related changes. Further, teacher ratings may also be used to determine whether skills or behaviors were transferred across settings and/or maintained over time. In using narrow-band measures, one must select appropriate outcome measures that are related to the skill targeted for change (e.g., academic measure if target is academic performance). Finally, some studies have shown a regression to the mean artifact when behavior ratings are completed on more than one occasion, even in the absence of treatment (Barkley, 1988). Thus, ratings should be completed on at least two occasions during baseline, with the latter results being compared to ratings collected during the treatment phase.

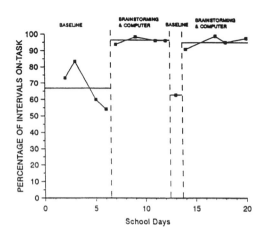

FIGURE 5. Results of intervention evaluation for Joey. Percentage of intervals without off-task behaviors are shown for writing class. Horizontal lines denote mean level of intervals without off-task behaviors during each condition. From Ervin et al., 1996.

When Intervention Doesn't Work

Due to the inherent variability of ADHD-related behaviors, there may be a plethora of reasons an intervention does not work initially. For example, the treatment may not be comprehensive enough, motivational factors may preclude client cooperation, or the treatment could be implemented with low treatment integrity. One plausible solution for an unsuccessful intervention is to modify the student's motivation level. More specifically, the reinforcement schedule may need to be modified, at least initially, to occur more frequently. A study conducted by Rapport, Tucker, DuPaul, Merlo, and Stoner (1986), for example, found that children with ADHD chose smaller, more immediate rewards, rather than waiting for two days to obtain larger rewards. Douglas (1984) posited that children with ADHD seek more continuous reinforcement, and when this frequency is decreased, these children become highly frustrated and their motivation to perform is thereby diminished. Reinforcer satiation may also occur. To address this issue, the practitioner should use a reinforcer menu developed mutually by the teacher and child wherein specific reinforcers are rotated periodically.

Fading the Program

Treatments that combine positive reinforcement with mild punishment strategies may be more easily faded than programs that include positive reinforcement alone. A study conducted by Sullivan and O'Leary (1990) found that response cost and token reinforcement both were effective in increasing on-task behavior among a small sample of children with ADHD. The researchers found, however, that the children who were rated as aggressive and hyperactive did not maintain gains during the withdrawal phases of the reward program. The authors noted that they employed a short fading period, and suggested that changes in the frequency of feedback may have contributed to these differences. Further, they found children who had received both response cost and reward were likely to maintain gains in on-task behavior when rewards were withdrawn.

A study conducted by Rosen, O'Leary, Joyce, Conway, and Pfiffner (1984) found that there was a decrease in on-task behavior and academic productivity when there was a cessation of negative consequences, whereas the withdrawal of positive reinforcers had no effect on performance. Past research has also demonstrated that children with ADHD typically perform better with a response cost program, rather than with the use of only positive reinforcement strategies. Although a program that exclusively relies on aversive procedures is certainly not advocated (by us or other researchers), mild punishing contingencies may be important to the fading process. Further, children with attention problems may also need more frequent "booster sessions" during the fading/generalization phase, with fading conducted over a long time period.

Treatment Integrity

With constraints on time and resources in the classroom, the teacher may eventually deviate from specific intervention procedures. To reduce nonadherence with treatment, the practitioner should devise a checklist of the intervention steps so that teachers can self-monitor their completion of intervention steps. To further ensure integrity, one must set up contacts with the teacher and conduct integrity checks, as described in the plan implementation section.

Social Validation

Social validation of the intervention is important to determine if treatment-related changes were of applied or clinical importance (Kazdin, 1982). Within the classroom, this can easily be done in two ways: by social comparison or by subjective evaluation. To employ a method of social comparison, data are collected on a target child who exhibits "typical" on-task behavior, work completion, etc. The typical child's behavior can then be used as a guide to determine whether the target student's behavior has changed to a level similar to his or her classroom peers. For example, if a child's on-task behavior increased from 30% to 60%, but the class norm was 80%, a discrepancy remains, and there is a need to continue and/or to modify the intervention.

A subjective evaluation can be used to determine whether the teacher or parents see qualitative differences in the behavior after the intervention and whether they are satisfied with the treatment outcomes and procedures. That is, if the person coming in contact with the child (i.e., teacher, parent) views the behavior change as sufficient and thinks that the goal of the intervention was attained, this serves to establish the social validity of the program. One way this can be accomplished is through the use of behavior rating scales. For example, if the intervention was to increase attentive behavior, the teacher could be given the Conners scale to complete before and after the intervention to see whether differences in behavior are perceived. A subjective evaluation can also be obtained through consumer satisfaction surveys completed by the teacher and child to determine how well they liked the intervention, if they would perform/participate in the intervention again, and whether they would recommend the intervention to others.

Maintenance and Generalization

Assessment of maintenance and generalization of the intervention effects should be conducted over time and across settings. Unfortunately, this step is often ignored; omitting this process results in short-term remedies with no evidence for long-term gains. In a literature review conducted by Abikoff (1985), only 30% of 23 studies of cognitive treatment for ADHD included follow-up or maintenance assessment. Similar findings were obtained by Du-Paul and Eckert (1995) in their meta-analysis of 77 studies of school-based interventions for students with ADHD. Practitioners should have a planned follow-up period wherein the intervention is evaluated approximately 1 or 2 months after the program is terminated. When assessing behavior over long follow-up periods, one must consider developmental changes as a possible variable accounting for maintenance or lack thereof.

Summary and Directions for Future Research

Difficulties with concentration and attention are among the most common problems exhibited by children and adolescents in classroom settings. In a small percentage of cases, attention difficulties are associated with significant impulsivity and overactivity (i.e., symptoms of ADHD). Given the typical chronicity of ADHD-related behaviors and their association with significant difficulties in academic and social functioning, it is important for practition-

ers to address these behaviors with a long-term plan that is implemented across settings. In this chapter, we have provided suggestions for assessment and intervention related to ADHD in the context of the four stages of behavioral consultation. The nature and extent of attention difficulties are delineated in the problem identification stage. Next, the function of ADHD-related behaviors relative to environmental antecedents and consequences is determined through problem analysis activities. Based on these assessment data, an intervention plan is designed and implemented. The most effective plans incorporate the manipulation of both antecedent and consequent events. Targets for treatment should include both behavior difficulties *and* academic performance, as enhancement of the latter often leads to reductions in the former. Finally, data are collected on an ongoing basis to determine whether the plan is effective and what modifications are necessary.

Most of the outcome studies examining interventions for ADHD-related behaviors have examined the utility of psychostimulant medications, with methylphenidate (Ritalin) being the most widely studied (Barkley, 1990). This research has documented quite clearly that methylphenidate can be effective for a majority of youngsters diagnosed with ADHD. Unfortunately, there is a dearth of research on the effectiveness of nonpharmacological treatments for this disorder. For example, while there are literally hundreds of studies examining the efficacy of methylphenidate, DuPaul and Eckert (1995) were able to locate only 77 investigations (conducted over a 29-year period from 1966 to 1995) of classroom-based interventions for ADHD. Thus, there is an obvious need for more research on psychosocial interventions. Further, the psychosocial intervention literature is dominated by studies of consequent-based interventions, such as token reinforcement programs. The few studies that have involved the manipulation of antecedent events (e.g., providing choices, instructional intervention) have yielded promising results; however, additional investigations in this area are sorely needed. From a practitioner's perspective, the need for development of effective antecedent-based interventions is particularly acute, given that token reinforcement and response cost strategies are difficult to implement with integrity in many school settings.

The most intractable attention difficulties will require a combination of intervention strategies that is implemented across home, school, and community settings. Yet, most outcome studies have evaluated a single intervention implemented in one setting for a short period of time. Empirical data are necessary to determine (a) the optimal method(s) for identifying environmental events to manipulate, (b) the best combination of antecedent- and consequent-based interventions to address the varying functions of attentional difficulties, (c) methods of introducing interventions sequentially across settings and caretakers, (d) ways of enhancing the treatment integrity among several individuals, all of whom are implementing multiple interventions, and (e) optimal strategies for modifying interventions over time to enhance maintenance and generalization. At a more general level, the time has come for researchers to go beyond showing that methylphenidate helps children to pay attention or that positive reinforcement and response cost can ameliorate disruptive behavior. Practitioners require empirical guidelines that can lead to effective, long-term, multimodal intervention plans to address the complexities of ADHD-related behavior difficulties exhibited across the lifespan.

APPENDIX: Problem Identification Interview (PII)

Consultant note: The purposes of the PII are to:

—Define the problem(s) in behavioral terms.

—Provide a tentative identification of behavior in terms of antecedent, situation, and consequent conditions.

—Provide a tentative strength of the behavior (e.g., how often or severe).

—Establish a procedure for collection of baseline data in terms of the sampling plan, what, who, how the behavior is to be recorded.

The consultant should question and/or comment in the following areas:

1. Opening salutation

2. General statement to introduce discussion:
   (e.g., "Describe Diane's hyperactive behavior."
     "Let's see, you referred Johnny because of his poor self-concept, lack of progress, and rebellious behavior. Which of these do you want to start with . . . ? Describe Johnny's rebellion [self-concept or lack of progress in the classroom].")

   Record responses:

   _____

   _____

   _____

3. Behavior specification:
   (e.g., "What does Charles do when he is hyperactive?"
     "What does Mary do when she is disrespectful?")
   (A precise description of the behavior of concern to the consultee/client; e.g., What does _____ do?)

   a. Specify examples: _____

   _____

   _____

   _____

   Important: Ask for as many examples of the problem behavior as possible.

   b. Specify priorities _____

   _____

   _____

   _____

   Important: After eliciting all the examples the consultant/client can give, ask which behavior is causing the most difficulty and establish a priority.

   (*Note*: To help prioritize problems, ask consultee/client, "On a scale of 0 to 10 [where 0 = no problem, 10 = severe problem], how severe is the problem for you [the client]?")

4. Behavior setting
(A precise description of the settings in which the problem behaviors occur; e.g., where does _____ do this?)

   a. Specify examples: (e.g., home, where in home, etc.) _____

   _____

   _____

   _____

   Important: Ask for as many examples of settings as possible.

   b. Specify priorities: _____

   _____

   _____

   _____

   Important: After eliciting all the examples the consultee/client can give, ask which setting is causing the most difficulty and establish priorities.

   (*Note*: Settings can be ranked in the same manner as behaviors.)

5. Identify antecedents
(What happens right before the problem behavior occurs?)
(e.g., "What happens before Mary makes an obscene gesture to the rest of the class?"
     "What happens before George begins to hit other children?")

Record responses: _____

_____

_____

_____

6. Sequential conditions analysis
(When during the day does the behavior occur and/or what is the pattern of antecedent–consequent conditions across several occurrences of the problem behavior?).
(e.g., "When does Mary . . . Who is Mary with . . . What is Mary supposed to be doing when . . . ?")

Record responses: _____

_____

_____

_____

7. Identify consequent conditions
(What happens after the problem behavior has occurred?)
(e.g., "What happens after Mary . . . ?")
     "What do the other students do when Charles climbs on the radiator?"
     "What do you do when George hits other children?")

Record responses: _____

_____

_____

_____

8. Summarize and validate antecedent, consequent, and sequential conditions
(e.g., "You've said that you and Timmy argue after you have asked him to do something, and he has refused. The argument continues as long as you try to talk to him. Is that correct?" "You've said that at bedtime you tell Ava that it is time for bed, and that she doesn't answer you. You tell her again, and she says, 'Oh, Mom.' You remind her a third time, and she asks for 10 more minutes. You get mad, threaten to tell her father, and take her physically down to her room. She leaves her room approximately twice, asks for a drink of water, and finally falls asleep. Is that how it goes?")

Record responses: _____

_____

_____

_____

9. Behavior strength
   a. *Frequency*—how often a behavior occurs
      (e.g., "How often does Kevin have tantrums?")
   b. *Duration*—length of time that a behavior occurs
      (e.g., "How long do Craig's tantrums last?")

   Record responses: _____

   _____

   _____

   _____

10. Summarize and validate behavior and behavior strength
    a. "You have said that Jason makes you angry and upset by wetting his bed."
    b. "That he wets his bed approximately four times a week."
    c. "Is that right?"

    Record responses: _____

    _____

    _____

    _____

11. Tentative definition of goal—question
    (e.g., "How often would Patrick have to turn in his work in order to get along OK?"
          "How frequently could Charles leave his seat without causing problems?")

    Record responses: _____

    _____

    _____

    _____

12. Assets question
    (to determine what student is good at)
    (e.g., "Is there something that Mary does well?")

    Record responses: _____

    _____

    _____

    _____

13. Question about approach to teaching or existing procedures
    (e.g., "How long are Charles and the other students doing seat-work problems?" "What kind of . . . ?")

    Record responses: _____

    _____

    _____

    _____

14. Summarization statement and validation
    (e.g., "Let's see, the main problem is that Charles gets out of his seat and runs around the room during independent work
          assignments. He does this about 4 times each day, and . . . , etc. Is that right?")

    Record responses: _____

    _____

    _____

    _____

15. Directional statement to provide rationale for data recording
    (e.g., "We need some record of Sarah's completion of homework assignments . . . how often assignments are completed, what assignments are completed . . . , to determine how frequently the behavior is occurring and it may give us some clues about the nature of the problem. Also, the record will help us decide whether any plan we initiate is effective or not.")

    Record responses: _____

    _____

    _____

    _____

16. Discuss data collection procedures
    (Data can be collected in four ways)—

    a. *Real-time recording:*
       Advantages:
           —provides unbiased estimates of frequency and duration.
           —data capable of complex analyses such as conditional probability analysis.
           —data susceptible to sophisticated reliability analysis.
       Disadvantages:
           —demanding task for observers.
           —may require costly equipment.
           —requires responses to have clearly distinguishable beginnings and ends.

    b. *Event or duration recording:*
       Advantages:
           —measures are of a fundamental response characteristic (i.e., frequency of duration).
           —can be used by participant-observers (e.g., parents or teachers) with low rate responses.
       Disadvantages:
           —requires responses to have clearly distinguishable beginnings and ends.
           —unless responses are located in real time (e.g., by dividing a session into brief recording intervals), some forms of reliability assessment may be impossible.
           —may be difficult with multiple behaviors unless mechanical aids are available.

    c. *Momentary time samples:*
       Advantages:
           —response duration of primary interest.
           —time-saving and convenient.
           —useful with multiple behaviors and/or children.
           —applicable to responses without clear beginnings or ends.
       Disadvantages:
           —unless samples are taken frequently, continuity of behavior may be lost.
           —may miss most occurrences of brief, rare responses.

    d. *Interval recording:*
       Advantages:
           —sensitive to both response frequency and duration.
           —applicable to wide range of responses.
           —facilitates observer training and reliability assessments.
           —applicable to responses without clearly distinguishable beginnings and ends.
       Disadvantages:
           —confounds frequency and duration.
           —may under- or overestimate response frequency and duration.

    Record responses: _____

    _____

    _____

    _____

17. Summarize and validate recording procedures
    (e.g., "We have agreed that you will record the amount of time that Doug's tantrums last by recording the start and stop times. You will do this for three days and you will use this form. You will also record what happens before the behavior occurs and what you do after it has occurred. Is this okay with you?")

Record responses: _____

_____

_____

_____

18. Establish a date to begin data collection

Record responses: _____

_____

_____

_____

19. Establish date of next appointment

Record responses: Date: _____

Day: _____

Time: _____

Place: _____

20. Closing salutation

From T.R. Kratochwill, unpublished manuscript, University of Wisconsin, Madison, WI, reprinted by permission of author.

References

Abikoff, H. (1985). Efficacy of cognitive training intervention in hyperactive children: A critical review. *Clinical Psychology Review, 5,* 479–512.

Abikoff, H., Gittelman-Klein, R., & Klein, D. (1977). Validation of a classroom observation code for hyperactive children. *Journal of Consulting and Clinical Psychology, 45,* 772–783.

Achenbach, T.M. (1991). *Manual for the Child Behavior Checklist and Revised Child Behavior Profile.* Burlington, VT: Author.

Achenbach, T.M., McConaughy, S.H., & Howell, C.T. (1987). Child/adolescent behavioral and emotional problems: Implications of cross-informant correlations for situational specificity. *Psychological Bulletin, 101,* 213–232.

American Psychiatric Association. (1994). *Diagnostic and statistical manual of mental disorders* (4th ed.). Washington, DC: Author.

Anastopoulos, A.D., & Barkley, R.A. (1988). Biological factors in attention-deficit hyperactivity disorder. *Behavior Therapist, 11,* 47–53.

Anastopoulos, A.D., & Barkley, R.A. (1990). Counseling and training parents. In R.A. Barkley (Ed.), *Attention deficit hyperactivity disorder: A handbook for diagnosis and treatment* (pp. 397–431). New York: Guilford.

Asher, S.R., & Dodge, K.A. (1986). Identifying children who are rejected by their peers. *Developmental Psychology, 22,* 444–449.

Barkley, R.A. (1981). *Hyperactive children: A handbook for diagnosis and treatment.* New York: Guilford.

Barkley, R.A. (1985). The social interactions of hyperactive children: Developmental changes, drug effects, and situational variation. In R. McMahon & R. Peters (Eds.), *Childhood disorders: Behavioral–developmental approaches* (pp. 218–243). New York: Brunner/Mazel.

Barkley, R.A. (1988). Attention-deficit hyperactivity disorder. In E.J. Mash & L.G. Terdal (Eds.), *Behavioral assessment of childhood disorders* (2nd ed., pp. 69–104). New York: Guilford.

Barkley, R.A. (Ed.) (1990). *Attention Deficit Hyperactivity Disorder: A handbook for diagnosis and treatment.* New York: Guilford.

Barkley, R.A., Copeland, A., & Sivage, C. (1980). A self-control classroom for hyperactive children. *Journal of Autism and Developmental Disorders, 10,* 75–89.

Barkley, R.A., Fischer, M., Edelbrock, C.S., & Smallish, L. (1990). The adolescent outcome of hyperactive children diagnosed by research criteria: I. An 8-year prospective study. *Journal of the American Academy of Child and Adolescent Psychiatry, 29,* 546–557.

Barkley, R.A., DuPaul, G.J., & Costello, A. (1993). Stimulants. In J.S. Werry & M.G. Aman (Eds.), *Practitioner's guide to psychoactive drugs for children and adolescents* (pp. 205–237). New York: Plenum.

Bergan, J.R., & Kratochwill, T.R. (1990). *Behavior consultation and therapy.* New York: Plenum.

Cantwell, D.P., & Baker, L. (1991). Association between attention-deficit hyperactivity disorder and learning disorders. *Journal of Learning Disabilities, 24,* 88–95.

Demaray, M.K., Ruffalo, S.L., Carlson, J., Busse, R.T., Olson, A.E., McManus, S.M., & Leventhal, A. (1995). Social skills assessment: A comparative evaluation of six published rating scales. *School Psychology Review, 24,* 648–671.

Douglas, V.I. (1984). The psychological processes implicated in ADD. In L.M. Bloomingdale (Ed.), *Attention deficit disorder: Diagnostic, cognitive, and therapeutic understanding* (pp. 147–162). New York: Spectrum.

Dunlap, G., Kern, L., dePerczel, M., Clarke, S., Wilson, D., Childs, K.E., White, R., & Falk, G.D. (1993). Functional analysis of classroom variables for students with emotional and behavioral disorders. *Behavioral Disorders, 18,* 275–291.

Dunlap, G., dePerczel, M., Clarke, S., Wilson, D., Wright, S., White, R., & Gomez, A. (1994). Choice making to promote adaptive behavior for students with emotional and behavioral challenges. *Journal of Applied Behavior Analysis, 27,* 505–518.

DuPaul, G.J. (1991). Parent and teacher ratings of ADHD symptoms: Psychometric properties in a community-based sample. *Journal of Clinical Child Psychology, 20,* 245–253.

DuPaul, G.J., & Barkley, R.A. (1992). Situational variability of attention problems: Psychometric properties of the revised home and school situations questionnaires. *Journal of Clinical Child Psychology, 21,* 178–188.

DuPaul, G.J., & Eckert, T.L. (1995, August). *Classroom intervention strategies for attention deficit hyperactivity disorder: A meta-analysis.* Paper presented at the annual convention of the American Psychological Association, New York.

DuPaul, G.J., & Henningson, P.N. (1993). Peer tutoring effects on the classroom performance of children with attention-deficit hyperactivity disorder. *School Psychology Review, 22,* 134–143.

DuPaul, G.J., & Stoner, G. (1994). *ADHD in the schools: Assessment and intervention strategies.* New York: Guilford.

DuPaul, G.J., Guevremont, D.C., & Barkley, R.A. (1991). Attention deficit hyperactivity disorder in adolescence: Critical assessment parameters. *Clinical Psychology Review, 11,* 231–245.

DuPaul, G.J., Rapport, M.D., & Perriello, L.M. (1991). Teacher ratings of academic skills: The development of the Academic Performance Rating Scale. *School Psychology Review, 20,* 284–300.

DuPaul, G.J., Anastopoulos, A.D., Power, T.J., Murphy, K., & Barkley, R.A. (1995). *ADHD Rating Scale-IV.* Unpublished manuscript, Lehigh University, Bethlehem PA.

DuPaul, G.J., Hook, C.L., Ervin, R., & Kyle, K. (1995, August). *Effects of Classwide Peer Tutoring on students with attention deficit hyperactivity disorder.* Paper presented at the annual convention of the American Psychological Association, New York.

Ervin, R., DuPaul, G.J., Kern, L., & Friman, P. (1996). *A functional assessment of the variables affecting classroom compliance for students with ADHD and ODD: Toward a proactive approach to classroom management.* Unpublished manuscript, Lehigh University, Bethlehem, PA.

Fiore, T.A., Becker, E.A., & Nero, R.C. (1993). Educational interventions for students with ADHD. *Exceptional Children, 60,* 163–173.

Goyette, C.H., Conners, C.K., & Ulrich, R.F. (1978). Normative data on Revised Conners Parent and Teacher Rating Scales. *Journal of Abnormal Child Psychology, 6,* 221–236.

Greenwood, C.R. (1991). Classwide peer tutoring: Longitudinal effects on the reading, language, and mathematics achievement of at-risk students. *Journal of Reading, Writing, and Learning Disabilities International, 7,* 105–123.

Greenwood, C.R., Delquadri, J., & Carta, J.J. (1988). *Classwide peer tutoring.* Seattle, WA: Educational Achievement Systems.

Gresham, F.M. (1989). Assessment of treatment integrity in school consultation and prereferral intervention. *School Psychology Review, 18,* 37–50.

Gresham, F.M., & Elliott, S.N. (1990). *Social skills rating system.* Circle Pines, MN: American Guidance Service.

Gresham, F.M., & Little, S.G. (1993). Peer-referenced assessment strategies. In T.H. Ollendick & M. Hersen (Eds.), *Handbook of child and adolescent assessment.* Boston: Allyn and Bacon.

Guevremont, D.C., DuPaul, G.J., & Barkley, R.A. (1990). Diagnosis and assessment of attention-deficit hyperactivity disorder in children. *Journal of School Psychology, 28,* 51–78.

Hinshaw, S.P. (1992). Academic under achievement, attention deficits, and aggression: Comorbidity and implications for intervention. *Journal of Consulting and Clinical Psychology, 60,* 893–903.

Hinshaw, S.P., Henker, B., & Whalen, C.K. (1984). Self-control in hyperactive boys in anger-inducing situations: Effects of cognitive–behavioral training and of methylphenidate. *Journal of Abnormal Child Psychology, 12,* 55–77.

Hoff, K.E., & DuPaul, G.J. (1996). *Reducing disruptive behavior in general education classrooms: The use of self-management strategies.* Unpublished manuscript, Lehigh University, Bethlehem, PA.

Hynd, G., Hern, K.L., Voeller, K.K., & Marshall, R.M. (1991). Neurobiological basis of attention-deficit hyperactivity disorder (ADHD). *School Psychology Review, 20,* 174–186.

Jacob, R.G., O'Leary, K.D., & Rosenblad, C. (1978). Formal and informal classroom settings: Effects on hyperactivity. *Journal of Abnormal Child Psychology, 6,* 47–59.

Kazdin, A.E. (1982). *Single-case research designs: Methods for clinical and applied settings.* New York: Oxford University Press.

Kazdin, A.E. (1984). *Behavior modification in applied settings* (3rd ed.). Homewood, IL: Dorsey.

Kazdin, A.E. (1992). *Research design in clinical psychology* (2nd ed.). Boston: Allyn & Bacon.

Kern, L., Dunlap, G., Clarke, S., & Childs, K.E. (1995). Student assisted functional assessment interview. *Diagnostique, 19,* 29–39.

Landau, S., Milich, R., & Widiger, T.A. (1991). Conditional probabilities of child interview symptoms in the diagnosis of attention deficit disorder. *Journal of Child Psychology and Psychiatry, 32,* 501–513.

Landau, S., & Moore, L.A. (1991). Social skill deficits in children with Attention-deficit hyperactivity disorder. *School Psychology Review, 20,* 235–251.

Lindsley, O.R. (1991). From technical jargon to plain English for application. *Journal of Applied Behavior Analysis, 24,* 449–458.

Loney, J., & Milich, R. (1982). Hyperactivity, inattention, and aggression in clinical practice. In D. Routh & M. Wolraich (Eds.), *Advances in developmental and behavioral pediatrics* (Vol. 3, pp. 113–147). Greenwich, CT: JAI.

McCarney, S.B. (1989). *The Attention Deficit Disorders Evaluation Scale: School Version.* Columbia, MO: Hawthorne.

McConnell, S.R., & Odom, S.L. (1986). Sociometrics: Peer referenced measures and the assessment of social compctence. In P. Strain, M. Guralnick, & H. Walker (Eds.), *Children's social behavior: Development, assessment, and modification.* Orlando, FL: Academic.

Milich, R., & Landau, S. (1982). Socialization and peer relations in hyperactive children. In K.D. Gadow & I. Bialer (Eds.), *Advances in learning and behavioral disabilities* (Vol. 1, pp. 283–339). Greenwich, CT: JAI.

Pelham, W.E., & Bender, M.E. (1982). Peer relationships in hyperactive children: Description and treatment. In K.D. Gadow & I. Bialer (Eds.), *Advances in learning and behavioral disabilities* (Vol. 1, pp. 365–436). Greenwich, CT: JAI.

Pelham, W.E., & Murphy, H.A. (1986). Attention deficit and conduct disorders. In M. Hersen (Ed.), *Pharmacological and behavioral treatment: An integrative approach* (pp. 108–148). New York: Wiley.

Peterson, L., Homer, A.L., & Wonderlich, S.A. (1982). The integrity of independent variables in behavior analysis. *Journal of Applied Behavior Analysis, 15,* 477–492.

Pfiffner, L.J., & Barkley, R.A. (1990). Educational placement and classroom management. In R.A. Barkley (Ed.), *Attention deficit hyperactivity disorder: A handbook for diagnosis and treatment* (pp. 498–539). New York: Guilford.

Platzman, K.A., Stoy, M.R., Brown, R.T., Coles, C.D., Smith, I.E., & Falek, A. (1992). Review of observational methods in attention deficit hyperactivity disorder (ADHD): Implications for diagnosis. *School Psychology Quarterly, 7,* 155–177.

Porrino, L.J., Rapoport, J.L., Behar, D., Sceery, W., Ismond, D.R., & Bunney, W.E., Jr. (1983). A naturalistic assessment of the motor activity of hyperactive boys. *Archives of General Psychiatry, 40,* 681–687.

Quay, H.C., & Peterson, D.R. (1983). *Interim manual for the Revised Behavior Problem Checklist.* Unpublished manuscript, University of Miami, Miami, FL.

Rapport, M.D., Murphy, A., & Bailey, J.S. (1982). Ritalin vs. response cost in the control of hyperactive children: A within subject comparison. *Journal of Applied Behavior Analysis, 15,* 205–216.

Rapport, M.D., Tucker, S.B., DuPaul, G.J., Merlo, M., & Stoner, G. (1986). Hyperactivity and frustration: The influence of size and control over rewards in delaying gratification. *Journal of Abnormal Child Psychology, 14,* 191–204.

Reynolds, C.R., & Kamphaus, R.W. (1992). *Behavior Assessment System for Children.* Circle Pines, MN: American Guidance Service.

Rhode, G., Morgan, D.P., & Young, K.R. (1983). Generalization and maintenance of treatment gains of behaviorally handicapped students from resource rooms to regular classrooms using self-evaluation procedures. *Journal of Applied Behavior Analysis, 16,* 171–188.

Rosen, L.A., O'Leary, S.G., Joyce, S.A., Conway, G., & Pfiffner, L.J. (1984). The importance of prudent negative consequences for maintaining the appropriate behavior of hyperactive students. *Journal of Abnormal Child Psychology, 12,* 581–604.

Scruggs, T.E., Mastopieri, M.A., & Casto, G. (1987). The quantitative synthesis of single-subject research: Methodology and validation. *Remedial and Special Education, 8,* 24–33.

Shapiro, E.S. (1989). *Academic skills problems: Direct assessment and intervention.* New York: Guilford.

Shapiro, E.S., & Cole, C.L. (1994). *Behavior change in the classroom: Self-management intervention strategies.* New York: Guilford.

Shelton, T.L., & Barkley, R.A. (1990). Clinical, developmental, and biopsychosocial considerations. In R.A. Barkley (Ed.), *Attention deficit hyperactivity disorder: A handbook for diagnosis and treatment* (pp. 209–231). New York: Guilford.

Sheridan, S.M. (1993). Models for working with parents. In J.E. Zins, T.R. Kratochwill, & S.N. Elliott (Eds.), *Handbook of consultation services for children: Applications in educational and clinical settings* (pp. 110–136). San Francisco: Jossey-Bass.

Shinn, M.R. (Ed.) (1989). *Curriculum-based measurement: Assessing special children.* New York: Guilford.

Stokes, T.F., & Baer, D.M. (1977). An implicit technology of generalization. *Journal of Applied Behavior Analysis, 10,* 349–367.

Stokes, T.F., & Osnes, P.G. (1989). An operant pursuite of generalization. *Behavior Therapy, 20,* 337–355.

Sullivan, M.A., & O'Leary, S.G. (1990). Maintenance following reward and cost token programs. *Behavior Therapy, 21,* 139–151.

Ullmann, R.K., Sleator, E.K., & Sprague, R.L. (1985). Introduction to the use of the ACTeRS. *Psychopharmacology Bulletin, 21,* 915–920.

Walker, H.M., & McConnell, S.R. (1988). *Walker-McConnell Scale of Social Competence and School Adjustment.* Austin, TX: Pro-Ed.

Weiss, G., & Hechtman, L. (1993). *Hyperactive children grown up: ADHD in children, adolescents, and adults* (2nd ed.). New York: Guilford.

Witt, J.C., & Elliott, S.N. (1985). Acceptability of classroom management strategies. In T.R. Kratochwill (Ed.), *Advances in school psychology* (Vol. 4, pp. 251–288). Hillsdale, NJ: Erlbaum.

Zagar, R., & Bowers, N.D. (1983). The effect of time of day on problem solving and classroom behavior. *Psychology in the Schools, 20,* 337–345.

Zentall, S.S., & Meyer, M.J. (1987). Self-regulation of stimulation for ADD-H children during reading and vigilance task performance. *Journal of Abnormal Child Psychology, 15,* 519–536.

Bibliography

Barkley, R.A. (Ed.) (1990). *Attention Deficit Hyperactivity Disorder: A handbook for diagnosis and treatment.* New York: Guilford. This book is the most comprehensive guide to ADHD currently available. Clinic-based procedures for assessment and treatment planning are covered in detail.

DuPaul, G.J., & Stoner, G. (1994). *ADHD in the schools: Assessment and intervention strategies.* New York: Guilford. Written for school psychologists and other support personnel, this book provides detailed coverage of school-based assessment and intervention strategies.

Fiore, T.A., Becker, E.A., & Nero, R.C. (1993). Educational interventions for students with ADHD. *Exceptional Children,*

60, 163–173. This article provides a relatively comprehensive review of school-based interventions for students with ADHD. Recommendations for intervention planning are provided.

Paine, S.C., Radicchi, J., Rosellini, L.C., Deutchman, L., & Darch, C.B. (1983). *Structuring your classroom for academic success.* Champaign, IL: Research Press. This classic text provides teachers with numerous ideas on how to promote effective management of classroom learning and behavior. One of the best features of this book is its emphasis on changing antecedent events (e.g., posting rules, arrangment of desks in classroom) to enhance the learning of all children, not just those exhibiting challenging behaviors.

Platzman, K.A., Stoy, M.R., Brown, R.T., Coles, C.D., Smith, I.E., & Falek, A. (1992). Review of observational methods in attention deficit hyperactivity disorder (ADHD): Implications for diagnosis. *School Psychology Quarterly, 7,* 155–177. This review article details the features of a variety of observational coding methods for use in assessing students exhibiting ADHD-related behaviors. The authors highlight three behaviors that best discriminate students with ADHD from their normal counterparts; these are off-task behavior, out-of-seat or fidgeting, and vocalizations.

Rapport, M.D., Murphy, A., & Bailey, J.S. (1982). Ritalin vs. response cost in the control of hyperactive children: A within subject comparison. *Journal of Applied Behavior Analysis, 15,* 205–216. This landmark study provides conclusive evidence supporting the use of response cost procedures to alter the disruptive behavior *and* academic productivity of students with ADHD. Changes in behavior and academics for two students in some instances surpassed treatment effects obtained with methylphenidate (Ritalin).

7

Speech Disfluencies

RAYMOND G. MILTENBERGER AND DOUGLAS W. WOODS

Introduction

Stuttering and cluttering are two prominent types of childhood speech fluency disorders. The disfluencies in cluttering may consist of excessive speed, articulation, phonological and language defects, and lack of awareness (Stansfield, 1988). Although the *Diagnostic and Statistical Manual of Mental Disorders,* third edition, revised (*DSM-III-R*) included cluttering (American Psychiatric Association, 1987), the *DSM-IV* no longer classifies it as a disorder (American Psychiatric Association, 1994). For this reason, and because of the relative paucity of research on cluttering, this chapter will focus on stuttering.

Stuttering (sometimes called stammering) consists of frequent repetitions of speech sounds, syllables, words, or phrases, prolongations of sounds, and/or hesitations in speech that disrupt its rhythmic quality (Leung & Robson, 1990). In addition, some stutterers exhibit secondary tension/struggle behaviors such as reduced eye contact, facial grimacing, head movements, rhythmic body movements, and fear/avoidance responses (Van Riper, 1982).

The incidence, or percentage, of people who have stuttered at any time in their lives, is approximately 10%. This is higher than the prevalence of the problem, which is approximately 1% for the general population (Bloodstein, 1981), and about 5% for preschool children (Leung & Robson, 1990). Stuttering usually begins between the ages of 2 and 6 years,

with the earliest age of onset being about 1.5 to 2 years (Andrews et al., 1983; Homzie & Lindsay, 1984). In childhood, male stutterers outnumber female stutterers 3 to 1. This difference increases with age, and adult male stutterers outnumber adult female stutterers 5 to 1 (Bloodstein, 1981).

Etiology

Physiologically, stuttering stems from a disruption of the airflow involved in speech production. Research suggests that laryngeal muscles tighten at the exact moment of the stutter (Healey, 1991), thus disrupting airflow and, subsequently, speech. Researchers suggest that a genetic component may underlie stuttering, although the means by which it causes the disfluent speech is unclear (Andrews, Morris-Yates, Howie, & Martin, 1991). Recent research also identifies neurological correlates of stuttering, such as problems with interhemispheric lateralization (Webster, 1985, 1986), although it is not clear whether these neurological findings are a cause or an effect of stuttering behavior.

Although there is a large volume of literature regarding the physiology of stuttering, perhaps of greater interest to the behavior analyst are the behavioral explanations which have dominated the theories of stuttering in the past few decades. In most behavioral theories of stuttering, anxiety plays a key role.

Role of Anxiety in Stuttering

Many people think of stutterers as nervous or anxious individuals (Ingham, 1984). However, trait anxiety (Spielberger, Gorsuch, Lushene, Vagg, &

RAYMOND G. MILTENBERGER • Department of Psychology, North Dakota State University, Fargo, North Dakota 58105. DOUGLAS W. WOODS • Department of Psychology, Western Michigan University, Kalamazoo, Michigan 49008.

Handbook of Child Behavior Therapy, edited by Watson and Gresham. Plenum Press, New York, 1998.

Jacobs, 1983), or the tendency to behave anxiously across situations, is not clearly related to stuttering. Some studies have found a relationship between self-reported trait anxiety and stuttering (Craig, 1990), whereas others have not (Blood, Blood, Bennett, & Simpson, 1994).

State, or situation-specific anxiety (Spielberger et al., 1983), seems to play a larger role in stuttering. For example, the stutterer who is asked to give a speech in front of the class may become anxious and stutter more frequently (Ingham, 1984). Likewise, certain speaking situations, such as speaking novel or difficult words or speaking to specific people, appear to be related to increased anxiety and a subsequent increase in the frequency of stuttering (Ingham, 1984).

However, establishing a link between state anxiety and stuttering has been difficult. Ingham and Andrews (1971) demonstrated that, although their treatment reduced stuttering by 99%, the subjects' self-reported state anxiety increased after treatment. The treatment involved delayed or synchronous auditory feedback in which the subject's voice was played back to the subject electronically as he or she spoke. The increase in anxiety following treatment may be attributed to the treatment procedures themselves or to the post hoc assessment of anxiety involving a subjective self-report measure. The apparent lack of a functional relationship between state anxiety and stuttering was also reported by Gray and England (1972).

It is likely that the failure to establish a relationship between stuttering and state or trait anxiety is due to problems with the definition and measurement of anxiety as a construct. However, a relationship between stuttering and anxiety can be established when anxiety is behaviorally defined as increased muscle tension as a component of autonomic arousal. It is clear that the occurrence of the speech disfluency is related to airflow disruption brought on by tension in the vocal musculature. Research has demonstrated that immediately prior to a disfluency, tension in the vocal musculature is increased, and immediately following the response, the tension is reduced. It is likely that stressful situations increase autonomic arousal, which leads to tension in the vocal musculature. Brutten and Shoemaker (1967) have suggested that stressful situations function as conditioned stimuli that elicit autonomic arousal as a conditioned response. When tension in the vocal musculature is a component of the autonomic arousal, the probability of stuttering is increased.

An Operant Model

We propose another model of stuttering etiology based on an operant paradigm. Most children stutter as their speech is developing, and, in fact, up to 10% do it with enough severity at one point in their lives to be classified as stutterers. When parents or others in the verbal community notice the child's disfluency, they may reprimand the child or respond in ways that increase the child's apprehension or physiological arousal in speaking situations. As discussed earlier, this increase in autonomic arousal and tension in the vocal region may result in the increased frequency of stuttering. The stuttering may then be negatively reinforced by the tension reduction in the laryngeal muscles that immediately follows the stutter. This model suggests that the vocal muscle tension functions as an establishing operation (Michael, 1982) that makes tension reduction more reinforcing and increases the momentary probability of stuttering as a behavior that results in tension reduction.

Although automatic negative reinforcement involving tension reduction is one possible explanation for the maintenance of stuttering, one cannot rule out the role of external contingencies in maintaining the behavior. Various studies have demonstrated the control of external stimuli over stuttering (e.g., Flanagan, Goldiamond, & Azrin, 1958, 1959). For example, James (1981) showed that punishment reduced stuttering, and Manning, Trutna, and Shaw (1976) showed that verbal or tangible reinforcement increased fluency rates. Knowing that stuttering can be modified through external contingency manipulation, it is not unreasonable to believe that the behavior may be maintained by similar factors in some children. For example, stuttering may be reinforced by the parent who completes the child's sentence, thereby allowing the child to escape the aversive speaking situation, or by the parent who responds to the child's stuttering with attention in the form of concern or disapproval. Social reinforcement is a possibility that should be considered in the assessment of stuttering.

Covariance with Other Problems

Although there is a belief that stutterers tend to be anxious or depressed individuals, this does not appear to be true (Miller & Watson, 1992). However, even though psychopathology is not more common in children who stutter, the clinician should be aware of problems the child may face as a result of his or her stuttering. First, because specific speaking situations are difficult for the child, the child may avoid such situations. Second, the child may be teased by peers and this reaction from peers could lead to social difficulties, aggressive or antisocial behavior, or increased anxiety or dysphoria.

Differential Diagnoses

Although stuttering is not typically related to organic pathology, hearing impairments and speech-motor impairments may cause stuttering in some cases (American Psychiatric Association, 1994). Before starting treatment, the clinician should seek appropriate assessments to determine the extent to which these may play a role in the stuttering behavior. If one of these problems is causing the stuttering, and if it can be ameliorated, then stuttering treatment would be unnecessary.

Prognosis

Most stutterers will spontaneously recover. In fact, 83% of children who stutter will stop stuttering by the time they are 8 years old (Dickson, 1971). However, even though the chance for spontaneous recovery is high, the child's stuttering should not be ignored. If the stuttering is ongoing for more than 6 to 12 months, it should be treated. Providing treatment early in childhood may prevent the behavior from becoming a chronic problem that would be likely to persist into adulthood.

Because there are so many different treatments for stuttering, it is difficult to provide an accurate relapse rate across all treatments. However, for the regulated breathing approach to be discussed in this chapter, the relapse rate for stuttering is low (e.g., Wagaman, Miltenberger, & Woods, 1995). Although there is little research about the effects of untreated stuttering, it is safe to assume that ignoring the child's speech problem will increase the likelihood of stuttering chronicity, and thus hinder

the child's ability to communicate effectively as an adult.

Problem Identification

Although a clinician may "know" when a child is a stutterer, the behavior analyst should not be satisfied with subjective assessment or clinical impression. To determine whether or not a stuttering problem exists and to judge the effectiveness of treatment, the clinician should collect adequate data, assessing not only speech disfluencies, but secondary struggle behaviors, stuttering duration, generalization effects, and social validity of treatment effects.

Diagnosis

In our opinion, the *DSM-IV* diagnostic criteria that distinguish fluent from disfluent speakers are not adequate. The *DSM-IV* (American Psychiatric Association, 1994) requires that the child meet the following criteria to be diagnosed as a stutterer. First, the child must exhibit frequent deviations from normal age-appropriate fluency and speech rhythms. This must include one or more of the following disfluencies: part-word repetitions, whole-word repetitions, prolongations, interjections, hesitations, blocking, circumlocutions, and/or words spoken with excessive physical tension. Second, the the individual's disfluency must interfere with academic, occupational, or communicative success. Finally, the disfluency should not be the result of a speech–motor impairment or sensory deficit (American Psychiatric Association, 1994).

The ambiguous aspects of this definition of stuttering lie in the first two criteria. Although the topographies of stuttering are adequately represented in the definition, the statement that the child must exhibit "frequent" deviations in fluency allows for much subjective variation in the diagnosis of stuttering. Gagnon and Ladouceur (1992) have found that normal adult speakers are disfluent on ≤ 3% of their syllables. Unfortunately, such normative data do not exist for children. Nevertheless, until such norms are established, it seems reasonable to also apply the 3% criterion to define stuttering in children (Caron & Ladouceur, 1989; Wagaman, Miltenberger, & Arndorfer, 1993).

The second criterion for diagnosing stuttering, that the disfluency must interfere with academic, occupational, or communicative success, also relies on a subjective judgment of the clinician or of the stutterer. We propose that this criterion may be strengthened through social validation in which speech naturalness or the severity of the disfluency is rated by parents and professionals (e.g., Wagaman et al., 1993, 1995). Peers might also participate in social validity assessments by rating the acceptance of their classmate who stutters or by rating the naturalness of the classmate's speech.

Once stuttering is determined to be a problem for the child, based on more objective criteria and systematic social validation assessments, the clinician can then focus on how stuttering behaviors are defined and reliably recorded so that informed treatment decisions can be made.

Defining Stuttering

The first step in assessing speech disfluencies is to operationally define stuttering. We suggest the following operational definitions. *Sound or syllable repetitions* involve repeating the same sound or syllable two or more times in a row. An example of this disfluency is "I p-p-p-ut a nail in the board." *Word repetitions* are defined as repeating the same word two or more times in a row. An example of a word repetition is "I put a nail nail nail in the board." The definition of a *phrase repetition* is repeating the same two or more words two or more times in a row. An example of this type of disfluency is "I put a nail in the in the board."

A *prolongation* is defined as an abnormal extension of a speech sound. Such a disfluency may sound like "I put a nnnnnnnail in the board." Finally, a *hesitation* or *block* in speech that disrupt its rhythmic quality is defined as a pause in speech that is accompanied by observable tension in the facial region. When the sound is emitted, it will often have a forced, explosive quality.

Defining Secondary Behaviors

Secondary behaviors often accompany disfluencies and seem especially prevalent in the presence of hesitations/blocks. Some of the behaviors include, but are not limited to, grimacing, hard extended blinking, and extending the neck. Re-

searchers have described these behaviors as giving the person the appearance of expressing such emotions as excitement, fear, or embarrassment (Webster, 1974).

The etiology of these behaviors and the reason for their persistence are unclear. They may be related to muscle tension in the facial region. Alternatively, they may be superstitious behaviors that have been reinforced by "getting the word out." Imagine a child who is stuttering. He cannot emit the word, but as he grimaces, the word comes out, which then reinforces the grimacing behavior, making it more likely to occur in similar circumstances in the future. Although this is only speculation, it is a conceptually sound explanation from a behavioral perspective.

It is important to assess secondary behaviors, because they may indicate stuttering severity. For example, consider a child who is still stuttering 7% of his words after treatment (as compared to 10% at baseline). By this measure alone, treatment does not appear successful. However, if assessment demonstrates frequent and severe struggle behaviors during baseline but shows no observable tension in the child at the time of the stutter during posttreatment, there is evidence for a beneficial treatment effect.

Collecting Data

We now turn our attention to how data on disfluencies, secondary behaviors, speech rate, and stuttering duration can be obtained and scored. The procedures described in this and the next section could be used in both problem identification and treatment evaluation. Data on all four categories (disfluencies, secondary behaviors, duration, and speech rate) can be obtained through videotaped assessments of the child in speaking situations. We suggest the use of video- over audiotape because the video medium makes it possible to obtain information on blocking and secondary behaviors.

Ideally, the clinician would assess the child's speech frequently (2–3 times per week). During each assessment session, the child should be asked to do two tasks. First, the child should hold a conversation with a parent or another adult on a topic that the child finds interesting and exciting. The assessment should continue until the child has spoken for 3 to 5 minutes (Andrews & Ingham, 1971). Second, in each assessment session, the child should read a book passage, appropriate for his or her reading level, for 3 to 5 minutes. Reading is an important assessment component because it will circumvent any possible attempt to engage in circumlocution of the words with which the child has the greatest problem. It is also important to remember that the assessor should not use the same reading passage repeatedly with the same child, because stutterers will exhibit a decrease in stuttering after repeated exposure to the same passage (Webster, 1974).

The aforementioned procedure is obviously time-consuming, and if done by a psychologist, expensive. The videotaping could be done by the parents at home or by a teacher at school. In both cases, we encourge the parents and/or teachers to (a) let the child do most of the talking by using open-ended questions and (b) try to record the child in the same situation or at the same time each day in which he or she stutters most frequently. This information should be determined in the functional assessment which will be described in the next section.

In the schools, we urge the teacher do the assessment in a way that would not further stigmatize the child. We suggest that the child be excused from the classroom to be recorded in a private room. Perhaps a good time to do this would be during a recess, lunch period, or study hall, so the child's absence will not be noticed by his or her peers.

Scoring Data

After the data are collected, each videotaped speech sample should be scored for percentage of words stuttered (%WS) or percentage of syllables stuttered (%SS), speech rate in words per minute (WPM), secondary behaviors, and duration of stuttering. To score for %WS, the clinician counts the number of stutters in the speech sample, divides that number by the total number of words spoken by the child during the sample, and multiplies by 100%. Likewise, to score for WPM, the clinician counts the number of words spoken during the assessment and divides that number by the number of minutes the child was speaking.

When scoring %WS, a situation could arise in which more than one stutter occurs on a given word. For example, the child could say "I want my b-b-b-bbbbbball." This could be counted as two stutters, a

sound repetition and a prolongation; the clinician probably would count it this way. However, for research purposes, it would be best to count such a situation as one stutter, so that the percentage of stuttered words is not artificially inflated.

We recommend two of the three subscales used by Riley (1972) in the Stuttering Severity Instrument (SSI) to assess secondary behaviors and stuttering duration. The SSI is a three-component measure designed to provide a gross estimate of stuttering severity. We recommend the Duration scale (Form 7.1) to assess stuttering duration and the Physical Concomitants scale (Form 7.2) to assess secondary behaviors.

To assess stuttering duration, the clinician estimates the length of the three longest blocks in each assessment using the standard durations given in the SSI. The three estimated durations are then averaged to produce a total duration score. The interrater reliability for this subtest is .91, even without the use of stopwatches to time the blocks. The simplicity of this test should be very appealing to the busy clinician.

The second subscale is used to assess secondary behaviors or physical concomitants. After watching the speech sample on videotape, the clinician rates four classes of behavior: distracting sounds, facial grimaces, head movement, and movement of the extremities, based on the salience of the behaviors. Although the clinician could count the frequency of the secondary behaviors, we see this as time-consuming and of little benefit to the clinician. The effect the behaviors have on the listener seems to be of greater importance.

FORM 7.1. Stuttering Severity Instrument Stuttering Duration Subscale*

Directions: Circle the appropriate task score, and place this number in the line marked "Total duration score."

Estimated mean length of three longest blocks	*Score*
Fleeting	1
One half second	2
One full second	3
2 to 9 seconds	4
10 to 30 seconds	5
30 to 60 seconds	6
More than 60 seconds	7
Total duration score	____

*From Riley (1972), p. 321.

FORM 7.2. Stuttering Severity Instrument Physical Concomitants Subscale*

Directions: Circle the appropriate values, sum across the four categories, and place the total score in the line marked "Total physical concomitant score."

0 = none   3 = distracting
1 = not noticeable unless looking for it   4 = very distracting
2 = barely noticeable to casual observer   5 = severe and painful looking

1. Distracting sounds. Noisy breathing, whistling, sniffing, blowing, clicking sounds.
      1   2   3   4   5
   List any examples _____

2. Facial grimaces. Jaw jerking, tongue protruding, lip pressing, jaw muscles tense.
      1   2   3   4   5
   List any examples _____

3. Head movement. Back, forward, turning away, poor eye contact, constant looking around.
      1   2   3   4   5
   List any examples _____

4. Extremities movement. Arm and hand movement, hands about face, torso movement, leg movements, foot tapping or
   swinging.
      1   2   3   4   5
   List any examples _____

                        Total physical concomitant score _____

---

*From Riley (1972), p. 321.

In assessing the four dependent variables (%WS, WPM, duration, and secondary behaviors), the clinician should have a colleague or a supervisee rate a portion of the same tapes for reliability. This is especially important for the %WS and WPM because these are the primary dependent variables. Although reliability assessment is typically considered a research activity, it is also important in good clinical practice. An interval system may be used in data collection to provide a more rigorous estimate of interrater reliability. In an interval system, both observers record the number of stuttered words in short time intervals (e.g., 10–30 seconds) and then compare their recording on an interval by interval basis to assess the percentage of agreement (e.g., Wagaman et al., 1993).

An alternative procedure for assessing the %WS and WPM consists of transcribing the child's conversation from the assessment tape into written form. The clinician then analyzes the transcription by circling each stuttered word, and easily counts the number of words spoken during the assessment. Although time is required for transcription, this method of assessment may have advantages such as time savings during scoring, increased interobserver reliability, and decreased difficulty inherent in interval scoring methods (Miltenberger, Elliott, Long, & Rapp, 1996).

In this section we have discussed how a clinician could approach the assessment and diagnosis of stuttering. If stuttering is to be classified as a problem (a) the child should be disfluent on >3% of his or her syllables, (b) this level of disfluency must be accompanied by observable or reported tension, (c) the disfluencies must be causing educational, occupational, or communicative distress as reported by the child or as indicated by the social validity assessments, and (d) the disfluency cannot be the result of an underlying speech–motor problem or sensory deficit. In terms of assessment, four types of speech variables are recorded, including %WS, WPM, secondary behaviors, and stuttering duration. We will make use of these assessment methods as we evaluate the effects of the environment on stuttering.

Problem Analysis

Because of the success of the regulated breathing method (Azrin & Nunn, 1974), there has been little emphasis on the functional assessment of social variables influencing stuttering. Nevertheless, we believe a thorough functional assessment of stuttering behavior is an important pretreatment activity. The focus of this section will be on the functional assessment methods used to identify antecedents that may elicit or evoke stuttering behavior and social consequences that may be involved in the maintenance of stuttering.

Assessing the Antecedents to Stuttering

Before beginning a treatment for stuttering, it is important to assess the most difficult speaking situations. This is important for a number of reasons. First, when possible, treatment should take place in the most difficult settings. Second, such an assessment may shed light on potential eliciting or evocative stimuli. Finally, these assessments may provide information suggesting that the behavior is being controlled by social contingencies.

The clinician should use indirect and direct methods in assessing the antecedents to stuttering (e.g., Arndorfer & Miltenberger, 1993). First, the clinician should interview the child, his or her parents, and teachers. The clinician should determine where the child stutters with the greatest frequency, what the child is discussing when this happens, with whom the child is speaking, and the nature of the speaking task. Any other antecedents that may predict an increase in stuttering should also be investigated. The clinician may find that stuttering is more frequent around peers, around a parent, in a specific class, talking about a certain topic, reading aloud, or when verbally fighting with a sibling, to name only a few possible antecedents.

To maximize clarity, it is important to obtain information on antecedents from a number of sources. For example, a parent and child may agree that the stuttering occurs primarily at school. However, five of the child's seven teachers may say that the child never stutters in their classes, while the other two teachers, who require daily oral recitation, say stuttering is frequent. If we interview only the child or parent, we would not have complete information about the antecedent situations most likely to evoke stuttering.

After developing hypotheses about various antecedents to stuttering, the clinician should, if possible, videotape the person on a number of occasions in these situations. When coded, these assessments will provide objective data to strengthen (or weaken) support for the hypotheses.

The clinician should also ask about antecedent events that are covert, such as feelings of excitement, nervousness, or being scared. It may be helpful to ask the child for information regarding tension in the vocal musculature, although in most cases the child will not be aware of the tension. Once the clinician has developed a hypothesis about the covert factors that may evoke stuttering, he or she might then develop brief experiments to determine the role of these reported private events and the environmental antecedents associated with them. Consider the following example.

Suppose our interview suggests that Billy stutters more when he is frustrated (e.g., unsuccessful performance on a difficult task), and when he is anxious. We would manipulate conditions that produce these private events and record the level of stuttering to see if it increased during these conditions. First, we find a frustrating situation that we can manipulate. For example, suppose Billy gets frustrated when doing math problems. We would record a conversation with Billy while he is doing math problems and one while he is working on a subject he completes successfully. We would also record his speech in conditions during which he is anxious and in conditions during which he is relaxed (e.g., doing a book report in front of class versus talking to his best friend). To the extent that we see an increased level of stuttering in the frustrated condition over the nonfrustrated condition, and in the anxious condition versus the relaxed condition, we could conclude that our hypothesis was supported. In other words, Billy is more likely to stutter when he is frustrated or anxious. Experimental evaluation of such a hypothesis may lead to the enhancement of Billy's treatment program with the inclusion of skills training to deal with frustrating situations and relaxation to address anxiety-provoking situations.

This section has discussed the basic assessment procedures for identifying antecedent stimuli that may evoke or elicit stuttering. Interview, observation, and, in some cases, experimental manipulations, are used to assess antecedents. We now turn our attention to the assessment of social consequences of stuttering.

Assessing the Consequences of Stuttering

As mentioned earlier, it may be possible for stuttering to be maintained by social consequences. Functional assessment methodology involving interview, observation, and brief experiments can be employed to identify social consequences of stuttering (e.g., Arndorfer & Miltenberger, 1993; Arndorfer, Miltenberger, Wooster, Rortvedt, & Gaffaney, 1994). Although stuttering treatment seems to be effective independent of problem function, the assessment of potential social contingencies should not be ignored, especially if standard treatments have failed.

The clinician should obtain interview information that could lead to the formation of hypotheses about social reinforcement of stuttering. The child, parents, teachers, and any other caretakers should be asked to describe what happens immediately after the child emits a stutter. Does someone finish the child's sentence? Does the child get removed from a task? Does the child get sympathy or attention from adults or peers? After the initial interview yields information regarding potential social reinforcers, the clinician should directly observe the child's stuttering in natural situations and record the consequences. Alternatively, a parent or teacher might be trained to conduct direct observation assessments. The results of direct observation of social consequences should provide support for the hypotheses developed from interview information. The final step in a thoroughgoing functional assessment is for the clinician to manipulate the consequences to test the hypotheses.

For example, suppose that our initial interview suggested that as Laurie stuttered, her parents finished her sentences. Based on this information, we would set up an ABAB experiment in which we first instruct Laurie's parents not to finish her sentences when she stutters. After a few sessions, we would then go to the B condition, in which the parents would finish the word or sentence she was trying to emit. After this phase, we would repeat the cycle. To the extent that we saw an increase in stuttering during the "B" phases (in which the parents finished the word or sentence), and a lower level of stuttering in the "A" phases (in which the parents did nothing), we may conclude that finishing the sentence or word negatively reinforced the stuttering behavior by allowing escape from the aversive block or speaking situation.

In this section, we have discussed the importance of assessing the antecedents and consequences of stuttering and the types of functional assessment methods used to generate this informa-tion. Although effective treatments for stuttering are often implemented without functional assessment information on the social variables related to stuttering, we suggest that the clinician always assess the antecedents and consequences of stuttering to establish the situations in which stuttering is most probable and to identify or rule out social reinforcement for the stuttering behavior.

Plan Implementation

In this section, we will discuss primarily the regulated breathing treatment developed by Azrin and Nunn (1974). Regulated breathing is just one of numerous treatments for stuttering that have been evaluated over the years. These treatments include procedures based on operant conditioning and involving punishment of disfluency and reinforcement of fluency (e.g., Berecz, 1973; Bloodstein, 1981; Flanagan et al., 1958, 1959; Goldiamond, 1965; James, 1981; Martin & Siegel, 1966a, b) and procedures based on respondent conditioning, such as systematic desensitization (e.g., Boudreau & Jeffrey, 1973; Tyre, Maisto, & Companik, 1973).

Although the treatments for stuttering based on either operant or respondent paradigms appear to be effective, there are concerns about their use. First, improvement does not appear to be maintained. Second, the procedures have not been widely used; this limits the conclusions that can be made about their use. Third, they do not directly address the airflow problem that underlies stuttering. Finally, one must question the use of punishment to treat stuttering, when other effective treatments are available. With these concerns in mind, we will now turn our discussion to the regulated breathing treatment, perhaps the best established behavioral treatment for stuttering.

Regulated Breathing

The regulated breathing treatment of stuttering (Azrin & Nunn, 1974) is based on habit reversal, a multicomponent treatment package developed by Azrin and Nunn (1973) to treat nervous habits and motor tics. The basic approach in both habit reversal and regulated breathing is to teach the client a new behavior that is incompatible with the problem response. For habit reversal, the competing response involves tensing the muscles isometric to those involved in the problem behavior, and in regulated breathing, the competing response is diaphragmatic breathing and gentle airflow in response to, or in anticipation of, a stutter. The original regulated breathing procedure is a complex multicomponent treatment package that includes 11 separate techniques grouped into four major categories.

Awareness Training

The first technique is called *response description.* The child is asked to give a detailed description of his or her stuttering while looking into a mirror; the description includes the secondary behaviors as well as the primary disfluencies. The second technique is called *response detection.* With this technique the child is taught to identify each instance of stuttering, with both positive and corrective feedback given by the therapist. The third technique is *early warning.* Here, the child is taught to recognize the cues that are associated with stuttering onset. For example, if the functional assessment indicated that stuttering is more likely when the child is excited, we would then teach the child to monitor his or her level of excitement, because it may signal a stuttering episode. In the fourth technique, *situation awareness training,* the child describes all the situations where the behavior occurs, and gives a detailed description of how he or she stutters in these situations. Collectively, these first four techniques are described as awareness training.

Competing Response Training

The fifth technique is the use of a competing response, a behavior incompatible with stuttering. The child is instructed to "(1) stop speaking, (2) take a deep breath by exhaling and then slowly inhaling, (3) consciously relax one's chest and throat muscles, (4) formulate mentally the words to be spoken, (5) start speaking immediately after taking a deep breath, (6) emphasize the initial part of a statement, (7) speak for shorter durations, and (8) eventually increase the duration of speech" (Azrin & Nunn, 1974, p. 282). This competing response is to be implemented by the child immediately upon the awareness of a disfluency, or when the child "feels" that he or she is about to stutter.

Motivation Training

The sixth technique in the treatment is the *inconvenience review.* The clinician asks the child to discuss all the problems caused by the stuttering. *Social support* is the seventh technique. Parents are asked to praise the child when they witness correct implementation of the competing response (breathing exercise). Parents are also asked to remind the child to use the breathing exercises when they detect a stutter and the child does not use the competing response. The eighth technique is *public display,* in which the child demonstrates control of his or her speech to family members and/or friends. Collectively, these last three techniques are known as motivation training.

Generalization Training

The ninth technique is *symbolic rehearsal,* in which the child imagines being in a situation where he or she is about to stutter, but then prevents the stutter with the competing response. This technique promotes generalization.

Azrin and Nunn (1973) included the preceding nine techniques in the original habit reversal treatment of habits and tics. However, Azrin and Nunn (1974) added two more techniques in the treatment of stuttering. *Positive practice* was achieved by having the child begin speaking or reading one word at a time, and then gradually building longer fluent phrases while maintaining the stutter-free speech, using the competing response. The final technique was *relaxation training,* in which the client was taught to relax in tense situations.

In the original study using regulated breathing, all eleven techniques were taught to the clients in a single 2-hour session. Two studies have used this multicomponent treatment to successfully treat stuttering in children (Azrin & Nunn, 1974; Ladouceur & Martineau, 1982). Combined, the studies demonstrated stuttering reductions ranging from 29% to 100%. A number of other studies have demonstrated the effectiveness of the regulated breathing treatment with adult stutterers as well (e.g., Azrin, Nunn, & Frantz, 1979; Cote & Ladouceur, 1982; Ladouceur & Saint-Laurent, 1986; Saint-Laurent & Ladouceur, 1987; Waterloo & Gotestam, 1988).

From the discussion on the full regulated breathing treatment package, the clinician can surmise that the treatment is complex, and perhaps contains unnecessary techniques. There has been a good deal of research demonstrating that not all of the techniques are necessary for treatment effectiveness (e.g., Caron & Ladouceur, 1989; Gagnon & Ladouceur, 1992; Wagaman et al., 1993). From these studies, a simplified regulated breathing procedure has been developed which is as effective as the original regulated breathing procedure.

Simplified Regulated Breathing

The simplified regulated breathing treatment consists of four techniques, including two awareness techniques (response detection and description); competing response training, consisting of diaphragmatic breathing and airflow modification, in which the child is taught to exhale slightly prior to speaking a word on the exhale; and social support. We recommend that the clinician use this simplified version instead of the full procedure. We will now describe the simplified treatment procedure in detail.

Response Description

Following the initial assessment session, the clinician should proceed with awareness training. For response description, we recommend that the child be asked to view videotapes of him or herself that were obtained during the initial assessment. The child should be asked to describe in detail what his or her stuttering looks like and sounds like, and what the secondary behaviors are that accompany the stuttering. If the child omits any of the types of stuttering or secondary behaviors, the clinician should point these out. When the child gives an accurate description of the behavior, the clinician should praise him or her.

Response Detection

Following response description, training in response detection should take place. First, the child and clinician view segments of videotape and the child identifies each stutter he or she emits on the tape. The clinician prompts the child when necessary and provides praise when the child correctly identifies each stutter. Next the clinician sits facing the child, engages the child in conversation (or reading), and instructs the child to raise a finger

contingent upon each disfluency. The child should be praised each time he or she correctly identifies a stutter and should be prompted for each disfluency missed. For example, if the child stutters but does not raise his finger, the clinician could say, "Greg, there was a stutter; let's try to catch those." Response detection training will teach the child to discriminate each stutter as it is being emitted.

Competing Response Training

After awareness has been established (i.e., the child is aware of at least 90% of his or her stutters), competing response training should be implemented. First, the clinician should teach diaphragmatic breathing by instructing the child to move his or her abdomen outward while inhaling, and to move the abdomen inward while exhaling. This can be practiced by having the child place a hand on his or her abdomen just below the rib cage, where the diaphragm muscle is located, and instructing him or her to make the hand go out while inhaling, and to make the hand go back in while exhaling.

The second part of the competing response is the airflow. The child should be taught to speak only after exhaling a small amount of air so that the air is already flowing across the larynx when speech is initiated. This can be accomplished by having the child take a mid-sized breath, exhale slightly, and then speak the word on the exhale. The clinician can detect the child's compliance by placing his or her fingers in front of the child's mouth and feeling for the breath. The child can put his or her fingers in front of the clinician's mouth as the clinician demonstrates the airflow. The child is then instructed to do the same as he or she exhales before speaking. The child should practice this technique until he or she is reliably exhaling a small amount of air prior to speaking.

The competing response technique will be completed when the diaphragmatic breathing and airflow components are combined and used contingent upon the beginning of a stutter, or in a situation where stuttering is more likely for that child. We have found it useful to call this competing response the "breathing exercise" when working with children. As soon as the child is aware of a stutter, he or she should start using the breathing exercise. Every time the child stutters in conversation with the therapist, the child should immediately stop speaking and begin the breathing exercise. The therapist should praise the child for correct implementation of the breathing exercise and prompt the child to use the breathing exercise when the child fails to stop the stuttering and start the competing response.

When first teaching the breathing exercise, it is useful to start slowly, having the child speak only one word while using the competing response. After the child has mastered one word utterances, the child is required to speak two-word phrases while using the breathing exercise. This process continues until the child is speaking full sentences fluently at a normal speech rate. The clinician should have the child practice the techniques with everyday words and phrases, but should also be aware of words that are difficult for the child, and should focus on these words. For example, when we first start working with Ted, we may ask him to practice the breathing exercise while speaking a word he has trouble with, such as "ball." After he is fluently speaking this word and using the exercises correctly, we would add another word, such as "play ball." We would practice these and other words containing sounds Ted has difficulty with until he could say them fluently.

Social Support

Social support should be implemented last. In training social support, the clinician should first model the social support behaviors. The clinician and later the parents should praise the child for stutter-free speech and for correct implementation of the breathing exercise. Likewise, the clinician, and later the parents, should remind the child to "use your breathing exercise" when he or she stutters, but fails to emit the competing response. For example, if Bryan forgets to do the exercise upon emitting a stutter, the parents should be instructed to respond by saying "Bryan, there was a stutter; don't forget to do your exercise." The parents should be taught not to respond in an aversive or condescending tone. The social support procedures should be practiced with the parent, and feedback given, until there is a high degree of compliance with the procedures.

The entire simplified treatment is typically implemented in one session lasting approximately two hours. We also recommend at least weekly one-hour visits with the child and parents to review the treatment procedures and to have them continue to practice the competing response. The clinician would decrease the frequency and length of sessions as the child and parents continue to use the procedures reliably and as the assessments indicate continued low levels of stuttering.

Programming for Generalization

As stated earlier in this chapter, it would be ideal for treatment to take place in situations where speech is most difficult. We understand that many times this is impossible. However, in an attempt to program for generalization, the child should be encouraged to use the competing response in all speaking situations. In the clinic, the child will practice with the therapist as they role-play some of the difficult situations and conversation topics. In the home or other natural settings, the child should use the breathing exercise with the parents as they provide social support. It is also useful to train the child's teacher(s) to act as a social-support person(s). The social-support technique is the primary way to facilitate generalization, as the parents and others will prompt the child to use the competing response across various situations and will provide social reinforcement for successful speech and accurate use of the breathing exercises across situations.

Treatment Modifications

As mentioned earlier, a functional assessment of antecedents and consequences of stuttering is an important pretreatment activity. If the simplified regulated breathing treatment package is ineffective, the clinician reassesses which antecedent conditions may be evoking stuttering and which consequent events may be maintaining the stuttering, such as escape from the aversive speaking situations, or attention received for the stuttering, respectively. The treatment is then modified to address the antecedents and consequences identified in the reassessment.

For example, suppose we implemented the regulated breathing treatment with an 8-year-old child, but found only modest decreases in stuttering. If, after conducting further assessment, we found that the child was more likely to stutter when he was anxious, we may then modify the treatment procedure to include relaxation training in stressful situations. Consider another example in which treatment modification would be warranted. Let us suppose the regulated breathing treatment with 15-year-old Julie was producing limited reductions in her stuttering. Subsequent analyses of environmental factors showed that when Julie stuttered, her mother paid a great deal of attention to her in the form of scolding, whereas during periods of fluent speech, her mother provided no attention. This finding would indicate that her mother was noncompliant with the use of social support procedures and was probably reinforcing stuttering with attention. A treatment modification would involve further intensive behavioral skills training with her mother to teach her to refrain from scolding and to implement the social support procedures as originally instructed.

Consider one other example. Let us suppose that the simplified treatment was ineffective with 12-year-old Ryan. We then conduct further functional assessment of social consequences and find that when Ryan is in a difficult speaking situation, his mother finishes his sentences. For example, Ryan may say, "Mom, can I have some s-s-s-s-s . . . ," and his mother finishes the word, "soda," and gets him a soda. In this example, one can see that Ryan need not finish the difficult word; in such a case, stuttering is reinforced by escape from the aversive situation (speaking) and possibly by the tangible reinforcement of getting what he was trying to ask for. To improve the success of treatment, we would modify the simplified regulated breathing package by asking his mother to refrain from completing difficult words for Ryan, to wait patiently as he speaks, and to respond to his successful communication with praise and other requested reinforcers.

In this section we reviewed the regulated breathing treatment of stuttering and provided explicit instruction about implementing the simplified regulated breathing treatment. We discussed the necessity of generalization programming via social support, and briefly identified what a clinician could do to address environmental factors contributing to the maintenance of stuttering if the standard simplified package is ineffective. We will now focus our attention on how to evaluate the effectiveness of treatment.

Plan Evaluation

It is our belief that any clinical intervention should be accompanied by a data collection strat-

egy. In this chapter, we have discussed a method for collecting data on stuttering behaviors. We now describe how to use the data to evaluate the treatment program and make decisions regarding treatment.

To determine treatment effectiveness, the clinician should look at three factors. First, the clinician should compare the %WS, WPM, secondary behaviors, and duration at baseline with the same measures at posttreatment. If there is a decrease in %WS, secondary behaviors, and/or duration from baseline to posttreatment, the clinician can conclude that the treatment is producing positive effects. For example, consider the graph in Figure 1 from Wagaman et al. (1993). This graph shows the %WS for four children who were treated with the simplified regulated breathing procedure. There are a number of important points about evaluation illustrated in this graph: (a) You can see that stuttering data (%WS) were collected on a number of occasions over time in baseline to establish the level of stuttering before treatment; (b) data were collected at home and at school to assess stuttering in multiple settings; (c) the level of stuttering decreased following treatment as determined by the data collected on numerous occasions over a 20-to 30-day period; (d) stuttering decreased at home and school, providing evidence of generalization; and (e) data collection then continued periodically in the posttreatment phase across months, to establish that the behavior change was maintained and that stuttering did not increase with the passage of time.

If stuttering had increased at any point after the treatment phase, the clinician would detect this increase in the data and would implement booster sessions. Further data collection would indicate whether stuttering decreased again or whether further booster sessions were needed.

The second factor the clinician should look at when assessing treatment effectiveness is the criterion measure. As stated earlier in the paper, normal speakers are disfluent on approximately 0–3% of their syllables. To the extent that the child is below this criterion at posttreatment, we can assume that our treatment has produced a level of fluency close to the range of normal speakers.

Social validity is the final factor in determining treatment effectiveness (e.g., Wagaman et al., 1993, 1995). The purpose of social validity as-

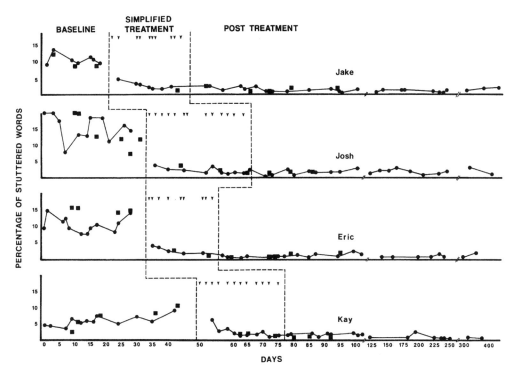

FIGURE 1. This graph, from Wagaman et al. (1993), shows the percentage of stuttered words from four children treated with a simplified habit reversal procedure. The round data points indicate home observations and the square data points indicate generalization data from the school setting. Each arrowhead in the simplified treatment phase indicates the day on which a treatment session was conducted. Treatment was implemented in a multiple baseline across subjects design.

sessment is to determine whether the results of treatment are evaluated positively by individuals other than the treatment agents. We have found it useful to take two to three 2-minute samples of videotape from randomly selected baseline assessments, and two to three 2-minute samples of videotape from randomly selected posttreatment assessments and have professionals, parents, or others rate them using the Social Validity Scale (see Form 7.3). The ratings for each item on the scale can be summed to obtain a social validity score.

The simplified regulated breathing treatment sessions should end when the child is at or below the 3% SS criterion for five or more assessments. It may also be useful to give follow-up booster sessions biweekly, and to eventually fade these out. During these booster sessions, the child should be asked to use the awareness procedures again if stuttering awareness has fallen below 90%. The child should also be asked to speak difficult words while

using the breathing exercise, to make certain that the competing response is being implemented correctly. Finally, during the booster sessions, the parents should be reminded how to do the social support technique, and should be asked to role-play social support in front of the clinician so that any problems can be addressed. The child should be encouraged to continue using the breathing exercise in all speaking situations outside the treatment sessions. The clinician may notice that at follow-ups, the child will report no longer using the breathing exercises, even though he or she is actually using the technique. At this point, the response has become part of the child's natural speaking repertoire. If treatment proves to be less effective than expected, further assessment is conducted to identify possible maintaining variables that may have been missed during previous assessments and to identify other variables that may account for the diminished treatment effectiveness (e.g., compliance problems).

FORM 7.3. Social Validity Inventory*

Directions: When listening to the speech segments, consider the child's speech in terms of disfluencies (stuttering). Do not consider other types of fluency problems such as lisps, grammar, or pronunciation.

1. How would you rate the subject's speech?

    1   2   3   4   5   6   7
   very impaired   somewhat impaired   unimpaired

2. How noticeable are the subject's disfluencies (stuttering)?

    1   2   3   4   5   6   7
   very noticeable   somewhat noticeable   not at all noticeable

3. How would you rate the subject's need for intervention? In other words, does this child need help in improving language production?

    1   2   3   4   5   6   7
   very much needed   somewhat needed   at all needed

4. How would you rate the naturalness of the subject's speech?

    1   2   3   4   5   6   7
   very unnatural   somewhat natural   very natural

5. Would you consider, from the speech sample you heard, this child to be a stutterer?

    1   2   3   4   5   6   7
    yes   maybe   no

Comments:

*From Wagaman, Miltenberger, and Arndorfer (1993).

Summary

This chapter has provided a discussion of stuttering, with an emphasis on the assessment and treatment of the disorder. We started the chapter by discussing the prevalence and etiology of stuttering, with special attention given to the relationship between anxiety and stuttering. It was suggested that, although there may not be a relationship between the constructs of state or trait anxiety and stuttering, a relationship between tension in the vocal musculature and stuttering may be supported. Further empirical support for this relationship would be beneficial and may provide information with which we can better evaluate the conceptualizations of stuttering described in this paper.

After presenting an operant model of stuttering, we addressed the assessment, diagnosis, and treatment of stuttering in children. We emphasized the importance of assessing a number of different areas, including stuttering frequency, speech rate, stuttering duration, and physical concomitants, as well as the importance of assessing for treatment validity and generalization. We provided methods and suggestions for adequate assessment.

We continued with a discussion of functional assessment of antecedent and consequences of stuttering behavior. Functional assessment information has not been used extensively in stuttering treatment. In fact, the regulated breathing approach was developed without regard to the possible operant contingencies that may influence stuttering behavior. We suggest that functional assessment information may enhance treatment development and is particularly important when treatment produces limited success.

Treatment was then discussed, with primary emphasis placed on a description of the simplified regulated breathing method. We also discussed potential modifications that could be made to the standard package if it failed to reduce stuttering. Such modifications would incorporate information from the functional assessment of operant contingencies. We concluded the chapter with a brief discussion on the importance of evaluating the treatment, and the different methods by which the clinician could evaluate treatment outcome.

To the perceptive reader, this chapter has not only presented a method for the assessment and treatment of stuttering, but has also implied a number of potential research questions. First, one must ask whether the simplified regulated breathing treatment could be further simplified. Would it be possible to treat stuttering through awareness training alone? Second, as stated earlier, more investigation should take place regarding the role of anxiety in the frequency of stuttering. Third, does the simplified regulated breathing treatment affect only stuttering frequency, or does it also decrease stuttering duration and physical concomitants? As yet, the evidence is unclear. Finally, to what extent is stuttering controlled by external contingencies? The regulated breathing treatment has been so effective that the role of social contingencies has largely been ignored. Such information would shed light on the social variables involved in the development and maintenance of stuttering. Even if this information is not useful in treating stuttering, because of the success of the regulated breathing treatment, such information may be useful in the prevention of the problem.

After reading this chapter, the practicing professional should be better prepared to diagnose, assess, and treat stuttering in children (with appropriate supervision as necessary). We have written the chapter from a decidedly behavior analytic viewpoint, and encourage the clinician who is treating stuttering to adhere to the rigorous scientific standards that accompany this viewpoint. It is our hope that, after reading this chapter, more psychologists will become involved in the research and treatment of stuttering.

References

American Psychiatric Association (1987). *Diagnostic and statistical manual of mental disorders* (3rd ed., rev.). Washington, DC: Author.

American Psychiatric Association (1994). *Diagnostic and statistical manual of mental disorders* (4th ed.). Washington, DC: Author.

Andrews, G., & Ingham, R.J. (1971). Stuttering: Considerations in the evaluation of treatment. *British Journal of Disorders of Communication, 6,* 129–138.

Andrews, G., Craig, A., Feyer, A.M., Hoddinott, S., Howie, P., & Neilson, M. (1983). Stuttering: A review of the research findings and theories circa 1982. *Journal of Speech and Hearing Disorders, 48,* 226–246.

Andrews, G., Morris-Yates, A., Howie, P., & Martin, N.G. (1991). Genetic factors in stuttering confirmed. *Archives of General Psychiatry, 48,* 1034–1035.

Arndorfer, R.E., & Miltenberger, R.G. (1993). Functional assessment and treatment of challenging behavior: A review with implications for early childhood. *Topics in Early Childhood Special Education, 13,* 82–105.

Arndorfer, R.E., Miltenberger, R.G., Woster, S.H., Rortvedt, A.K., & Gaffaney, T. (1994). Home-based descriptive and experimental analysis of problem behaviors in children. *Topics in Early Childhood Special Education, 14,* 64–87.

Azrin, N.H., & Nunn, R.G. (1973). Habit reversal: A method of eliminating nervous habits and tics. *Behaviour Research and Therapy, 11,* 619–628.

Azrin, N.H., & Nunn, R.G. (1974). A rapid method of eliminating stuttering by a regulated breathing approach. *Behaviour Research and Therapy, 12,* 279–286.

Azrin, N.H., Nunn, R.G., & Frantz, S.E. (1979). Comparison of regulated breathing versus abbreviated desensitization on reported stuttering episodes. *Journal of Speech and Hearing Research, 44,* 331–339.

Berecz, J.M. (1973). The treatment of stuttering through precision punishment and cognitive arousal. *Journal of Speech and Hearing Disorders, 38,* 256–267.

Blood, G.W., Blood, I.M., Bennett, S., & Simpson, K.C. (1994). Subjective anxiety measurements and cortisol responses in adults who stutter. *Journal of Speech and Hearing Research, 37,* 760–768.

Bloodstein, O. (1981). *A handbook on stuttering.* The National Easter Seal Society: Chicago, IL.

Boudreau, L.A., & Jeffrey, C.J. (1973). Stuttering treated by desensitization. *Journal of Behavior Therapy and Experimental Psychiatry, 4,* 209–212.

Brutten, E.J., & Shoemaker, D.J. (1967). *The modification of stuttering.* Englewood Cliffs, NJ: Prentice-Hall.

Caron, C., & Ladouceur, R. (1989). Multidimensional behavioral treatment for child stutterers. *Behavior Modification, 13,* 206–215.

Cote, C., & Ladouceur, R. (1982). Effects of social aids and the regulated breathing method. *Journal of Counseling and Clinical Psychology, 50,* 450.

Craig, A. (1990). An investigation into the relationship between anxiety and stuttering. *Journal of Speech and Hearing Disorders, 55,* 290–294.

Dickson, S. (1971). Incipient stuttering and spontaneous remission of stuttered speech. *Journal of Communication Disorders, 4,* 99–110.

Flanagan, B.I., Goldiamond, I., & Azrin, N.H. (1958). Operant stuttering: The control of stuttering behavior through response contingent consequences. *Journal of the Experimental Analysis of Behavior, 1,* 173–177.

Flanagan, B.I., Goldiamond, I., & Azrin, N.H. (1959). Instatement of stuttering in normally fluent individuals through operant procedures. *Science, 130,* 979–981.

Gagnon, M., & Ladouceur, R. (1992). Behavioral treatment of child stutterers: Replication and extension. *Behavior Therapy, 23,* 113–129.

Goldiamond, I. (1965). Stuttering and fluency as manipulatable operant response classes. In L. Krasner & L. Ullman (Eds.), *Research in behavior modification: New developments and implications.* New York: Holt, Rinehart, & Winston.

Gray, B.B., & England, G. (1972). Some effects of anxiety deconditioning upon stuttering frequecy. *Journal of Speech and Hearing Research, 15,* 114–122.

Healy, E.C. (1991). *Readings on research in stuttering.* White Plains, NY: Longman.

Homzie, M.J., & Lindsay, J.S. (1984). Language and the young stutterer: A new look at old theories and findings. *Brain and Language, 22,* 232–252.

Ingham, R.J. (1984). *Stuttering and behavior therapy: Current status and experimental foundations*. San Diego, CA: College Hill Press.

Ingham, R.J., & Andrews, G. (1971). The relation between anxiety reduction and treatment. *Journal of Communication Disorders, 4,* 289–301.

James, J.E. (1981). Punishment of stuttering: Contingency and stimulus parameters. *Journal of Communication Disorders, 14,* 375–386.

Ladouceur, R., & Martineau, G. (1982). Evaluation of regulated-breathing method with and without parental assistance in the treatment of child stutterers. *Journal of Behavior Therapy and Experimental Psychiatry, 13,* 301–306.

Ladouceur, R., & Saint-Laurent, L. (1986). Stuttering: a multi-dimensional treatment and evaluation package. *Journal of Fluency Disorders, 11,* 93–103.

Leung, A., & Robson, W.L. (1990). Stuttering. *Clinical Pediatrics, 29,* 498–502.

Manning, W.H., Trutna, P.A., & Shaw, C.K. (1976). Verbal versus tangible reward for children who stutter. *Journal of Speech and Hearing Disorders, 41,* 52–62.

Martin, R., & Siegel, G. (1966a). The effects of response contingent shock on stuttering. *Journal of Speech and Hearing Research, 9,* 340–352.

Martin, R., & Siegel, G. (1966b). The effects of simultaneously punishing stuttering and rewarding fluency. *Journal of Speech and Hearing Research, 9,* 466–475.

Michael, J. (1982). Distinguishing between the discriminative and motivational functions of stimuli. *Journal of the Experimental Analysis of Behavior, 37,* 149–155.

Miller, S., & Watson, B.C. (1992). The relationship between communication attitude, anxiety, and depression in stutterers and nonstutterers. *Journal of Speech and Hearing Research, 35,* 789–798.

Miltenberger, R.G., Elliott, A., Long, E., & Rapp, J. (1996). *Improving the accuracy and reliability of stuttering assessment.* Manuscript submitted for publication.

Riley, G.D. (1972). A stuttering severity instrument for children and adults. *Journal of Speech and Hearing Disorders, 37,* 314–322.

Saint-Laurent, L., & Ladouceur, R. (1987). Massed versus distributed application of the regulated breathing method for stutterers and its long term effect. *Behavior Therapy, 18,* 38–50.

Spielberger, C.D., Gorsuch, R.L., Lushene, R., Vagg, P.R., & Jacobs, G.A. (1983). *State-trait anxiety inventory for adults.* Palo Alto, CA: Consulting Psychologists.

Stansfield, J. (1988). Stuttering and cluttering in the mentally handicapped population: A review of the literature. *British Journal of Mental Subnormality, 34,* 54–61.

Tyre, T.E., Maisto, S.A., & Companik, P.J. (1973). The use of systematic desensitization in the treatment of chronic stuttering behavior. *Journal of Speech and Hearing Disorders, 38,* 514–519.

Van Riper, C. (1982). *The nature of stuttering* (2nd ed.). Englewood Cliffs, NJ: Prentice-Hall.

Wagaman, J.R., Miltenberger, R.G., & Arndorfer, R.E. (1993). Analysis of a simplified treatment for stuttering in children. *Journal of Applied Behavior Analysis, 26,* 53–61.

Wagaman, J.R., Miltenberger, R.G., & Woods, D.W., (1995). Long term follow-up of a simplified treatment for stuttering in children. *Journal of Applied Behavior Analysis, 28,* 233–234.

Waterloo, K.K., & Gotestam, K.G. (1988). The regulated breathing method for stuttering: An experimental evaluation. *Journal of Behavior Therapy and Experimental Psychiatry, 19,* 11–19.

Webster, R.L. (1974). A behavioral analysis of stuttering treatment and theory. In K.S. Calhoun, H.E. Adams, & K.M. Mitchell (Eds.), *Innovative treatment methods in psychopathology psychopathology* (pp. 17–61). New York: Wiley.

Webster, W.G. (1985). Neuropsychological models of stuttering—I: Representation of sequential response mechanisms. *Neuropsychologia, 23,* 263–267.

Webster, W.G. (1986). Neuropsychological models of stuttering—II: Interhemispheric interference. *Neuropsychologia, 24,* 737–741.

Bibliography

Azrin, N.H., & Nunn, R.G. (1973). Habit reversal: A method of eliminating nervous habits and tics. *Behaviour Research and Therapy, 11,* 619–628.

Azrin, N.H., & Nunn, R.G. (1974). A rapid method of eliminating stuttering by a regulated breathing approach. *Behaviour Research and Therapy, 12,* 279–286.

Azrin, N.H., Nunn, R.G., & Frantz, S.E. (1979). Comparison of regulated breathing versus abbreviated desensitization on reported stuttering episodes. *Journal of Speech and Hearing Research, 44,* 331–339.

Bloodstein, O. (1981). *A handbook on stuttering.* Chicago: National Easter Seal Society.

Goldiamond, I. (1965). Stuttering and fluency as manipulatable operant response classes. In L. Krasner & L. Ullman (Eds.), *Research in behavior modification: New developments and implications.* New York: Holt, Rinehart, & Winston.

Ingham, R.J. (1984). *Stuttering and behavior therapy: Current status and experimental foundations.* San Diego, CA: College Hill Press.

Van Riper, C. (1982). *The nature of stuttering* (2nd ed.). Englewood Cliffs, NJ: Prentice-Hall.

Wagaman, J.R., Miltenberger, R.G., & Arndorfer, R.E. (1993). Analysis of a simplified treatment for stuttering in children. *Journal of Applied Behavior Analysis, 26,* 53–61.

8

School Attendance

CHRISTOPHER A. KEARNEY AND CHERYL A. TILLOTSON

Introduction

School attendance in childhood and adolescence is an aspect of life that many people take for granted, but problems in this area may result in some of the most intransigent difficulties of the developmental period. Although such problems have been referred to in various historical terms, we prefer the term "school refusal behavior" to include any child-motivated refusal to attend school or to remain in class for an entire day. Specifically, school refusal behavior refers to youngsters aged 5 to 17 years who either (1) are completely absent from school, and/or (2) initially attend, then leave school during the course of the day, and/or (3) go to school following behavior problems such as morning temper tantrums, and/or (4) display unusual distress during school days that precipitates pleas for future nonattendance (Kearney & Silverman, 1996). School refusal behavior is differentiated from school withdrawal, referring to parents who deliberately prevent their children from attending school (Kahn & Nursten, 1962).

The term "school refusal behavior" is meant to coalesce narrowly focused concepts such as (1) school phobia, referring to youngsters who are specifically fearful of some school-related stimulus, (2) separation anxiety, referring to typically younger children who are fearful of being away from parents or home, and (3) truancy, referring to typically older adolescents who miss school and display various conduct-related problems (Hersov, 1985). School refusal behavior, as defined above, provides better coverage for those with difficulties attending school (Kearney, Eisen, & Silverman, 1995). Problematic absenteeism affects about 5% of youth (Granell de Aldaz, Vivas, Gelfand, & Feldman, 1984).

Symptomatology and Covariance

School refusal behavior is marked by considerable heterogeneity with respect to symptomatology. Common internalizing symptoms include general and social anxiety, fear, depression, social withdrawal, and somatic complaints (particularly headache, stomachache, and abdominal pain; Last, 1991; Last & Strauss, 1990). Common externalizing symptoms include aggression, running away from home or school, noncompliance, and tantrums (Cooper, 1986). The clinical picture of school refusal behavior is thus mixed, and subtle covariance with other behaviors often leads to problems in differential diagnosis.

Such covariance is most often displayed in one of three ways. The first involves youngsters who display school refusal behavior in addition to conduct problems such as disruptive behavior, drug use, breaking curfew, and stealing. In this case, the clinician must determine whether school refusal behavior is the primary problem and whether the initial resolution of nonattendance will lead to a generalized therapeutic response regarding the other behaviors.

Two other problems that often covary with school refusal behavior are depression and poor

CHRISTOPHER A. KEARNEY AND CHERYL A. TILLOTSON • Department of Psychology, University of Nevada–Las Vegas, Las Vegas, Nevada 89154-5030.

Handbook of Child Behavior Therapy, edited by Watson and Gresham. Plenum Press, New York, 1998.

academic performance. Oftentimes, it is difficult to say whether these problems contributed to later school refusal behavior or vice versa. For example, many adolescents are depressed about social interactions and subsequently avoid school, whereas others initially refuse school and later develop depression at the prospect of having to return (Kearney, 1993). Similarly, youngsters with poor academic competence are certainly at risk for school dropout (Zigler, Taussig, & Black, 1992), whereas youngsters with primary school refusal behavior usually fall behind in their classwork. In each case, clinicians must make a determined effort to identify the temporal link between these behaviors and decide which problems require more immediate and intensive treatment.

Etiology and Prognosis

Like symptomatology, the etiology of school refusal behavior is mixed, and the primary proximal factors that initiate and maintain the behavior are described later in this chapter. Distal variables that affect attendance include level of school violence, availability of drugs, quality of the educational setting, homelessness, marital conflict and divorce, abuse, and problematic family dynamics. With respect to the latter, Kearney and Silverman (1995) described four familial subtypes that seem intricately related to school refusal behavior: enmeshed, conflictive, detached, and isolated. For example, enmeshed families are often characterized by over-involved family interactions that spur attention-seeking school refusal behavior in youngsters. Similarly, conflictive, detached, and isolated family dynamics appear related to other functions of school refusal behavior to be discussed.

The prognosis of school refusal behavior may be best linked to the length of the problem. Approximately 25% of all cases of school refusal behavior remit spontaneously or are self-corrective in nature. This generally refers to youngsters who miss a few days of school following an illness or an extended vacation, but the behavior is usually quashed by parents soon after it begins or the child simply returns to school on his or her own (Kearney, 1995). Although this behavior may recur later, most of these children do not show any significant long-term problems.

Acute school refusal behavior may be defined as problematic school attendance for at least two weeks but less than one year, whereas chronic school refusal behavior refers to cases lasting longer than one year. The latter implies generalized nonattendance across two academic years, a condition associated with severe resistance to treatment. The development of serious problems is directly related to the increased duration of absenteeism, and includes poor academic performance, impaired social development, depression and suicidal ideation, school dropout, and, in adulthood, a greater likelihood of alcohol abuse, criminal behavior, and marital, occupational, and psychiatric difficulties (Berg, 1970; Berg & Jackson, 1985; Flakierska, Lindstrom, & Gillberg, 1988; Hibbett & Fogelman, 1990; Hibbett, Fogelman, & Manor, 1990; Robins & Ratcliffe, 1980).

Problem Identification

Problem identification at our clinic for youngsters with school refusal behavior begins during the screening process. Our referral sources typically involve those who first encounter the problem (i.e., parents and school officials such as school psychologists, teachers, principals, guidance counselors, and nurses). During this initial screening process, the identification of school refusal behavior is both simple and complex. Identifying whether the youngster physically attends school is relatively easy, but identifying the surrounding clinical picture often is not. Clinicians should note that parents and teachers are not very accurate observers of covert child behavior (Harris & Ferrari, 1983), and the crisis-like atmosphere of acute school refusal behavior sometimes exacerbates this situation. For example, many children report an overall dread (negative affectivity) about attending school, but initial referral sources tend to emphasize overt, immediate problems such as breaking curfew and refusing to complete homework. Clinicians should be sensitive to this tendency and probe as well for internalizing problems such as anxiety and depression. Following this process, a formal assessment session is scheduled if school refusal behavior is sufficiently severe. This is defined by the parameters described earlier and excludes youngsters with self-corrective school refusal behavior (i.e., child-motivated absenteeism that remits spontaneously within two weeks of onset).

The initial assessment session generally consists of standardized semistructured interviews, self-report measures, and parent checklists. When the family arrives for assessment, we separately address the child and parents for two main reasons. First, separation allows for a brief but direct observation of whether the child can appropriately detach from his or her parents. Careful attention should be paid to behaviors such as excessive reassurance-seeking, complaining, noncompliance, and tantrums. Second, separation allows for an early explanation about confidentiality and helps build rapport with the child, who has likely been identified as the central antagonist (Eisen & Kearney, 1995). The therapist may wish to assure the child that his or her report will be taken as seriously as any other and, as partial evidence of this, interview the child first.

Interview

A commonly used semistructured interview for youngsters who refuse school is the Anxiety Disorders Interview Schedule (ADIS), which has child and parent versions (Silverman & Eisen, 1992; Silverman & Nelles, 1988). The ADIS covers a variety of behavior problems in children and adolescents, with a particular focus on anxiety disorders. The overall reliability of the ADIS is good, with kappa coefficients of .75–.78 (Silverman & Eisen, 1992; Silverman & Nelles, 1988). These flexible interviews, now revised to reflect *DSM-IV* diagnostic criteria (Silverman & Albano, 1996), allow clinicians to gather data from different sources, assess informant variance, and pursue various avenues of information. With respect to the latter, for example, clinicians may determine whether medical conditions (e.g., gastrointestinal disorders, viruses) have been ruled out as a possible primary cause of school refusal behavior. If not, this should be done immediately. During the interview, the clinician should concentrate on defining the history, extent, and clinical picture of school refusal behavior and develop hypotheses about the variables maintaining the problem.

Self-Report Measures

Self-report measures are also useful for understanding the clinical picture of youngsters with school refusal behavior. Measures often used to assess this population are described here, although the School Refusal Assessment Scale (Kearney & Silverman, 1993) is described in the next section. Measures of negative affectivity are especially pertinent to cases of school refusal behavior that involve substantial levels of anxiety and depression, and include the (1) Negative Affect Self-Statement Questionnaire (NASSQ; Ronan, Kendall, & Rowe, 1994), an inventory of anxious and depressive self-statements with child and adolescent versions, (2) Revised Children's Manifest Anxiety Scale (RC-MAS; Reynolds & Paget, 1981) and State–Trait Anxiety Inventory for Children (STAIC; Spielberger, 1973), measures of general, situation-specific, and physiological anxiety and worry, and (3) Children's Depression Inventory (CDI; Kovacs, 1992), an instrument designed to assess recent cognitive and behavioral symptoms of negative affective states.

In addition to these, the Fear Survey Schedule for Children–Revised (FSSC–R; Ollendick, 1983) is particularly useful in cases where a child refuses school due to fears of failure or criticism. Likewise, the Social Anxiety Scale for Children–Revised (SASC–R; La Greca & Stone, 1993) is helpful in assessing youngsters, especially adolescents, who refuse school to escape aversive social or evaluative situations. Other self-report measures that we commonly use include the (1) Piers-Harris Self-Concept Scale (Piers, 1984) to measure self-esteem, (2) Daily Life Stressors Scale (Kearney, Drabman, & Beasley, 1993) to measure common but specific areas of stress at home and school, and (3) Children's Anxiety Sensitivity Index (Silverman, Fleisig, Rabian, & Peterson, 1991) to measure perceptions of one's anxiety symptoms. Each self-report measure mentioned here displays good psychometric quality and is applicable to youngsters in a wide age range.

Parent Checklists

Parent checklists are frequently used to help define the clinical picture of school refusal behavior. The most common is the Child Behavior Checklist (Achenbach, 1991a), a 118-item measure that elicits parent ratings of various internalizing and externalizing behaviors. Narrow-band factors that are most salient in the assessment of school refusal behavior include withdrawn, somatic complaints, anxious/depressed, and delinquent and aggressive behavior. The Conners Parent Rating Scale (Conners, 1990) is shorter (48 items) and may be helpful if time is limited. Each scale has a teacher version as well, i.e., the Teacher's Report Form (Achenbach, 1991b) and Conners Teacher Rating Scale (Conners, 1990). However, the reader should note that, in many cases of school refusal behavior (see parts 1, 3, 4 of the definition provided earlier), school officials have little knowledge of the child outside of his or her school attendance rate and may shed little light on the clinical picture.

Other parent checklists are also useful for assessing youth with school refusal behavior. For example, the Family Environment Scale (FES; Moos & Moos, 1986) measures various family dynamics that, as mentioned earlier, may distally affect a child's refusal to attend school. Pertinent subscales include cohesion, expressiveness, conflict, independence, and control. In addition, the Parental Expectancies Scale (Eisen, Spasaro, Kearney, Albano, & Barlow, 1996) is partially designed to measure unusual or stringent parent attitudes about their child's social, academic, and athletic performance. Finally, the Dyadic Adjustment Scale (Spanier, 1976) may be used if the clinician suspects that marital conflict is problematic and contributes to a child's school refusal behavior (Kearney, 1995).

Baseline Measures

Following the formal assessment session, the clinician should establish measures of baseline performance. In our clinic, children and parents are asked to maintain daily logbooks (see Forms 8.1 and 8.2). These logbooks elicit ratings of anxiety, depression, overall distress, noncompliance, disruption to the family's daily life routine, and school attendance. Training for completing the logbooks is brief but intensive. Each party is instructed as to the correct procedures, shown a sample completed logbook, asked to complete ratings for that day to assure comprehension, and solicited for any questions they may have. In addition, families are often contacted within two days of the assessment session to update the status of their case and identify and remedy any problems with the logbook procedure. Children and parents are asked to separately maintain their logbooks except for cases involving young children (aged 5–7 years), where parents are allowed to assist their child with the procedure without providing feedback regarding the child's answer.

Baseline measures should be completed for at least five days, after which they may be closely examined by the clinician. If family members fail to produce the logbooks or deliver incomplete measures at this time, the clinician should be extremely wary, as failure to complete this task is often pre-

FORM 8.1. Child Daily Logbook

Participant: _____

Please rate the following every day on a 0–10 scale where 0 = none, 2 = mild, 4 = moderate, 6 = marked, 8 = severe, and 10 = extreme (for younger children: 0–10 scale where 0 is none and 10 is very much). Feel free to use any number 0–10.

Date	Anxiety	Depression	Distress
————	————	————	————
————	————	————	————
————	————	————	————
————	————	————	————
————	————	————	————
————	————	————	————
————	————	————	————
————	————	————	————

Please list any problems you have had at home or school in the past days:

FORM 8.2. Parent Daily Logbook

Participant: _____

Please rate the following *child* behaviors every day on a 0–10 scale where 0 = none, 2 = mild, 4 = moderate, 6 = marked, 8 = severe, and 10 = extreme. Feel free to use any number 0–10.

Date	Anxiety	Depression	Distress	Noncompliance	Disruption
————	————	————	————	————	————
————	————	————	————	————	————
————	————	————	————	————	————
————	————	————	————	————	————
————	————	————	————	————	————
————	————	————	————	————	————
————	————	————	————	————	————
————	————	————	————	————	————

Please list number of hours missed from school on each school day:

Please list specific problems your child has had at home or school in the past days:

dictive of noncompliance by family members in later sessions and must be addressed promptly (Kearney, 1995). Specifically, one should explore the reasons for failure to comply and reemphasize the importance of collecting daily data to evaluate treatment effectiveness. Under these conditions, the clinician may wish to reassign the task and follow up with daily telephone calls to assess compliance. In cases of chronic school refusal behavior, compliance is typically poor. As a result, treatment may need to focus initially on building rapport and motivation to help change negative attitudes about the perceived effectiveness of the upcoming intervention (see Thompson & Rudolph, 1988).

Finally, problem identification may be enhanced by employing direct observations of behavior. A formal protocol is presented in Forms 8.3 and 8.4. A less formal observational process, however, might involve two in vivo observations. One might involve driving the child to school on a school day and/or observing him/her in a classroom (or other problematic) setting. This can be done to confirm reports of excess (e.g., tantrums, threats to run away) or deficit (e.g., social withdrawal) behavioral problems when attending school. A second observation may be scheduled when school is not in session (e.g., weekend) or when few people are in the school building. A comparison of the two observations is desirable to determine whether refusal to attend school is truly due to avoidance of specific stimuli (e.g., classroom activity) or to social/evaluative situations (e.g., meeting people). Finally, an analogue behavioral observation may also be set up to role-play potentially problematic social interactions or performances (e.g., speaking in front of others).

Problem Analysis

Given the heterogeneity of this population, several researchers have argued that it may be more profitable to explore the function rather than the form of school refusal behavior. Kearney and Silverman (1990, 1993) delineated four primary functions of school refusal behavior that may be helpful in this regard. First, youngsters may refuse school to avoid stimuli that provoke negative affectivity. Such stimuli can be varied, but often include school buses, fire alarms, teachers, classrooms, gymnasiums, hallways, cafeterias, and playgrounds. In many cases, children report an ill-defined dread of these places; however, a small subset of children have a specific phobic reaction that may be subsumed under this functional condition. Second, youngsters may refuse school to escape aversive social or evaluative situations. Such situations most commonly involve meeting new people, daily social

FORM 8.3. Behaviorial Approach Test for School Refusal Behavior

Client's Name: _____   Date: _____

Assessor: _____   Assessment point: _____

Needed:
Scheduled home visit, stopwatch, rating scale forms

Instructions for the recorder (follow these instructions step by step):
Prior to the home visit, discuss the 0–10 rating scale with the child and parents. Describe in detail the constructs of negative affectivity (i.e., general negative mood, including anxiety and depression) and noncompliance (i.e., refusal to comply with parental commands/requests). Distribute to each party a copy of the rating scale form for review.

Schedule a time to meet with the family in their home setting on a school day. Determine the child's rising time (e.g., 6:30 A.M.) and schedule to arrive 15 minutes earlier. Using a stopwatch, record the amount of time the child resists activities that would serve to prepare him/her for school attendance.

Specifically, record time in minutes taken for the following:
(1) *Verbal/physical resistance to rise from bed at the prespecified time*
   Verbal/physical resistance in this situation is defined as any verbalization, vocalization, or physical behavior that serves to contradict school attendance. In this situation, such behaviors might include (but are not limited to) verbal and physical noncompliance, clinging to bed, locking oneself in a bedroom, or refusal to move.
(2) *Verbal/physical resistance to dressing, washing, and eating*
   Verbal/physical resistance in this situation is defined as any verbalization, vocalization, or physical behavior that serves to contradict school attendance. In this situation, such behaviors might include (but are not limited to) verbal and physical noncompliance, clinging, screaming, crying, throwing objects, aggressive behavior, locking oneself in a room, running away, or refusal to move.
(3) *Verbal/physical resistance to riding in a car/bus to school*
   Verbal/physical resistance in this situation is defined as any verbalization, vocalization, or physical behavior that serves to contradict school attendance. In this situation, such behaviors might include (but are not limited to) verbal and physical noncompliance, screaming, crying, aggressive behavior, running away, or refusal to move.
(4) *Verbal/physical resistance to entering the school building*
   Verbal/physical resistance in this situation is defined as any verbalization, vocalization, or physical behavior that serves to contradict school attendance. In this situation, such behaviors might include (but are not limited to) verbal and physical noncompliance, clinging, screaming, crying, aggressive behavior, running away, or refusal to move.

In addition, record the child's rating of negative affectivity on the 0–10 scale where 0 = none, 2 = mild, 4 = moderate, 6 = marked, 8 = severe, and 10 = extreme. Use any number 0–10. *Remind the child to use the entire range of ratings.*

Record this rating twice:
(1) In the middle of morning preparation activities, and
(2) Upon entering the school building (if applicable).

In addition, record the parent's rating of child negative affectivity and noncompliance on the 0–10 scale where 0 = none, 2 = mild, 4 = moderate, 6 = marked, 8 = severe, and 10 = extreme. Use any number 0-10. *Remind the parent to use the entire range of ratings.*

Record this rating twice:
(1) In the middle of morning preparation activities, and
(2) Upon entering the school building (if applicable).

Contact the school attendance officer at the child's school to record any time missed during that school day. Complete all remaining sections of the recording sheet for the behavioral approach test.

interactions, tests, recitals, athletic performances, speaking/writing in front of others, and potentially embarrassing events such as being lost or sent to the principal. These two functional conditions describe school refusal behavior maintained by negative reinforcement. In other words, school refusal behavior may be a response reinforced by the reduction of anxiety or aversive somatic states.

Third, youngsters may refuse school to obtain verbal or physical attention from others (e.g., parents, teachers, peers). This functional condition is most analogous to the traditional notion of separa-

FORM 8.4. Recording Sheet for Behavioral Approach Test

Date/time: _____

All participants: _____

Assessment period: _____

  1. Record total verbal/physical resistance time for rising from bed:

     Total minutes: _____

  2. Record total verbal/physical resistance time for dressing, washing, and eating:

     Total minutes: _____

  3. Record child rating (0–10) of negative affectivity at midpoint of morning preparation activities:

     Rating: _____

  4. Record parent rating (0–10) of child's (a) negative affectivity and (b) noncompliance at midpoint of morning preparation activities:

     Negative affectivity rating: _____

     Noncompliance rating: _____

  5. Record total verbal/physical resistance time for riding in a car or bus to school:

     Total minutes: _____

  6. Record total verbal/physical resistance time for entering the school building:

     Total minutes: _____

  7. Record child rating (0–10) of negative affectivity upon entering school building (if applicable):

     Rating: _____

  8. Record parent rating (0–10) of child's (a) negative affectivity and (b) noncompliance upon entering school building (if applicable):

     Negative affectivity rating: _____

     Noncompliance rating: _____

  9. Record total amount of time missed during the school day:

     Total minutes: _____

 10. Record total amount of resistance time plus time missed during the school day:

     Total minutes: _____

 11. Record total time between rising time and end of school day:

     Total minutes: _____

 12. Calculate percentage of resistance/missed time to total time between rising time and end of school day:

     Percentage: _____

tion anxiety, but is broader in scope. Specifically, this refers to youngsters who wish to remain home with their parents or who create disruptions at school to receive attention from teachers and peers and expulsion from class to home. Finally, youngsters may refuse school to obtain positive tangible reinforcement. Such reinforcement often comes in the form of watching television at home, attending day parties with friends, drug use, or other stimulation (e.g., casinos) that increases the attractiveness of missing school. These two functional conditions describe school refusal behavior maintained by positive reinforcement.

Youngsters may also refuse school for a combination of these reasons. Approximately one-quarter of our clients with school refusal behavior display such a mixed functional profile (Kearney, Silverman, & Eisen, 1989). For example, it is not unusual for children to initially miss school to avoid a particular stimulus and subsequently discover the many positive advantages of staying home. Similarly, it is not unusual for children to initially miss school for positive tangible reinforcement and subsequently dread the prospect of returning to school and facing new social interactions. Any functional analysis and treatment for this population will be complicated by these scenarios, and clinicians should be sensitive to their presence in this population.

An exploration of these functions should be an integral part of the assessment process and may be accomplished in several interlocking phases. The first phase involves hypothesizing about the function of behavior, whereas the second and third phases involve a descriptive and experimental functional analysis, respectively. Each phase is described separately in this section.

Hypothesized Function of Behavior

Clinicians may initially hypothesize about the function of school refusal behavior by asking certain questions during the screening and formal assessment process. In the screening process, for example, the child's age should be ascertained. In general, younger children tend to refuse school to avoid general negative affectivity and/or to obtain attention; adolescents tend to refuse school to escape aversive social/evaluative situations and/or to obtain positive tangible reinforcement. These are general rules, however, that do not necessarily pertain to one particular case.

In the interview process, specific questions may also help reveal a primary functional condition for school refusal behavior. For youngsters, questions should surround some of the major stimuli (noted above) that dampen school attendance or attract one to an outside setting. Patterns of answers and stimuli should be noted and compared to the functional conditions described earlier. For example, a child's consistent reports of dread about attending a crowded classroom may provide support for an assumption of negative reinforcement function. Conversely, a child who consistently reports that he or she is bored with school, daydreams about events outside of school, and is substantially tempted by peer offers to miss school may provide

support for a hypothesis of positive reinforcement function.

Parents should be asked similar questions about their child, but care should be taken to note informant variance and incomplete parent reports. Because flaws in verbal reports are common, we recommend that clinicians initially hypothesize about whether school refusal behavior is motivated by simply negative and/or positive reinforcement. In some cases, however, the specific function will become quite clear during this process.

Self-report measures and parent/teacher checklists may also be helpful in developing a hypothesis about the functions of school refusal behavior. Data from our clinic reveal certain patterns of behavior that parallel these functions (Wadiak, Kearney, & Nagel, 1994). For example, children who refuse school to avoid stimuli provoking negative affectivity often display moderate to severe fear and general anxiety, mild depression and social anxiety, and good self-esteem. Parent reports indicate moderate levels of internalizing problems and very low levels of externalizing problems. In addition, the families of these children tend to be healthy in nature (i.e., high cohesion, expressiveness; low conflict). Children who refuse school to escape aversive social/evaluative situations often display moderate fear and general anxiety, severe depression and social anxiety, and poor self-esteem. Such children are characterized by high levels of internalizing but low levels of externalizing behavior, and their families are generally isolated in nature (i.e., low activity and intellectual–cultural orientation; Kearney & Silverman, 1995).

Children who refuse school for attention often display severe fear and general anxiety, moderate depression and social anxiety, and average self-esteem. Parent reports indicate high levels of internalizing but moderate levels of externalizing behavior as well as families characterized by enmeshment (i.e., low independence). Finally, children who refuse school for positive tangible reinforcement often display low fear and general anxiety, mild depression and social anxiety, and poor self-esteem. Parent reports indicate moderate levels of internalizing but high levels of externalizing behavior as well as families characterized by detachment (i.e., low cohesion; Kearney & Silverman, 1995). Before proceeding to a formal descriptive functional analysis, the clinician may wish to utilize these broad profiles to formulate an initial hypothesis about the variables that maintain school refusal behavior.

Descriptive Functional Analysis

A descriptive functional analysis of school refusal behavior may be accomplished by employing the one assessment measure specifically designed for this population. The School Refusal Assessment Scale (SRAS; Kearney & Silverman, 1993) is an instrument designed to solicit child (SRAS–C) and parent (SRAS–P) ratings to indicate the relative influence of the four functional conditions of school refusal behavior described earlier. The SRAS is modeled after the Motivation Assessment Scale (Durand & Crimmins, 1988), a device used to evaluate the function of problematic behavior in persons with severe handicaps. Specifically, children and parents complete separate versions of the SRAS, and item ratings are averaged to determine the primary motivating condition for school refusal behavior. In the original version of the SRAS, four items are devoted to each of the four functional conditions. Each item is scored on a 0–6 scale from "never" to "always." The SRAS, available from the first author, has been found to demonstrate sound interrater and test–retest reliability as well as concurrent and construct validity (see Kearney & Silverman, 1993, for items and scoring).

To conduct a descriptive functional analysis of school refusal behavior, the clinician solicits SRAS ratings from the child and two parents if possible. In most cases, we merge these reports into a single functional profile. For example, if mean item ratings on the (1) SRAS–C were 5.00 (avoidance of stimuli provoking negative affectivity), 4.25 (escape from aversive social/evaluative situations), 6.00 (attention), and 2.25 (positive tangible reinforcement), (2) mother SRAS–P were 5.00, 1.00, 6.00, and 2.75, and (3) father SRAS–P were 3.00, 3.00, 3.25, and 1.75, then the overall means for the functional profile would be 4.33, 2.75, 5.08, and 2.25, respectively. The primary functional condition for school refusal behavior is defined as the highest overall rating, in this case the third condition (5.08; attention), that is at least 0.25 points above the second-highest scoring condition. Ratings within this 0.25 point window (e.g., 4.50 and 4.33) are equivalent; two or more functional conditions could therefore be considered equally influential on school refusal behavior.

Such a functional profile allows the clinician to examine the primary motivating condition of school refusal behavior as well as secondary and tertiary influences. For example, a functional profile of 3.25, 3.50, 1.50, and 5.50 would indicate that a youngster is primarily refusing school to obtain positive tangible reinforcement (condition four). However, the clinician can also note that, to some lesser extent, the youngster is refusing school to avoid aversive negative affectivity and social/evaluative situations (conditions one and two). These latter influences may become important at some point during treatment, and the clinician can thus be forewarned about their presence.

During this descriptive analytic process, the clinician should watch for certain anomalies that may arise. The most critical is substantial informant variance, during which the child endorses one functional condition of school refusal behavior as the parent endorses another. This is most often due to one party who (1) is not well informed about the child's school refusal behavior, or (2) believes his or her "position" will be enhanced by a particular way of scoring the SRAS. With respect to the latter, for example, parents who feel guilty about their role in causing the child's behavior may produce misleading ratings indicating that school refusal behavior is primarily child based.

For these cases, we make several suggestions. One is to readminister the SRAS and evaluate the new ratings for convergence. A second suggestion is to look for inconsistencies among data from each family member's interviews, checklists, and SRAS ratings. In cases where such inconsistencies are common, we suggest that the clinician meet with each family member and gently derive an explanation. Should the problem involve one party not well informed of the behavior, then his or her particular SRAS rating should be deemphasized.

Another problem during this descriptive functional analysis is that children aged five to seven years sometimes cannot provide optimally useful ratings. In these cases, the clinician may administer the SRAS verbally or rely on parent reports. Should the latter be done, clinicians are encouraged to modify the functional profile in accordance with the youngster's verbal reports and other behaviors. For example, parent ratings indicating that school refusal behavior is primarily motivated by attention should be viewed cautiously in light of child reports that several school stimuli are upsetting to him or her.

Experimental Functional Analysis

To confirm initial hypotheses and descriptive functional analyses, clinicians should, if possible, conduct a more formal, experimental functional analysis. Specifically, a set of in vivo and analogue procedures may be established to validate a particular functional profile. In this section, we explore some recommended procedures for confirming the relative strength of each functional condition of school refusal behavior.

For children who may be refusing school to avoid stimuli provoking negative affectivity, the clinician may first establish two situations that either contain or do not contain the specific stimuli. For example, if a child is highly anxious about attending a playground setting, school attendance and ratings should be closely monitored under two conditions. The first may involve an extension of baseline measures, in that the child will be expected to attend school and the playground for one week (or shorter time depending on the severity of the case). During the subsequent week, a second, manipulated situation could be established so that the child would not be required to attend the playground. Should school attendance and ratings of negative affectivity from multiple sources improve demonstrably from the first week, then such evidence would appear to support the initial, descriptive functional analysis.

The reader should note, however, that in cases where aversive stimuli are not readily determined, such a process will require alternative methodologies. For example, many children report an ill-defined dread of the entire school building without identifying specific problems. In such cases, we recommend that the manipulated situation involve another building with similar features (e.g., narrow hallways, many rooms, crowded spaces). This may involve another school building or a business facility. In addition, should the child's aversion to a specific stimulus be so intense that approach to the school building is not initially possible, the clinician may set up an analogue behavioral approach task in the office. For example, a child reportedly terrified of fire alarms could be asked to approach as much as possible a smoke or intruder alarm that is currently sounding. Again, such an approach

should be compared to baseline performance to confirm or refute a descriptive functional analysis.

Similar scenarios may be used to conduct an experimental functional analysis for children refusing school to escape aversive social/evaluative situations. For example, baseline approach to school and ratings of behavior (e.g., social anxiety) may be compared to performance in manipulated situations such as an empty school building, recitals without an audience, exemption from physical education class, and allowing one to eat outside alone. Similarly, analogue situations may be contrived in the office. A common scenario in our practice involves youngsters who feel they cannot speak publicly. In this situation, we ask the youngster to read a newspaper article in front of a small group of unknown people; we gauge his or her avoidance, anxiety, and performance accordingly.

For youngsters who refuse school for positive reinforcement, experimental functional analysis may take place in or outside of school. With respect to children refusing school for attention, for example, the manipulated situation could involve allowing the parent to attend school with the child. However, home- or office-based tasks may also be established to see if the child consistently tries to achieve physical proximity to the parents or to seek reassurance from others. With respect to youngsters refusing school for positive tangible reinforcement, the manipulated situation may involve a short-term, substantial increase of incentives to attend school or a substantial curtailment of activities if the child is home from school.

Following descriptive and experimental functional analyses, the clinician should have a fair grasp of the primary motivating condition(s) for school refusal behavior. In addition, such analyses should provide a rich set of treatment targets that can be addressed in short-term fashion. In our model of school refusal behavior, we encourage clinicians to closely link descriptive and experimental functional analysis results with individualized, step-by-step treatment plans. The next section of this chapter describes these prescriptive treatment plans.

Plan Implementation

Traditional treatments for school refusal behavior include family therapy to increase distance between a mother and child (Eisenberg, 1958), enhancing child self-esteem (Levanthal & Sills, 1964), forced school attendance (Kennedy, 1965), residential treatment (Church & Edwards, 1984), systematic desensitization (Lazarus, Davison, & Polefka, 1965), and pharmacotherapy (e.g., imipramine; Gittelman-Klein & Klein, 1971), among others. Although each treatment has been found to be moderately effective in reducing school refusal behavior for some youngsters, none have shown efficacy for all those with problematic absenteeism. For example, Kennedy's (1965) forced school attendance approach often works well for young children with initial school refusal behavior, but is generally not effective for older children and adolescents with longer histories of the problem.

A potentially more effective strategy for addressing this heterogeneous population may be to employ a prescriptive treatment approach or the assignment of different, circumscribed treatments to different subtypes of youngsters with school refusal behavior. We employ a prescriptive treatment approach that follows the functional analytic process described above. In this section, we present an outline of our treatment procedures for each designated function, as well as information about treatment integrity and generalization of treatment effects. These procedures have been found to be effective with different subsets of youngsters with school refusal behavior (e.g., Ayllon, Smith, & Rogers, 1970; Leal, Baxter, Martin, & Marx, 1981; Morris & Kratochwill, 1991; O'Reilly, 1971; Vaal, 1973). In addition, the procedures have been found to be effective on a preliminary basis when prescriptively assigned on the basis of the functional analysis described above (Kearney, 1992; Kearney & Silverman, 1990).

Avoidance of Stimuli Provoking Negative Affectivity

For children who refuse school to avoid stimuli that provoke general negative affectivity, we employ a child-based treatment approach utilizing relaxation training and gradual exposure to the school setting. For children who are fearful of a specific stimulus regarding the school setting, the fuller process of systematic desensitization is implemented. A key goal is to provide the child with a behavior that serves as an antagonist to the feeling of dread experienced at school. As a result, the reintegration of the child into the school setting should be more easily facilitated.

Various relaxation procedures are available, although we prefer the tension-release technique refined for children by Ollendick and Cerny (1981). Initially in the office setting, the youngster is asked to systematically tense different muscle groups (e.g., hands, face, stomach), hold the muscles in place, and release the tension quickly. Youngsters are urged to concentrate on the difference between a relaxed and a tense muscle, and identify those muscle groups that are most rigid in a stressful situation. Typically, the therapist conducts the relaxation sesson using a verbalized script, which is audiotaped and given to the client. We ask our clients to practice the relaxation procedure twice per day and during any daily situations that produce stress.

When the youngster is adept at inducing relaxation, some form of imaginal exposure is introduced. For children who report general negative affectivity at school, an overall description of the school setting (e.g., classroom, gymnasium, hallways, playground) may be conveyed during relaxation. In cases where a specific stimulus is feared, the formal construction of an anxiety hierarchy is made with the client prior to imaginally pairing relaxation with each successive item on the hierarchy (Wolpe, 1990). If the child is already attending school but with substantial dread, then these treatment processes can start in vivo almost immediately. If the child is not going to school regularly, then a schedule should be established to gradually reintroduce the child to a full-time attendance routine. In vivo practice may then begin as the child gradually increases his or her school attendance.

A treatment example of this function from our clinic involved a nine-year-old male who reported an ill-defined dread of school and unease about returning to school following an extended absence. In this case, we initially taught the child relaxation training and engaged in imaginal exposure to a variety of school-related stimuli (e.g., bus, teacher, in-school assignments). Following proficiency at this task, we worked closely with the school officials to (1) allow the child to refamiliarize himself with the school surroundings and meet the teacher when school was not in session, and (2) gradually reintroduce the child into the classroom setting. We initially began by asking the child to sit in the library under supervision for a half day and then a full day. We subsequently reintegrated the child into the classroom for one hour per day and then added one hour each day. Over a two-month period, anxiety was significantly reduced and the child attended school full-time.

Escape from Aversive Social and Evaluative Situations

For children who refuse school to escape aversive social/evaluative situations, we employ a child-based treatment approach utilizing modeling, role-play, and cognitive restructuring. The overall goal is to enhance a child's social skill, reduce social anxiety, and/or modify interfering cognitive distortions that impede school attendance. The achievement of these goals should facilitate school reattendance behavior.

Initially, about 5–10 social or evaluative situations are identified that make school attendance most problematic. Each situation, beginning with the least aversive, is initially role-played in the office setting. A common scenario involves a youngster who refuses school to avoid assigned oral presentations in class. In this situation, the youngster is asked to give an oral presentation in a contrived setting with a small audience. Following the performance, feedback is given regarding strengths and areas that require improvement (Cartledge & Milburn, 1995). A model for sound performance is provided if appropriate. This performance and feedback process is continued repeatedly until the therapist and client are relatively confident of the latter's efficacy and reduced anxiety in the situation. Increasingly aversive social/evaluative situations are subsequently addressed.

Following this process, the youngster is asked to practice these newly refined skills in the school setting. A partial schedule for attending school may also be established at this time. In this case, for example, the youngster could be required to attend school except for the one class that is most problematic. Eventually, however, the child would be expected to complete the modeled task and report his or her performance level to the therapist. An expansion of modeled tasks to other real-life situations would ensue (e.g., initiating conversations with peers).

In addition to these procedures, we employ cognitive restructuring to modify maladaptive thought patterns that interfere with reexposure to the school setting. Although various cognitive therapy procedures have been utilized for youngsters in recent years, we tend to focus on three in particular. Decatastrophizing, or the "what if" strategy, involves subjecting unrealistic conclusions about one's environment to logical analysis (Beck & Emery, 1985). For example, a youngster may state that he will stumble over his words during a presentation, provoking laughter from the entire class. Such a statement should be thoroughly examined and reframed more positively. Similarly, decentering may be used for youngsters convinced that others are closely evaluating their behavior. In this case, one should examine whether the client is always as aware of others as others are allegedly aware of the client. Finally, youngsters may be taught appropriate coping skills such as distraction or actively examining alternatives to rigid thoughts. These techniques often begin early in treatment and continue through follow-up. In using these techniques, however, the clinician should assess the cognitive developmental level of the child. If such development cannot support these treatment procedures, then an emphasis should be placed on the modeling and role-playing methods.

A treatment example of this function from our clinic involved a 15-year-old female who was upset about speaking in front of others in a classroom setting. New to the school, the adolescent was not yet surrounded by a supportive social network and had begun to leave school in the middle of the day. Modeling and role-play treatment focused on refining social skills so that the youngster could approach others and potentially develop new friendships. In addition, such treatment was used to practice in-session oral presentations. A schedule for presenting in class was set up with the adolescent's teacher in concert with the therapeutic regimen. Therefore, a timely "real-life" practice of therapy procedures could occur. Cognitive restructuring was also utilized to combat depressive and self-destructive thoughts. Full-time school attendance was achieved within four weeks, and social anxiety was reduced 75% in six weeks.

Attention-Getting Behavior

For children who refuse school to obtain verbal or physical attention from others, we employ a parent-based treatment approach utilizing contingency management procedures. The overall goal is to strengthen the parents' ability to provide effective commands to the child and appropriate consequences to adaptive and maladaptive behavior. Following such an approach, parents should be better equipped to address the child's school refusal behavior and facilitate school attendance on their own.

Specifically, we first ask the parents to establish a regular morning routine for the child (e.g., specific times for rising, washing, dressing, eating, leaving home). This routine should be explained to the child before the end of the session and implemented the next day. An evening schedule should also be designed if the child engages in several excess school refusal behaviors (e.g., reassurance-seeking) prior to bedtime. This scheduling allows parents to note specific deviations in the routine and assign later contingencies accordingly.

Various problematic morning behaviors are subsequently identified and parents are provided with suggestions for responding to them. For example, we encourage parents to respond in an emotionally neutral manner to somatic and other complaints raised by the child. In addition, we encourage parents to reframe negative child self-statements and indicate their confidence in the child's ability to go to school on his or her own (e.g., "I know you can do it; it's time to go now"). Finally, parents are urged to provide terse and clear commands to the child prior to school. Any excess verbal or physical attention is discouraged, although we allow the parents to physically bring the child to school under certain predefined circumstances. The latter applies particularly to situations where two parents can work in tandem to facilitate the child's school attendance.

A critical aspect of this process is developing appropriate contingencies for positive as well as negative behavior (Barkley, 1989). Should the child attend school in the absence of the previously defined school refusal behaviors, we recommend that parents provide substantial verbal praise that evening after school. Should this behavior continue for one full school week, parents should provide a more substantial reinforcer, involving interaction with the child (e.g., staying up an extra half-hour to read with parents).

If the child demonstrates some school refusal behavior but eventually goes to school, we recommend that some negative contingency be applied when the child returns home. This generally consists of being grounded (for double the amount of time that school is missed) and/or having to stay in one's room until bedtime. During this time, the child should work on homework and studying without television or other amenities. If the child demonstrates severe school refusal behavior and successfully stays home from school, we recommend that he or she sit in a chair under parental supervision during school hours. Extra verbal or physical attention should be avoided, and the setting should be as dull as possible. Following the end of normal school hours, the contingencies noted above should be implemented and the child should work on homework solicited from the teacher. Should this behavior continue for a majority of the school week, then appropriate weekend contingencies should be applied.

The overall purpose of this strategy is to empower the parents and establish clear rules and consequences regarding maladaptive behavior. Specifically, the amount of verbal and physical attention awarded to the child should be redirected toward more appropriate behaviors. The child should be told of the upcoming contingencies and informed that compliance to the rules remains their choice. In addition, parents should be reminded of the importance of consistency during this process.

A treatment example of this function from our clinic involved a seven-year-old girl who displayed severe acting-out behaviors, such as tantrums and clinging, from 6:30 to 8:15 A.M. on school days. No other difficulties were evident, and the child did not present problems once in school. Here, parental contingency management began by delineating a specific morning routine. The child would get out of bed at 6:30, attend the bathroom and wash until 6:45, dress and prepare schoolwork until 7:15, eat until 7:45, brush teeth and put on shoes and coat until 8:00, and then be driven to school by both parents. The parents were instructed to attend only to positive behavior and physically prompt the completion of the morning routine even if it took half a day. Verbal rewards were provided for good days and consequences similar to those outlined above were provided for disruptions. The child initially presented with an increased severity of behavior for four days, but school refusal declined suddenly thereafter. Within one month, the child had gone to school for two consecutive weeks with no morning problems. Sporadic recurrences were reported on some Monday mornings in following months, but these were effectively rectified.

Positive Tangible Reinforcement

For children who refuse school to obtain positive tangible reinforcement, we employ a family-based treatment approach that focuses on contingency contracting. The overall goal is to reduce the substantial reinforcers for missing school and increase incentives for attending school. Following such an approach, the family should have, and be able to generate, a problem-solving strategy to maintain school attendance and address related problems across time. In many cases, for example, family conflict serves to exacerbate a child's school nonattendance or trigger unauthorized absence from home. Almost invariably, this leads to further disruption and punishment. As an alternative, family members may be taught to recognize potentially volatile situations and defuse them in a more diplomatic, cohesive, and productive manner via contracting.

In our clinic, contracting is essentially a negotiation process in which the clinician acts as mediator. Specific goals as well as proposed methods of achieving such goals are solicited from each relevant party. In most instances, parents wish for a resumption of full-time school attendance and compliance with household rules, whereas youngsters tend to demand more independence and recognition for accomplishments at home and school.

Our most successful contracts usually involve an agreed-upon return to school in response to clear-cut parental reactions to certain behaviors. Specifically, youngsters are offered the opportunity to earn compensation by going to school and by completing various household chores. The opportunity to complete the chores for compensation is provided only, however, if the child maintains adequate school attendance. If not, then the chores must be completed without compensation. In this case, we allow the parents to maintain "veto" power over the quality of the chore (i.e., the option of asking the child to repeat the task). School attendance is also monitored on a daily basis. Conversely, we ask the youngsters to identify any areas of the contract that the parents have not upheld. Additional concerns are then imbedded into later contracts, in-

volving curfew time, homework, activities with friends, and other relevant contingencies (including additional ones levied for absenteeism).

As part of the negotiation process, we emphasize to both parties that no contract will be signed unless each fully consents with all provisions. Any reservations should be completely addressed by the time of signing. In addition, each party should monitor the compliance of the other and alert the therapist immediately should any problems arise. We recommend that initial contracts last only two or three days at most and be circumscribed in nature to enhance early success. Later contracts can be designed more broadly and incorporate longer timespans. By the end of treatment, school attendance should be steady and family members should be able to initiate and complete contracts without substantial therapist guidance.

A treatment example of this function from our clinic involved a 14-year-old male who had missed school 67% of the time during the past five months. His mother, a single parent, worked during the day and could not supervise him at all times. A contract between the adolescent and mother increased the time the teen could spend with his father if school was attended without absence. This was done with the father's agreement. Also, both parents were instructed to contact the school daily and establish a strict monitoring schedule. Any missed school time was punished via grounding. No substantial change in school attendance occurred until the parents agreed to take their son to school and walk him from class to class. After seven school days, the adolescent asked for a new contract that involved the chores and financial incentives mentioned previously. Although daily monitoring of school attendance via telephone remained necessary, the teen did attend school regularly for the next four months.

Special Considerations

Some special circumstances may arise during prescriptive treatment of school refusal behavior. One circumstance involves children who refuse school primarily for two or more of the functions described earlier. Many children, for example, refuse school to avoid negative affectivity-provoking stimuli *and* aversive social/evaluative situations. In these cases, combined prescriptive treatment would be appropriate.

Special considerations also apply to each prescriptive treatment. During reexposure to the school setting in desensitization and modeling or cognitive therapy, for example, a key element of success is the cooperation of school officials. In many cases, we find it necessary to ask a librarian, guidance counselor, or principal to supervise a child in a substitute setting while gradual reintegration into the classroom takes place. To improve cooperation, we suggest that clinicians involve all relevant school officials in the treatment process as soon as possible and solicit recommendations from them at each therapeutic step.

During parent training, a key consideration is an "extinction burst" often displayed by children. In essence, a child may increase the severity of his or her problematic behavior immediately after the parents implement the contingency management procedures. This is done to induce acquiescence to the previous status quo. In this situation, we find it helpful to inform parents about this process and provide suggestions for addressing excess problems (e.g., taking off work in the morning for the next few days). In related fashion, a special consideration of family contracting is the exploitation of unforeseen loopholes. This is typically seen in a youngster who wishes his or her parents to hold up their end of the contract without having to fully complete his or her own responsibilities. In this case, we recommend that clinicians strictly define all contract terms and further assure that all parties are completely content with the document before signing.

Special considerations also apply to every prescriptive treatment. These include the family's financial resources, dynamics, and noncompliance with the treatment regimen. We have found noncompliance to be most damaging to the treatment process. Should the clinician encounter substantial difficulties in treatment compliance, it may be helpful to contact the family daily to address problems immediately, monitor school attendance, and anticipate upcoming periods that are highly predictive of relapse. Such periods most often include Mondays and days following extended holidays. We recommend that clinicians contact family members during these times (e.g., call on Sunday night) and assess for (1) increased child anxiety, and (2) weakened child or parental resolve to follow through on treatment procedures.

Treatment Integrity

In related fashion, treatment integrity regarding children and parents is best accomplished by constantly monitoring compliance with the therapeutic regimen and completion of the daily logbooks. A similar process may also be employed with teachers and other school officials, who can supply daily report cards regarding class behavior, tardiness, homework, and peer interactions. With respect to clinicians, we audiotape a subset of all treatment sessions and subject the conversation to ratings made by independent observers. These observers are trained to indicate whether the clinician transacted the key elements of each prescriptive treatment (i.e., relaxation, modeling, contingency management, contracting). Any deviation from the prescriptive treatment protocol is then immediately addressed and rectified.

Generalization of Treatment Outcome

Generalization of treatment outcome regarding school refusal behavior is best accomplished by (1) expanding the foci of treatment during therapy, and (2) scheduling several follow-up sessions. With respect to the former, we try to address several problematic behaviors that are sometimes predictive of relapse once the child has achieved full-time school attendance. For example, fear and anxiety are targeted in school-related situations such as coming home from school, attending school functions at night, and meeting school friends outside of academic settings. In addition, the child is asked to model appropriate social responses to a variety of extracurricular interactions such as dating, meeting new people, and performing in front of others outside of school. With respect to parent training and contracting, we provide each relevant family member with hypothetical, problematic scenarios to test the appropriateness of their responses (e.g., development of new contingencies and contract).

Scheduling follow-up sessions is also critical to generalization. We recommend frequent telephone contact with clients at least four weeks after treatment termination, and formal follow-up sessions three and six months later. In addition, some contact should be made with the family just prior to the start of the next academic year. Preferably, the child should be exposed to the new school building and related situations prior to the start of classes to reduce anticipatory anxiety and prevent other problems. Specific areas of concern include one's bus, locker, homeroom, cafeteria, library, and gymnasium.

Plan Evaluation

When treating youngsters with school refusal behavior, we define positive end-state functioning as at least two weeks of continuous, full-time school attendance (excluding legitimate physical illness) and/or a 75% reduction in distress. Given this criterion, the effectiveness of treatment for school refusal behavior can be determined in several ways. The most straightforward way is to monitor school attendance from formal assessment to follow-up. In our clinic, we encourage parents to monitor and record daily the number of hours the child is in school. This is done to identify improvement and incorporate parental monitoring into an everyday routine. As a result, the child knows that his or her behavior is being closely supervised and any deviations in school attendance can be addressed immediately.

The criterion for positive end-state functioning also applies to children who go to school but tolerate it with great dread. In these cases, we focus more intently on child and parent ratings of anxiety, depression, and overt behavior problems. Specifically, baseline ratings are compared to ongoing treatment data to quantify patterns of change and help determine whether treatment should be terminated. To support or refute these findings, familial responses to the hypothetical problem scenarios mentioned previously are carefully scrutinized and graded by the therapist. If the family's response to these scenarios is inadequate or contradicts the daily ratings, then the therapist should explore the reasons for this variance and decide whether treatment should continue.

Pretreatment behavioral observations and questionnaires are also readministered. These are compared to earlier findings as well as to daily ratings. If treatment has successfully resolved school refusal behavior, substantial discrepancies between pre- and posttreatment measures should be evident. In addition, the posttreatment results should parallel those found from the daily ratings. If this is not the case, the clinician should, again, explore reasons

for the variance and decide whether treatment should continue.

Plan Evaluation for Specific Functions

With respect to youngsters who refuse school for negative reinforcement (i.e., to avoid stimuli provoking negative affectivity or to escape aversive social/evaluative situations), clinicians should concentrate on pre- and posttreatment comparisons that are most pertinent to these conditions. For example, an emphasis should be placed on child self-reports of anxiety and depression (e.g., NASSQ, RCMAS, CDI, SASC–R), behavioral approach to school in general and social interactions in particular, and heart rate if possible. With respect to youngsters who refuse school for positive reinforcement (i.e., attention or tangible reinforcement), clinicians may wish to concentrate on more parent- and family-focused variables. For example, an emphasis should be placed on pre- and posttreatment comparisons of parent reports of child behavior problems, family members' ability to design contingency management protocols and contracts, and measures of problematic family dynamics (e.g., FES).

Social Validation

Another key element in evaluating the treatment plan for school refusal behavior is social validation. In our clinic, we solicit parent ratings of the effectiveness of treatment during the posttreatment process. Parents are asked to answer the question, "How much would you attribute the changes in your child's behavior to the treatment procedure?" The question is answered both anecdotally and by providing a rating on a 0–10 scale where zero is "completely not due to the treatment procedure" and 10 is "completely due to the treatment procedure." This measure of treatment credibility is extended to youngsters and teachers if possible. Ratings of six or above are acceptable; ratings less then six should prompt the clinician to examine extraneous variables (e.g., change of classrooms by the principal) that may have spurred the final outcome. This should be done to help assess the client's risk of relapse and alert the clinician about circumstances (e.g., difficulty carrying out a treatment assignment) that may affect the treatment progress of similar, future clients.

Plan Evaluation During and After Treatment

The effectiveness of different treatments for school refusal behavior may also be determined at different points in the therapeutic process. This is most applicable to youngsters who refuse school for an influential but secondary reason. For example, a child may refuse school to primarily escape aversive social situations and, secondarily, to obtain positive tangible reinforcement. Initial treatment in this case should focus on the social function, and appropriate measures to gauge progress (those noted previously) should be taken. Treatment may then focus, however, on reducing the tangible reinforcers for missing school. Gauging treatment progress regarding this function should continue, with some assessment measures protracted from earlier therapy (e.g., school attendance) and other measures subsequently brought to the fore (e.g., parent reports of compliance to contracts). During the final posttreatment process, however, behaviors specific to all relevant functions should be assessed.

Monitoring the effectiveness of treatment for school refusal behavior should continue during the follow-up sessions noted previously. In these sessions, we focus on general parent and child reports, data regarding school attendance, and readministration of questionnaires. More in-depth measurement is utilized if the family engages in a booster session designed to improve the effectiveness of techniques and skills learned during treatment. In this situation, for example, a greater emphasis should be placed on behavioral observation during analogue procedures (e.g., oral presentation in an office). Finally, the effectiveness of treatment should be gauged at the beginning of the following academic year, when the child may be most at risk for relapse. We have found that child reports of significant anticipatory anxiety are often predictive of such relapse; as a result, we rely on such reports to decide if further intervention is warranted.

Summary and Directions for Further Research

Given the heterogeneity of school refusal behavior in children and adolescents, the assessment and treatment of this population may best be accomplished by pursuing a functional analytic process in various phases. Specifically, the assessment process should involve a variety of sources and empirically derived measures. Such measures should be used to initiate and later confirm a clinician's hypothesis that school refusal behavior is motivated by avoidance of stimuli that provoke negative affectivity, escape from aversive social or evaluative situations, attention, and/or positive tangible reinforcement. Treatment for this population is likely to be most effective when prescriptively assigned from the results of this functional analysis.

In this chapter, we have tried to present a basic formula for utilizing a functional analytic process in assessing and treating youngsters with school refusal behavior. However, we also recognize that further research is needed to refine and validate the process. Specifically, the functional profiles that characterize this population need to be more carefully defined. For example, it would be quite helpful to clinicians to know exactly what symptomatology, family dynamics, and developmental patterns are embedded in each functional condition. In addition, descriptive functional analytic processes (e.g., the School Refusal Assessment Scale) may be further developed and expanded to include teachers. Finally, more extensive outcome studies are required to fully assess the treatment validity of the model we have expounded upon here. Overall, the assessment and treatment of school refusal behavior, traditionally a neglected area of social clinical practice, remains still an open field for clinical and theoretical development. We therefore encourage clinical practitioners and researchers to be innovative when addressing this population.

References

Achenbach, T.M. (1991a). *Manual for the Child Behavior Checklist/4-18 and 1991 profile.* Burlington: University of Vermont, Department of Psychiatry.

Achenbach, T.M. (1991b). *Manual for the Teacher's Report Form and 1991 profile.* Burlington: University of Vermont, Department of Psychiatry.

Ayllon, T., Smith, D., & Rogers, M. (1970). Behavioral management of school phobia. *Journal of Behavior Therapy and Experimental Psychiatry, 1,* 125–138.

Barkley, R.A. (1989). Attention-deficit hyperactivity disorder. In E.J. Mash & R.A. Barkley (Eds.), *Treatment of childhood disorders,* (pp. 39–72). New York: Guilford.

Beck, A.T., & Emery, G. (1985). *Anxiety disorders and phobias: A cognitive perspective.* New York: Basic.

Berg, I. (1970). A follow-up study of school phobic adolescents admitted to an inpatient unit. *Journal of Child Psychology and Psychiatry, 11*, 37–47.

Berg, I., & Jackson, A. (1985). Teenage school refusers grow up: A follow-up study of 168 subjects, ten years on average after inpatient treatment. *British Journal of Psychiatry, 147*, 366–370.

Cartledge, G., & Milburn, J.F. (1995). *Teaching social skills to children and youth: Innovative approaches* (3rd. ed.). Boston: Allyn & Bacon.

Church, J., & Edwards, B. (1984). Helping pupils who refuse school. *Special Education: Forward Trends, 11*, 28–31.

Conners, C.K. (1990). *Conners' rating scales manual.* North Tonawanda, NY: Multi-Health Systems.

Cooper, M. (1986). A model of persistent absenteeism. *Educational Research, 28*, 14–20.

Durand, V.M., & Crimmins, D.B. (1988). Identifying the variables maintaining self-injurious behavior. *Journal of Autism and Developmental Disorders, 18*, 99–117.

Eisen, A.R., & Kearney, C.A. (1995). *Practitioner's guide to treating fear and anxiety in children and adolescents: A cognitive–behavioral approach.* Northvale, NJ: Aronson.

Eisen, A.R., Spasaro, S.A., Kearney, C.A., Albano, A.M., & Barlow, D.H. (1996). Measuring parental expectancies in a child anxiety disorders sample: The Parental Expectancies Scale. *Behavior Therapist, 19*, 37–38.

Eisenberg, L. (1958). School phobia: A study in the communication of anxiety. *American Journal of Psychiatry, 114*, 712–718.

Flakierska, N., Lindstrom, M., & Gillberg, C. (1988). School refusal: A 15–20-year follow-up study of 35 Swedish urban children. *British Journal of Psychiatry, 152*, 834–837.

Gittelman-Klein, R., & Klein, D.F. (1971). Controlled imipramine treatment of school phobia. *Archives of General Psychiatry, 25*, 204–207.

Granell de Aldaz, E., Vivas, E., Gelfand, D.M., & Feldman, L. (1984). Estimating the prevalence of school refusal and school-related fears: A Venezuelan sample. *Journal of Nervous and Mental Disease, 172*, 722–729.

Harris, S.L., & Ferrari, M. (1983). Developmental factors in child behavior therapy. *Behavior Therapy, 14*, 54–72.

Hersov, L. (1985). School refusal. In M. Rutter & L. Hersov (Eds.), *Child and adolescent psychiatry: Modern approaches* (pp. 382–399). Boston: Blackwell Scientific.

Hibbett, A., & Fogelman, K. (1990). Future lives of truants: Family formation and health-related behaviour. *British Journal of Educational Psychology, 60*, 171–179.

Hibbett, A., Fogelman, K., & Manor, O. (1990). Occupational outcomes of truancy. *British Journal of Educational Psychology, 60*, 23–36.

Kahn, J.H., & Nursten, J.P. (1962). School refusal: A comprehensive view of school phobia and other failures of school attendance. *American Journal of Orthopsychiatry, 32*, 707–718.

Kearney, C.A. (1992, November). *Prescriptive treatment for school refusal behavior.* Symposium presented at the meeting of the Association for the Advancement of Behavior Therapy, Boston.

Kearney, C.A. (1993). Depression and school refusal behavior: A review with comments on classification and treatment. *Journal of School Psychology, 31*, 267–279.

Kearney, C.A. (1995). School refusal behavior. In A.R. Eisen, C.A. Kearney, & C.E. Schaefer (Eds.), *Clinical handbook of anxiety disorders in children and adolescents* (pp. 19–52). Northvale, NJ: Aronson.

Kearney, C.A., & Silverman, W.K. (1990). A preliminary analysis of a functional model of assessment and treatment for school refusal behavior. *Behavior Modification, 14*, 340–366.

Kearney, C.A., & Silverman, W.K. (1993). Measuring the function of school refusal behavior: The School Refusal Assessment Scale. *Journal of Clinical Child Psychology, 22*, 85–96.

Kearney, C.A., & Silverman, W.K. (1995). Family environment of youngsters with school refusal behavior: A synopsis with implications for assessment and treatment. *American Journal of Family Therapy, 23*, 59–72.

Kearney, C.A., & Silverman, W.K. (1996). The evolution and reconciliation of taxonomic strategies for school refusal behavior. *Clinical Psychology: Science and Practice, 3*, 339–354.

Kearney, C.A., Silverman, W.K., & Eisen, A.R. (1989, October). *The function of school refusal behavior: Loathing school or loving home?* Paper presented at the meeting of the Berkshire Association for Behavior Analysis and Therapy, Amherst, MA.

Kearney, C.A., Drabman, R.S., & Beasley, J.F. (1993). The trials of childhood: The development, reliability, and validity of the Daily Life Stressors Scale. *Journal of Child and Family Studies, 2*, 371–388.

Kearney, C.A., Eisen, A.R., & Silverman, W.K. (1995). The legend and myth of school phobia. *School Psychology Quarterly, 10*, 65–85.

Kennedy, W.A. (1965). School phobia: Rapid treatment of 50 cases. *Journal of Abnormal Psychology, 70*, 285–289.

Kovacs, M. (1992). *Children's Depression Inventory manual.* North Tonawanda, NY: Multi-Health Systems.

La Greca, A.M., & Stone, W.L. (1993). Social Anxiety Scale for Children–Revised: Factor structure and concurrent validity. *Journal of Clinical Child Psychology, 22*, 17–27.

Last, C.G. (1991). Somatic complaints in anxiety disordered children. *Journal of Anxiety Disorders, 5*, 125–138.

Last, C.G., & Strauss, C.C. (1990). School refusal in anxiety-disordered children and adolescents. *Journal of the American Academy of Child and Adolescent Psychiatry, 29*, 31–35.

Lazarus, A.A., Davison, G.G., & Polefka, D.A. (1965). Classical and operant factors in the treatment of school phobia. *Journal of Abnormal Psychology, 70*, 225–229.

Leal, L.L., Baxter, E.G., Martin, J., & Marx, R.W. (1981). Cognitive modification and systematic desensitization with test anxious high school students. *Journal of Counseling Psychology, 28*, 525–528.

Leventhal, T., & Sills, M. (1964). Self-image in school phobia. *American Journal of Orthopsychiatry, 34*, 685–695.

Moos, R.H., & Moos, B.S. (1986). *Family Environment Scale manual* (2nd ed.). Palo Alto, CA: Consulting Psychologists Press.

Morris, R.J., & Kratochwill, T.R. (1991). Childhood fears and phobias. In T.R. Kratochwill & R.J. Morris (Eds.), *The practice of child therapy* (2nd ed., pp. 76–114). New York: Pergamon.

Ollendick, T.H. (1983). Reliability and validity of the revised Fear Survey Schedule for Children (FSSC–R). *Behaviour Research and Therapy, 21*, 685–692.

Ollendick, T.H., & Cerny, J.A. (1981). *Clinical behavior therapy with children.* New York: Plenum.

O'Reilly, P.P. (1971). Desensitization of fire bell phobia. *Journal of School Psychology, 9,* 55–57.

Piers, E.V. (1984). *Piers-Harris Children's Self-Concept Scale: Revised manual 1984.* Los Angeles: Western Psychological Services.

Reynolds, C.R., & Paget, K.D. (1981). Factor analysis of the Revised Children's Manifest Anxiety Scale for blacks, whites, males, and females with a national normative sample. *Journal of Consulting and Clinical Psychology, 49,* 352–359.

Robins, L.N., & Ratcliffe, K.S. (1980). The long-term outcome of truancy. In L. Hersov & I. Berg (Eds.), *Out of school* (pp. 65–83). New York: Wiley.

Ronan, K.R., Kendall, P.C., & Rowe, M. (1994). Negative affectivity in children: Development and validation of a self-statement questionnaire. *Cognitive Therapy and Research, 18,* 509–528.

Silverman, W.K., & Albano, A.M. (1996). *Anxiety Disorders Interview Schedule for DSM-IV: Parent and child version (ADIS-P&C).* San Antonio, TX: The Psychological Corporation.

Silverman, W.K., & Eisen, A.R. (1992). Age differences in the reliability of parent and child reports of child anxious symptomatology using a structured interview. *Journal of the American Academy of Child and Adolescent Psychiatry, 31,* 117–124.

Silverman, W.K., & Nelles, W.B. (1988). The Anxiety Disorders Interview Schedule for Children. *Journal of the American Academy of Child and Adolescent Psychiatry, 27,* 772–778.

Silverman, W.K., Fleisig, W., Rabian, B., & Peterson, R.A. (1991). The Child Anxiety Sensitivity Index. *Journal of Clinical Child Psychology, 20,* 162–168.

Spanier, G.B. (1976). Measuring dyadic adjustment: New scales for assessing the quality of marriage and similar dyads. *Journal of Marriage and the Family, 38,* 15–28.

Spielberger, C.D. (1973). *Manual for the State–Trait Anxiety Inventory for Children.* Palo Alto, CA: Consulting Psychologists Press.

Thompson, C.L., & Rudolph, L.B. (1988). *Counseling children* (2nd. ed.). Pacific Grove, CA: Brooks/Cole.

Vaal, J.J. (1973). Applying contingency contracting to a school phobia: A case study. *Journal of Behavior Therapy and Experimental Psychiatry, 4,* 371–373.

Wadiak, D., Kearney, C.A., & Nagel, H.E. (1994, April). *The functional profiles of school refusal behavior.* Symposium presented at the meeting of the Rocky Mountain Psychological Association, Las Vegas, NV.

Wolpe, J. (1990). *The practice of behavior therapy* (4th. ed.). Boston: Allyn & Bacon.

Zigler, E., Taussig, C., & Black, K. (1992). Early childhood intervention: A promising preventative for juvenile delinquency. *American Psychologist, 47,* 997–1006.

Bibliography

Blagg, N.R., & Yule, W. (1984). The behavioural treatment of school refusal: A comparative study. *Behaviour Research and Therapy, 22,* 119–127.

Broadwin, I.T. (1932). A contribution to the study of truancy. *American Journal of Orthopsychiatry, 2,* 253–259.

Flakierska, N., Lindstrom, M., & Gillberg, C. (1988). School refusal: A 15–20-year follow-up study of 35 Swedish urban children. *British Journal of Psychiatry, 152,* 834–837.

Gittelman-Klein, R., & Klein, D.F. (1971). Controlled imipramine treatment of school phobia. *Archives of General Psychiatry, 25,* 204–207.

Granell de Aldaz, E., Vivas, E., Gelfand, D.M., & Feldman, L. (1984). Estimating the prevalence of school refusal and school-related fears: A Venezuelan sample. *Journal of Nervous and Mental Disease, 172,* 722–729.

Hersov, L. (1985). School refusal. In M. Rutter & R. Hersov (Eds.), *Child and adolescent psychiatry: Modern approaches* (2nd. ed., pp. 382–399). Oxford, England: Blackwell Scientific.

Johnson, A.M., Falstein, E.I., Szurek, S.A., & Svendsen, M. (1941). School phobia. *American Journal of Orthopsychiatry, 11,* 702–711.

Kearney, C.A., & Silverman, W.K. (1993). Measuring the function of school refusal behavior: The School Refusal Assessment Scale. *Journal of Clinical Child Psychology, 22,* 85–96.

Kennedy, W.A. (1965). School phobia: Rapid treatment of 50 cases. *Journal of Abnormal Psychology, 70,* 285–289.

King, N.J., Ollendick, T.H., & Tonge, B.J. (1995). *School refusal: Assessment and treatment.* Boston: Allyn and Bacon.

Last, C.G., & Strauss, C.C. (1990). School refusal in anxiety-disordered children and adolescents. *Journal of the American Academy of Child and Adolescent Psychiatry, 29,* 31–35.

Lazarus, A.A., Davison, G.G., & Polefka, D.A. (1965). Classical and operant factors in the treatment of school phobia. *Journal of Abnormal Psychology, 70,* 225–229.

III

Home-Based Problems

The problems included in this section are those that occur primarily in the home environment and are treated through home-based programs. Although some problems, like elimination, are usually first diagnosed in a medical setting, almost all the treatment occurs in the home with the parents as change agents. Because parents are the agents of change in many treatment programs, we have included a chapter on teaching parenting skills (Chapter 9). Shriver illustrates a step-by-step, empirically tested parent training protocol for teaching parents basic child management skills.

Child abuse and neglect are serious concerns, not only at the individual level but at the social and cultural levels as well. Donohue, Ammerman, and Zelis, in Chapter 10, present an ecological model for understanding and treating child abuse and neglect. Sleep disturbances, as most parents will verify, are common during early childhood. If left untreated, sleep problems can persist into adolescence and even into adulthood. Durand, Mindell, Mapstone, and Gernert-Dott, Chapter 11, cover some of the most common sleep problems in children and the most effective assessment and intervention strategies for each. Chapter 12, "Injury Prevention," by Saldana and Peterson, is a unique chapter among the other chapters in this book. Preventing injuries in children is not about treating one type of behavior, but rather about altering an entire class of stimulus conditions, and therefore making injuries significantly less likely to occur. Friman and Jones (Chapter 13), in addressing enuresis and encopresis, deviate a bit from the other chapters because the behaviors of concern (i.e., urinating and defecating) are not readily amenable to a traditional functional assessment/analysis like many other behaviors (e.g., school attendance, stereotypy).

9

Teaching Parenting Skills

MARK D. SHRIVER

Introduction

Many types of child therapy provide direct psychological services to the child (e.g., play therapy). These child-directed therapies typically evaluate child outcome based on parent report of child behavior change (e.g., child appears happier, child less angry) or parental satisfaction (i.e., parent believes child getting the help child needs). Parent report, however, is biased in a positive direction for child outcome *regardless* of the type of therapy/ treatment utilized (Patterson & Narrett, 1990). Therefore, it is necessary to evaluate child therapy based not only on parent report, but also on actual child behavior change. Most current forms of psychotherapy for children, however, do not have empirical support demonstrating actual child behavior outcomes (Patterson & Narrett, 1990).

In contrast, measuring behavior change is one of the defining characteristics and an essential component of the therapeutic process in behavior analysis (Martin & Pear, 1992). In child behavior therapy, the behaviors of parents and other adult caregivers are the most important ecological factors to consider in producing meaningful child behavior change. As demonstrated throughout this text, effective child behavior therapy utilizes parents and other caregivers (e.g., grandparents, foster parents, teachers) frequently to produce measurable child behavior change. Teaching parents skills to change child behavior is often referred to as parent training.

Parent training may be called an indirect model of service delivery for children (Gutkin & Conoley, 1990), as the child professional is not working directly or solely with the child to change the child's behavior. The child treatment professional, however, will provide direct services to the parent with the goal of changing parent behavior that will influence child behavior. It is this direct service delivery component of child behavior therapy that is the focus of this chapter. Specifically, this chapter will discuss how parents are effectively taught skills to change child behavior.

There are many methods discussed in the literature on how to teach parents skills in changing child behavior, as evidenced by the PsychLit database, which contains more than 700 articles and chapters including the topic of parent training published between January 1990 and December 1995. Much of the parent training research, however, does not report data on parent behavior change or child outcomes (Rogers Wiese, 1992). Similarly, there are numerous parent training programs or packages (e.g., STEP, Dinkmeyer & McKay, 1977; PET, Gordon, 1970) and numerous books in the popular press claiming to teach parenting skills. However, there is little or no empirical data supporting the effectiveness of many packaged parent training programs in changing parent or child behavior. The lack of empirical research on parent and child outcomes resulting from parent training has direct implications for child professionals, especially in this age of managed health care and accountability, as stated by Kramer (1990):

> What if we were to seek out our physician for a particular ailment and she or he were to suggest the use

MARK D. SHRIVER • Division of Pediatric Psychology, Munroe-Meyer Institute for Genetics and Rehabilitation, and University of Nebraska Medical Center, Omaha, Nebraska 68198-5450.

Handbook of Child Behavior Therapy, edited by Watson and Gresham. Plenum Press, New York, 1998.

of a treatment procedure for which there were no data indicating that this technique worked for our ailment. Our "treatment" would consist of two-and-a-half-hour sessions one night a week for 6 weeks and would cost $50. If we were to become aware of information indicating that the best we could hope for would be an increase in our knowledge of the disorder (but no "cure"), would we be upset? Would we demand to know the reason for our physician's behavior? Would we feel cheated and would we suggest incompetence on the part of our physician? At present, the most popular parent training programs (e.g., STEP, Active Parenting, PET) exist without any convincing data suggesting that they ever result in productive behavior change in either parents or children. What reasons can be advanced for the continued use of such procedures? (p. 697)

This chapter will draw heavily from parent training models that *have* empirically demonstrated positive changes in parent and child behavior (e.g., Forehand & McMahon, 1981; Hembree-Kigin & Bodiford McNeil, 1995; Patterson, 1976; Patterson & Forgatch, 1987). Historically, these parent training models are based on the work of Hanf (1969), who utilized a two-stage model of parent training including differential reinforcement and time-out. Variations of parent training have been used successfully for a wide variety of child problems, including oppositional behavior (Eyberg & Boggs, 1989; Forehand & McMahon, 1981), conduct disorder and juvenile delinquency (Bank, Marlowe, Reid, Patterson, & Weinrott, 1991; Doll & Kratochwill, 1992), attention-deficit/hyperactivity disorder (Barkley, 1987a; Newby, Fischer, Roman, 1991), feeding problems (Stark, Powers, Jelalian, Rape, & Miller, 1994; Werle, Murphy, & Budd, 1993), pain management (Allen & McKeen,1991; Beames, Sanders, & Bor, 1992), phobias (Yule, 1989), developmental disabilities (Lutzker, 1992; L.E. Powers, Singer, Stevens, & Sowers, 1992), medical compliance and chronic illness (Matthews, Spieth, & Christophersen, 1994), weight management (Epstein, 1985), and many others (Graziano & Diament, 1992; Sisson & Taylor, 1993).

This chapter will not discuss specific child problems nor focus exclusively on the content of a particular parent training model. It will provide the practitioner with a framework for training or teaching parents skills for changing child behavior. This framework is derived from a problem solving or behavioral consultative approach to parent training and consists of specific activities that promote ef-

fective information gathering and utilization (Bergan & Kratochwill, 1990; Carrington Rotto & Kratochwill, 1994). This chapter will discuss the activities involved in teaching parents skills during each step of the problem-solving process. Although, typically, the ultimate goal of parent training is child behavior change, this chapter will primarily discuss issues related to changing parent behavior. Teaching parents skills to change child behavior means changing parent behavior. This requires knowledge and skill in behavior analysis. Similarly, it requires an understanding of the eco-behavior variables affecting parent–child interaction.

Behavioral and Ecological Considerations in Parent–Child Interaction

Figure 1 provides an illustration of parent and child behavioral interaction and examples of potential ecological considerations. The parent and child are each a culmination of his or her unique learning

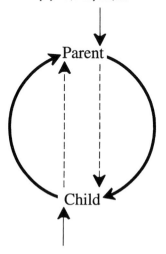

Parent–Child Interaction

Ecological Considerations

SES, Marital Relationship
Depression, Social Support,
Employment, Family Size, etc.

Parent

Child

Ecological Considerations

House Rules, Nutritional Status,
Family Size, Sibling Interaction, etc.

FIGURE 1. Model of parent–child interaction.

history brought to the behavioral interaction and influenced by individual and shared ecological variables. The parent and child each serve as discriminative stimuli and reinforcing or punishing stimuli for the other's behavior in the interaction. Following approximately 30 years of research with parents and children, investigators at the Oregon Social Learning Center have developed an empirical data-based model describing problematic parent and child interaction termed the Coercion Model (Patterson, 1982; Patterson, Reid, Dishion, 1992). The Coercion Model was developed within the context of a social interactional theory of child development directly influenced by work in behavior analysis. Patterson and colleagues describe coercive parent–child interactions as characterized over time by higher levels of negative reinforcement relative to positive reinforcement. In other words, negative behaviors by the parent or the child, or both (e.g., arguing), are reinforced by escaping (e.g., either the child or the parent "gives in") aversive parent–child interactions (Patterson et al., 1992).

The ecological considerations described in Figure 1 refer to temporally distant events and stimuli that are not immediately connected to the parent–child interaction but which may influence parent's behavior (i.e., ability to monitor the child and dispense effective discipline) and subsequent parent–child interaction. These variables have been termed setting events and may include the total number of life stressors (e.g., familial, financial, employment, housing) affecting a parent or family, the level of social support, and the quality of the parents' relationship (Wahler & Hann, 1986). Setting events may serve as establishing operations (Michael, 1993) which influence subsequent reinforcer valence in parent–child interactions. Other variables that may also serve as establishing operations or setting events to affect parent behavior and subsequent parent–child interaction include maternal depression, parental psychopathology, father involvement, and SES (Forehand, 1993; Graziano & Diament, 1992). Setting events and establishing operations that directly affect child behavior may include family size, nutritional status, opportunities for positive family interaction, consistent rules and structure/schedule, parent availability, sibling interaction, and so on.

Due to biological, developmental, and legal considerations, it is the parent who typically has most control (or the potential for most control) over the contingencies affecting the parent–child interaction. Note, however, that the model of parent–child interaction illustrated in Figure 1 does not blame or fault the parent for problem child behavior. The model does, however, illustrate that the parent is often in a position to effectively change child behavior. Teaching parents skills to effectively utilize antecedent stimuli and provide contingent positive reinforcement and punishment to change child behavior is the goal of parent training.

Effectively changing parent behavior and subsequent parent–child interaction is hypothesized to have positive long-term effects on child behavior (Patterson et al., 1992). If not changed, coercive or problematic parent–child interactions are believed to contribute to future antisocial behavior and problems in adulthood (Patterson et al., 1992). Currently, there is promising support for the long-term positive effects of parent training (e.g., Long, Forehand, Wierson, & Morgan, 1994). Before long-term impact is possible, however, the child behaviors of concern must be identified, along with the parent's current skill level and the relevant reinforcing and punishing contingencies in the parent–child interaction.

Problem Identification

Accurate identification of the problem is an important step in effective consultation and in parent training (Bergan & Kratochwill, 1990). In parent training, there are two concurrent problem identification processes: (1) identifying the child problem, and (2) identifying the parent problem. The child problem refers to the parent's primary concerns regarding child behavior. This process involves working with the parent to identify problematic child behaviors in terms that are observable and measurable. Identification of child behavior problems may also include prioritizing child behavior problems with the parent and/or identifying a class of target behaviors. Prioritizing child behavior problems will assist in making intervention decisions, such as what child behaviors to target first. Identifying a class of behaviors refers to identifying behaviors that serve a similar function. For example, throwing tantrums, not following directions, and physical aggression may belong to a class of behaviors termed noncompliance in which parental attention maintains each of the behaviors. Noncompliance is frequently targeted in parent training as a class of child behaviors to be changed (Forehand & McMahon, 1981).

Identifying the parent problem refers to identifying parent behaviors/skills (verbal and nonverbal) that impact child behavior. Identifying current parent behaviors that affect child behavior overlaps substantially with problem analysis of child behavior (see the following discussion). In parent training, however, the purpose of identifying current parent behaviors affecting child behavior is to assist in targeting parent behaviors for change and to help parents understand their influence on child behavior. Problem identification in parent training utilizes multiple sources of information, including previous records, behavior checklists and rating forms, parent interview, child interview, informal and formal observations, and baseline data collection.

Record Review

Records are often the only objectively written permanent product of a parent and/or child's learning history available to the child professional. These records may include the child and parents' developmental, medical, and educational history. In addition, records may sometimes include information on the child's and parent's social, economic, legal, and psychological history. A review of records typically occurs prior to the initial meeting with parent(s) and child or as soon as records are available following the first meeting and after release forms have been signed by parents. The child professional will review records specifically for information about the child's age, family constellation, SES, medical history, previous contact with psychological services, previous treatments and outcomes, and current reason for referral.

Behavior Rating Forms

Behavior checklists or rating forms are useful to acquire a parent's perspective on his or her child's behavior. This perception is often compared with other parents' perceptions of their children of the same chronological age (i.e., normative data). Although based on parent report, behavior rating forms are useful in assisting in the initial identification of child behaviors of concern and as part of the ongoing assessment process to determine parent training effectiveness. The Child Behavior Checklist (Achenbach, 1991), Conners Behavior Rating Scale (Conners, 1990), and Eyberg Behavior Inventory (Robinson, Eyberg, & Ross, 1980) are common behavior checklists utilized to assess parent perceptions of child behavior. All three behavior inventories include a teacher form that may be useful for identifying school concerns and evaluating generalization of parent training treatment effects to the school setting (e.g., McNeil, Eyberg, Eisenstadt, Newcomb, Funderburk, 1991). The child behavior professional using behavior rating scales should be aware of the psychometric qualities (e.g., Kramer & Conoley, 1992), sensitivity to behavior change, and treatment utility (Hayes, Nelson, Jarrett, 1987) of the particular instruments. Typically, personality inventories are not useful for problem identification or treatment evaluation because they do not hold up well when evaluated against these criteria.

Parent Interview

During the first meeting between the child professional and parent(s), the parents are interviewed to obtain information regarding parent and child background (i.e., ecological variables) and parent perceptions regarding child behavior. Table 1 presents areas of questioning during the parent interview. Specific questions will vary dependent on the particular parent and child. The areas included often overlap with information that already may have been obtained in record review. However, the interview allows the child professional an opportunity to validate information, fill in missing information, informally assess parents' ability to communicate information, and build rapport. It is during the parent interview that specific child behavior problems are identified, goals for parent training identified (e.g., fewer tantrums, more frequent compliance) and child problem behavior analysis is initiated. The parent interview includes the parent's description of the antecedents

TABLE 1. Parent Interview

I.   Parent(s) primary concerns

II. Parent(s) goals

III. Family background
  A. Immediate family
  B. Current employment status and schedules
  C. Family members' level of functioning
    1. Mental health
    2. Parents relationship
    3. Financial stressors
    4. Other (e.g., sibling relationships, extended family)

IV. Developmental history

V.   Medical history

VI. Educational history

VII. Functional assessment of presenting child problem(s)

and consequences surrounding child behaviors of concern.

Child Interview

Depending on the child's developmental status, a child interview can also be informative. In addition to providing an opportunity to develop rapport with the child and assess the child's ability to communicate information, the child interview provides an additional source of information regarding the parent–child interaction. Information obtained from the child may assist in confirming or disconfirming parent perceptions of child behavior. For example, the child may identify the parent yelling as a consequence for the child's hitting a sibling, whereas the parent identified time-out as the consequence. A child may indicate that occasionally she or he is allowed to stay up later after repeated requests to stay up, whereas the parent indicates that the child is never allowed to stay up. In addition, the child is often the best source of information regarding potential reinforcers to utilize in treatment.

Behavior Observation

Observation of actual child and parent behavior is critical to evaluating parent and child outcomes of parent training. Without observation of parent and child interaction, the child treatment professional must rely on parent report to determine the effectiveness of the parent training. Most important, behavior observation provides the professional an opportunity to observe parent–child interaction, form hypotheses regarding the mechanism maintaining child behavior problems (in conjunction with other sources of information), and conduct functional analyses (i.e., experimental manipulation) to validate hypotheses. Behavior observation will also be an ongoing part of the parent training process and will provide opportunities to observe parent and child progress. Although behavior observation is too large an area to consider in detail (cf. Foster, Bell-Dolan, & Burge, 1988), two critical types of observation necessary in evaluating outcomes in parent training are informal and formal observation.

Informal Observation

Informal observation will occur throughout the parent training process, and this primarily consists of observing parent and child interaction in situations not formally set up as part of the parent training program. Informal observation is typically anecdotal, but may occasionally include quantitative information. Informal behavior observation occurs whenever the professional makes note of parent and child interaction, such as during the parent interview, waiting in an outer office area, putting on a coat, picking up toys, and/or leaving the session. Informal observation provides a source of information for the child behavior professional regarding the generalization of skills being taught in parent training and the impact on child behavior. For example, it may be that the parent states that she or he is consistently utilizing time-out following the presentation of one command and one warning, but informal observation in the waiting room prior to the session indicates that the parent asked the child at least four times to pick his or her coat off the floor. Additional examples of information that informal observation can provide include the level of a child's independent play skills (e.g., during parent interview), the frequency of the child's interruptions and how the parent responds, the child's developmental level of play, and how the parent responds when the child is behaving appropriately.

Formal Observation

Formal behavior observations occur when the professional arranges situations to observe parent and child interaction. Formal behavior observations may include functional analysis, compliance protocols, reinforcer assessment, or other structured observation procedures. Given that compliance is often an identified target behavior in parent training, the parent trainer will often observe the parent and child during a compliance protocol. Compliance protocols may take many forms (e.g., S.W. Powers & Roberts, 1995; Roberts & Powers, 1988), but primarily consist of observing the parent provide the child with commands and watching subsequent child and parent interactions. Useful recording forms for coding parent and child behaviors during compliance protocols include Barkley (1987b) and Forehand and McMahon (1981). In addition, parent and child interactions may be videotaped for later coding or for subsequent training purposes with the parents. Formal behavior observations during the first contact with a parent and child provide a baseline of parent behavior (e.g., proportion of alpha to beta commands) to judge the effectiveness of parent training.

Baseline Data Collection

Following the collection of information as outlined above, the parent will begin collecting data on their child's behavior or on their own behavior. Data collection in parent training can serve any or all of three purposes: (1) Data collection teaches parents to monitor their children's behavior, a necessary parent skill in effectively providing reinforcement and/or discipline (Patterson et al., 1992); (2) data collection can be used to help the parent monitor his or her own behavior, to assist with completing homework assignments given, and/or to assist with teaching parents about how their behavior affects their children's behavior; and (3) data collected prior to, during, and following parent training are necessary to adequately judge the effectiveness of the training.

Whether the parent collects data on child behavior or on parent behavior will be a clinical decision based on the parent interview and presenting problems. Typically, child behaviors are targeted for baseline data collection. Child behaviors targeted should reflect the parent's primary concern and goals for intervention. In addition, the targeted behavior should be one that is not cumbersome for the parent to observe/monitor. For example, for children who are frequently noncompliant, it may be easier for the parent to collect data on the frequency of child compliance to parent commands in contrast to collecting data on noncompliance. For high-frequency behaviors (e.g., hand mouthing), it may be better for the parent to collect samples of behavior (e.g., hand mouthing) at scheduled intervals (e.g., every hour for five minutes) throughout the day. It is important for the parent trainer to assess the parent's ability to collect data, and that means asking the parent what is reasonable for them to do given their family situation and child concerns. There are a variety of behavior data observation/collection techniques and forms available. An example of one form is provided in Form 9.1.

Monitoring/observing and collecting behavior data is one of the first skills taught to parents during parent training. The child (or parent) behavior to be observed/monitored will need to be operationally defined. For example, noncompliance may be defined as an episode of tantrum behavior, physical aggression, or failure to follow through with a parent command. Each, or all, of these child behaviors need to be further defined with the parent so that the behavior is directly observable and measurable by the parent. The recording form to be used in behavior data collection will need to be ex-

FORM 9.1. Antecedent, Behavior, Consequence (ABC) Recording Form

BEHAVIOR (Define): ————————————   WHOSE BEHAVIOR? ————————————

INSTRUCTIONS:
1. BEFORE: Record who was present, where the behavior occurred, and what was happening at the time.
2. BEHAVIOR: Describe the behavior exactly.
3. AFTER: Record who did what and how the child responded.

DATE	TIME	BEFORE (A)			BEHAVIOR (B)	AFTER (C)	
		Who?	Where?	What?		Who?	What?

plained to the parent and didactic teaching of data collection must be conducted. The child professional should model appropriate observation and recording procedures during the session if possible. In addition, the parent should practice behavior observation and data collection prior to leaving the session so that feedback may be provided by the parent trainer and reliability of observations (i.e., whether parent and parent trainer are talking about and observing the same child behavior) may be established between the parent and parent trainer. It may be necessary for the professional to call the parent at home prior to the next session, to prompt data collection and to assess and/or answer any problems or concerns that have arisen regarding data collection.

Summary of Problem Identification

Through historical records, behavior checklists and rating forms, parent and child interviews, behavior observations, and baseline data, the child professional will identify child behaviors of con-

cern and conduct a problem analysis of child behaviors. As part of the problem analysis of the child behavior, specific parent behaviors will be identified that can be targeted for intervention. Before we discuss intervention, however, we need to further consider the analysis of problem behavior.

Problem Analysis

As indicated in the preceding discussion, child problem behavior analysis overlaps substantially with identifying parent problem behaviors. Effective problem analysis is necessary to effective consultation and parent training (Gresham, 1991). There are typically two concurrent, and frequently overlapping, processes in parent training problem analysis: (1) identification of the function of child behavior, and (2) identification of the parent behaviors that function to maintain child behaviors. Less acknowledged, but of equal importance, are two other processes in parent training problem analysis: (1) identification of the function of parent behavior, and (2) identification of child behaviors that function to maintain parent behaviors.

Identifying the Function of Child Behavior

Identifying the function of child behavior may take place at any of three levels of problem analysis: hypothetical, descriptive, or experimental. Intervention (i.e., teaching parenting skills) may occur following completion of any of the three levels. The probability of successful identification of the function of the child behavior problem, and successful intervention, however, will increase with use of higher levels of analysis. The first level of problem analysis is most cursory and consists of hypothesizing functional relationships between parent and child behavior based on previous empirical research. For example, if a child presents as primarily oppositional or noncompliant with parent commands, it may be hypothesized that a coercive relationship is in effect, involving a high degree of negative reinforcement. This level of analysis requires the least time, but the greatest inference, and is usually used only as a first step in child behavior problem analysis. This level of problem analysis is probably most commonly used in teaching parenting skills in group contexts.

The second level is that of a descriptive functional analysis. This was briefly described in the problem identification section and it consists of identifying environmental variables, specifically parent behaviors, that correlate highly with the onset and maintenance of child behavior. Problem analysis at this level occurs during behavior observations, from baseline data collection, and during the parent interview, when parents are asked to describe what happens before and after child behavior. It is following this level of problem analysis that further teaching of parenting skills usually begins. Specific skills related to identifying the antecedents and consequences of behavior during consultation (e.g., parent interview) can be found in Kratochwill and Bergan (1990) and O'Neill, Horner, Albin, Storey, and Spraque (1989). In addition, there is an impressive literature on the utility of descriptive functional analysis for intervention planning (e.g., Lalli, Browder, Mace, & Brown, 1993; Taylor & Romanczyk, 1994).

There is also an impressive literature supporting the treatment utility of the third level of problem

analysis—experimental functional analysis (Neef, 1994). An experimental functional analysis (also termed analogue analysis) typically follows the first two steps, and consists of actually manipulating variables believed to function to maintain problematic child behavior. In essence, a functional analysis involves observing the parent differentially respond to child behavior given different antecedent events or contexts, such as having frequent demands placed on the child or the child being left alone to play in a room. The parent may then ignore problematic child behavior that occurs, may attend to the behavior, or may allow the child to escape a demand contingent on problematic behavior. The parent and child are observed during these interactions, to determine what parent behavior may be maintaining child behavior and/or what antecedent conditions predict the occurance of the problematic child behavior. This step requires more time, but allows the parent trainer and parent to specifically observe how the parent's behavior affects child behavior. This level of analysis is used to confirm hypotheses from the first two steps. It should be noted that this step or level of problem analysis occurs naturally (at a basic level) during the teaching of parenting skills if the parent trainer is including ongoing observation of parent–child interaction.

Identifying the function of the child behavior problem, with emphasis on parent behavior, will identify those parent behaviors that need to be changed or taught. Like all behavior, however, parent behavior also is determined by a learning history of reinforcement contingencies. It is useful for the child behavior professional, therefore, to have an understanding of the reinforcing variables that may function to maintain parent behavior and, specifically, child behaviors that may maintain parent behavior.

Identifying the Function of Parent Behavior

An extensive part of problem analysis is identifying parent behaviors that function to maintain child behaviors. Child professionals, however, should be aware that parent behavior is susceptible to the same reinforcement parameters as is child behavior. For example, parents attending to a child's tantrum may be negatively reinforced by decreasing the duration or intensity of the tantrum.

In addition, parents are likely to exhibit behaviors requiring less response effort (Friman & Poling, 1995). It is assumed in parent training that parent behavior will be reinforced by child compliance and other appropriate behavior. If the response effort is too high, given the parent's ability or environmental situation/setting events, then child compliance may not be as reinforcing for the parenting behaviors being taught, when compared with the parent's current inappropriate (and lower response effort) behaviors. For example, the consequent effect of a child quieting after a parent yells "shut up (a low response effort behavior) may be more reinforcing to the parent than the continued yelling that may result when the child is put in time-out (a relatively higher response effort), regardless of the long-term positive effects of the latter technique on the child's behavior. These considerations are all important in teaching parenting skills and are part of problem analysis. Reinforcement parameters (such as response effort) and competing reinforcement contingencies affect parent implementation of treatment. Parent behavior operating on these schedules has often been termed resistance. Resistance is discussed more fully in the following section on plan implementation.

Plan Implementation: Teaching Parenting Skills

The child behavior professional will begin to teach parenting skills once she or he is confident that specific child behavior problems have been targeted for intervention and specific parent behaviors have been identified as targets for change to affect child behavior. This section will briefly outline how parenting skills are taught to parents, how to increase treatment integrity, and the clinical skills needed in parent training that are particularly related to reducing parent resistance.

Parent Training

There are two primary skills taught to parents during parent training. All other aspects of parent training are conducted to facilitate these two skills. The first skill is to reinforce child behavior that the parent wishes to increase, and the second is to punish child behavior the parent wishes to decrease. Typically, the punishment or discipline procedure consists of some type of time-out procedure con-

tingent on the inappropriate target behavior. These are the basic steps in the Hanf model of parent training (1969), and the basic components of the currently better empirically supported parent training programs (e.g., Forehand & McMahon, 1981; Hembree-Kigin, & Bodiford McNeil, 1995). In addition, parent training programs often include teaching parents skills to increase the probability of success in providing effective reinforcing and punishing consequences for their children. These skills generally consist of setting up antecedent conditions and/or establishing stimulus control through the use of effective child monitoring, use of direct (alpha) commands, problem-solving skills, and effective negotiation and communication skills, particularly with adolescents. Effective use of antecedent skills (including rules) are important parenting skills, but reliance on these skills without use or acknowledgement of the effective use of consequences is less likely to change child behavior. The parent is at the mercy of the child contacting naturally occurring consequences that may or may not reinforce or punish the targeted child behavior. A reliance on antecedent skills without strategic and effective use of consequences may be the problem contributing to the lack of empirical support for many packaged parent training programs that focus largely on talking or reasoning with the child and/or parent–child negotiation and communication skills.

A generic parent training process is presented in Table 2. Obviously, the number and even the order of sessions will change dependent on the child and parent's identified problems and problem analysis. For example, it is not necessary to present time-in components prior to time-out components (Hembree Eisenstadt, Eyberg, Bodiford McNeil, Newcomb, & Funderburk, 1993), although that typically is done to promote positive parent–child interaction and to increase contrast with the time-out component (Shriver & Allen, 1996). In addition, some cases will move faster, some more slowly than others, and some therapists may move faster or more slowly depending on their experience and style. The basic components of each session remain the same, however, and will include information gathering/ review, didactic teaching, modeling, and practice or role-playing of the parenting skill with feedback on parent performance.

TABLE 2. Teaching Parenting Skills

SESSION ONE	√ Parent interview
	√ Child/adolescent interview
	√ Review behavior checklists
	√ Observation of parent–child interaction
	√ Teach parent data collection
	√ Provide parent homework to collect baseline data
SESSION TWO	√ Review baseline data collected
	√ Conduct further parent interview regarding problem identification and/or analysis if needed
	√ Teach effective reinforcement of targeted child behavior (didactic, model, practice)
	√ Provide homework assignment (i.e., practice reinforcement procedure)
	√ Continue to have parent collect data
SESSION THREE	√ Review data collected
	√ Observe parent–child interaction with focus on skills being learned
	√ If criterion not met for successful demonstration of reinforcement continue practice and feedback
	√ If criterion met for successful demonstration of reinforcement begin teaching time-out skills (didactic, modeling, practice)
	√ Provide parent homework
	√ Continue data collection
SESSION FOUR	√ Review data collected
	√ Observe parent–child interaction
	√ Determine if criterion met for successful demonstration of parenting skill being taught
	√ Continue practice as needed
	√ Provide relevant homework
	√ Continue data collection
SESSION FIVE	√ Review data collected
	√ Teach problem-solving and/or generalization skills (didactic, modeling, practice)
	√ Re-administer behavior rating forms
	√ Determine how follow-up will be conducted

Note: Each Session is assumed to be approximately one hour in duration.

Session One

This session primarily includes information gathering to assist with problem identification and begin problem analysis. Parent and possibly child/adolescent interview comprise the majority of this session. It is during session one that behavior checklists may be reviewed or presented and initial observations of parent–child interaction conducted. To begin encouraging parent cooperation with the parent-training process, the parent is taught to collect data on child behavior or to self-monitor parent behavior. As noted above, teaching parents to collect data involves explaining the procedure, modeling the data collection procedure with the parent and child, and having the parent practice data collection before leaving the session. The initial homework assignment may involve minimal response effort by the parent, in order to increase the probability of follow-through. This initial teaching process and expectations for the parent to complete homework helps the professional assess the parent's willingness and ability to follow through with recommendations. Provided that the child behavior professional has not yet provided treatment recommendations to the parent, the data collected initially provides baseline information to assist in determining the subsequent effects of parent training.

In addition, it is during session one that the child behavior professional begins to establish rapport with the parent and the child. Often parents are looking for the reason their child is exhibiting a problem. The professional must communicate to the parents a reason or rationale for the child's problem and provide an overview of the treatment or parent training process. It is important to help the parent understand how he or she is to be involved in treating the child's problem. With training and experience, the child behavior professional develops effective rationales for parents regarding child problems and treatment. Obviously, the rationale used is dependent on the presenting child problem and the parent's level of cognitive functioning. It is incumbent upon the parent trainer to be knowledgeable about behavior analytic principles to the extent that child behavior may be explained to parents in terms that are easily understood and devoid of technological terminology. Excerpts of one rationale commonly used in a child and family psychological services clinic for parents with children exhibiting oppositional behavior is provided in Figure 2.

Session Two

The second session begins by reviewing baseline data collected or discussing barriers or problems that prevented the parent from collecting data. Further parent interview and behavior observations are conducted as needed to continue information gathering for problem identification and to continue the problem analysis phase. It is during this session that the parent is taught skills of effectively reinforcing targeted child behavior. Didactic teaching on effective reinforcement, modeling by the professional with the parent and child, and practice or role-play with the parent and child with immediate feedback by the child behavior professional are conducted. Parents are taught how to identify reinforcers for their child (e.g., "What does your child like to do? What do you see your child doing during their play or free time?") and how to present reinforcement (e.g., immediately following or during behavior when possible).

Excerpts from "How Children Learn" or [Why Current Parent Discipline Isn't Working]

"First, let me tell you what we know about how children don't learn. Young children, up through preadolescence do not learn well through language and logic. Lectures, rationale, and talking typically do not help children change their behavior very well. I'm sure you've heard the old saying 'In one ear and out the other.' In fact, you have probably found yourself telling your child something like, 'don't jump on the furniture', and the child quits jumping for a short period of time, but soon you find the child again jumping on the furniture. At some point, you may even find yourself shouting 'How many times do I have to tell you . . .' [parent trainer may bang the table at this point]. The child hears you, may nod his head in understanding, but his behavior doesn't change.

". . . How children do learn is by the effect that they make happen around them. Children are looking to make things happen, to produce effect either with a toy, another object, a peer, or an adult. They are looking to push buttons around them that make things happen. In fact, your child probably knows very well which of your buttons to push to create some effect. When children find a behavior that will produce effect they will tend to stick with that behavior, repeat it over time. If a behavior does not produce any effect for them, nothing happens, the child will typically not repeat that behavior.

". . . What we will do is work together to learn how you can provide positive effect for your child when he is doing what you want him to do, and how to provide no effect for the child when he is not doing what you want him to do. This will involve practice here in the clinic and practice at home. There may be some trial and error involved and we will keep track of your child's behavior so that we can make sure that what we recommend is most effective for your child and family."

Note: These are excerpts from one example of a rationale for child behavior and treatment that is used with parents of oppositional children. Obviously, this should be adapted to the individual child and family and other points will be included (e.g., children prefer predictability, children learn through repetition).

FIGURE 2. Excerpts from rationale provided to parents with oppositional children.

For example, if a child who frequently fights with his or her siblings is observed by the parent to play appropriately with his or her siblings, the parent should take a brief moment to physically touch the child (e.g., pat on back) and provide verbal praise for appropriate behavior. This parenting skill is practiced during parent training, as the parent trainer frequently prompts the parent to touch and praise the child during the session whenever the child plays appropriately without interrupting the adults, or plays appropriately with siblings. The parent trainer's prompting of parents to reinforce child behavior may even occur as the parent trainer and parent are talking to each other. The child behavior professional also demonstrates effective reinforcement by frequently approaching the child and providing verbal praise and positive touch for appropriate behavior, again, even while talking with the parent. This helps demonstrate for the parent that reinforcement can be brief and may occur during parent-oriented activities without interrupting the parent activity, yet still provide the child the feedback she or he needs in order to learn to behave appropriately. Regardless of the actual reinforcement procedure used, and the child behavior to be reinforced, it is important that the professional model the reinforcement procedure, provide opportunity to practice it, and give immediate feedback.

The parent trainer recommends a homework assignment that focuses on practicing the reinforcement procedure and continued data collection. Homework provided throughout parent training is aimed at parents' practicing the parenting skills they are taught, and at assessing the degree of effort the parents are willing to put forth. Without practice and use of skills outside the clinical context, change in child behavior is not expected. With practice and continued monitoring of child behavior through data collection, the impact of changes in parent behavior may be assessed.

The reader should note the emphasis on the parent practicing skills with his or her child and collecting data on actual child (or parent) behavior change. Not all parents follow through with data collection or completing homework assignments. The child behavior professional should continuously assess the parent's ability and willingness to follow through with recommendations and should work with the parent to remove any impediments to following through with recommendations. The

earlier in the process the professional demonstrates the importance of parent follow-through, the more likely the parent will be to continue following recommendations and practicing parenting skills as the skills become more complex and difficult.

Session Three

Session three consists of data review from the previous week. Additional observation of the parent–child interaction is conducted to assess the parent's acquisition of the skills being taught (e.g., differential reinforcement) and the impact on child behavior, particularly in comparison with previous observations of parent and child behavior. In addition, the child professional may have a specific behavioral criterion the parent is expected to meet to demonstrate competence with the parenting skills being taught (e.g., provides 15 specific verbal praises for targeted child behavior during a 5-minute child-directed parent–child activity). The parent can then be provided with feedback on specific parenting skills and progress toward meeting the criterion established. The behavioral criterion established and used by the clinician is dependent on the particular parent skill being taught. The criterion should be objective enough that the parent is aware of what constitutes mastery of the behavior. If the parent is not demonstrating effective mastery of the parenting skills being taught according to the established criterion, additional practice with feedback, problem solving of barriers in implementing the skills in clinic and at home, additional modeling, and some additional didactic teaching are indicated.

As the parent demonstrates adequate mastery of parenting skills, and changes in child behavior are observed in the clinic and in data collected by the parent, additional parenting skills are taught to the parent (e.g., time-out procedure). After each session, the parent is provided homework to practice particular skills and collect data on child behavior outcomes.

As the number and order of sessions varies from the generic format presented here, in respect to individual parents and children, so too may the order of events within sessions vary depending upon emphasis needed for each individual parent and child. For example, it may be that, rather than starting with data review, the child behavior professional begins a session immediately with parent–child observation and parenting skill practice. This order of events may be especially useful for parents who tend to talk in session rather than follow clinician prompts to practice skills. As indicated earlier, although the components for each session do not vary, the order of presentation may vary depending on the case, the clinician's style, and parent feedback.

Sessions Four and Five

Typically, parent training does not continue beyond eight to ten sessions, and may often be completed within four to six sessions depending on the problem identified, problem analysis, and parent follow-through (i.e., data collection, homework completion). As indicated above, following time-in procedures (i.e., differential reinforcement), time-out procedures typically are taught to parents. There may be many procedural components involved in structuring an effective time-out for a particular family situation (Brantner & Doherty, 1983). However, time-out is essentially about creating a contrast between a time-in environment (i.e., providing reinforcement for appropriate child behavior) and the time-out situation (i.e., removing reinforcement for targeted child behavior) (Shriver & Allen, 1996). The child behavior professional should be knowledgeable about behavioral technology so as to implement effective child interventions and flexible enough to adapt the interventions to the specific ecological considerations presented by the parents and family of the child. For an intervention such as time-out, that means not relying on any particular procedure for every family, but, rather, teaching the parent how to effectively remove reinforcement from the child contingent on targeted child behavior, taking into account the family's situation (e.g., family size, floor plan of house, marital status of parent). In addition, the use of effective commands, parent–child communication skills, and negotiation skills may be taught to parents to facilitate the effective presentation and withdrawal of reinforcement contingent on targeted child behaviors.

Generalization and Maintenance

The final parent training sessions (e.g., session five in Table 2), consists of teaching parents problem-solving skills utilized in the parent training process (i.e., problem identification, analysis, intervention, evaluation) and generalization of specific skills learned (e.g., reinforcement and time-out) to other child problems (Chamberlain & Baldwin, 1988). At this point, the professional may become less directive about what needs to be done regarding child problems, in order to discover whether parents can problem-solve independently. How follow-up will occur between the child professional and parent is also determined; this may consist of phone contact, increasing the time interval between sessions, and/or occasional "booster" sessions (i.e., short-term consultation) to assist in maintenance of skills learned and generalization of parenting skills to other child problems.

Treatment Integrity

Treatment integrity refers to the accuracy with which an intervention is actually implemented in an applied setting (Gresham, Gansle, & Noell, 1993). A primary point throughout this chapter is that if parent behavior does not change, there is little reason to expect child behavior to change. The role of the child professional is to teach parents skills to change child behavior. Although effective parent training may occur in groups or individually (Grazianao & Diament, 1992), training should be individualized to some extent to increase effectiveness (e.g., L.E. Powers et al., 1992). In addition, clinician-directed training encouraging active parent participation is more effective in changing parent and child behavior than is passive parent participation or didactic training (Graziano & Diament, 1992; Knapp & Deluty, 1989; Webster-Stratton, 1990).

To encourage active parent participation, parents are expected to practice skills in the clinic and demonstrate mastery before implementing parenting skills at home. The child behavior professional is modeling skills, setting up situations for observations, observing parent–child interaction, and providing frequent feedback to the parents. Feedback may be provided verbally, through a communication device called "bug-in-the-ear," and/or through videotape. Active parent participation requires the professional also to be active. The child behavior professional rarely sits during parent training!

Clinical Skills

Knowledge of parent-training content (e.g., behavior analysis principles, ecological considerations) is important for effective teaching of parenting skills; however, clinical skills also are required (Webster-Stratton & Herbert, 1993). The relationship between the child behavior professional and the parent is often described as collaborative, but the professional functions as the expert in parent training content and in controlling the process, albeit respectful of parent needs, skills, and rate of progress. The child behavior professional must possess effective communication skills (verbal and nonverbal) to establish rapport with the parent. Rapport may be defined as having a positive relationship with the parent as demonstrated by the parent's honesty and attempts to follow recommendations. Combined with previous experience with many different parents, adequate rapport with a parent will allow the child behavior professional to confront the parent when necessary (e.g., parent exhibiting resistance) and also allow the professional to know when to reduce expectations for a parent's ability to follow through.

In addition, the professional should be knowledgeable of behavior analytic principles so that flexibility may be demonstrated to match individual parent and child ecological situations. The child behavior professional should be adept in behavioral assessment, particularly observation and data collection, and should have developed a cognitive portfolio of effective examples/stories to provide parents to promote understanding of effective parenting skills. Chamberlain and Baldwin (1988) provide examples of responses to parent questions they have developed over the years in teaching parenting skills (e.g., proper discipline response, bribery). Clinical skill development requires training and professional supervision and feedback, and it is necessary to promote treatment integrity (parents do as recommended) and reduce parent resistance (parents do not do as recommended).

Resistance

Resistance was briefly described previously and may occur for many reasons related to parent ability and/or parent eco-behavioral considerations (e.g., competing reinforcement contingencies, setting events, response effort). Referring to Figure 1, there is research indicating that parents with a greater number of ecological considerations typically considered negative or more stressful in current society are less likely to be successful with parent training. These ecological considerations include low level of social support, lower socioeconomic status, minority status, single parenting status, and depression (Graziano & Diament, 1992).

Parent resistance will frequently occur approximately during mid-treatment, which is often the time of greatest expectation regarding parent behavior change (Chamberlain & Baldwin, 1988). As demonstrated in Table 2, it is often approximately during mid-treatment that the focus of parent training shifts from teaching differential reinforcement skills to teaching discipline skills. This changes the focus of parent training from positive child behaviors to targeted negative behaviors and may require more complex or effort-laden responses by the parents. Child resistance to changes in discipline or use of punishment is not uncommon. It is at this point that the child behavior professional will utilize many clinical skills regarding use of examples/stories, rapport, reframing of difficulties, problem solving, and persistence (Chamberlain & Baldwin, 1988). In addition, through earlier reinforcement of parent efforts to complete less cumbersome homework and data collection, the professional will have prevented many difficulties regarding parent resistance to treatment implementation. It may be necessary for the professional to videotape parent–child interactions to emphasize changes in child behavior and effective use of parenting skills. Home visits to model intervention and problem-solve difficulties may also prove beneficial when possible.

Summary of Plan Implementation

Teaching parenting skills involves behavior data collection/monitoring, didactic teaching, modeling, and practice of skills with performance feedback. It is an active treatment process that requires clinical skill and a strong knowledge base of behavior analysis to effectively meet individual parent and child needs. To judge the effectiveness of parent training, the child behavior professional evaluates treatment throughout the process of teaching parenting skills, and utilizes information obtained in problem identification, problem analysis, and plan implementation.

Plan Evaluation

The primary question to be answered during plan evaluation is whether the parent's goals identified during the problem identification phase are being attained. This is evaluated in behavioral parent training by measures assessing parent behavior outcomes and child behavior outcomes. These measures include the parent's ongoing data collection regarding parent and/or child behavior, observation of parent–child interaction, behavior rating forms, and parent report. Note that evaluation is ongoing throughout parent training via data collection, behavior observation, and parent interview. The child behavior professional should be continuously aware of her or his impact on parent and child behavior. If changes in parent or child behavior toward the parent's goal are not occurring, then the child professional will need to conduct additional analyses of parent–child interaction, of any competing reinforcement contingencies, and/or of other ecological events that may be barriers to parent implementation of skills.

For example, it may be that observation of parent–child interaction in the clinic indicates that the parent is demonstrating mastery of a specific parenting skill (e.g., time-out); however, data collected by the parent on child behavior at home indicates that the child continues to exhibit frequent tantrums not significantly different from baseline. Additional parent interview and/or child feedback indicates that the parent is not practicing the skill at home. Further analysis through parent interview indicates that the parent has recently lost a job, is looking for a new job, is looking for a new residence, and is having difficulty finding adequate child care. These additional stressors in the parent's life have made implementation or practice of parenting skills more difficult (e.g., "I don't have time to think about how to respond to the tantrums; I just get angry"). The child behavior professional must now utilize clinical judgment to decide whether to reduce expectations for parent follow-through with this skill and perhaps focus on parent coping skills with current stressors, or to increase structure for parent follow-through with parenting skills, perhaps via home visits.

If the parent training is having a positive impact on parent and child behavior outcomes, the child behavior professional will begin to work with the parent to fade the professional's role in using the parenting skills. This is often done by increasing time between parent training sessions. In addition, a greater proportion of contact between the professional and parent may occur by phone and/or future "booster" sessions. The child behavior professional will work with the parent to teach a problem-solving process, as outlined in this chapter, and generalization of the process to other child behaviors. The parent's ability to generalize skills, however, will be tested only through exposure to new child behaviors of concern. Therefore, it is important to let the parent know that future contact with the child behavior professional is available.

Summary

Children are brought to psychologists, social workers, counselors, and other child behavior professionals for a wide range of behavioral, emotional, cognitive/academic, medical, and social problems. Helping children requires that professionals attend not only to the individual child, but also to the child's ecological context. A child's parent often controls the essential reinforcement contingencies influencing child behavior and thus the parent is a primary ecological variable in a child's life. Child therapy that does not utilize parents or other caregivers in changing child behavior will likely have little impact on child behavior. Teaching parents skills can be an effective method of changing child behavior, if done properly. As indicated throughout this chapter, parent training programs following the Hanf model of differential reinforcement and time-out have been found effective in changing child behavior. It is incumbent upon the parent trainer, however, to ensure that parents are taught these behavior management skills effectively. This requires knowledge and skill in behavior change principles. Behavior change requires that the child behavior professional teach the parent using didactic interaction, modeling, practice with feedback, and behavior assessment to monitor behavior change. If parent behavior is not changed, it is highly unlikely the child behavior will be changed. Therefore, it is also important to be cognizant of behavioral–ecological considerations affecting parent behavior, including response effort, competing reinforcement contingencies, and setting events.

Although there is substantial research on effective parent training techniques, more research is needed regarding the specifics of parent training. This includes the role of commands, the role of problem-solving skills, the timing of time-out, effective parent training with resistant or hard-to-train parents, and long-term follow-up of parent training effectiveness. In addition, more research on how to train child behavior professionals to do effective parent training is necessary. Continuing research in these areas will provide information to professionals about how to most effectively teach parents skills: the crux of child behavior therapy.

ACKNOWLEDGMENT

The author would like to thank Jack J. Kramer, Ph.D., for his review and helpful comments on an earlier draft of the manuscript.

References

Achenbach, T.M. (1991). *Manual for the Child Behavior Checklist/4-18 and 1991 Profile*. Burlington: University of Vermont, Department of Psychiatry.

Allen, K.D., & McKeen, L.R. (1991). Home-based multicomponent treatment of pediatric migraine. *Headache, 31,* 467–472.

Bank, L., Marlowe, J.H., Reid, J.B., Patterson, G.R., & Weinrott, M.R. (1991). A comparative evaluation of parent-training interventions for families of chronic delinquents. *Journal of Abnormal Child Psychology, 19,* 15–33.

Barkley, R.B. (1987a). *Defiant children: A clinician's manual for parent training*. New York: Guilford.

Barkley, R.B. (1987b). *Defiant children: Parent-teacher assignments*. New York: Guilford.

Beames, L., Sanders, M.R., & Bor, W. (1992). The role of parent training in the cognitive behavioral treatment of children's headaches. *Behavioural Psychotherapy, 20,* 167–180.

Bergan, J.R., & Kratochwill, T.R. (1990). *Behavioral consultation and therapy*. New York: Plenum.

Brantner, J.R., & Doherty, M.A. (1983). A review of timeout: A conceptual and methodological analysis. In S. Axelrod & J. Apsche (Eds.), *The effects of punishment on human behavior* (pp. 87–132). New York: Academic.

Carrington Rotto, P., & Kratochwill, T.R. (1994). Behavioral consultation with parents: Using competency-based training to modify child compliance. *School Psychology Review, 23,* 669–693.

Chamberlain, P., & Baldwin, D.V. (1988). Client resistance to parent training: Its therapeutic management. In T.R. Kratochwill (Ed.), *Advances in School Psychology VI* (pp. 131–171). Hillsdale, NJ: Lawrence Erlbaum.

Conners, C.K. (1990). *Conners' Rating Scales manual*. North Tonawanda, NY: Multi-Health Systems.

Dinkmeyer, D., & McKay, G. (1977). *Systematic training for effective parenting*. Circle Pines, MN: American Guidance Service.

Doll, B., & Kratochwill, T.R. (1992). Treatment of parent–adolescent conflict through behavioral technology training: A case study. *Journal of Educational and Psychological Consultation, 3,* 281–300.

Epstein, L.H. (1985). Family-based treatment for pre-adolescent obesity. *Advances in Developmental and Behavioral Pediatrics, 6,* 1–39.

Eyberg, S., & Boggs, S.R. (1989). Parent training for oppositional-defiant preschoolers. In C.E. Schaefer & J.M. Briemeister (Eds.), *Handbook of parent training: Parents as co-therapists for children's behavior problems*. New York: Wiley.

Forehand, R.L. (1993). Twenty years of research on parenting: Does it have practical implications for clinicians working with parents and children? *Clinical Psychologist, 46,* 169–176.

Forehand, R.L., & McMahon, R.J. (1981). *Helping the noncompliant child: A clinician's guide to parent training*. New York: Guilford.

Foster, S.L., Bell-Dolan, D.J., & Burge, D.A. (1988). Behavioral observation. In A.S. Bellack & M. Hersen (Eds.), *Behavioral Assessment* (pp. 119–160). New York: Pergamon.

Friman, P.C., & Poling, A. (1995). Making life easier with effort: Basic findings and applied research on response effort. *Journal of Applied Behavior Analysis, 28,* 583–590.

Gordon, T. (1970). *Parent effectiveness training*. New York: David McKay.

Graziano, A.M., & Diament, D.M. (1992). Parent behavioral training: An examination of the paradigm. *Behavior Modification, 16,* 3–38.

Gresham, F.M. (1991). Whatever happened to functional analysis in behavioral consultation? *Journal of Educational and Psychological Consultation, 2,* 387–392.

Gresham, F.M., Gansle, K.A., & Noell, G.H. (1993). Treatment integrity in applied behavior analysis with children. *Journal of Applied Behavior Analysis, 26,* 257–263.

Gutkin, T.B., & Conoley, J.C. (1990). Reconceptualizing school psychology from a service delivery perspective: Implications for practice, training, and research. *Journal of School Psychology, 28,* 203–223.

Hanf, C. (1969). A two-stage program for modifying maternal controlling during mother–child (m–c) interaction. Paper read at the meeting of the Western Psychological Association, Vancouver, British Columbia, Canada.

Hayes, S.C., Nelson, R.O., & Jarret, R.B. (1987). The treatment utility of assessment: A functional approach to evaluating assessment quality. *American Psychologist, 42,* 963–974.

Hembree Eisenstadt, T., Eyberg, S., Bodiford McNeil, C., Newcomb, K., & Funderburk, B. (1993). Parent–child interaction therapy with behavior problem children: Relative effectiveness of two stages and overall treatment outcome. *Journal of Clinical Child Psychology, 22,* 42–51.

Hembree-Kigin, T.L., & Bodiford McNeil, C. (1995). *Parent–child interaction therapy*. New York: Plenum.

Knapp, P.A., & Deluty, R.H. (1989). Relative effectiveness of two behavioral parent training programs. *Journal of Clinical Child Psychology, 18,* 314–322.

Kramer, J.J. (1990). Training parents as behavior change agents: Successes, failures, and suggestions for school psychologists. In T.B. Gutkin & C.R. Reynolds (Eds.), *The handbook of school psychology*. New York: Wiley.

Kramer, J.J., & Conoley, J.C. (Eds.). (1992). *The eleventh mental measurements yearbook.* Lincoln: University of Nebraska Press.

Kratochwill, T.R., & Bergan, J.R. (1990). *Behavioral consultation: An individual guide.* New York: Plenum.

Lalli, J.S., Browder, D.M., Mace, F.C., & Brown, D.K. (1993). Teacher use of descriptive analysis data to implement interventions to decrease students' problem behaviors. *Journal of Applied Behavior Analysis, 26,* 227–238.

Long, P., Forehand, R., Wierson, M., & Morgan, A. (1994). Does parent training with young noncompliant children have long-term effects? *Behavior Research and Therapy, 32,* 101–107.

Lutzker, J.R. (1992). Developmental disabilities and child abuse and neglect: The ecobehavioural imperative. *Behavior Change, 9,* 149–156.

Martin, G., & Pear, J. (1992). *Behavior modification: What it is and how to do it.* Englewood Cliffs, NJ: Prentice-Hall.

Mathews, J.R., Spieth, L.E., & Christophersen, E.R. (1994). Behavioral compliance in a pediatric context. In M.C. Roberts (Ed.), *Handbook of pediatric psychology* (2nd ed.). New York: Guilford.

McNeil, C.B., Eyberg, S., Eisenstadt, T.H., Newcomb, K., & Funderburk, B. (1991). Parent–child interaction therapy with behavior problem children: Generalization of treatment effects to the school setting. *Journal of Clinical Child Psychology, 20,* 140–151.

Michael, J. (1993). Establishing operations. *Behavior Analyst, 16,* 191–206.

Neef, N.A. (Ed.). (1994). Functional analysis approaches to behavioral assessment and treatment [Special issue]. *Journal of Applied Behavior Analysis, 27* (2).

Newby R.F., Fischer, M., & Roman, M.A. (1991). Parent training for families of children with ADHD. *School Psychology Review, 20,* 252–265.

O'Neill, R.E., Horner, R.H., Albin, R.W., Storey, K., & Spraque, J.R. (1989). *Functional analysis: A practical assessment guide.* Eugene: University of Oregon, Research and Training Center on Community-Referenced Nonaversive Behavior Management.

Patterson, G.R. (1976). *Living with children: New methods for parents and teachers.* Champaign, IL: Research Press.

Patterson, G.R. (1982). *Coercive family process.* Eugene, OR: Castalia.

Patterson, G.R., & Forgatch, M.S. (1987). *Parents and adolescents living together—Part I: The basics.* Eugene, OR: Castalia.

Patterson, G.R., & Narrett, C.M. (1990). The development of a reliable and valid treatment program for aggressive young children. *International Journal of Mental Health, 19,* 19–26.

Patterson, G.R., Reid, J.B., & Dishion, T.J. (1992). *Antisocial boys.* Eugene, OR: Castalia.

Powers, L.E., Singer, G.H., Stevens, T., & Sowers, J. (1992). Behavioral parent training in home and community generalization settings. *Education and Training in Mental Retardation, 27,* 13–27.

Powers, S.W., & Roberts, M.W. (1995). Simulation training with parents of oppositional children: Preliminary findings. *Journal of Clinical Child Psychology, 24,* 89–97.

Roberts, M.W., & Powers, S.W. (1988). The compliance test. *Behavioral Assessment, 10,* 375–398.

Robinson, E.A., Eyberg, S.M., & Ross, A. W. (1980). The standardization of an inventory of child conduct problem behaviors. *Journal of Clinical Child Psychology, 9,* 22–28.

Rogers Wiese, M.R. (1992). A critical review of parent training research. *Psychology in the Schools, 29,* 229–236.

Shriver, M.D., & Allen, K.D. (1996). The time-out grid: A guide to effective discipline. *School Psychology Quarterly, 11,* 67–75.

Sisson, L.A., & Taylor, J.C. (1993). Parent training. In A.S. Bellack & M. Hersen (Eds.), *Handbook of Behavior Therapy in the Psychiatric Setting* (pp. 555–574). New York: Plenum.

Stark, L.J., Powers, S.W., Jelalian, E., Rape, R.N, & Miller, D.L. (1994). Modifying problematic mealtime interactions of children with cystic fibrosis and their parents via behavioral parent training. *Journal of Pediatric Psychology, 19,* 751–768.

Taylor, J.C., & Romanczyk, R.G. (1994). Generating hypotheses about the function of student problem behavior by observing teacher behavior. *Journal of Applied Behavior Analysis, 27,* 251–265.

Wahler, R.G., & Hann, D.M. (1986). A behavioral systems perspective in childhood psychopathology: Expanding the three-term operant contingency. In N. Krasnegor, J. Anasteh, & M. Cataldo, (Eds.), *Child Health Behavior* (pp. 146–167). New York: Wiley.

Webster-Stratton, C. (1990). Enhancing the effectiveness of self-administered videotape parent training for families with conduct-problem children. *Journal of Abnormal Child Psychology, 18,* 479–492.

Webster-Stratton, C., & Herbert, M. (1993). What really happens in parent training? *Behavior Modification, 17,* 407–456.

Werle, M.A., Murphy, T.B., & Budd, K.S. (1993). Treating chronic food refusal in young children: Home-based parent training. *Journal of Applied Behavior Analysis, 26,* 421–433.

Yule, W. (1989). Parent involvement in the treatment of the school phobic child. In C.E. Shaffer & J.M. Briesmeister (Eds.), *Handbook of parent training: Parents as co-therapists for children's behavior problems* (pp. 223–244). New York: Wiley.

Bibliography

Dangle, R.F., & Polster, R.A. (Eds.). (1984). *Parent training.* New York: Guilford. Although this book is over a decade old, it is still one of the best compilations of work by leaders in the field of behavioral parent training. This book describes conceptual underpinnings of the training and specific programs successfully applying it.

Forehand, R.L., & McMahon, R.J. (1981). *Helping the noncompliant child: A clinician's guide to parent training.* New York: Guilford. This book describes in detail the parent training program developed by Forehand and McMahon. The reader is provided with step-by-step directions on the process, as well as methods of monitoring behavior change and coding parent–child interaction. Forehand and Mc-

Mahon present a data-based approach to parent training that is currently widely used.

Hembree-Kigin, T.L., & Bodiford McNeil, C. (1995). *Parent–child interaction therapy.* New York: Plenum. This book describes the parent training program developed by Sheila Eyberg and colleagues termed Parent–Child Interaction Therapy (PCIT). This book also provides data-based, step-by-step procedures for conducting parent training.

Patterson, G.R. (1986). Performance models for antisocial boys. *American Psychologist, 41,* 432–444. This article describes the coercion model of parent–child interaction and its development by Patterson and colleagues at the Oregon Social Learning Center. Although more updated readings are available, this article is a well-written summary of the coercion model.

Patterson, G.R., Reid, J.B., & Dishion, T.J. (1992). *Antisocial boys.* Eugene, OR: Castalia. This is one of the more recent publications from the Oregon Social Learning Center. It describes in detail the development, research and applications of the coercion model.

Wahler, R.G., & Hann, D.M. (1986). A behavioral systems perspective in childhood psychopathology: Expanding the three-term operant contingency. In N. Krasnegor, J. Anasteh, & M. Cataldo (Eds.), *Child Health Behavior* (pp. 146–167). New York: Wiley. This chapter provides a well-written presentation of ecological considerations in behavior analysis, specifically related to child problems. It provides a clear conceptual base for the consideration of ecological variables in parent–child interactions.

10

Child Physical Abuse and Neglect

BRAD DONOHUE, ROBERT T. AMMERMAN, AND KATHLEEN ZELIS

Introduction

Maltreatment of children has become endemic in our society. In a recent summary of statistics on child abuse and neglect in the United States, Curtis, Boyd, Liepold, and Petit (1995) reported the following physical consequences to the approximately 3 million children maltreated in 1993: 2,000 fatalities, 18,000 serious disabilities, and 141,700 serious injuries. In 1993, the incidence of reported maltreatment was 43 per thousand children, up from 28 per thousand in 1984. Among substantiated and indicated reports of maltreatment, 45% involved neglect, 22% physical abuse, 13% sexual abuse, 5% emotional maltreatment, 2% medical neglect, and 13% other. It is generally believed that these official reports are underrepresentations of the actual incidence of maltreatment, given that some types of abuse (e.g., psychological mistreatment) are difficult to identify and document. The human and financial costs of child maltreatment are unfathomable, although research has clearly documented that the consequences of child maltreatment are potentially devastating (see Briere, Berliner, Bulkley, Jenny, & Reid, 1996).

The causes of maltreatment are varied and multifactorial. In the case of neglect, drug and alcohol abuse has been implicated as the largest single contributor. Additional and concomitant risk factors

BRAD DONOHUE AND **KATHLEEN ZELIS** • Center for Psychological Studies, Nova Southeastern University, Fort Lauderdale, Florida 33314. **ROBERT T. AMMERMAN** • Allegheny General Hospital, Department of Psychiatry, MCP♦ Hahnemann School of Medicine, Allegheny University of the Health Sciences, Pittsburgh, Pennsylvania 15212.

include poverty, cognitive limitations, social isolation, and some forms of psychiatric disorder, to name a few. Etiologic factors contributing to physical abuse include poverty, poor community resources, substance abuse, social isolation, having been maltreated as a child, and inadequate coping and parenting skills. Variations of the ecological model of child development have been put forward to account for the etiology of abuse (e.g., Ammerman, 1990; Belsky, 1993). According to this model, child development emerges and progresses within four systems, each of which is nested hierarchically within the other: child, family, community, and society. Influences from these systems are reciprocal. Development is affected by the complex interactions and synergistic relationships among variables. Some variables are conducive to positive development (e.g., responsive caregiving), whereas others undermine optimal adjustment and adaptation (e.g., inconsistent parenting). Children may display characteristics that promote resilience (e.g., good coping skills) in the face of adversity, or they may be more vulnerable to poor parenting (e.g., cognitive limitations). Some variables are transient in nature (e.g., intermittent unemployment), and others are stable and relatively unchangeable (e.g., low IQ). As a result, according to the ecological model, development is a dynamic process in which multiple variables compete and combine to affect the child's social, emotional, and behavioral functioning.

There are several implications of the ecological model for understanding child abuse and neglect. First, abuse and neglect are caused by multiple variables, and the pathways through which families become maltreating are diverse and unique. It is for

Handbook of Child Behavior Therapy, edited by Watson and Gresham. Plenum Press, New York, 1998.

this reason that no one factor or even a consistent constellation of factors have been found that generally account for abuse and neglect. Second, etiologic influences emanate from several sources, some of which (e.g., community, society) are difficult to change at the level of the individual clinician. The impact of individual and family-based interventions is likely to be affected by other factors in the community that undermine family functioning and child development. Finally, the interplay of risk and protective factors over time affects whether or not the child is likely to be maltreated at any given point (Wolfe, 1987). In other words, the child and family often move in and out of risk, and interventions must be adjusted accordingly to reflect treatment designed to stop ongoing abuse and neglect or to prevent future mistreatment.

Behavioral interventions are the treatment of choice for child abuse and neglect. The behavioral approach, with its emphasis on functional assessment and individually tailored interventions, fits well conceptually with the ecological model. Moreover, it is the only form of intervention that has been repeatedly evaluated empirically, and found to be relatively efficacious, at least in the short term. However, a caveat is necessary. Child abuse and neglect in general, and chronic maltreatment of children in particular, is often minimally responsive to intervention (Ammerman, Hersen, & Lubetsky, 1996; Daro, 1988). Recidivism is common, and bringing about long-term change in family functioning can be a daunting task. Intervention with child abuse and neglect, therefore, must involve the use and coordination of multiple services, of which behavior therapy is a significant part. Long-term management and intervention is essential to bringing about and maintaining meaningful improvements in functioning.

Problem Identification

Identification and Confirmation of Physical Abuse and Neglect

Other than reports of abusive behavior, physical appearance and manifestation of behaviors highly correlated with abusive behavior are the two most common methods of identifying child maltreatment. Physical injury which is unexplained or does not account for the type of injury present may be a result of physical abuse. Indeed, injuries sustained from play are often distinct from injuries resulting from physical abuse. Suspicious marks include bruises on the arm or neck that look like "grab" marks, bite marks, and lash marks from whips or straps (see Johnson, 1996). Burn marks that have identifiable patterns such as those from curling irons and cigarettes should always bring about further investigation. Children are sometimes immersed in hot water as punishment. Usually a child who is accidentally exposed to hot water will quickly pull the exposed body part away from the water, leaving splash marks. A child who is immersed in hot water may have no splash marks, and accounts of the incident may be inconsistent with the burn marks. Nonetheless, even if unintentional, burns are often a sign of neglect (i.e., not putting the heat source out of child's reach). Bone fractures, particularly cranial fissures, that are at different stages of healing can be detected by x-rays and are indicative of abuse. Children who have been physically abused may demonstrate hypervigilance or "startle reflexes" in response to abrupt external movements or loud noises.

A consistently disheveled child (e.g., dirty body and clothing, clothes that are too small or in need of repair, unkempt hair) or home (e.g., unwashed dishes, dog feces on kitchen floor) may be a sign of neglect. Other indications of neglect include caregiver delays in obtaining professional medical assistance for physical injuries or medical conditions of their children. Common hazards associated with neglect which may be identified from home visits include access to medications, electric wires, alcohol, drugs, toxins, weapons, sharp and/or heavy objects, animal feces on the floor, no running water, extreme temperature, and lack of nutritional foods.

Hallmark correlates of child abuse that warrant exploration of abusive behavior include negative caregiver–child interaction, chronic caregiver frustration with child, child misconduct or noncompliance, difficult child characteristics, child fears of suspected perpetrator, poor child management skills of caregiver, unrealistic caregiver expectations of child's behavior or development, previous history of violence in family, and abrupt changes in child's mood or behavior (Ammerman, Cassisi, Hersen, & Van Hasselt, 1986). Familial stress is a frequent correlate of child maltreatment, including various transitional changes. In fact, one study (Justice & Justice, 1975) reported that 85% of a sample of abusing parents moved within the year prior to assessment. Other child abuser characteristics include social isolation, single status, poor understanding of child development, unemployment, substance abuse, history of being abused as a child, and lack of social support. Moreover, family constellation often changes. Indeed, many victims of child maltreatment have several caregivers, with length of residency in each caregiver's home being somewhat unpredictable (e.g., victim's mother dies due to drug overdose and the child is placed in custody of the grandmother who subsequently states that she is unable to raise the child due to his noncompliance; the child is then placed in foster care).

Mandated Reporting of Suspected Incidents of Child Abuse

Once child maltreatment is suspected, it is necessary to confirm abuse. In most states professionals are required to report suspected incidents of child maltreatment to state child protective service agencies. After receiving an alleged report of abuse, a child protective service caseworker is assigned to conduct an investigation and make referrals to appropriate agencies, if necessary. If suspected abuse is founded, a protective service caseworker is assigned to monitor the welfare and rehabilitation of the victim(s). Protective service assessments are oftentimes inadequate, due to many factors, including time constraints, inadequate training, victim recantation of abuse, and intimidation by, and uncooperativeness of, family being investigated. Therefore, the court often mandates that confirmed cases of child abuse undergo a comprehensive psychological assessment to be performed by a clinician familiar with child abuse issues. The duration of case monitoring usually depends on progress in therapy, and is determined by the court with assistance from professionals assigned to the case (most notably therapist or caseworker). Thus, even after the child protective service investigation, a thorough confirmation and assessment is warranted.

Correlates of Child Abuse

The purpose of this section is to provide an appreciation of the importance of assessing problem correlates of child abuse during intervention, in light of their functional relationship with abusive behavior. It is well established that caregivers of abused children often do not have accurate expectations of the developmental capabilities of their children (Azar & Rohrback, 1986; Wolfe, 1985). For example, they may expect their children to be more cognitively advanced, to have longer attention spans, to sit still for extended periods of time, or to have larger vocabularies than what is normal for the child's age. When children are unable to meet lofty expectations, abusive caregivers often feel that the child is being deliberately disobedient or spiteful, and do not accept the undesired behavior as a normal process of learning (Azar, 1988). Negative attributions may lead to frustration and subsequent abuse.

Consistent with most studies, Chaffin, Kelleher, and Hollenberg (1996) found that substance abuse was the most prevalent disorder associated with the onset of both child neglect and physical abuse. Frequent substance abuse in child abusive caregivers may lower inhibitions to hit when the parent is angry. Indeed, rapid mood changes are common in substance abuse, and irritability associated with withdrawal symptoms may lead to limited patience and understanding regarding child mishaps. The effects of substance intoxication (e.g., apathy, forgetfulness) negatively influence caretaking behaviors such as supervision (e.g., toddler walks into street via open front door, child left in car while caregiver is in bar). With certain drugs (i.e., "crack" cocaine) addicted caregivers may buy the substance rather than food or other items necessary for the child's well-being and development (e.g., heat for home, medical attention). In extreme cases, children may be prostituted, or influenced to do so, in order for the caregiver to obtain money for drugs. Parties involving substance use may promote exposure of children to age-inappropriate experiences such as foul and sexual language.

Marital problems and violence between caregivers is also a strong predictor of child abuse (e.g., Stark and Flitcraft, 1988). Indeed, children are especially vulnerable to abuse when caregivers are abusive to one another. It is not uncommon for children to become physically abused while attempting to separate caregivers from physical or verbal abusive interactions. Sometimes battered women resort to physically abusive behavior with their children in attempts to prevent child behavior problems that may lead to more severe violence from angry male perpetrators (McKernan-McKay, 1994). Even if children are not physically abused themselves, witnessing family violence can be very traumatic (see Carroll, 1994).

Behavioral Assessment of Physical Abuse and Neglect

The method of assessment utilized to confirm and understand the function of abusive behavior and its remediation is largely dictated by the nature of the referral, and reasons for referral are diverse. For example, sometimes assessment is conducted to determine if the alleged perpetrator did indeed act abusively or to determine if the victim is safe remaining in the home of the perpetrator. In this case, it would be prudent to thoroughly assess the perpetrator and perpetrator–victim relationship, among other areas. At other times, perpetrator–victim remediation is highly unlikely due to the severity of the abuse. In these cases, assessment will usually exclude the perpetrator and focus on the victim and relevant family members, foster-care parents, friends, and so on. Assessment methods are also influenced by the type of abuse to be assessed and numerous diversity issues (e.g., age, IQ, sex, socio-economic status, religion).

Nonetheless, all referrals have in common assurance of future safety and well-being of the victim. Thus, in determining whom to assess, clinicians should include any persons who assume (or may later assume) caregiver duties, the perpetrator (if remediation is likely), the victim, and if time allows, significant family or friends.

Methods of assessment should be selected in view of the specific problem behaviors evinced in the homes of abused children. Child maltreatment includes a plethora of problem behaviors with unique and complicated etiologies and referrals often involve multiple victims and perpetrators. Indeed, it is sometimes the case that the identified perpetrator is actually less abusive than a previously unidentified offender. Furthermore, presence and severity of abusive and nonabusive behaviors differ widely among families, and across time within each family. In addition to problem behaviors of the victim, family and friends of the victim often exhibit psychological symptoms and functional impairments that negatively affect the target victim. Thus, it is necessary to assess a wide array of behaviors across various situations (e.g., school, home, play) using a multidimensional assessment. Areas worthy of formal assessment in children typically include compliance/conduct at school and home, fears, relationship with target family members, depression, anxiety, anger, aggression, and social skills and self-protection skills. Caregivers should be formally assessed in the areas of stress, mood, relationship with target child, social functioning and support, expectations of child, parent disciplinary practices and beliefs, substance abuse, home cleanliness and hazards (if home-based) and child abuse potential. In this endeavor, it is a good idea to implement a standard and comprehensive assessment battery initially, and later add assessment tools as idiosyncratic problem areas are revealed. Selected instruments should of course target problem areas specific to the referral. We will now delineate frequently used assessment methods that have demonstrated efficacy in child maltreated populations. Although it is necessary to assess a wide array of problem domains, we will emphasize instruments developed to assess physical abuse and neglect.

Interview Techniques

It is generally helpful to begin interviews with small talk about the interviewee's interests and one or two comments about any positive caretaking behaviors that may have been observed or implied (e.g., "You really seem to care about your children; I notice they look up to you"). It is important to objectively review state laws governing specific abusive behaviors prior to conducting the interview, including differentiation of these behaviors from corporal punishment. The major disadvantage of such disclosure is that perpetrators may be less inclined to report behaviors that are reportable to child protective services, whereas benefits may include increased trust in the interviewer and greater inclination to disclose undesired behaviors that are nonreportable. In interviewing the victim, leading questions should be avoided whenever possible, as these questions will influence the interviewee (Powell, 1991). Instead, the interviewer should use open-ended questions, with initial questions being more peripheral to abuse than later questions (e.g., "What do you and your uncle do after school that you like?" "What kinds of things do you do with your uncle before bedtime that you don't like?"). It is equally important to avoid comments which may disconfirm abuse during the interview (e.g., "Are you sure it was your uncle?"). A more accurate strategy is to include relevant significant others in the interview process and note inconsistencies in their reports across time and between interviewees. All interviewees should be evaluated separately.

Content of the interview should include a thorough exploration of abusive behaviors (e.g., type and history of abuse, consequences/precursors/concomitants of present abusive behaviors, including feelings, behaviors, and thoughts), relationships within family (e.g., who lives in home, custody issues, marital problems, family activities), extent of alcohol and drug use (e.g., type of substances used, frequency, concomitants, severity, antecedents, consequences, relation to child abuse), employment and academic history, mental status and medical history. Disciplinary practices used by caregiver across various situations (e.g., disciplines used by caregiver's parents and caregiver's beliefs about such disciplines, disciplines used with child in various situations, response of child before, during and after various disciplines), child's problematic and nonproblematic behaviors (e.g., failure to perform homework or chores, noncompliance, athletic events and abilities) should also be explored in order to identify excessive discipline practices by parents as possible targets for intervention. In addition, questions regarding caregiver expectations of child, caregiver's understanding of child developmental milestones, recreational events and interests of family (e.g., sports, hobbies, community involvement), safety skills of child (e.g., child's response to aggressive behavior, awareness of home hazards), sexually deviant behaviors of family members (e.g., juvenile sex offenses, exposure of child to pornography), social skills of caregiver and child, including relations with others (e.g., assertiveness skills with landlord, number and quality of friendships, type of social activities engaged in), psychopathology in family (e.g., depression, fears), and environmental stressors (e.g., unemployment, inadequate housing) should be presented so that the clinician may begin to assess the social environment of the child and identify variables that may interfere with treatment . To gain an understanding of the functions of abusive behaviors across various develop-

mental stages and situations that change over time, it is beneficial to assess abusive behaviors in a chronological fashion, beginning with premorbid functioning.

Structured and Semistructured Interviews

Structured interviews generally utilize standardized questions to assess specific presenting problems. These interviews are generally more reliable than unstructured interviews and help the interviewer avoid contamination due to bias. B. Wood, Orsak, Murphy, and Cross (1996) suggest that semistructured interviews are the preferred interview format with child victims of abuse because structured interview formats often do not allow the interviewer to accommodate developmental and attentional differences between children, and unstructured interviews are unreliable. Semistructured interviews generally include a greater number of questions to assess specific target areas (as compared with structured interviews). However, the interviewer is usually free to select listed questions that appear most appropriate given the child's unique circumstances. An example of a semistructured instrument is the Child Abuse and Neglect Interview Survey (CANIS; Ammerman, Hersen, & Van Hasselt, 1987), which assesses the presence of maltreatment and factors related to abuse and neglect.

Direct Observation

Monitoring marks on the body each session is one method for detecting abuse. However, this procedure may be intrusive as removal of clothing is often necessary in order to identify most marks possibly resulting from abuse. Furthermore, identified marks are often the result of accidents (e.g., falling off bike) or may be reported as such. It is also possible that increased attention to marks might result in greater reports from children stating that these marks were consequent abusive behaviors when in actuality they were not. Nevertheless, for obvious reasons, clinicians must always inquire about observed marks on the bodies of victims of suspected child abuse.

Recognizing that caregivers of abused children tend to demonstrate minimal and negative interaction with their children (see Burgess, Anderson, & Schellenbach, 1981), Schellenbach, Trickett, and Susman (1991) assessed several dimensions of parent–child interaction in a set of physically abused twins using behavioral observation techniques. In one procedure, trained observers recorded whether or not each twin was interacting with a family member for specified time periods, and if so, who initiated the interaction to whom, the nature of the behavior (e.g., sociability, nurturance, conflict), the style of the interaction (e.g., pleasant, irritable, passive, humorous), and the intensity of that style (i.e., mild, moderate, strong). Despite the valuable data gleaned from such an observation procedure, training of raters is not practical in nonresearch settings and the external validity of this method is undetermined.

In a different approach, Lutzker and his colleagues (1988) developed the Home Accident Prevention Inventory (HAPI) to assess and monitor common hazards in the homes of maltreated children. The HAPI consists of a list of common home hazards covering five categories (fire and electrical hazards, mechanical suffocation, ingested object suffocation, firearms, and poisons) which are assessed during a tour of the child's home. For each list (category), an absolute number may be obtained corresponding to the number of hazards in the home. Benefits of this instrument include its ability to assess neglectful behaviors in the home via direct observation, and its clinical utility (e.g., the HAPI may be utilized at regular intervals to educate caregivers in the remediation of hazards and to provide opportunities to reinforce improvements in home safety). As reported by Tertinger, Greene, and Lutzker (1988), mean interobserver reliability on frequency of hazards for each separate category is poor. However, agreement on the overall number of hazards (collapsing across categories) is good. Thus, although raters may identify different hazards, they do appear to agree about the frequency of hazards in the home. Lutzker and his colleagues are currently revising the HAPI and further establishing its psychometric properties. Of clinical importance, utilization of the HAPI as an ongoing assessment tool during intervention will not likely be aversive if the clinician is careful to reinforce the caregiver for home safety and cleanliness behaviors prior to identifying hazards.

A measure similar to the HAPI, the Checklist for Living Environments to Assess Neglect (CLEAN; Watson-Perczel, Lutzker, Greene, and McGimpsey, 1988), was developed to objectively assess home cleanliness. For each room in the home, a specific area is assessed for cleanliness. Ratings are derived for presence of (1) dirt or organic matter, (2) number of clothes or linens, and (3) nonorganic matter and items other than clothes.

Caregiver Self-Report Measures of Physical Abuse and Neglect

Milner (1986) developed the Child Abuse Potential Inventory (CAPI) to detect children at risk for maltreatment. Administered to caregivers of abused children, the CAPI yields an Abuse Potential scale as well as three validity scales. Factor scores for several domains related to child abuse are also derived (distress, rigidity, unhappiness, loneliness, problems with others, problems with one's child and one's self, and problems with one's family). CAPI items include "Children should never be bad," "I always try to check on my child when it's crying." Cutoff scores may be used to predict whether the parent is at high risk for abuse (i.e., abuse-risk cutoff = 215). Psychometric properties of the CAPI (e.g., reliability, convergent and predictive validity) are good (Kaufman & Walker, 1986; Milner, 1986), and the instrument is widely used. Although the CAPI is lengthy (i.e., 160 items), its clinical utility and strong psychometric properties justify its inclusion. Moreover, computer scoring is available. Surprisingly, a study by Holden and Banez (1996) found that nonperpetrating caregivers of child victims scored significantly higher on the Problems with the Family subscale than did perpetrating caregivers prior to treatment, and these populations responded similarly in all other domains. The findings by Holden and Banez (1996) stress the need to assess all caregivers of abused children, regardless of their perpetrator or nonperpetrator status.

O'Keefe (1994) modified the Conflict Tactics Scale (CTS; Straus, 1979) to accommodate greater frequencies of aggression typically experienced by child witnesses of violence. Her version may be completed by parents to assess degree of violence in the relationship (i.e., husband to wife, wife to husband, parent to child). Items assess how often specific acts of violence have occurred during the past year on a scale ranging from 0 (never) to 8 (100 times). For each item, the parent is additionally asked: "How often has this occurred in front of your child?" Thus, differently from the original scale, the modified version includes an expanded frequency of violence (i.e., 100 times per year instead of 20), and specific items were added to assess whether each violent behavior was witnessed by the child. Normative data are available for a population of 185 children in families of battered women; the relationship between amount of marital violence witnessed and Child Behavior Checklist scores was positive (O'Keefe, 1994).

Specifically related to neglectful behavior, the Childhood Level of Living Scale (urban version) (Halley, Polansky, & Polansky, 1980) is a 99-item self-report instrument completed by caregivers to assess child care and neglect. The instrument targets children aged 4 to 7 and provides an indication of emotional, cognitive, and physical care. Although the instrument is time-consuming to complete in its entirety, selected subscales can be administered separately and independently evaluated. A rural version is also available.

Caregiver Self-Report Measures of Problems Related to Physical Abuse and Neglect

The Treatment Outcome Questionnaire (TOQ; Brunk, Henggeler, & Whelan, 1987) was developed to quantify severity of treatment needs and evaluate changes in these needs over time in families of maltreated children. In this procedure, therapists and abusive parents separately complete a list of at least four specific problem areas believed to contribute to abuse in the home. These problems are then rated in severity using a 10-point Likert-type scale, and classified into one of three categories: (1) individual (e.g., parent's alcoholism, child's noncompliance); (2) family (e.g., marital discord, poor child management skills); and (3) social (e.g., unemployment, academic problems, poor relations with neighbors). An average score may be obtained for each category by dividing the sum of the severity ratings by the number of problems in that category. Interrater reliability for the classification of problems on the TOQ is excellent.

The parent version of the Child Behavior Problem Checklist (CBCL; Achenbach & Edelbrock, 1983) is a 133-item checklist that contains 20 social competence items and 113 behavior problem items. The instrument generates two primary subcategories of problem behaviors: internalizing behavioral disorders and externalizing behavioral problems in children ages 4 to 16 years. Significant positive correlations between parent scores on the Externalizing factor and ratings of physical and emotional abuse have been found in child maltreated populations (Kaufman, Jones, Stieglitz, Vitulano, & Mannarino, 1994).

The Eyberg Child Behavior Inventory (Eyberg & Ross, 1978) is a 36-item inventory that describes parental perceptions of specific problem behaviors, and has demonstrated its clinical utility in child abusive populations (e.g., Acton & During, 1992, Koverola, Manion, & Wolfe, 1985). Benefits of this instrument, as compared to other child behavior checklists, include its ability to assess a younger age range (2–16 years), quick and easy administration, and provision of overall Intensity (frequency) and Problem (degree to which parent sees behavior as a problem) scores. Moreover, for each problem behavior the clinician may compare Intensity and Problem scores to obtain a rough estimate of the parent's tolerance of the behavior.

A method of assessing the appropriateness of parental expectations of child behavior is the Parent Opinion Questionnaire (POQ; Twentyman, Plotkin, Dodge, & Rohrbeck, 1981). Subscales of the POQ include self-care, punishment, family responsibility and care of siblings, leaving children alone, proper behavior and feelings, and help and affection to parents. The POQ has discriminated child-abusive mothers from nonabusive mothers, as well as abusive mothers from nonabusive mothers with abusive partners (Azar, Robinson, Hekimian, & Twentyman, 1984; Azar & Rohrbeck, 1986).

Other scales that may be helpful in assessing variables related to abusive behavior include the Family Environment Scale-Revised (FES-R; Moos & Moos, 1981), the Index of Parenting Attitudes (IPA; Hudson, 1982), the Parenting Stress Index– Short Form (PSI/SF; Abidin, 1990), and the Family Life Stress Form, adapted from the Parenting Stress Index (Abidin, 1990). As social support is often lacking in abusive families, the Interpersonal Support Evaluation List (ISEL; Cohen, Mermelstein, Kamarck, & Hoberman, 1985), the Network Orientation Scale (Vaux, Burda, & Stewart, 1986), and the Community Interaction Checklist (Wahler,

Leske, & Rogers, 1979) are available to measure support, willingness to use social support, and the frequency and type of social contacts.

Child Self-Report Measures

Measures of child physical abuse and neglect are conspicuously absent from the empirical literature as most child instruments measure abuse-related domains. The Social Support Questionnaire (SSQ-6; Sarason, Sarason, Shearin, & Pierce, 1987) consists of six items that measure perceived social support. Internal consistency of the SSQ-6 is adequate, although the measure of satisfaction with social support derived from the SSQ-6 tends to be unstable. Brevity of the SSQ-6 is certainly a benefit. In a retrospective study by Grist-Litty, Kowalski, and Minor (1996), it was found that physically abused individuals with high SSQ-6 scores were significantly less likely to perpetrate abuse than individuals with low SSQ-6 scores. Interestingly, when social support was high (according to SSQ-6 scores), abused and nonabused individuals did not differ in potential to perpetrate abuse.

A measure to assess quality in the relationship is the depth and conflict subscales of the Quality of Relationships Inventory (QRI; Pierce, Sarason, & Sarason, 1991). The instrument may be used to assess a variety of relationships (i.e., parent–child, significant other–child, perpetrator–victim). The depth subscale consists of only 6 items that assess perceived commitment in the relationship, value of the relationship, and feelings of security in the relationship. The conflict subscale includes 12 items that assess anger and ambivalence in the relationship. Grist-Litty et al. (1996) averaged responses to items specific to each subscale and obtained adequate internal consistency. These researchers found that individuals who had been physically abused demonstrated lower scores in depth and higher scores in conflict than their nonabused peers.

Other standardized scales that may be useful in assessing corollary behaviors include the Revised–Children's Manifest Anxiety Scale (RCMAS; Reynolds & Richmond, 1985), the Fear Survey Schedule for Children–Revised (FSSC–R; Ollendick, 1983), and the Children's Depression Inventory (CDI; Kovacs, 1983). The Fear of the Unknown and Fear of Failure and Criticism subscales of the FSSC–R appear particularly relevant in child abuse populations.

Medical Evaluation

Medical professionals should be routinely involved in the assessment of abuse. Physicians may identify/corroborate vaginal/anal penetration and sexually transmitted diseases, and assess and treat lacerations, bruises, and damage to internal organs due to physical abuse. Physicians may also conduct nutritional assessments, intervening when necessary. When referrals are made to medical professionals it is important to encourage and assist the caregiver in scheduling an appointment, as caregivers of abused children are often negligent in this endeavor (e.g., identifying physician that caregiver can afford, assuring transportation). To prevent repeated questions and unnecessary discomfort of caregiver and child, the referral should be made to a physician who is familiar with child maltreatment, and the physician should be informed of important details of the alleged abuse prior to the examination, if possible (e.g., when and how abuse was reported to occur).

Involving Significant Others in Problem Identification

In attempting to utilize significant others in the assessment of child maltreatment, it should be emphasized that abusive behaviors are against the law, and denial and failure to report such actions by members in the abusive family (and professionals to a lesser extent; see Watson and Levine, 1989) are both well established. Thus, to improve quality of information derived from assessment measures, a useful strategy is to instruct persons to monitor behaviors and events that are related to abusive behavior (e.g., frequency of tantrums, spankings). Protective service caseworkers and teachers are the professionals most commonly used in the provision of information to clinicians, whereas nonprofessional informants include relatives and friends of caregiver and victim. For example, Koverola et al. (1985) instructed subjects to complete the Daily Events Checklist (DEC), a checklist consisting of 35 stressful events from categories of family, economic, household, transportation, health and legal problems. On a random basis, research assistants phoned significant others who maintained daily contacts with the subjects in the study to obtain their estimates of the subject's daily stress as a reliability check. Interrater agreement between the subject and significant other was good. Along similar lines, clinicians can create recording formats which indicate the date and time specific target behaviors occur, and then instruct clients and significant others to monitor these behaviors.

Problem Analysis

Graziano and Mills (1992) argued that because research indicates that maltreated children suffer psychopathological and behavioral problems in virtually all areas of development, no single profile can adequately describe all maltreated children, and therefore there is a need to individualize evaluations and interventions. Indeed, after abusive and related nonabusive behaviors have been identified in the assessment process, it is necessary to understand their function and plan treatment accordingly.

Prior to performing a functional analysis, it is necessary to review the materials obtained from assessment (e.g., interviews, questionnaires, role-play interactions). Clinical notes should be reviewed first to form preliminary hypotheses regarding the factors causing and maintaining abusive behavior. Standardized instruments may then be administered, with particular emphasis given to measures designed to confirm or disconfirm the clinician's initial hypotheses gained from the interview. Analysis of assessment instruments should involve a review of elevated overall and factor scores. For each elevated factor scale, its individual items should be read and compared to initial presumptions. If further assessment of a particular domain or domains appears warranted (e.g., an item reflecting frequent fights in school may suggest the need to assess social skills) it is a good idea to administer other measures targeting this domain, review significantly elevated factor scale items, and so on.

In the last phase, assessment information is integrated to identify the function of abusive behavior in environmental context. The first step is to generate a list of specific "abusive" behaviors which are considered contributory to harm of the target victim(s) (e.g., striking with objects, hands, or feet; derogatory or obscene statements; leaving toxins in baby's reach). Variables contributing to, and maintaining, these behaviors should be listed next to each abusive behavior (antecedent behavior, for ex-

ample, illicit substance intoxication, child noncompliance, destruction of property; consequences, for example, compliance, termination of yelling; and environmental stressors, for example, unemployment, developmental disabilities). These variables are obvious targets for therapy, with priority given to the variables thought to be most contributory to abuse and for which treatment is thought likely to bring about immediate positive change.

In conducting functional analyses of child abusive behavior it is important to realize that (1) many controlling variables relevant to abusive behavior will not be identified in the assessment process (e.g., substance abuse typically preceding violence may be denied), (2) the function of target abusive behaviors change as other behaviors change (e.g., elimination of cocaine abuse may initially increase irritability and use of critical comments), (3) abusive behaviors reciprocally interact with other behaviors across various situations (e.g., caregiver may discipline child's noncompliance with loss of privileges while on school grounds, due to presence of teacher, but may use excessive corporal punishment at home), and (4) the impact of controlling variables will vary over time and across developmental stages (e.g., spanking a 3-year-old with a paddle may bring about crying and consequent compliance, whereas spanking an 11-year-old may elicit laughter).

Plan Implementation

Selecting Target Behaviors in Therapy

Prior to choosing a package of interventions to address the problem behaviors identified as contributory to abuse, a useful strategy is to separate problems that are specific to victim, caregiver, or other appropriate family members. For each person, behaviors should be clustered into specific categories/domains (e.g., behaviors related to child misconduct: noncompliance to parental directives, failure to perform household chores, truancy, failure to perform homework). The therapist may then present a list of corresponding, positively stated, target behaviors to family members (e.g., behaviors related to child conduct: compliance to parental directives, performance of household chores, attendance at school, completion of homework). Family members may then define each target behavior so that it may be objectively monitored during intervention (e.g., take out garbage by 4 P.M. Friday, attend school six hours daily, complete homework assignments by 8:00 P.M. each night). Although each family member should be prompted to commit to the amelioration of each target behavior, the clinician must remember that verbal promises may not be predictive of actual changes in behavior.

Research on Effective Interventions

The next phase involves matching target behaviors to efficacious interventions. To assist with the selection of interventions, we will now highlight studies appearing in the last 15 years that appear to have demonstrated treatment efficacy with child maltreated populations and that have utilized relatively adequate experimental designs. The behavioral clinician should remember, whenever possible, to match the intervention strategy with the function (either antecedent or consequent) of the abusive behavior. For example, the interventions directed at adults can be considered antecedent interventions because lack of management skills, maladaptive responses to stress, or inappropriate expectations for children are often establishing operations for abuse or maltreatment. The resulting changes in management skills may then lead to positive consequences in the form of compliant child behavior and avoidance of abusive behavior. Thus, clinicians should select the appropriate intervention for the specific establishing operation/antecedent.

Adult Child Management Skills

Most child management strategies for use with caregivers of maltreated children include components from Hanf-Forehand's parent training program (see Forehand & McMahon, 1981, for description) and the Oregon Learning Parent Training and Family Management Program (Patterson, Reid, Jones, & Conger, 1975). The former program uses a highly structured two-step process. In the first step, caregivers learn to attend and reinforce prosocial behavior and to ignore minor misbehaviors. The second step involves teaching the caregiver to give clear and concise directives and warnings, as well as time-out procedures. Parents are instructed to perform therapy assignments to facilitate generalization to the home

environment. Program efficacy is extensive with nonabused populations (e.g., Wells & Egan, 1988).

Similarly, the Oregon Social Learning Parent Training and Family Management Program has demonstrated treatment outcome success with nonabused populations (e.g., Patterson, 1974). As in Hanf-Forehand's program, parents are required to pass minimum skill criteria in order to progress through each stage. In the first stage, parents learn rudiments of social learning theory via a textbook. After successfully passing an examination which targets their understanding of these concepts, the caregiver is taught to define and monitor two deviant and two prosocial child behaviors for three days. Parents learn to develop an intervention program in the last stage, targeting three behaviors utilizing point systems, daily rewards, social reinforcers, time-out, and other consequences. The program also includes training in problem-solving skills (i.e., defining problem, generating solutions to problematic situation, evaluating pros and cons of each solution).

Wolfe and colleagues (1982) utilized a "bug-in-the-ear" device to instruct, prompt, and provide immediate feedback in teaching a child-abusive mother child management strategies. The mother was prompted to increase her frequency of positive behavior (hugs, praise, pats) and decrease her use of hostile verbal and physical behaviors. Results demonstrated improvements in targeted parenting behaviors up to two months follow-up.

J.R. Lutzker, Megson, Webb, and Dachman (1985) demonstrated positive results in teaching an abusive parent to increase her intonation during delivery of directives, leveling (talking with child at eye level), smiling, and other affective behaviors. Noncompliance decreased for the target child. Interestingly, noncompliance of a nontargeted sibling also decreased. This is particularly relevant, as multiple victims of abuse are sometimes present in these homes.

In a controlled study, Wolfe, Edwards, Manion, and Koverla (1988) randomly assigned thirty mother– child dyads at risk for child abuse and neglect to either an information group offered by child protective services or a behavioral parent training group plus the information group. The parent training group was based on Hanf-Forehand's program. However, parents also (1) watched videotaped sessions of their parenting practices and engaged in subsequent self-analysis with therapists, (2) were provided opportunities to practice relaxation and coping skills related to child management in the presence of their children, and (3) received periodic home visits from protective service caseworkers, including the aforementioned information groups. Standardized measures indicated that the behavioral child management group demonstrated greater improvements in parenting risk and child behavior problems at posttest and three-month follow-up.

In one of the few standardized programs to differentially treat neglect and physical abuse in the same condition, Brunk and colleagues (1987) randomly assigned 43 child maltreating families to either parent training or multisystemic therapy. Seventy-seven percent of the subjects completed treatment and were thus included in the study (N = 33). Parent training (similar to Wolfe, Sandler, & Kaufman, 1981) was conducted in groups (parents only), and focused on parental instruction in human development and child management techniques (e.g., contingent positive reinforcement). Unlike Wolfe's program, competency training and rehearsal in the home was excluded. Multisystemic Therapy was provided in the home with all family members and included systems interventions (e.g., joining, reframing). Most families also received informal education in child management and appropriate expectations for child; some received coaching in relationship enhancement (i.e., marital, peer); physically abusive families received training in flexibility; and neglectful families were trained to perform executive functions in the home. Results of this study are difficult to interpret, as multisytemic therapy involved many child management techniques and the child management program was not implemented in the home. However, parents in the child management group demonstrated significant decreases in their perceived social problems (i.e., social isolation), whereas the systemic group significantly improved several parent–child behavioral interactions.

Support for contingency contracting in child-abusive populations was provided in a study by Wolfe and Sandler (1981). These researchers found long-term benefits after training parents in contingency contracting and other child management strategies (i.e., reading about child management and using problem solving to assist with rearing of children). Reductions in maladaptive parent–child interactions were maintained at one-year posttreatment.

As mentioned earlier, caregivers of victims of child abuse are many times ignorant of developmental milestones and physical limitations of their children and are unable to assume caregiver management responsibilities such as handling prolonged crying, feeding and sleep problems, and soiling (Herrenkohl, Herrenkohl, & Egolf, 1983). Therefore, interventions targeting child management skills of caregivers should also teach caregivers about child development (particularly for teenage parents). Such a program has been used in combination with cognitive restructuring and problem-solving training (Azar, 1989). Indeed, outcome support, although preliminary, suggests a decrease in parents' negative biases and improvements in problem-solving ability (Azar, 1989).

Adult Stress Management and Self-Control Skills Training

Stress management interventions with caregivers of abused children are typically oriented to solving major problems with sudden onset (e.g. helping evicted families secure shelter, securing food from Protective Services), or learning techniques to manage stress on a long-term basis (e.g., relaxation training, anger management, problem-solving techniques). Stress-management techniques involve identification of stressors and subsequent alteration of the environment to eliminate these stressors. This method typically necessitates professional assistance, because caregivers lack awareness and access to many community services. For example, caregivers may be unaware of cost-free child-care services while they seek employment, or crisis nurseries that may be used for temporary breaks from children who are whiny, colicky, or who have multiple handicaps. Moreover, they may not know how (or have the influence) to involve themselves in these programs. Therapists may alleviate stress by encouraging, facilitating, and reinforcing family membership in community groups and formal social networks (e.g., churches, home associations, boys' and girls' clubs), including informal social contact with neighbors, family members and friends. Parents Anonymous is a support group for parents who are abusive toward their children. Similar to Alcoholics Anonymous, this group provides support and opportunities to learn from others. Testing and referrals for children and adolescents to assist with specialized school placements (e.g., teenage mothers, severe emotional/behavioral problems) are often warranted. Encouraging and facilitating the child's involvement with a qualified guardian ad litem volunteer is usually beneficial, as these legal advocates for children have great influence in court and often engage the child in social activities (e.g., trips to movies, museums). However, the aforementioned programs consist largely of nonprofessionals who sometimes err in their opinions. As pointed out by Azar and Siegel (1990), the use of stress-reducing adjuncts must be considered carefully, as empirical support of such interventions is lacking and negative effects are certainly possible (e.g., child feels unloved after being sent to day care because his mother says she "needs a break"). Nevertheless, uncontrolled investigations suggest that therapeutic day treatment programs may relieve stress of caregivers and improve children's self-concept, cognitive and physical development, and social skills (Culp, Heide, & Richardson, 1987; Culp, Richardson, & Heide, 1987).

In a controlled evaluation, Gaudin, Wodarski, Arkinson, and Avery (1990) compared 34 neglectful caregivers receiving social network enhancement strategies to 17 caregivers receiving standard child welfare services. Social network strategies consisted of personal networking, mutual aid groups, volunteer linking, employing neighborhood helpers, and skills training relevant to establishing social networks. Postintervention, perceptions of the home environment and parenting practices and attitudes were greater for caregivers in the social network condition. Nevertheless, until more controlled studies are conducted to evaluate stress-reducing adjuncts, these interventions must be used with caution.

The second method of stress management consists largely of teaching caregivers to reduce (or control) negative emotional states and solve problems that often occur during stressful events. These interventions include cognitive–behavioral interventions such as relaxation training, anger management, problem solving, and coping skills training procedures. Such strategies appear to have great promise in child abusive populations, particularly with perpetrators of violence. For example, Campbell, O'Brien, Bickett, and Lutzker (1983) implemented child management and relaxation training procedures with a mother who suffered from mi-

graine headaches. Treatment resulted in improvements in her child's compliance. The relaxation procedures appeared to alleviate her pain and subsequently helped her to learn child management techniques in an environment perceived to be less stressful.

Acton and During (1990) developed an anger-management program to assist perpetrators of child physical abuse. The goal of treatment is to teach caregivers to recognize and consequently reduce physiological arousal, which may be an antecedent for abusive behavior. After anger is diminished, caregivers are taught to utilize communication and problem-solving skills to improve child management. Importantly, caregivers are also taught to respond with empathy. The program has empirical support in terms of reducing risk of physical abuse and negative parental expectations and improving perceptions of improvements in parent–child relationship at posttreatment (Acton & During, 1992). Moreover, results indicate reductions in disruptive childhood behaviors and improvements in caregiver satisfaction with their children.

In a controlled treatment outcome study, stress-management skills training was found to be more effective compared with a control group at a six-month follow-up (Schinke et al., 1986). Similar to the Acton and During (1992) study, the stress-management skills program focused on self-control, communication, and child-management skills training. The program also included a social support component. Those who were trained demonstrated significantly improved attitudes toward their children, and anger-management/coping skills. Caregivers were also found to have improved rates of positive behaviors when their children misbehaved.

Egan (1983) compared stress-management training, child-management training, and a wait-list control condition. Caregivers who received stress-management training had improved parental feelings, while those receiving child-management skills training demonstrated better parenting skills (Egan, 1983). These results supported the claim that treatment in child-abusive populations should include multiple interventions.

A controlled multi-intervention program was developed and evaluated for maltreating parents with infants and toddlers (Barth, Blythe, Schinke, Stevens, & Schilling, 1983). This comprehensive cognitive–behavioral program (self-control training) includes identification of self-statements that often preclude abuse, relaxation skills to decrease anger, brainstorming nonabusive alternatives to solve problems, and self-reinforcement for engaging in these alternatives. Videotaped scenarios and other behavioral techniques (e.g., role-playing, feedback) are emphasized. Relative to a control group of parents who enrolled their children in a "well-baby clinic," parents in the self-control group demonstrated improvements in target behavior and self-praise and decreases in blaming statements.

Whiteman, Fanshel, and Grundy (1987) randomly assigned 55 caregivers (15 abusive, 40 judged to be potential perpetrators) to cognitive restructuring (N = 8), relaxation (N = 12), problem solving (N = 11), agency control (N = 13), or combined (i.e., cognitive restructuring, relaxation, problem solving; N = 11). Results indicated that the combined treatment was superior in decreasing anger and increasing empathy. However, the low number of subjects per group, lack of follow-up, and very short duration of treatment (appeared to be 6 weeks, 6 sessions) do not permit definitive conclusions regarding generalization of improvements over time. Nevertheless, the results support the contention that comprehensive programs consisting of multiple self-control strategies are more effective than when applied alone.

Child Therapies

Treatment outcome studies investigating individual therapies for use with abused children has been neglected in the literature for many reasons (see Fantuzzo, 1990). Indeed, we could find only one well-controlled treatment outcome study that targeted the child's behavioral reactions to violence. In this study (Kolko, 1996), 38 physically abused children were randomly assigned to cognitive behavior treatment (CBT) or family therapy. In the CBT condition, parents and children had separate therapists, but similar protocols involving both clinic and home visits. CBT visits included discussion, rehearsal, feedback, and home practice instructions. Child CBT included discussion of family stressors and violence, constructive thinking and relaxation, and later interpersonal skills training designed to minimize the child's risk for harsh punishment (e.g., using social supports, assertion, social skills). The first half of parent CBT consisted

of discussion of stress and use of physical punishment (e.g., parental views on violence), attributions (e.g., child development, expectations), anger control, and cognitive restructuring. The second half consisted of behavioral principles training (e.g., attending/ignoring), and contingency management training (e.g., time-out, response cost). Family therapy (FT) clinic visits consisted of discussions of family issues, queries regarding family interactions, and behavioral rehearsal of specific skills. FT home visits mostly consisted of reviewing clinic material and progress, applying session content to family issues, and identifying clinical concerns. Three phases of FT were implemented: (1) assessing family structural roles and interactions, reframing to shift negative attributions of blame, positive engagement of family (e.g., family treatment contract, educating family about effects of abuse), (2) developing a family problem list, problem solving, communication training, and identified individual family responsibilities, and (3) applying problem solutions and establishing problem-solving family routines in interactions likely to precipitate physical punishment. Problems related to spouse/partner relationship and school were also addressed to a lesser extent. Results indicated that parent reports of anger and use of physical discipline/force (according to Likert ratings) were significantly lower in the CBT group throughout treatment, and child self-reports indicated a greater reduction of family problems throughout treatment. Importantly, the average length of time reported until the first use of any physical discipline/force was nearly twice as long for CBT. Weaknesses of this study include the lack of standardized assessment measures and post-treatment assessment. However, the study supports use of specific behavioral skills training programs in the amelioration of child abuse and provides a strong reminder of the importance of individual therapy for children, which is so often overlooked.

Ecobehavioral Approach

The ecobehavioral approach views child abuse and neglect as a multifaceted problem requiring multifaceted behavioral assessment and intervention (J.R. Lutzker, 1990). According to the tenets of Project 12-Ways, behavioral intervention is conducted in the child's environment (e.g., home, school, medical facilities, shelters) to facilitate generalization of treatment results. Although treatment outcome data for the ecobehavioral approach is largely uncontrolled, support is clear and dramatic. The ecobehavioral approach has been extensively evaluated in child abusive and at-risk populations to treat a wide array of problem behaviors, including teaching maltreating parents to stimulate their infants (S.Z. Lutzker, Lutzker, Braunling-McMorrow, & Eddleman, 1987), to reduce home hazards and improve home cleanliness via identification of home stressors, and to install home safety equipment (Tertinger, Greene, & Lutzker, 1984). The ecobehavioral approach has also been used to improve parenting skills and subsequent child compliance (J.R. Lutzker et al., 1985), to alleviate child conduct and migraine headaches/stress via relaxation training and child management skills training (Campbell et al., 1983), to teach abusive parents to plan and budget meals to improve child nutrition (Delgado & Lutzker, 1985), to improve child hygiene skills with contingent reinforcement (Lutzker, Campbell, & Watson-Perczel, 1984), and to help caregivers identify symptoms of illness in their children and appropriately intervene (Sarber, Halasz, Messmer, Bickett, & Lutzker, 1983).

Clinic vs. Home-Based Intervention

Therapy is typically conducted in the target child's environment (i.e., home, foster home, shelter) or in the clinic office. The clinic is certainly more cost-effective, as expenses related to travel and outside distractions (e.g., phone calls, unexpected visitors) are minimized. Clinic-based therapy is also safer for the counselor, as home-visits are often provided in dangerous areas. Another advantage in utilizing clinic-based therapy is access to basic aids that are often missing in the child's home. However, unlike home visits, clinic visits do not provide opportunities to assess home hazards and cleanliness or to observe interpersonal interactions in the child's natural environment. We recommend the use of home-based therapy whenever feasible, particularly during assessment and periodically throughout intervention. Indeed, Kolko (1996) reported that home visits facilitated generalization of their treatment program. In their study, clinic and home visits were both provided, with home visits occurring after every one or two clinic sessions (depending upon client progress and availability).

Several guidelines appear useful when providing therapy in the child's environment. When the child lives in an area that is known to have high crime rates, we recommend that counselors provide therapy in pairs (preferably male–female dyads), and drive to homes together and prior to dusk. This procedure appears effective for several reasons: (1) safety is enhanced, (2) one counselor can intervene with caregiver(s) while the other simultaneously treats the child(ren), (3) it is less stressful for counselors, and (4) it assists with treatment protocol adherence. We also recommend that counselors obtain a commitment from each family member to be at their home 30 minutes prior to session to verify session via phone call (if caregiver denies having phone she or he can call from neighbor's home), meet counselor(s) outside home when in dangerous areas, turn off television and radios during sessions, and inform friends and relatives not to phone or visit during sessions.

Improving Attendance

As mentioned earlier, attendance and promptness at sessions, both home and clinic-based, is often poor with child abusive families. Although research is lacking, methods to improve attendance with child abusive families include reminders (i.e., phone calls prior to session, posting next appointment on refrigerator), contingent rewards (e.g., faster program advancement, cleaning supplies, safety devices, self-help and child-development books, coupons, money, gift certificates), praise, contingent letters to protective services or court, and monetary deposits to be returned consequent to session attendance/completion (see Hansen & Warner, 1994).

Treatment Integrity

Treatment integrity (treatment protocol adherence) refers to the clinician's implementation of therapy as its protocol dictates. "Therapist drift" is a common problem in child maltreated families, as problems are often perceived by clinicians and family members as overwhelming and in need of additional therapies (usually resulting in spur-of-the-moment advice). In addition, caregivers are many times scrutinized for their parenting practices by others (e.g., protective investigation officers, lawyers, judges, relatives), and this contributes to defensiveness and anxiety that may be manifested in reluctance to perform role-playing or review of therapy assignments. Indeed, structured therapy procedures typically reveal skill deficits that may be perceived by the caregiver to result in detrimental consequences (e.g., reports to case managers or court, loss of custody, reminder of their inadequacies). Thus, caregivers often attempt to discuss issues that do not allow performance evaluation and that elicit empathy from the therapist (e.g., talk about how difficult their children are to manage).

Provision of frequent compliments to the target individual for any competencies or efforts related to compliance with the target intervention, and statements that remove blame, will usually reduce interruptions and/or disruptions from standardized protocol procedures such as role-playing and review of therapy assignments. Another method to enhance treatment integrity involves the use of standardized treatment manuals which clearly depict treatment protocol. Of course, sufficient training in the use of the treatment manual is necessary prior to implementation. Indeed, if a clinician is not sufficiently comfortable with the intervention, she or he will be more likely to rely on skills that have been reinforced in the past (e.g., long-winded discussions similar to day-to-day conversation). Training usually involves role-playing the targeted intervention with the training instructor until minimum level of proficiency is achieved. Practice role-plays should include difficult scenarios that often lead to therapist drift. Clinicians must be aware that caregivers sometimes attempt to divert from protocol because they perceive a lack of empathy or support from the clinician. In these cases, genuine statements of empathy may be sufficient to allow treatment to resume as planned.

Monitoring/rating session content in vivo (or from audio- or videotapes of session) is an excellent method to enhance treatment protocol adherence. For example, in Kolko's (1996) outcome study, clinicians reviewed their session tapes with a supervisor each week. Clinicians were also instructed to use a 5-point Likert-type scale to rate the degree to which primary concepts or tasks in each protocol were correctly presented in cases in which they were not involved (i.e., 1 = not reviewed, 2 = partially reviewed, 3 = completely/clearly reviewed).

Planning for Generalization

Generalization of acquired skills to the natural environment is of primary importance. The selection of empirically derived assessment tools and interventions will likely facilitate generalization of treatment gains because these procedures were specifically evaluated for this purpose. However, there are methods to enhance generalization that are sometimes not emphasized in treatment outcome studies. First, interventions targeting specific behavioral and/or cognitive skills in child maltreated families should be implemented sequentially and cumulatively. That is, the most pressing problem (or group of related problems) should be addressed first with a specific intervention (attends/praise/ignoring to address child noncompliance). Demonstrated client proficiency in the skills being taught should then result in the implementation of a new intervention (e.g., addition of time-out). However, the first intervention would still be reviewed during subsequent sessions to a lesser degree. This process would continue with all additional interventions, fading extent of review (and homework) of each specific intervention with the passage of time and the competency of person targeted. Thus, during the last treatment session, several interventions would be reviewed. Of course, reviews should include therapy assignments and role-playing to further facilitate generalization.

We recommend that the target individual initially be seen alone when conducting skills training to alleviate audience control (e.g., perceptions of parent that child will think she or he is an inadequate disciplinarian). After skill mastery is achieved via role-play with the therapist, it is very important to practice the technique in vivo whenever possible. For example, if a child was noncompliant during session, the therapist might instruct the caregiver to practice the newly learned time-out procedure. Indeed, when these opportunities come up during sessions, we instruct our therapists to temporarily terminate their agenda whenever possible and immediately prompt the target individual to utilize the skills they have mastered. For example, if a child suddenly punched her little brother while the therapist was teaching a caregiver problem solving, the therapist might prompt the caregiver to discipline the behavior using a recently mastered skill such as positive practice. Other procedures to improve generalization include extensive role-playing and positive feedback when evaluating therapy assignments in session. We also enlist into therapy almost any family member or close friend in the child's environment. If a close friend visits during a home-based session, our therapists will usually encourage their participation upon caregiver approval. The extent of significant-other involvement in therapy is generally consistent with their involvement in the child's life, which may include imitating a problematic child during a role-play, encouraging the target child to teach the friend a particular technique, or involving a friend in a social skills game with target children. We have informally found the latter procedure to be particularly effective in generalizing skill acquisition and improving rapport with our families, particularly in poor communities that are closely integrated (e.g., neighbor comes over to borrow sugar during session, elderly woman down the hall informs caregiver that his child "sassed" her and requests permission to discipline the child if a repeated offense should occur).

Plan Evaluation

Determining Treatment Completion

At some point, the therapist must decide when to terminate therapy. Treatment outcome studies have generally conducted about 12 intervention sessions. However, given the large number of problems evidenced in child abusive homes, it seems that intervention should typically include many more sessions whenever possible. Indeed, most treatment outcome studies are conducted to evaluate specific interventions targeting a relatively limited number of problem behaviors. Treatment length is often determined by extra-therapist variables such as court mandates, dropouts, excessive no-shows, frequent tardiness to scheduled sessions, change in residency, and change of custody. Therapist decisions to terminate therapy should be based on demonstrated competence in targeted areas. Perhaps the most valid method of evaluation is examination of objective, ongoing, performance indicators (i.e., session attendance and punctuality, absence of abuse via self-report from relevant persons and observation, compliance/performance during role-

playing, therapy assignment completion/performance). The therapist should also compare baseline measures with scores obtained at subsequent time periods to determine whether current functioning warrants termination of intervention. At least one or two measures should include a "lie scale" (i.e., Child Abuse Potential Inventory) in this endeavor to assess the target individual's attempt to deny pathological responses. Unfortunately, criteria do not exist specifying the magnitude of effect necessary for successful therapy termination. Thus, the clinician must rely on "clinical lore" and the factors mentioned earlier when planning termination.

What to Do when Treatment Is Ineffective

Of course, intervention will sometimes fail to bring about significant positive change in target domains. Failure in therapy is usually preceded by noncompliance to therapy protocol. Indeed, compliance to treatment protocol is strongly associated with treatment success (see Hansen & Warner, 1994). Thus, therapists must continuously attend to the various objective measures of treatment progress such as attendance, tardiness, participation in role-plays, and skill acquisition. One method of early detection is to objectively review progress indicators/goals at the start of each session, including feedback from family members (e.g., "Johnny seems to be hitting his sister more often, would you like to modify the disciplines we've been practicing?"). Another method involves administering consumer satisfaction inventories consisting of standardized questions of satisfaction/progress in therapy usually rated on a Likert-type scale. To alleviate inhibitions, an objective rater may administer the scale via telephone. The therapist may then modify intervention to accommodate family concerns.

A written agreement may also be recorded with targeted family members at the start of therapy, delineating objective indicators of program success (i.e., attendance, punctuality, completion of therapy assignments, compliance with role-plays) to be reported to the child's protective service caseworker or court (if appropriate) every month. It is important to emphasize effort and not performance, as established contingencies of performance may result in later noncompliance to performance evaluation situations (e.g., role-playing). When failure to progress in treatment appears to be related to cognitive limitations, mental illness, or failure of the above procedures, the therapist may change therapy emphasis or goals, modify intervention, make adjunct referral(s), arrange a court hearing to determine appropriate custody of child, switch emphasis of treatment to only motivated family members, and/or discontinue therapy.

Fading the Program

Although formal evaluation of treatment duration with child abusive families has yet to be evaluated and is variable across outcome studies, it is probably best to attempt at least two 90-minute sessions per week initially and gradually diminish session length and frequency according to objective progress indicators. Booster sessions are recommended when necessary. A written contract, specifying these paramets, completed prior to intervention is especially helpful in this endeavor.

Social Validity

Most programs should include consumer satisfaction scales to assess social validity upon completion of therapy. Social validity is usually assessed by having knowledgeable persons judge whether the individual's functioning following therapy is adaptive or acceptable. Persons other than the therapist should administer these questions, although professionals may be instructed to return information via sealed letter. O'Brien, Lutzker, and Campbell (1993), for example, surveyed families, agency personnel, and professionals regarding process and outcome of their treatment program. Questions were rated using Likert-type scales and an open-ended format to assess areas worthy of future emphasis or improvement (e.g., "What do you think was most useful to your child about our program?").

Follow-up

After sufficient time has elapsed (usually 3, 6, and 12 months), a follow-up assessment should be conducted with target family members. Again, assessment measures should be readministered. Progress indicators and skills targeted during therapy should be reviewed (role-played), and effort and progress should be descriptively praised. Last, booster sessions should be scheduled, if necessary.

Summary and Directions for Future Research

During the last two decades, controlled treatment outcome studies of child abuse and neglect have increased exponentially. Indeed, established measures of abuse-related domains have been normed in child maltreated populations and innovative assessment tools to identify extent and severity of child maltreatment have been developed. Although controlled treatment outcome research in child maltreatment is in its very early stages, cognitive–behavioral interventions particularly have demonstrated efficacy in several target domains. Results seem to indicate that intervention in child maltreatment should involve multiple members in the child victim's environment (e.g., see Bavolek & Comstock, 1983), separating individuals whenever appropriate. Comprehensive home-based interventions targeting multiple problem domains appear particularly promising. Although each family has a unique set of problems requiring a set of specific interventions, it seems that most caregivers benefit from child-management skills training, particularly programs that educate the caregiver about developmental child norms and possible physical and cognitive limitations of their child. Relationship enhancement training such as planning pleasant family activities, training children in the identification and prevention of high-risk situations, communication training, encouragement and training in home cleanliness and elimination of home hazards, problem solving and conflict resolution appear to improve quality and attachment in target relationships and should probably be stressed in every family to some degree. Other interventions appear more applicable to various subpopulations (e.g., anger/stress management to treat caregivers who have problems controlling their anger/stress, anxiety-management training or cue-controlled relaxation to assist children with anxiety or specific phobias). Moreover, given the large number of additional problem behaviors sometimes present in these homes, it may be necessary to borrow interventions derived from treatment outcome studies of other clinical populations (e.g., Azrin's dry-bed training for nocturnal enuresis).

It appears there is a sound foundation of child abuse research on which to build. However, we still have a long way to go. Characteristics of perpetrators and victims of child abuse need to be specified more fully in outcome studies in order to delineate choice interventions for specific populations within child maltreatment. Although it may be difficult to differentially examine subgroups of abuse (e.g., neglect only) in treatment outcome research due to overlap of these conditions, given the growing sophistication of assessment instruments, it is possible to categorize groups based on standard cutoff scores. At the very least, subjects should be selected for outcome studies based on clearly specified criteria. Interventions targeting child abusive subgroups (e.g., spouse and substance abusers, juvenile sex offenders, developmentally delayed caregivers and victims) need to be evaluated in controlled treatment outcome studies. We also know little about differential responsiveness of various subgroups to specified interventions and very little research has been conducted regarding the additive benefits of home-based intervention.

References

Abidin, R. (1990). *Parenting Stress Index*. Charlottesville, VA: Pediatric Psychology Press.

Achenbach, T.M., & Edelbrock, C.S. (1983). *Manual for the Child Behavior Checklist and Child Behavior Profile.* Burlington: University of Vermont.

Acton, R., & During, S. (1990). The treatment of aggressive parents: An outline of a group treatment program. *Canada's Mental Health, 38,* 2–6.

Acton, R., & During, S. (1992). Preliminary results of aggression management training for aggressive parents. *Journal of Interpersonal Violence, 7,* 410–417.

Ammerman, R.T. (1990). Etiologic models of child maltreatment: A behavioral perspective. *Behavior Modification, 14,* 230–254.

Ammerman, R.T., Cassisi, J.E., Hersen, M., & Van Hasselt, V.B. (1986). Consequences of physical abuse and neglect in children. *Clinical Psychology Review, 6,* 291–310.

Ammerman, R.T., Hersen, M., & Van Hasselt, V.B. (1987). *Child Abuse and Neglect Interview Schedule*. Unpublished manuscript, Western Pennsylvania School for Blind Children, Pittsburgh.

Ammerman, R.T., Hersen, M., & Lubetsky, M.J. (1996, November). *Difficulties in implementing interventions in chronic maltreatment*. Paper presented at the Association for Advancement of Behavior Therapy, New York.

Azar, S.T. (1988). Methodological considerations in treatment outcome research in child maltreatment. In J.T. Hotaling, D. Finkelhor, J.T. Kirkpatrick, & M. Straus (Eds.), *Coping with family violence: Research and policy perspectives*. Newbury Park, CA: Sage.

Azar, S.T. (1989). Training parents of abused children. In C.E. Schafer and J.M. Briesmeister (Eds.), *Handbook of parent training: Parents as cotherapists for children's behavior problems*. New York: Wiley.

Azar, S.T., & Rohrbeck, C.A. (1986). Child abuse and unrealistic expectations: Further validation of the parent opinion questionnaire. *Journal of Consulting and Clinical Psychology, 54,* 867–868.

Azar, S.T., & Siegel, B.R. (1990). Behavioral treatment of child abuse: A developmental perspective. *Behavior Modification, 14,* 279–300.

Azar, S.T., Robinson, D.R., Hekimian, E., & Twentyman, C.T. (1984). Unrealistic expectations and problem-solving ability in maltreating and comparison mothers. *Journal of Consulting and Clinical Psychology, 52,* 687–691.

Barth, R.P., Blythe, B.J., Schinke, S.P., Stevens, P., & Schilling, R.F. (1983). Self control training with maltreating parents. *Child Welfare, 62,* 313–323.

Bavolek, S.J., & Comstock, C. (1983). *Nurturing program for parents and children*. Eau Claire, WI: Family Development Resources.

Belsky, J. (1993). Etiology of child maltreatment: A development–ecological analysis, *Psychological Bulletin, 114,* 413–434.

Briere, J., Berliner, L., Bulkey, J.A., Jenny, C., & Reid, T. (Eds.). (1996). *The APSAC handbook on child maltreatment*. Thousand Oaks, CA: Sage.

Brunk, M., Henggeler, S.W., & Whelan, J.P. (1987). Comparison of multisystemic therapy and parent training in the brief treatment of child abuse and neglect. *Journal of Consulting and Clinical Psychology, 55,* 171–178.

Burgess, R.O., Anderson, E.A., & Schellenbach, C.J. (1981). Child abuse: A social interactional analysis. In B. Lahey, and A. Kazdin (Eds.), *Advances in clinical child psychology II*. New York: Plenum.

Campbell, R.V., O'Brien, S., Bickett, A., & Lutzker, J.R. (1983). In-home parent-training, treatment of migraine headaches, and marital counseling as an ecobehavioral approach to prevent child abuse. *Journal of Behavior Therapy and Experimental Psychiatry, 14,* 147–154.

Carroll, J. (1994). The protection of children exposed to marital violence. *Child Abuse Review, 3,* 6–14.

Chaffin, M., Kelleher, K., & Hollenberg, J. (1996). Onset of physical abuse and neglect: Psychiatric, substance abuse, and social risk factors from prospective community data. *Child Abuse and Neglect, 20,* 191–203.

Cohen, S., Mermelstein, R., Kamarck, T., & Hoberman, H.M. (1985). Measuring the functional components of social support. In I.G. Sarason and B.R. Sarason (Eds.), *Social support: Theory, research and applications* (pp. 73–94). The Hague: Martinus Nijhoff.

Culp, R.E., Heide, J., & Richardson, M.T. (1987). Maltreated children's developmental scores: Treatment versus nontreatment. *Child Abuse & Neglect, 11,* 29–34.

Culp, R.E., Richardson, M.T., & Heide, J.S. (1987). Differential developmental progress of maltreated children in day treatment. *Social Work, 32,* 497–499.

Curtis, P.A., Boyd, J.D., Liepold, M., & Petit, M. (1995). *Child abuse and neglect: A look at the states*. Washington, DC: Child Welfare League of America.

Daro, D. (1988). *Confronting child abuse: Research for effective program design.* New York: Free Press.

Delgado, A.E., & Lutzker, J.R. (1985, November). *Training parents to identify and report their children's illness.* Paper presented at the annual convention of the Association for Advancement of Behavior Therapy, Houston, TX.

Egan, K. (1983). Stress management and child management with abusive parents. *Journal of Clinical Child Psychology, 12,* 292–299.

Eyberg, S.M., & Ross, A.W. (1978). Assessment of child behavior problems: The validation of a new inventory. *Journal of Clinical Child Psychology, 7,* 113–116.

Fantuzzo, J.W. (1990). Behavioral treatment of the victims of child abuse and neglect. *Behavior Modification, 14,* 316–339.

Forehand, R.L., & McMahon, R.J. (1981). *Helping the noncompliant child: A clinician's guide to parent training.* New York: Guilford Press.

Gaudin, J.M., Jr., Wodarski, J.S., Arkinson, M.K., & Avery, L.S. (1990). Remedying child neglect: Effectiveness of social network interventions. *Journal of Applied Social Sciences, 15,* 97–123.

Graziano, A.M., & Mills, J.R. (1992). Treatment for abused children: When is a partial solution acceptable? *Child Abuse & Neglect, 16,* 217–228.

Grist-Litty, C., Kowalski, R., & Minor, S. (1996). Moderating effects of physical abuse and perceived social support on the potential to abuse. *Child Abuse & Neglect, 20,* 305–314.

Halley, C., Polansky, N.F., & Polansky, N.A. (1980). *Child neglect: Mobilizing services* (DHHS Publication No. OHDS 80-30257). Washington, DC: U.S. Government Printing Office.

Hansen, D.J., & Warner, J.E. (1994). Treatment adherence of maltreating families: A survey of professionals regarding prevalence and enhancement strategies. *Journal of Family Violence, 9,* 1–19.

Herrenkohl, R.C., Herrenkohl, E.C., & Egolf, B.P. (1983). Circumstances surrounding the occurrence of child maltreatment. *Journal of Consulting and Clinical Psychology, 51,* 424–431.

Holden, E.W., & Banez, G.A. (1996). Child abuse potential and parenting stress within maltreating families. *Journal of Family Violence, 11,* 1–12.

Hudson, W.W. (1982). *The clinical measurement package: A field manual.* Chicago: Dorsey.

Johnson, C.J. (1996). Abuse and neglect. In R.E. Behrman, R.M. Kliegman, & A.M. Arvin (Eds.), *Nelson textbook of pediatrics* (15th ed., pp. 112–121). Philadelphia: Saunders.

Justice, B., & Justice, R. (1975). *The abusing family.* New York: Human Sciences Press.

Kaufman, J., Jones, B., Stieglitz, E., Vitulano, D., & Mannarino, A.P. (1994). The use of multiple informants to assess children's maltreatment experiences. *Journal of Family Violence, 9,* 227–248.

Kaufman, K.L., & Walker, C.E. (1986). Review of the Child Abuse Potential Inventory. In J.D. Keyser & R.C. Sweetland (Eds.), *Test critiques.* Kansas City, MO: Westport.

Kolko, D.J. (1996). Clinical monitoring of treatment course in child physical abuse: Psychometric characteristics and treatment comparisons. *Child Abuse & Neglect, 20,* 23–43.

Kovacs, M. (1983). *The Children's Depression Inventory: A self-rated depression scale for school-aged youngsters.* Unpublished manuscript, University of Pittsburgh School of Medicine, Pittsburgh, PA.

Koverola, C., Manion, I., & Wolfe, D. (1985). A microanalysis of factors associated with child-abusive families: Identifying individual treatment priorities. *Behavior, Research and Therapy, 23,* 499–506.

Lutzker, J.R. (1990). Behavioral treatment of child neglect. *Behavior Modification, 14,* 301–315.

Lutzker, J.R., Campbell, R.V, & Watson-Perczel, M. (1984). Utility of the case study method in the treatment of several problems of a neglectful family. *Education and Treatment of Children, 7,* 315–333.

Lutzker, J.R., Megson, D.A., Webb, M.E., & Dachman, R.S. (1985). Validating and training adult–child interaction skills to professionals and to parents indicted for child abuse. *Journal of Child and Adolescent Psychotherapy, 2,* 91–104.

Lutzker, S.Z., Lutzker, J.R., Braunling-McMorrow, D.G., & Eddleman, J. (1987). Prompting to increase mother–baby stimulation with single mothers. *Journal of Child and Adolescent Psychotherapy, 4,* 3–12.

McKernan-McKay, M.M. (1994). The link between domestic violence and child abuse: Assessment and treatment considerations. *Child Welfare, 18,* 29–39.

Milner, J.S. (1986). *The Child Abuse Potential Inventory: Manual* (2nd ed.). Webster, NC: Psytec.

Moos, R.H., & Moos, B.S. (1981). *Family Environment Scale manual.* Palo Alto, CA: Consulting Psychologist Press.

O'Brien, M., Lutzker, J.R., & Campbell, R.V. (1993). Consumer evaluation of anechobehavioral program for families with developmental disabilities. *Journal of Mental Health Administration, 20,* 278–284.

O'Keefe, M. (1994). Linking marital violence, mother–child/father–child aggression, and child behavior problems. *Journal of Family Violence, 9,* 63–78.

Ollendick, T.H. (1983). Reliability and validity of the Revised Fear Survey Schedule for Children (FSC–R). *Behaviour Research and Therapy, 21,* 685–692.

Patterson, G.R. (1974). Intervention for boys with conduct problems: Multiple settings, treatments, and criteria. *Journal of Consulting and Clinical Psychology, 42,* 471–481.

Patterson, G.R., Reid, J.B., Jones, R.R., & Conger, R.E. (1975). *A social learning approach to family intervention: Families with aggressive children.* Eugene, OR: Castalia.

Pierce, G.R., Sarason, I.G., & Sarason, B.R. (1991). General and relationship-based perceptions of social support: Are two constructs better than one? *Journal of Personality and Social Psychology, 61,* 1028–1039.

Powell, M.B. (1991). Investigating and reporting child abuse: Review and recommendations for clinical practice. *Australian Psychologist, 26,* 77–83.

Reynolds, C.R., & Richmond, B.O. (1985). *Revised Children's Manifest Anxiety Scale (RCMAS) Manual.* Los Angeles, CA.: Western Psychological Services.

Sarason, I.G., Sarason, B.R., Shearin, E.N., & Pierce, G.R. (1987). A brief measure of social support: Practical and theoretical implications. *Journal of Social and Personal Relationships, 4,* 497–510.

Sarber, R.E., Halasz, M.M., Messmer, M.C., Bickett, A.D., & Lutzker, J.R. (1983). Teaching menu planning and grocery shopping skills to a mentally retarded mother. *Mental Retardation, 21,* 101–106.

Schellenbach, C.J., Trickett, P.K., & Susman, E.J. (1991). A multimethod approach to the assessment of physical abuse. *Violence and Victims, 6,* 57–73.

Schinke, S.P., Schilling, R.F., Kirham, M.A., Gilchrist, L.D., Barth, R.P., & Blythe B. J. (1986). Stress management skills for parents. *Journal of Child and Adolescent Psychotherapy, 3,* 293–298.

Stark, E., & Flitcraft, A. (1988). Women and children at risk: A feminist perspective on child abuse. *International Journal of Health Services, 18,* 97–118.

Straus, M.A. (1979). Measuring intrafamily conflict and violence: The conflict tactics (CT) scales. *Journal of Marriage and the Family, 41,* 75–88.

Tertinger, D.A., Greene, B.F., & Lutzker (1984). Home safety: Development and validation of one component of an ecobehavioral treatment program for abused and neglected children. *Journal of Applied Behavior Analysis, 17,* 159–174.

Tertinger, D.A., Greene, B.F., & Lutzker (1988). Home Accident Prevention Inventory. In M. Hersen and A.S. Bellack (Eds.) *Dictionary of behavioral assessment techniques.* New York:Pergamon.

Twentyman, C.T., Plotkin, R., Dodge, D., & Rohrbeck, C.A. (1981, November). *Inappropriate expectations of parents who maltreat their children: Initial descriptive survey and cross-validation.* Paper presented at the Association for the Advancement of Behavior Therapy Convention, Toronto, Ontario, Canada.

Vaux, A., Burda, P., & Stewart, D. (1986). Orientation toward utilization of support resources. *Journal of Community Psychology, 14,* 159–170.

Wahler, R.G., Leske, G., & Rogers, E.S. (1979). The insular family: A deviance support system of oppositional children. In L.A. Hamerlynck (Ed.), *Behavioral systems for the developmentally disabled: I. School and family environments.* New York: Brunner-Mazel.

Watson, H., & Levine, M. (1989). Psychotherapy and mandated reporting of abuse. *American Journal of Orthopsychiatry, 59,* 249–256.

Watson-Perczel, M., Lutzker, J.R., Greene, B.F., & McGimpsey, B.J. (1988). Assessment and modification of home cleanliness among families adjudicated for child neglect. *Behavior Modification, 12,* 57–81.

Wells, K.C, & Egan, J. (1988). Social learning theory and systems family therapy for childhood oppositional disorder: Comparative treatment outcome. *Comprehensive Psychiatry, 29,* 138–146.

Whiteman, M., Fanshel, D., & Grundy, J.F. (1987). Cognitive–behavioral interventions aimed at anger of parents at risk of child abuse. *Social Work, 32,* 469–474.

Wolfe, D. (1985). Child-abusive parents: An empirical review and analysis. *Psychological Bulletin, 97,* 462–482.

Wolfe, D. (1987). *Child abuse: Implications for child development and psychopathology.* Newbury Park, CA: Sage.

Wolfe, D., & Sandler, J. (1981). Training abusive parents in effective child management. *Behavior Modification, 5,* 320–335.

Wolfe, D.A., Sandler, J., & Kaufman, K. (1981) A competency based parent training program for abusive parents. *Journal of Consulting and Clinical Psychology, 49,* 633–640.

Wolfe, D.A., St. Lawrence, J., Graves, K., Brehony, K., Bradlyn, D., & Kelly, J. (1982). Intensive behavioral parent training for a child abusive mother. *Behavior Therapy, 13,* 438–451.

Wolfe, D.A., Edwards, B., Manion, I., & Koverla, C. (1988). Early intervention for parents at risk of child abuse and neglect: A preliminary investigation. *Journal of Consulting and Clinical Psychology, 56,* 40–47.

Wood, B., Orsak, C., Murphy, M., & Cross, H.J. (1996). Semi-structured child sexual abuse interviews: Interview and child characteristics related to credibility of disclosure. *Child Abuse & Neglect, 20,* 81–92.

Bibliography

Ammerman, R.T., & Hersen, M. (Eds.) (1992). *Assessment of family violence: A clinical and legal sourcebook.* New York: Wiley.

Ammerman, R.T., & Hersen, M. (Eds.). (1990). *Treatment of family violence: A sourcebook.* New York: Wiley.

Briere, J., Berliner, L., Bulkey, J.A., Jenny, C., & Reid, T. (Eds.). (1996). *The APSAC handbook on child maltreatment.* Thousand Oaks, CA: Sage.

Walker, C.E., Bonner, B.L., & Kaufman, K.L. (1988). *The physically and sexually abused child: Evaluation and treatment.* New York: Pergamon.

Wolfe, D.A. (1987). *Child abuse: Implications for child development and psychopathology.* Newbury Park, CA: Sage.

11

Sleep Problems

V. MARK DURAND, JODI MINDELL, EILEEN MAPSTONE,
AND PETER GERNERT-DOTT

Introduction

Sleep refreshes and restores us. There is evidence that sleep is necessary for learning and remembering (Smith & Lapp, 1991), as well as physical processes such as restoring our immune system (Palmblad, Petrini, Wasserman, & Akerstedt, 1979). Disruption in sleep can negatively influence our ability to concentrate, can make us irritable, and can increase health problems. Children often experience sleep problems and are equally susceptible to the difficulties that arise as a consequence. In addition to the deleterious effects on these children, parents can be significantly affected by their child's difficulties. Some research suggests, for example, that marital dissatisfaction and depression can occur in some parents as an outcome of disturbed child sleep (Durand & Mindell, 1990). There is ample reason to be concerned with the disturbed sleep of children.

Sleep problems in children are not usually considered within the province of psychologists or other nonmedical professionals. Typically, the parent of a child who experiences difficulty with various aspects of sleep will turn to a medical specialist, usually a pediatrician, for help. However, it is becoming increasingly clear that medical interventions for many sleep problems are limited and in some cases may be inappropriate for children.

In addition, there are exciting new developments in the nondrug treatment of sleep problems that require a degree of involvement and training that may be beyond the purview of most medical professionals. As a result, psychologists and special educators are increasingly called upon to intervene with children displaying a range of problems involving sleep. Unfortunately, many nonmedical professionals lack sufficient knowledge of the phenomenon of sleep itself, the problems of sleep and their causes, and appropriate intervention strategies.

This chapter will introduce the reader to several of the more common sleep problems displayed by children, their causes, and a range of intervention strategies. Because of the sheer number of sleep disorders (more than 80 are listed in the *International Classification of Sleep Disorders*—American Sleep Disorders Association, 1990), and the range of potential psychological (e.g., stress, parenting practices) and biological (e.g., obstructed airways, pain) influences on these problems, we can provide here only an introduction to this area. Additional information can be found in the readings provided at the end of the chapter.

Prevalence and Course

General estimates of the number of otherwise healthy children with some form of sleep problem usually are on the order of 25% (Mindell, 1993). One of the most common sleep disturbances exhibited by children is frequent night waking, a difficulty in maintaining sleep. Night wakings

V. MARK DURAND, EILEEN MAPSTONE, AND PETER GERNERT-DOTT • Department of Psychology, University at Albany, State University of New York, Albany, New York 12222. JODI MINDELL • Department of Psychology, St. Joseph's University, Philadelphia, Pennsylvania 19131-1395.

Handbook of Child Behavior Therapy, edited by Watson and Gresham. Plenum Press, New York, 1998.

occur in approximately 20% of one- to two-year-olds, 14% of three-year-olds, and 8% of four-year-olds (Jenkins, Bax, & Hart, 1980; Richman, 1981; Richman, Stevenson, & Graham, 1975), and are frequently found in combination with other sleep problems such as bedtime disturbances (Richman, Douglas, Hunt, Lansdown, & Levere, 1985). Bedtime disturbances, a difficulty in initiating sleep, are only slightly less common, occurring in 12.5% of 3-year-olds and 5% of 4-year olds (Richman, 1981). Salzarulo and Chevalier (1983) note changes in prevalence rates associated with age for night wakings (39% of 2- to 5-year-olds, 24% of 6- to 10-year-olds, and 14% of 11-year-olds) and for bedtime disturbances (17% of 2- to 5-year-olds, 29% of 6- to 10-year-olds, and 22% of 11-year-olds).

Night wakings have been estimated to occur at rates of between 21% (Clements, Wing, & Dunn, 1986) and 57% (Bartlett, Rooney, & Spedding, 1985) among children with developmental disabilities. Bedtime disturbances have been estimated as high as 56% in this population (Bartlett et al., 1985). DeMyer (1979) describes the sleeping patterns of almost all children with autism as disturbed at some point in their lives, and almost 50% of the $5\frac{1}{2}$-year-olds she studied exhibited severe sleeping problems. These findings point to the pervasive nature of sleep problems in children with autism and other developmental disabilities.

Although sleep disturbances tend to decrease with age, most children do not appear to "grow out of" these problems as was once commonly thought. Bernal (1973) noted that one-year-old children who exhibited night waking were more likely to have been wakeful as newborns. Bixler, Kales, Scharf, Kales, and Leo (1976) found that sleep problems in older children were associated with sleep disturbances in the first years of life and that children with early sleep problems tended to show multiple sleep problems later on. In addition, Richman and colleagues (1975) reported that 40% of their sample of eight-year-old children with night wakings had experienced this disturbance for five years or more. It has been noted that the prevalence rates of sleep disorders in adults and children are similar, which may suggest that many people who experienced sleep disturbances as children are still at risk for experiencing them in some form as adults (Durand, Mindell, Mapstone, & Gernert-Dott, 1995).

Overview of Sleep

Before moving to a discussion of sleep difficulties, it is important to understand the phenomenon of sleep. During sleep the brain is not "shut off" but is instead going through much the same type of cyclical process our bodies do when we are awake. This cycle of sleep is divided into two broad categories; *rapid eye movement* or REM sleep (what we commonly refer to as dream sleep), and *non-rapid eye movement* or NREM sleep (Hauri, 1982). The brain cycles through these stages of sleep throughout the night in a pattern that is similar across all human beings.

The NREM sleep is usually divided into four stages (referred to as stages 1–4), and these stages are based on different brain wave patterns seen during different points in NREM sleep. The stages of sleep roughly correspond to how deeply we sleep. For example, stage 1 represents "light" sleep, stage 2 would be a "deeper" sleep, and stages 3 and 4 represent the "deepest" levels of sleep. Stage 1 sleep is a transitional stage between sleep and wakefulness. People tend to feel that they are awake during this time, although their thoughts begin to drift, and in research in which volunteers had their eyes taped open, they could not recall pictures presented to them while they were in this sleep stage (Rechtschaffen & Foulkes, 1965). As the brain runs through its cycle and shifts back from the deeper stages of sleep into the light sleep of stage 1, we go through what are called "partial arousals" or "partial wakenings" (Anch, Browman, Mitler, & Walsh, 1988). Difficulties during this transition in sleep stages appear at least partially responsible for night waking among children as well as adults.

Stage 2 is the first true sleep state and includes two characteristic brain wave patterns called *sleep spindles* and *K-complexes*. Researchers often consider stages 3 and 4 sleep together and refer to them collectively as *slow wave* or *delta sleep* (for the type of brain wave pattern), or *deep sleep*. It is very difficult to awaken someone in deep sleep, and, even if successful, it can take some time before the person is fully alert. Sleep begins in NREM sleep and progresses through stages 1 through 4, with a complete "cycle" of the four stages of NREM sleep taking about 90 minutes in adults and about 60 minutes in infants (Hauri, 1982).

A number of the sleep disorders that people experience occur primarily during NREM sleep. A partial list of these NREM sleep disorders includes sleepwalking, sleep terrors (a disorder that is characterized by extreme emotional distress while sleeping, but that does not occur during dream or REM sleep), and nocturnal bruxism (teeth grinding during sleep) (Giles & Buysse, 1993). The purpose of NREM sleep is still unknown, although some preliminary research indicates that one function of these states of sleep may be related to our immune system—possibly signaling the rebuilding of this system (Blakeslee, 1993; Palmblad et al., 1979).

Following this progression of sleep stages (from stages 1 to 4), the brain transitions to rapid eye movement, or REM, sleep. This is the period of time when we dream. We know this because if someone is awakened during REM sleep, about 80% of the time the person will report very vivid dreams (Dement, 1960; Snyder, 1971). Our eyes periodically move in a rapid succession during this time, yet our body is "atonic" or does not move. The eye movements can be seen if you look at the movement of a person's closed eyelids while he or she is in REM sleep or from using an *electrooculograph* (EOG), which can detect the activity of the muscles that are responsible for eye movement. REM sleep is often characterized as a time when the brain is active but the body is not; in contrast, NREM sleep can be characterized as a time during sleep when our brain is relatively inactive, but our body is not. The brain progresses through NREM and REM stages of sleep several times during the night (Carskadon & Dement, 1989).

Some sleep disturbances occur primarily during REM sleep. Nightmares, for example, are reported when people are in this sleep stage. Another predominantly REM sleep phenomenon, *sleep paralysis,* involves the inability to move arms or legs, and is often accompanied by brief but intense fear. A number of the other disorders occur during either NREM or REM sleep, and include urination while asleep (called *nocturnal enuresis),* snoring, and sleep talking.

A "normal" amount of sleep varies considerably from person to person; for some people 5 or 6 hours of sleep per night is enough to be fully rested, whereas others may need as much as 9 hours of sleep per night. Sleep needs also change as we age. Infants sleep as much as $16^{1}/_{2}$ hours per day, whereas college age students sleep an average of 7 or 8 hours per day. Past the age of 50, total hours of sleep per day drops below 6 hours. Understanding how and why we sleep provides the context for understanding when sleep is disturbed. We next turn to identifying and assessing some of the more common disorders of sleep.

Problem Identification

The first step in an assessment of sleep problems involves compiling a complete sleep history. All aspects of the sleep–wake cycle need to be reviewed. Areas that should be addressed include evening activities such as television watching, intake of caffeinated beverages, bedtime, and bedtime routines. Areas to be evaluated during the night include latency to sleep onset, the number and duration of nighttime awakenings, and behaviors during the night. Details about abnormal nighttime events should be collected such as night terrors, confusional arousals, respiratory disturbances, seizures, and enuresis. In the morning, the time of awakening, sleepiness, and initial behaviors upon arising should be evaluated. During the day, sleepiness, naps, and behavior problems should be assessed. A review of psychological symptoms during the day is also important. Symptoms of anxiety and depression can be the result of lack of sleep, as can fatigue, irritability, and sluggishness. Medication intake should also be reviewed, as many drugs affect sleep.

As a first step, we have parents or caregivers complete a screening device that helps us identify some of the major areas of difficulty (see Form 11.1). This sleep problems scale highlights problems that may be the result of insomnia (difficulty initiating, maintaining, or gaining from sleep), hypersomnia (excessive sleepiness), narcolepsy (irresistible attacks of sleep), breathing-related sleep disorders, circadian rhythm sleep disorders (sleep difficulties due to a mismatch between the sleep–wake schedule desired and the current schedule), nightmares, sleep terrors (a disruption in sleep that begins with a panicky scream), as well as other sleep difficulties.

FORM 11.1. Albany Sleep Problems Scale (ASPS)

Name: _____ Date of birth: _____

Diagnoses: _____ Sex: _____

Name of respondent: _____ Date adm: _____

Instructions: Circle *one* number that best represents the frequency of the behavior.

0 = never

1 = less than once per week

2 = one to two times per week

3 = three to six times per week

4 = nightly

1. Does the person have a fairly regular bedtime and time that he or she awakens?	0	1	2	3	4
2. Does the person have a bedtime routine that is the same each evening?	0	1	2	3	4
3. Does this person work or play in bed often right up to the time he or she goes to bed?	0	1	2	3	4
4. Does this person sleep poorly in his or her own bed but better away from it?	Yes			No	
5. Does this person smoke, drink alcohol, or consume caffeine in any form?	0	1	2	3	4
6. Does this person engage in vigorous activity in the hours before bedtime?	0	1	2	3	4
7. Does the person resist going to bed?	0	1	2	3	4
8. Does the person take more than an hour to fall asleep but does not resist?	0	1	2	3	4
9. Does the person awaken during the night but remain quiet and in bed?	0	1	2	3	4
10. Does the person awaken during the night and is he or she disruptive (e.g., tantrums, oppositional)?	0	1	2	3	4
11. Does the person take naps during the day?	0	1	2	3	4
12. Does this person often feel exhausted during the day because of lack of sleep?	0	1	2	3	4
13. Has this person ever had an accident or near accident because of sleepiness from not being able to sleep the night before?	Yes			No	
14. Does this person ever use prescription drugs or over-the-counter medications to help him or her sleep?	0	1	2	3	4
15. Has this person found that sleep medication doesn't work as well as it did when he or she first started taking it?	Yes			No/NA	
16. If he or she takes sleep medication does this person find that he or she can't sleep on nights without it?	Yes			No/NA	
17. Does the person fall asleep early in the evening and awaken too early in the morning?	0	1	2	3	4
18. Do the person have difficulty falling asleep until a very late hour and difficulty awakening early in the morning?	0	1	2	3	4
19. Does this person wake up in the middle of the night upset?	0	1	2	3	4
20. Is the person relatively easy to comfort from these episodes?	Yes			No/NA	

FORM 11.1. (*Continued*)

21. Does the person have episodes during sleep where he or she screams loudly for several minutes but is not fully awake?	0	1	2	3	4
22. Is the person difficult to comfort during these episodes?	Yes			No/NA	
23. Does the person experience sleep attacks (falling asleep almost immediately and without warning) during the day?	0	1	2	3	4
24. Does the person experience excessive daytime sleepiness that is not accounted for by an inadequate amount of sleep?	0	1	2	3	4
25. Does this person snore when asleep?	0	1	2	3	4
26. Does this person sometimes stop breathing for a few seconds during sleep?	0	1	2	3	4
27. Does this person have trouble breathing?	0	1	2	3	4
28. Is this person overweight?	Yes			No	
29. Has this person often walked when asleep?	0	1	2	3	4
30. Does this person talk while asleep?	0	1	2	3	4
31. Are this person's sheets and blankets in extreme disarray in the morning when he or she wakes up?	0	1	2	3	4
32. Does this person wake up at night because of kicking legs?	0	1	2	3	4
33. While lying down, does this person ever experience unpleasant sensations in the legs?	Yes			No	
34. Does this person rock back and forth or bang a body part (e.g., head) to fall asleep?	0	1	2	3	4
35. Does this person wet the bed?	0	1	2	3	4
36. Does this person grind his or her teeth at night?	0	1	2	3	4
37. Does this person sleep well when it doesn't matter, such as on weekends, but sleep poorly when he or she "must" sleep well, such as when a busy day at school is ahead?	Yes			No	
38. Does this person often have feelings of apprehension, anxiety, or dread when he or she is getting ready for bed?	0	1	2	3	4
39. Does this person worry in bed?	0	1	2	3	4
40. Does this person often have depressing thoughts, or do tomorrow's worries or plans buzz through the person's mind when they want to go to sleep?	0	1	2	3	4
41. Does this person have feelings of frustration when he or she can't sleep?	0	1	2	3	4
42. Has this person experienced a relatively recent change in eating habits?	Yes			No	
43. Does the person have behavior problems at times other than bedtime or upon awakening?	Yes			No	
44. When did this person's primary difficulty with sleep begin?					

(*continued*)

FORM 11.1. (*Continued*)

45. What was happening in the person's life at that time, or a few months before?		
46. Is this person under a physician's care for any medical condition? (If yes, indicate condition below)	Yes	No

OTHER COMMENTS: _____

_____

_____

_____

_____

_____

_____

_____

_____

_____

_____

The second step in the evaluation of sleep problems is keeping sleep diaries (see Form 11.2). Sleep diaries typically include information on bedtime, latency to sleep onset, number and duration of night wakings, time awake in the morning, total sleep time, and time and duration of naps. Two weeks of baseline data are the most useful in clearly evaluating sleep patterns. Clinicians are cautioned, however, about relying solely on reports from parents for sleep problems. Recent data suggest that parents, whether through fatigue or other factors, may underreport the sleep problems of their children (Sadeh, 1994).

In cases in which there is a concern about a specific underlying physiological problem, such as with sleep apnea (interrupted breathing), narcolepsy, epilepsy, or periodic limb movements, a polysomnogram (PSG) is an essential component of assessment. Polysomnography typically consists of an overnight sleep study in which recordings of oxygen saturation, nasal and oral airflow, thoracic and abdominal respiratory movements, limb muscle activity, and electroencephalogram (EEG) are taken. Even in some cases in which the child does not report any physiological symptoms, it may be important to completely evaluate the person's sleep. For example, many parents are unaware of their child's snore arousals or sleep apnea which may be interrupting sleep and resulting in complaints of insomnia, frequent night wakings, and daytime sleepiness. As an adjunct to a PSG, a multiple sleep latency test (MSLT) may be conducted which evaluates the child's level of daytime sleepiness. The MSLT consists of four 20-minute nap opportunities given at two-hour intervals throughout the day following the overnight study. Measures of latency to sleep onset are obtained as an index of sleepiness. Norms are available for this test by age, and this information is used to objectively determine the restorative quality of the child's sleep. Most PSGs and MSLTs are conducted at accredited sleep disorders centers.

Another important aspect of assessment of sleep disorders is a thorough evaluation of daytime functioning and other psychological problems. Behavioral or psychological problems may be contributing factors to a sleep disorder. For example, significant life stressors may be related to acute sleep problems. Failure in school, death in the family, or a recent move can all contribute to a sleep problem that resembles insomnia. A thorough evaluation should include questioning about school performance, social functioning, and family functioning. A recent change in a family's financial sta-

FORM 11.2. Sleep Diary

Day	Date	A.M. Midnight	2:00	4:00	6:00	8:00	10:00	Noon	2:00	4:00	P.M. 6:00	8:00	10:00	Midnight
SUN														
MON														
TUE														
WED														
THU														
FRI														
SAT														
SUN														
MON														
TUE														
WED														
THU														
FRI														
SAT														
SUN														

tus can result in problems sleeping in children even if the parents do not believe that the child is aware of these financial problems. Often children, and especially adolescents, are much more aware of tensions in a family than are the parents. It is important, therefore, that a complete assessment of all aspects of sleep and daytime functioning be conducted.

Regarding differential diagnosis, the presenting complaints for many of the sleep disorders are similar. For example, excessive daytime sleepiness may be the result of insomnia, sleep apnea, or narcolepsy. Night wakings may be a sleep onset association disorder, the result of sleep apnea, periodic limb movements in sleep, or night terrors. It is clear, then, that a focus on differential diagnosis in the area of sleep disorders is essential.

Differentiation between a sleep disorder and other medical or psychological problems is also im-portant. A child with what looks like night terrors may actually be having seizures during sleep. In other cases, difficulties at bedtime may be symptomatic of more general problems with noncompliance. Nighttime fears may be just one aspect of a child's extensive fears. Furthermore, delayed sleep phase syndrome (a shift in the sleep pattern such that the child falls asleep late and has difficulty waking in the morning) should always be assessed before a diagnosis of school refusal is made. Given the similar characteristics of each disorder, it is likely that delayed sleep phase disorder may present as school refusal, especially among adolescents, who constitute the majority of individuals with this sleep disorder.

Finally, a brief review of parental expectations of their child's sleep is also important. The "sleep culture" of the family—beliefs about appropriate bedtimes, where the child will sleep (alone, in bed with the parent), the appropriateness of naps—will often affect the sleep problem itself as well as the outcome of treatment approaches. Sometimes minor problems can be resolved by educating parents about the range of sleep needs among children (i.e., not all children need eight or more hours of sleep) and about options for nighttime routines, appropriate bedtimes, naps, and so on.

Problem Analysis

Conducting a differential diagnosis should accomplish two important goals. First, it should help to identify the nature of the sleeping difficulty. At the same time, however, it should also provide information about the processes involved with the continued presence of the sleep disturbance. Several sleep disturbances, for example, have clear biological origins and may be less influenced by factors such as parental reactions. Sleep terrors—which are characterized by piercing screams during sleep—is a sleep problem that arises during NREM sleep and usually runs its course without the person waking. It is clear, then, that sleep terrors are not maintained by parental attention, and as a result they are not amenable to efforts such as extinction. In another example, the sleep difficulties of a child with insomnia that displays itself as a failure to get restful sleep may also have biological origins. If the child has apnea (interrupted breathing) during sleep, then this will disturb sleep and not provide the refreshment we typically expect after eight hours asleep. Again, psychosocial influences may not influence such a sleep disturbance in any significant way.

On the other hand, a number of the sleep problems children exhibit do seem to involve both biological and psychosocial influences. For example, bedtime disturbances, which are a significant difficulty for many families, may have many overlapping causes. Initially, a child may be a "light" sleeper and may have difficulty falling asleep soon after going to bed. At the same time, environmental disturbances such as the noise from a television or people talking in another room may contribute to a failure to fall asleep quickly. Parental reactions to such difficulties vary as well, and will influence whether or not this expands into a more severe problem. If the parent is caught in the unfortunately

common cycle of attending to efforts on the part of the child to leave the bedroom and/or engage other family members in interactions (e.g., "I need a drink of water," "Would you tell me one more story?"), the bedtime problems can continue for many months.

A functional assessment of sleep problems will therefore require an analysis of possible maintaining factors. In the example of bedtime disturbances, an interview with the parents and the child (if the child is older) can help identify some of these factors. We have also used videotapes—either by our staff or by the parents themselves—to help us recognize important influences. In one instance, a parent told us in an interview that she had a full bedtime ritual for her daughter, an intervention that can sometimes resolve bedtime disturbances by itself (Weissbluth, 1982). However, when we observed a video of two nights of this interaction, it was obvious that the routine was much shorter than the 30 minutes the mother reported and that it was often unpleasant, with the mother yelling at her daughter throughout. We were able to modify this routine and significantly improve the little girl's ability to go to bed without incident.

Night waking is another common childhood sleep problem. Here again, biologically based sleep problems may interact with psychosocial factors to create sleeping difficulties. Recall that people experience partial wakings when their sleep patterns transition from the deeper stage 3 and 4 sleep to stage 1 sleep. Typically, this awakening is brief (a few seconds) and is not remembered the next day. However, in some children the awakening is accompanied by crying and/or getting out of bed. If parents attend too much to these nighttime disturbances, they may further reinforce the pattern of night waking. As you can see, biological factors can interact with psychosocial influences in a reciprocal way to cause chronic sleep disturbances (Durand et al., 1995).

A functional assessment of night waking typically involves obtaining a detailed description of each incident. We ask parents to use the back of the sleep diary to describe what the child did upon waking as well as how the family responded. It is important to know, for example, whether the parent goes into the child's room, whether the child climbs into the parent's bed, whether the child is fed, whether music is played, and so forth. As implied previously, we look for evidence that the child has difficulty falling back to sleep alone after waking and whether parental attention in some form is further waking the child and contributing to the maintenance of this problem. We also assess the parent's emotional reaction to such events. In other words, how upset are they when they hear their child cry, and how difficult is it for them to ignore disruptions in the middle of the night? This becomes important later during treatment when we are determining whether some form of extinction can or should be used.

It is important to note at this point that we rarely perform an experimental analysis of factors potentially maintaining sleep problems—otherwise known as a functional analysis. There are several reasons for this. First, the nature of sleep problems is such that the environmental influences on disturbed sleep are often cumulative. For example, taking a nap one day may not influence the next night's sleep, yet taking naps over several days might begin to influence a child's ability to fall asleep at bedtime. Therefore, clear findings from a series of manipulations would take several weeks or months to assess, creating a hardship on the whole family. There are also ethical concerns centered on such analyses. Deliberately making a child's sleep worse in the name of assessment is difficult to justify, especially if nonmanipulative assessment strategies appear adequate.

One common problem in both children and adults that is often confused with insomnia is circadian rhythm disorder. At first glance, the sleep problem may resemble bedtime disturbances. A child may not fall asleep within 30 minutes of bedtime and may be disruptive. However, the child may also have difficulty waking in the morning and feel tired throughout the day. Here the problem may be that the child's sleep cycle does not match the expected sleep pattern. In delayed sleep phase syndrome, the child falls asleep late (e.g., 1 A.M.) and if left alone awakens late (e.g., 10 A.M.). In advanced sleep phase syndrome, the child has the opposite problem, falling asleep early (e.g., 8 P.M.) but also waking early (e.g., 4:30 A.M.). In both cases the child will have an adequate amount of sleep if left undisturbed, but because of demands such as school schedules or parental needs, these patterns are unacceptable. Here the sleep diaries are useful for assessing these patterns. Especially useful is observing weekend sleep patterns, when the child is often left to sleep as desired, or noting any naps the child is taking. The intervention for circadian rhythm problems differs from the intervention for a simple bedtime disturbance problem, so it is important to differentially assess what is causing problems at bedtime.

Plan Implementation

Given the often complex nature of sleep problems exhibited by children, a single approach is usually not appropriate for treating all sleep problems (see Mindell & Durand, 1993 for a possible exception). Intervention often takes place on multiple aspects of the problem simultaneously. Therefore, a clinician must be familiar with the range of approaches used to intervene specifically on sleep problems as well as on the associated issues that surround the sleep problems (e.g., unrealistic expectations by parents, cultural differences in sleeping arrangements, anxiety-related concerns). Because of the range of approaches available, we are unable to fully explore all of the possible intervention approaches. For a more complete description of these interventions, readers are referred to a number of other, more comprehensive sources (e.g., Durand, 1997; Ferber, 1985). Table 1 provides an overview of some of these efforts, and a brief description how and when to use them.

The table illustrates the importance of matching the function of the sleep problem with the specific intervention plan. For example, if assessment suggests that anxiety over daily concerns such as schoolwork or family difficulties is contributing to problems in falling asleep at night, then an intervention such as *progressive relaxation* or *cognitive relaxation* may be warranted. One additional factor must be considered when choosing an intervention; namely, the developmental level of the child. Certain interventions such as cognitive relaxation may not be appropriate for younger children. Understanding and following through on instructions may be difficult for these children, and therefore the intervention strategy should be tailored not only to the nature of their sleep problem but also to their ability to assist in treatment.

Bad "sleep habits" often contribute to sleep problems, and several of the interventions are de-

TABLE 1. Selected Interventions for Sleep Disorders

Sleep treatment	Description
Bedtime fading	For bedtime disturbances or sleep–wake schedule difficulties, using this intervention the parent establishes a time in which the child consistently falls asleep with little difficulty (e.g., 11:30 P.M.), then systematically makes bedtime 15 minutes earlier until child is falling asleep at the desired time.
Cognitive	This approach focuses on changing the sleeper's unrealistic expectations and beliefs about sleep ("I must have 8 hours of sleep each night," "If I get less than 8 hours of sleep it will make me ill"). Therapist attempts to alter beliefs and attitudes about sleeping by providing information on topics such as normal amounts of sleep and a person's ability to compensate for lost sleep. *More appropriate for older children or adolescents.*
Cognitive relaxation	Because some people become anxious when they have difficulty sleeping, this approach uses meditation or imagery to help with relaxation at bedtime or after a night waking. *More appropriate for older children or adolescents.*
Establishing bedtime routines	Creating a consistent and unchanging routine lasting about 30 minutes just prior to bedtime, including soothing activities (e.g., bath, reading a story), that always leads to bed. *Can be useful for difficulties initiating sleep for children of all ages.*
Graduated extinction	Used for children who have tantrums at bedtime or wake up crying at night, this treatment instructs the parent to check on the child after progressively longer periods of time, until the child falls asleep on his or her own.
Paradoxical intention	This technique involves instructing individuals in the opposite behavior from the desired outcome. Telling poor sleepers to lie in bed and try to stay awake as long as they can is used to try to relieve the performance anxiety surrounding efforts to fall asleep.
Progressive relaxation	This technique involves relaxing the muscles of the body in an effort to introduce drowsiness.
Scheduled awakening	Used for children who wake frequently during the night, this treatment involves waking the child approximately 60 minutes before he or she usually awakens at night. This helps teach children to fall back to sleep on their own while they are aroused from a deeper stage of sleep.
Sleep hygiene	Some people's daily habits can interfere with their nighttime sleeping. This approach involves instructing the sleeper about the negative effects of caffeine, nicotine, alcohol, exercise too close to bedtime, certain foods, and medications, on their sleep.
Sleep restriction	This consists of limiting a person's time in bed to the actual amount slept. This is done to help the sleeper associate time in bed only with sleeping, and not with tossing and turning, trying to fall asleep.
Stimulus control	This approach includes instructions to go to bed only when sleepy, use the bedroom only for sleep (not for reading, TV watching, or eating), get out of bed when unable to fall asleep, get out of bed in the morning at the same time each day regardless of the amount of time you slept.

signed to improve a child's involvement in his or her own sleep problems. *Sleep hygiene,* for example, involves assessing how a person's daily habits such as eating, drinking, or physical activity interfere with sleep. Caffeine in soft drinks can remain in our systems for up to eight hours. It is not uncommon for children to consume these drinks at dinnertime or shortly before bedtime; this can obviously cause difficulties falling asleep. *Stimulus control* is useful when the bed has become associated with activities incompatible with sleep, as in the case of children who do homework or play video games in bed. Using the bed only for sleep can help reduce the anxieties and tensions associated with other activities. A thorough assessment is needed to identify the factors influencing sleep problems for each child, and to design a treatment strategy that matches the child's sleep needs.

Treatment Research

An increasing number of both biological and behavioral strategies are used to intervene with children's sleep problems. We next briefly review the research on some of the more widely used of these interventions, and their effects on a variety of sleep problems experienced by children.

Pharmacological Interventions

The most widely used treatment strategy for sleep problems is medical. For example, Ounsted and Hendrick (1977) report that by 18 months, 25% of firstborn children have been prescribed sedatives. An extensive literature exists concerning the pharmacological treatment of sleep disorders in adults, yet few studies have involved treating children with drugs affecting sleep. Many sources (e.g., American Academy of Child and Adolescent Psychiatry, 1991; Kales, Soldatos, & Kales, 1987; McDaniel, 1986) recommend drug therapy as an adjunct to behavioral treatments only when sleep problems are extreme and chronic.

The sedating effect of the antihistamine diphenhydramine has been used to reduce sleep onset latency. In a sample of 50, 2- to 12-year-old children, Russo, Gururaj, and Allen (1976) found that diphenhydramine reduced sleep latency significantly more than placebo and was associated with (minimal) side effects in only 4% of the sample. In addition, treatment with diphenhydramine was associated with a significant reduction in the number of night wakings in children with this sleep difficulty (Russo et al., 1976). Diphenhydramine has also been suggested for treating nightmares and night terrors in children (Herskowitz & Rosman, 1982). However, evidence exists that it does not significantly reduce the frequency of these disturbances when compared to placebo (Russo et al., 1976). Hollister (1978) cautions that, although diphenhydramine may be an effective hypnotic, it is associated with some unpleasant anticholinergic side effects and is difficult to manage in the event of an overdose. In many cases, benzodiazepines may be more appropriate.

The primary use of benzodiazepines with children has been in the treatment of night terrors. These drugs tend to suppress stage 4 non-REM sleep, the stage when night terrors most often occur (Herskowitz and Rosman, 1982). In a placebo-controlled study of 15 hospitalized 6- to 15-year-olds, Popoviciu and Corfariu (1983) suppressed night terrors in all but one of their subjects using midazolam. The authors also noted an overall decrease in

the frequency of nocturnal arousals and no reported side effects. Unfortunately, follow-up data were not available. Effective reduction of night terrors has also been observed with alprazolam (Cameron & Thyer, 1985) and diazepam (Fisher, Kahn, Edwards, & Davis, 1973; Glick, Schulman, & Turecki, 1971). Noting relatively few side effects, McDaniel (1986) considers diazepam to be "the drug of first choice" (p. 71) in the pharmacological treatment of night terrors.

Unfortunately, the use of benzodiazepines has several drawbacks. Discontinuation of drug treatment is often associated with a recurrence of sleep disturbances (American Academy of Child and Adolescent Psychiatry, 1991; Fisher et al., 1973; Glick et al., 1971; Kales, Bixler, Tan, Scharf, & Kales, 1974). Adverse side effects including daytime sedation, cognitive and performance deficits, abuse, or dependence, may occur in children treated with benzodiazepines (Coffey, 1993). Among adults, rebound effects, the exacerbation of sleep disturbance above baseline levels, have been reported following drug discontinuation (Kales, Scharf, Kales, & Soldatos, 1979). Suppression of REM sleep increases with intermediate and long-term use of benzodiazepines, although the REM duration eventually returns to baseline levels after discontinuation (Kales et al., 1974). In light of the generally short duration of therapeutic effects and the potential side effects, the efficacy of benzodiazepine treatment remains controversial.

Imipramine (a tricyclic antidepressant) has been associated with a temporary reduction of sleep terrors in children (Pesikoff & Davis, 1971). Reduction of sleep terrors is also reported using a combined treatment with imipramine, relaxation, and self-hypnosis (Kohen, Mahowald, & Rosen, 1992). However, the authors noted similar success when imipramine was excluded from the treatment protocol. Pesikoff and Davis (1971) warned that the risk of overdose with imipramine is considerable and must be assessed carefully before prescribing the drug.

The hypnotic trimeprazine tartrate has been used as a treatment for sleep disturbances in children. France, Blampied, and Wilkinson (1991) reported an abrupt decrease in sleep disturbances for children receiving a combination of drug treatment and behavioral extinction. Children receiving extinction with placebo or extinction alone did not respond as quickly but reached the same low frequency of nightly disturbance as the drug group. Trimeprazine tartrate alone was shown to be superior to placebo in reducing the frequency of night wakings in a sample of one- to three-year-old children (Simonoff & Stores, 1987). In a double-blind study of children treated with this drug, Richman (1985) reported a significant but "not clinically striking" (p. 596) decrease in the number of night wakings in 66% of her subjects. One-third showed no improvement and a six-month follow-up of all subjects revealed no significant decreases in night waking from baseline. Richman went on to suggest that hypnotic drugs are of limited usefulness and should be used only in short-term (two to three weeks), carefully monitored treatments.

A different class of pharmacological interventions has recently been explored as an alternative to the hypnotic drugs previously reviewed. Melatonin is a hormone produced in the pineal gland that appears to be involved in the regulation of our sleep–wake cycle (Illnerova, 1991). The production of melatonin is stimulated by the onset of darkness, and appears to be involved in bringing on sleep (Lewy, Ahmed, Jackson, & Sack, 1992). A number of recent studies with adults suggest that melatonin may be a more benign alternative to the hypnotic drugs for helping people with insomnia and circadian rhythm sleep disorders (Dahlitz et al., 1991) although the long-term effects of its use are not yet known.

Many other drugs have been suggested for the treatment of sleep disorders. Unfortunately, research regarding their efficacy with children is sparse. The studies reviewed above highlight the controversial nature of drug treatment in childhood sleep disorders. It is clear, however, that certain medications may provide short-duration symptom relief. In certain situations, a combination of medication and behavioral methods (to be reviewed next) may be the optimal solution for intractable sleep problems.

Behavioral Interventions

Extinction procedures (e.g., ignoring the cries of the child) are often recommended as a first effort at treating bedtime disturbances or disruptive night waking. In a classic extinction study (Williams, 1959), these procedures were used to effectively eliminate the bedtime disturbances of a four-year-old boy. The treatment involved the withdrawal of parental attention during nighttime tantrums. The tantrums were successfully eliminated until the boy's grandmother attended to his disruptive behavior. The tantrums were subsequently reduced after parental attention was again withdrawn. Unfortunately, an obstacle in the use of extinction is that caretakers frequently find it difficult to ignore the cries of children for an extended period of time (Milan, Mitchell, Berger, & Pierson, 1981; Rolider & Van Houten, 1984).

An alternative to extinction that is often recommended for bedtime disturbances is *graduated extinction* (Ferber, 1985). As with extinction, graduated extinction is appropriate when either the bedtime disturbance or night waking appears to be maintained by parental attention. In a study by Rolider and Van Houten (1984), parents were trained to use a graduated extinction procedure to decrease crying at bedtime. The procedure consisted of delaying parental attention when the child cried for a specified amount of time and then briefly attending to the child. The duration of time spent ignoring their child increased by five minutes in each subsequent interval, but the parents were allowed to attend to their child after waiting the specified amount of time. This graduated extinction procedure resulted in a decrease of the children's crying. In addition, it enabled the parents to attend to their children without reinforcing the crying. Similar graduated extinction procedures have also been used to effectively reduce night waking in children (Durand & Mindell, 1990; Mindell & Durand, 1993; Rolider & Van Houten, 1984).

Scheduled awakenings have also been used to successfully reduce night wakings in children (Johnson, Bradley-Johnson, & Stack, 1981; Johnson & Lerner, 1985; Rickert & Johnson, 1988). Scheduled awakenings entail having the parents wake the child 15 to 60 minutes before a spontaneous awakening and doing what they normally do when the child wakes them (e.g., give backrubs, hugs, bottles). As the frequency of spontaneous wakings decrease, the scheduled wakings are eliminated. This intervention for night waking is sometimes recommended over procedures such as graduated extinction when parents are unwilling to ignore the cries of their child for even a brief period of time. When this intervention is successful, night waking is essentially prevented from occurring and the intervention can be faded to avoid the unpleasant nighttime events.

Other behavioral interventions that have been used to treat sleep disorders include time-out and social reinforcement (Ronen, 1991), the establishment of stable bedtime and wake-up routines (Weissbluth, 1982), relaxation training (Anderson, 1979), and shaping of an earlier bedtime (Piazza & Fisher, 1991). Adams and Rickert (1989) found that graduated extinction and positive bedtime routines (initiating a relatively invariant sequence of activities such as a bath, dressing, and reading a book that always leads to bedtime) were equally effective in reducing bedtime disturbances in a group of 36 young children.

Treatment of multiple sleep disorders frequently combines many of the previously mentioned interventions. Ronen (1991) treated a four-year-old girl with bedtime disturbances and night wakings using extinction, time-out, social reinforcement, and immediate rewards. Durand and Mindell (1990) used graduated extinction to successfully treat both night wakings and bedtime disturbances in a 14-month-old girl. Richman and colleagues (1985) used graduated extinction, positive reinforcement, shaping (making a gradually earlier bedtime), and establishing a stable bedtime routine to successfully treat night wakings and bedtime disturbances.

The treatment literature has usually focused on one disorder at a time (Durand & Mindell, 1990; Ronen, 1991). However, in one recent exception, we have found that intervention designed to help one problem may effectively resolve other sleep problems. We examined the multiple sleep problems displayed by six young children whose average age at intervention was approximately three years (Mindell & Durand, 1993). Each of these children exhibited bedtime disturbances characterized by tantrums and other efforts to resist going to sleep. The children also displayed frequent instances of night waking, averaging 1.5 per night. A combination of interventions was used to improve the bedtime problems, including establishing bedtime routines and using graduated extinction (gradually fading attention to tantrums). This package of treatments was successful in reducing the bedtime disturbances of all of the children, and importantly, also resulted in a near elimination of night waking for five of the six children. Although night waking was not specifically targeted, the improvement of

bedtime disturbances appeared to lead to improvements in this second sleep disturbance.

Several explanations may account for the success of this intervention for multiple sleep disturbances. It is possible, for example, that the establishment of bedtime routines and the reduction of behavior problems helped "normalize" sleep patterns in the children. At the same time, although parents reported no change in their handling the children during night waking, the training given to them surrounding bedtime problems may have influenced how they reacted to the children waking at night. It should be noted that it may be premature to speculate too much on the mechanisms involved in this finding. Future treatment research should address how interventions affect sleep-related behavior across a spectrum of problem areas.

Treatment Integrity

Treatment for sleep problems is, by its very nature, a relatively inaccessible activity. The problems themselves occur at times that are difficult for most clinicians to observe. Bedtime disturbances obviously occur in the early to late evening, and most other sleep problems manifest themselves in the middle of the night. Treatment is therefore carried out by parents or other caregivers outside the view of behavior therapists. Clearly, assessing treatment integrity can be a daunting task. In our work we have videotaped bedtime routines to assess any difficulties that arise but that go unreported by parents. For example, watching the videotape of bedtime for one young girl pointed out to us that her bedroom was adjacent to the family room, and that the television could be clearly heard in her room—a potentially important factor in her sleep difficulty that was not mentioned by her parents in our interviews. These videotapes are also used to assess how well parents carry out the agreed-upon intervention plan, and can be used for feedback sessions.

We also use the sleep diaries to assess treatment integrity for nighttime problems. In a recent study, for example, we had the mother of a young girl who engaged in frequent night waking indicate when and whether she followed through on the intervention each night (Durand, Gernert-Dott, & Mapstone, 1996). We observed a negative correlation between treatment compliance and night wakings such that on the weeks the mother followed the plan, there were fewer nights with wakings. This helped us determine that the intervention itself was successful, but that an additional goal was to assist the mother in her efforts to carry out the plan. Although it is difficult to assess the reliability of such measures (especially with the self-report data such as with the sleep diaries), they are useful in many situations.

Planning for Generalization

Because intervention is typically carried out by the parents (or by the child in partnership with the parents), efforts at generalization begin immediately. Parents are instructed in the proper intervention techniques over several sessions. Highlighted in these sessions are potential obstacles to implementing the plan. One important consideration that was mentioned previously is the level of emotionality experienced by the parent during difficult sleep interactions (e.g., bedtime tantrums, screaming during night waking). We assess these emotional reactions to try to determine whether the parent will be capable of fully carrying out the intervention. For example, one mother we worked with made it clear that she would not be able to tolerate any of her child's cries, and that she would have to comfort her daughter immediately. In fact, this had resulted in having her daughter sleep in her bed so that the mother could instantly respond when the daughter awoke during the night. We began by asking the mother to delay responding by seconds instead of minutes. This was followed by instructing the mother to systematically move her daughter out of her bed by placing a mattress next to her own, then moving it farther away, then down the hall into her daughter's room over several weeks. Such modifications are essential if parents are to be able to carry out our plans and thus generalize the intervention to the home.

Plan Evaluation

Data from the sleep diaries form the basis for our evaluation of the effectiveness of most sleep interventions. We request that parents complete a minimum of two weeks of diaries so that we can determine any pattern of sleep difficulties. The sleep diaries are structured so that we can assess the frequency of any sleeping difficulties (e.g., number of night wakings per evening) as well as more subtle measures such as the delay in falling asleep or the duration of nighttime disturbances. These latter measures take on importance especially in the initial stages of the intervention. Often, for example, the frequency of night waking may not decrease, but the time spent crying can be drastically reduced. One little girl who screamed when she awoke during the middle of the night kept her family awake for hours each evening. After two weeks of an intervention, she continued to wake up each evening, but her mother only needed to say, "Go back to sleep," and the daughter stopped making noises and went back to bed. Although it required several months of intervention to significantly reduce the number of night wakings, the family was delighted about the early changes in her sleep patterns.

This example illustrates the need to assess the social validity of the intervention itself along with the effects of the intervention. Pediatricians often recommend ignoring (extinction) for the sleep difficulties of young children. Although this can be an effective intervention for many families, we pointed out previously that many others have a great deal of difficulty listening to the plaintive cries of their children. We typically describe in detail the intervention for the parents and identify any potential difficulties in implementation. Fortunately, as we have seen, these plans can often be modified in ways that can accommodate the needs of the parents as well as the child.

Assessing the social validity of the results of the intervention is also essential. Sometimes the intervention may be "successful" such that the number of problem episodes has been reduced, but the child continues to experience daytime difficulties or the parents are still disturbed by the child's behavior. This issue is of particular importance for sleep difficulties. In fact, part of the criteria for determining if sleep is disturbed is an estimation of its effect on the person experiencing the difficulty (APA, 1994). For example, if someone sleeps only six hours per night, but this results in no negative effects and the person is not bothered by this amount of sleep, then it is not considered a sleep disorder. However, if a second person sleeps only six hours per night but is disturbed by this pattern, then it may be considered a sleep difficulty. The definition of a sleep disorder includes the subjective experience of the person affected.

The combination of the objective data from the sleep diaries and the family's subjective impressions of the course of the intervention is used to assess the progress of the plan. Oftentimes, it is the subjective impression of change that is more instrumental in determining the success of the intervention. For example, we had one family whose daughter had no consistent bedtime and who sometimes stayed awake until the early morning. We had the parents implement a graduated extinction procedure to reduce the daughter's resistance at bedtime and were hoping for a relatively early bedtime. It soon became apparent, however, that the parents were pleased at the daughter's improved compliance, and didn't really care what time she went to bed. Thus, although her bedtime remained erratic and averaged about the same time as it had prior to intervention, her parents didn't care to continue intervention in an effort to make further changes, because they were happy that she stopped arguing at bedtime.

Follow-up for sleep problems is essential. We typically try to gather data for a year or more following our intervention. This lengthy follow-up is necessary because sleep difficulties are prone to resurface from time to time. This makes sense when one considers that individuals have different biological predispositions to sleep problems, and that, despite our success in using behavioral interventions for certain problems, we are probably not successful in completely "normalizing" sleep for all children. We often observe relapse in sleep difficulties for children after some change in their routine, such as a vacation or other changes at home or school (e.g., a new sibling, marital difficulties). We attempt a form of *relapse prevention* by alerting parents to the likelihood of these relapses, and by encouraging them to reintroduce the previously successful intervention should this problem arise again. This serves to reassure parents that any regression is normal and is not a sign that the problem is intractable.

Conclusions

Significant advances have been made in our understanding and treatment of children's sleep disturbances. What is unfolding from this improved knowledge of sleep problems is an appreciation of the dynamic nature of the interplay between biology and the environment in these disorders. Only if we address all aspects of these problems will we be able to design appropriate and successful treatments for these children. The integrative-multidimensional view of sleep disturbances presented in this chapter provides a guideline for identifying the varied influences contributing to sleep disturbances among children. Especially when multiple sleep problems are present, it is important to assess and intervene on a number of different aspects of the child's and family's life.

Future research efforts in this area will need to firmly establish the prescriptive approach outlined. In other words, we need more specific guidelines for clinicians as to which factors identified during our assessments lead to which interventions. Because of the tremendous variability in biological, psychological, and social factors that differentiate each child, we do not anticipate the development of a "cookbook" approach to intervention. However, more research is needed to assist us in linking assessment and treatment for sleep disorders. We stress the integration of both biological and psychological intervention efforts to fully address the multifaceted problems surrounding sleep disturbances. Clearly, more work is needed to develop this view and its implications for treatment. However, we anticipate that, through this work, improved care for children with sleep problems will be forthcoming.

References

Adams, L.A., & Rickert, V.I. (1989). Reducing bedtime tantrums: Comparison between positive routines and graduated extinction. *Pediatrics, 84,* 756–761.

American Academy of Child and Adolescent Psychiatry. (1991). *Textbook of child and adolescent psychiatry.* (J.M. Wiener, Editor). Washington, DC: American Psychiatric Press, Inc.

American Psychiatric Association (APA). (1994). *Diagnostic and statistical manual of mental disorders* (4th ed.). Washington, DC: Author.

American Sleep Disorders Association. (1990). *The International classification of sleep disorders: Diagnostic and coding manual.* Rochester, MN: Author.

Anch, A.M., Browman, C.P., Mitler, M.M., & Walsh, J.K. (1988). *Sleep: A scientific perspective.* Englewood Cliffs, NJ: Prentice Hall.

Anderson, D. (1979). Treatment of insomnia in a 13-year-old boy by relaxation training and reduction of parental attention. *Journal of Behavior Therapy and Experimental Psychiatry, 10,* 263–265.

Bartlett, L.B., Rooney, V., & Spedding, S. (1985). Nocturnal difficulties in a population of mentally handicapped children, *British Journal of Mental Subnormality, 31,* 54–59.

Bernal, F. (1973). Night waking in infants during the first 14 months. *Developmental Medicine and Child Neurology, 15,* 760–769.

Bixler, E.O., Kales, J.D., Scharf, M.B., Kales, A., & Leo, L.A. (1976). Incidence of sleep disorders in medical practice: A physician survey. *Sleep Research, 5,* 62.

Blakeslee, S. (1993, August 3). Mystery of sleep yields as studies reveal immune tie. *New York Times,* p. C1.

Cameron, O.G., & Thyer, B.A. (1985). Treatment of pavor nocturnus with alprazolam. *Journal of Clinical Psychiatry, 46,* 504.

Carskadon, M.A., & Dement, W.C. (1989). Normal human sleep: An overview. In M.H. Kryer, T. Roth, & W.C. Dement (Eds.), *Principles and practice of sleep medicine* (pp. 3–13). Philadelphia: Saunders.

Clements, J., Wing, L., & Dunn, G. (1986). Sleep problems in handicapped children: A preliminary study. *Journal of Child Psychology and Psychiatry, 27,* 399–407.

Coffey, B.J. (1993). Review and update: Benzodiazepines in childhood and adolescence. *Psychiatric Annals, 23,* 332–339.

Dahlitz, M., Alvarez, B., Vignau, J., English, J., Arendt, J., & Parkes, J.D. (1991). Delayed sleep phase syndrome response to melatonin. *Lancet, 337,* 1121–1124.

Dement, W. (1960). The effect of dream deprivation. *Science, 131,* 1705–1707.

DeMyer, M. (1979). *Parents and children: Autism.* New York: Wiley.

Durand, V.M. (1997). *Sleep better!: A guide to improving sleep for children with special needs.* Baltimore: Paul Brookes.

Durand, V.M., & Mindell, J.A. (1990). Behavioral treatment of multiple childhood sleep disorders. *Behavior Modification, 14,* 37–49.

Durand, V.M., Mindell, J.A., Mapstone, E., & Gernert-Dott, P. (1995). Treatment of multiple sleep disorders in children. In C.E. Schaefer (Ed.), *Clinical handbook of sleep disorders in children* (pp. 311–333). Northvale, NJ: Jason Aronson.

Durand, V.M., Gernert-Dott, P., & Mapstone, E. (1996). Treatment of sleep disorders in children with developmental disabilities. *Journal of the Association for Persons with Severe Handicaps, 21,* 114–122.

Ferber, R. (1985). *Solve your child's sleep problems.* New York: Simon and Schuster.

Fisher, C., Kahn, E., Edwards, A., & Davis, D.M. (1973). A psychophysiological study of nightmares and night terrors: The suppression of Stage 4 night terrors with diazepam. *Archives of General Psychiatry, 28,* 252–259.

France, K.G., Blampied, N.M., & Wilkinson, P. (1991). Treatment of infant sleep disturbance by trimeprazine in combination with extinction. *Journal of Developmental and Behavioral Pediatrics, 12,* 308–314.

Giles, D.E., & Buysse, D.J. (1993). Parasomnias. In D.L. Dunner (Ed.), *Current psychiatric therapy* (pp. 361–372). Philadelphia: Saunders.

Glick, B.S., Schulman, D., & Turecki, S. (1971). Diazepam (Valium) treatment in childhood sleep disorders: A preliminary investigation. *Diseases of the Nervous System, 32,* 565–566.

Hauri, P. (1982). *The sleep disorders* (2nd ed.). Kalamazoo, MI: Upjohn.

Herskowitz, J., & Rosman, N.P. (1982). *Pediatrics, neurology, and psychiatry: Common ground.* New York: Macmillan.

Hollister, L.E. (1978). *Clinical pharmacology of psychotherapeutic drugs.* New York: Churchill Livingstone.

Illnerova, H. (1991). The suprachiasmatic nucleus and rhythmic pineal melatonin production. In D.C. Klein, R.Y. Moore, & S.M. Reppert (Eds.), *Suprachiasmatic nucleus: The mind's clock.* New York: Oxford University Press.

Jenkins, S., Bax, M., & Hart, H. (1980). Behavior problems in preschool children. *Journal of Child Psychology and Psychiatry, 21,* 5–17.

Johnson, C.M., & Lerner, M. (1985). Amelioration of infant's sleep disturbances: II. Effects of scheduled awakenings by compliant parents. *Infant Mental Health Journal, 6,* 21–30.

Johnson, C.M., Bradley-Johnson, S., & Stack, J.M. (1981). Decreasing the frequency of infant's nocturnal crying with the use of scheduled awakenings. *Family Practice Research Journal, 1,* 98–104.

Kales, A., Bixler, E.O., Tan, T.L., Scharf, M.B., & Kales, J.D. (1974). Chronic hypnotic drug use: Ineffectiveness, drug withdrawal insomnia, and dependence. *Journal of the American Medical Association, 5,* 573–577.

Kales, A., Scharf, M.B., Kales, J.D., & Soldatos, C.R. (1979). Rebound insomnia: A potential hazard following withdrawal of certain benzodiazepines. *Journal of the American Medical Association, 241,* 1691–1695.

Kales, A., Soldatos, C.R., & Kales, J.D. (1987). Sleep disorders: Insomnia, sleepwalking, night terrors, nightmares, and enuresis. *Annals of Internal Medicine, 106,* 582–592.

Kohen, D.P., Mahowald, M.W., & Rosen, G.M. (1992). Sleep-terror disorder in children: The role of self-hypnosis in management. *American Journal of Clinical Hypnosis, 34,* 233–244.

Lewy, A.J., Ahmed, S., Jackson, J.M.L., & Sack, R.L. (1992). Melatonin shifts human circadian rhythms according to a phase-response curve. *Chronobiology International, 9,* 380–392.

McDaniel, K.D. (1986). Pharmacologic treatment of psychiatric and neurodevelopmental disorders in children and adolescents (Part 1). *Clinical Pediatrics, 25,* 65–71.

Milan, M.A., Mitchell, Z.P., Berger, M.I., & Pierson, D.F. (1981). Positive routines: A rapid alternative to extinction for elimination of bedtime tantrum behavior. *Child Behavior Therapy, 3,* 13–25.

Mindell, J.A. (1993). Sleep disorders in children. *Health Psychology, 12,* 151–162.

Mindell, J.A., & Durand, V.M. (1993). Treatment of childhood sleep disorders: Generalization across disorders and effects on family members. *Journal of Pediatric Psychology, 18,* 731–750.

Ounstead, M.K., & Hendrick, A.M. (1977). The first-born child: Patterns of development. *Developmental Medicine and Child Neurology, 19,* 446–453.

Palmblad, J., Petrini, B., Wasserman, J., & Akerstedt, T. (1979). Lymphocyte and granulocyte reactions during sleep deprivation. *Psychosomatic Medicine, 41,* 273–278.

Pesikoff, R.B., & Davis, P.C. (1971). Treatment of pavor nocturnus and somnambulism in children. *American Journal of Psychiatry, 129,* 134–137.

Piazza, C.C., & Fisher, W.W. (1991). A faded bedtime with response cost protocol for treatment of multiple sleep problems in children. *Journal of Applied Behavior Analysis, 24,* 129–140.

Popoviciu, L., & Corfariu, O. (1983). Efficacy and safety of midazolam in the treatment of night terrors in children. *British Journal of Clinical Pharmacology, 16,* 97S–102S.

Rechtschaffen, A., & Foulkes, D. (1965). Effect of visual stimuli on dream content. *Perceptual and Motor Skills, 20,* 1149–1160.

Richman, N. (1981). A community survey of characteristics of one- to-two-year-olds with sleep disruptions. *Journal of the American Academy of Child Psychiatry, 30,* 281–291.

Richman, N. (1985). A double-blind drug trial of treatment in young children with waking problems. *Journal of Child Psychology and Psychiatry, 26,* 591–598.

Richman, N., Stevenson, J.E., & Graham, P.J. (1975). Prevalence of behaviour problems in three-year-old children: An epidemiological study in a London borough. *Journal of Child Psychology and Psychiatry, 16,* 277–287.

Richman, N., Douglas, J., Hunt, H., Lansdown, R., & Levere, R. (1985). Behavioural methods in the treatment of sleep disorders: A pilot study. *Journal of Child Psychology and Psychiatry, 26,* 581–590.

Rickert, V.I., & Johnson, C.M. (1988). Reducing nocturnal awakening and crying episodes in infants and young children: A comparison between scheduled awakenings and systematic ignoring. *Pediatrics, 81,* 203–212.

Rolider, A., & Van Houten, R. (1984). Training parents to use extinction to eliminate nightime crying by gradually increasing the criteria for ignoring crying. *Education and Treatment of Children, 7,* 119–124.

Ronen, T. (1991). Intervention package for treating sleep disorders in a four-year-old girl. *Journal of Behavior Therapy and Experimental Psychiatry, 22,* 141–148.

Russo, R., Gururaj, V., & Allen, J. (1976). The effectiveness of diphenhydramine HCl in paediatric sleep disorders. *Journal of Clinical Pharmacology, 16,* 284–288.

Sadeh, A. (1994). Assessment of intervention for infant night waking: Parental reports and activity-based home monitoring. *Journal of Consulting and Clinical Psychology, 62,* 63–68.

Salzarulo, P., & Chevalier, A. (1983). Sleep problems in children and their relationship with early disturbances of the waking–sleeping rhythms. *Sleep, 6,* 47–51.

Simonoff, E.A., & Stores, G. (1987). Controlled trial of trimeprazine tartrate for night waking. *Archives of Disease in Childhood, 62,* 253–257.

Smith, C., & Lapp, L. (1991). Increases in number of REMS and REM density in humans following an intensive learning period. *Sleep, 14,* 325–330.

Snyder, F. (1971). Psychophysiology of human sleep. *Clinical Neurosurgery, 18,* 503–536.

Weissbluth, M. (1982). Modification of sleep schedule with reduction of night waking: A case report. *Sleep, 5,* 262–266.

Williams, C.D. (1959). The elimination of tantrum behavior by extinction procedures. *Journal of Abnormal Social Psychology, 59,* 269–273.

Bibliography

Bootzin, R.R., Epstein, D., & Wood, J.M. (1991). Stimulus control instructions. In P.J. Hauri (Ed.), *Case studies in insomnia* (pp. 19–28). New York: Plenum.

Coates, T.J., & Thoresen, C.E. (1977). *How to sleep better: A drug-free program for overcoming insomnia.* Englewood Cliffs, NJ: Prentice-Hall.

Czeisler, C.A., Richardson, G.S., Coleman, R.M., Zimmerman, J.C., Moore-Ede, M.C., Dement, W.C., & Weitzman, E.D. (1981). Chronotherapy: Resetting the circadian clocks of patients with delayed sleep phase insomnia. *Sleep, 4,* 1–21.

Durand, V.M. (1997). *Sleep better!: A guide to improving sleep for children with special needs.* Baltimore: Paul Brookes.

Ferber, R. (1985). *Solve your child's sleep problems.* New York: Simon and Schuster.

Hauri, P., & Linde, S. (1990). *No more sleepless nights.* New York: Wiley.

Hauri, P.J. (1991). Sleep hygiene, relaxation therapy, and cognitive interventions. In P.J. Hauri (Ed.), *Case studies in insomnia* (pp. 65–84). New York: Plenum.

Lacks, P. (1987). *Behavioral treatment for persistent insomnia.* New York: Pergamon.

12

Preventing Injury in Children

The Need for Parental Involvement

LISA SALDANA and LIZETTE PETERSON

Introduction

What was once called an "accident" is now labeled by researchers as an "unintentional injury" (Robertson, 1983). What was once thought of as a simple twist of fate is now acknowledged as the leading cause of preventable death in children in industrialized nations (Division of Injury Control, 1990). Even further, hundreds of nonfatal injuries occur each year that leave children disfigured, physically and mentally handicapped, emotionally disturbed, and permanently brain damaged (Roberts & Brooks, 1987). Given the serious threat of unintentional injuries to every child in our country, prevention of childhood injuries is a topic of paramount importance for the child behavior therapist.

Childhood Injury

Defining the Problem

Perhaps the biggest misnomer in the study of childhood injuries has been the labeling of injury as an accident. As defined by Webster's dictionary (Patterson, 1989), the term accident implies "an unfortunate event occurring casually [or] happening by chance." Such an implication leads to the belief that injuries are not caused by avoidable environ-

mental hazards and behaviors and that they cannot be prevented. As this chapter will outline, with as many as 23,000 children suffering fatal injuries, 30,000 children suffering permanent disability, and 16 million children requiring emergency medical care each year due to injury (Division of Injury Control, 1990; Guyer & Ellers, 1990; Rodriguez, 1990), it is time for the lay public, child specialists, and researchers to recognize childhood injuries as preventable and to give up the notion of "accidental" injury.

For the remainder of this chapter, we will label our topic *unintentional injuries*. We need to note here, however, that we believe the intentional/unintentional dichotomy is a false one for conceptualizing injury (Peterson & Brown, 1994), but given the previous chapter in this book on child abuse, we will confine our focus to the area of research typically labeled unintentional injury. The term *injury* simply describes tissue damage which occurs as a result of extreme exposure to chemical or physical elements (Haddon & Baker, 1981), and does not presuppose its causes.

In addition, it is important to realize that injuries occur in varying degrees of severity. For example, skinned knees or burned fingers involve tissue damage and may limit a child's running and playing or use of fingers for a period of time. The extent to which the etiology of minor injuries resembles that of more severe injuries is unclear, as is the question of how risky behaviors that result in no injury or minor injury are maintained. Such minor injuries are not reported to medical

LISA SALDANA and LIZETTE PETERSON • Department of Psychology, University of Missouri–Columbia, Columbia, Missouri 65211.

Handbook of Child Behavior Therapy, edited by Watson and Gresham. Plenum Press, New York, 1998.

personnel and their prevalence is unknown at present. The majority of databases available for research involve only injuries that are severe enough to cause the parent or child to seek medical attention. Therefore, the epidemiological data presented in this chapter typically refer only to severe injuries.

Children at the Greatest Risk

All children are at risk for injury. There are, however, characteristics of children and particular activities that increase the chance for unintentional injury. Age is perhaps the most influential variable, as children under the age of four are at greatest risk for fatal injury (Baker, O'Neill, & Ginsburg, 1992). Boys are at greater risk than girls for almost all kinds of injuries (Rivara, Bergman, LoGerfo, & Weiss, 1982). Boys who are involved in sports, ride bicycles, use playground equipment, and use motorized vehicles are at greatest risk (Rivara & Mueller, 1987). The ratio between male and female injuries increases with age for children of both White and non-White populations (Irwin, Cataldo, Matheny, & Peterson, 1992). Furthermore, children from low-income and single-parent households have an increased chance for injury (Durkin, Davidson, Kuhn, O'Connor, & Barlow, 1994). Children who engage in antisocial behaviors, including aggressiveness and behavioral management difficulties, are at even greater risk (Davidson, 1987). And not surprisingly, children who have parents who engage in high-risk taking behaviors are more likely than other children to perform activities that increase their chance for injury (Williams, 1976).

Incidence/Prevalence

The prevalence of unintentional injury differs by the level of severity of the injury, the age and sex of the child, the geographical area and the season of the year. The number of occurring injuries, then, differs for different types of injuries. The following sections will discuss the six most frequently occurring injuries in descending order (Baker et al., 1992). In addition, we consider two injury categories because of their increasing prevalence: bicycle injuries and injuries due to firearms.

Motor Vehicle Injuries

Injuries involving motor vehicles are the number one killer of children, with a reported 2,331 children under the age of 13, and 6,354 children between the ages of 13 and 19 dying in 1990 (Insurance Institute for Highway Safety, 1991). The youngest children were at the greatest risk; 634 children were reported to be under the age of 5, 70% of whom were unrestrained in the car (Centers for Disease Control and Prevention, 1991). Of adolescents above the age of 13, males have twice as many fatalities as females, and nearly half of those fatalities involve alcohol (Rosenberg, Rodriguez, & Chorba, 1990). Furthermore, adolescents between the ages of 13 and 19 have been reported to be the least likely individuals to use seat belts, and only 25.1% observed seat-belt use in 1987 (Agran, Castillo, & Winn, 1990).

Other motorized vehicles account for an additional portion of childhood injuries. In 1985, there were 240 individuals who received fatal injuries due to all-terrain vehicles (ATVs) and an additional 85,900 individuals who received treatment in emergency rooms due to ATVs (National Committee for Injury Prevention and Control, 1989). More than half of these ATV injuries were in male children under the age of 16 (Jones, 1992).

Drownings

Death due to drowning is a leading cause of injury fatality for children birth to 5. Children under the age of 5 and adolescent boys are at highest risk for drowning fatalities (Wintemute, 1990). Large buckets filled with water, and bathtubs, pose a particular risk of drowning for infants (Consumer Product Safety Commission, 1989). Swimming pool drownings are responsible for a majority of fatal drownings for children under the age of 14, with additional incidents occurring in rivers and reservoirs (Rivara, 1985). Drowning rates are highest among Black males (Rosenberg et al., 1990) and White children aged 1 to 3 years (Zins, Garcia, Tuchfarber, Clark, & Laurence, 1994). In addition, the incidence of drownings is influenced by geographic location, with the highest number occurring in California, Arizona, and Florida (Hazinkinski, Francescutti, Lapidus, Micik, & Rivara, 1993). Overall, drownings account for 9.2% of childhood fatalities (Division of Injury Control, 1990).

Burns

In 1986, there were 1,619 childhood deaths as a result of fires or burns. The majority of these injuries resulted from house fires (80%; Division of Injury Control, 1990). In 1985, there were 23,638 children hospitalized for burn-related injuries (McLoughlin & McGuire, 1990). Seventy-five percent of all burn injuries occur to children under the age of 10 years, with children under the age of 4 at greatest risk (Guyer & Ellers, 1990). As with most injuries, male children are at greater risk for burn injuries than female children. In addition, geographic location influences childhood risk for burn fatalities, with children who live in the South at greatest risk for suffering injuries from fires.

Falls

Among very young children, there are a large number of injuries resulting from falls (Guyer & Ellers, 1990). One example of a common nonfatal fall injury for children under the age of 2 is a fall from a bunk bed (Selbst, Baker, & Shames, 1990) or other elevated platform where the infant's ability to roll off is unexpected by the caregiver. One of the most common circumstances in which toddlers sustain fatal injuries from a fall is a fall from a window above the first floor of a housing complex (Rivara, 1985). Despite the frequent occurrence of falls among toddlers (Martin, Langley, & Coffman, 1995), the number of deaths resulting from falls actually increases with age, with adolescents between the ages of 15 and 19 showing the greatest number of deaths (Scheidt, 1988). This may be due in part to the type of falls that occur at varying ages, the increased use of alcohol in high-risk environments in adolescents, and the distance of the fall.

Suffocation

For children under the age of 5, suffocation is a major cause of death (Rivara, 1985). Suffocation due to the obstruction of the air pathway is second only to motor vehicle injuries in children under the age of one year and is the fourth leading cause of death in children aged one to four years (Scheidt, 1988). As children reach ages beyond the preschool years, they are less likely to put inappropriate objects in their mouths and are more likely to be able to swallow or cough up an obstruction. In addition, older children are not as likely to suffocate from an inability to roll over and breathe, as are infants. Therefore suffocation decreases in its incidence as children increase in age.

Poisoning

Although the incidence of childhood poisonings has decreased nearly 50% since the development of child-resistant containers (Walton, 1982), unintentional poisoning continues to be a preventable cause of death in children. In 1984, seventy-seven children aged 1 to 4 years, 56 children aged 5 to 14, and 184 adolescents aged 15 to 19 died from poisoning. The higher rate of poisonings in adolescents may be due to intentional chemical ingestions as in suicide, or from ingesting more of a chemical than intended, such as an "accidental" drug overdose. Although the fatality number is not as large as some of the previously mentioned injury categories, it is important to note that for each poisoning death that occurs in a child under the age of 6, there are 20,000 reports made to poison control centers (Losh, 1994).

Bicycle Injuries

Bicycle injuries are the most common forms of tissue damage seen in emergency rooms (Rivara, 1985), and are among the leading killers of children in the United States (Baker & Waller, 1989). Of individuals killed as a result of bicycle injuries during the years 1984 to 1988, 62% were due to head injury; males between the ages of 10 and 14 had the highest rate (Sacks, Holmgreen, Smith, & Sosin, 1991). Similarly, in 1991, there were an estimated 492,000 bicycle-related injuries seen in emergency rooms, 61,000 of which were due to head injuries (Losh, 1994). Furthermore, males sustain a higher number of nonfatal bicycle injuries than do females; again, with the highest rate occurring between the ages of 10 and 14 (Freide, Azzara, Gallagher, & Guyer, 1985; Thompson, Thompson, & Rivara, 1990; Zavoski, Lapidus, Lerer, & Banco, 1995). Unlike many forms of injury, bicycle injuries become more likely as children increase in age and gain competence (Peterson, Gillies, Cook, Schick, & Little, 1994) and thus, are able, allowed to, and inclined to engage in more risk-taking behaviors on bicycles.

Firearm-Related Injuries

Another leading cause of death in the United States is firearm-related injuries (Zins et al., 1994). Suicide rates have doubled over the past 30 years, mostly due to the increased availability of guns (Koop & Lundberg, 1992). Although one may argue that suicide is not an unintentional injury, the increase in self-inflicted fatalities in adolescence may in part be due to the use of firearms removing the possibility of using suicide as a "cry for help." For children ages 10 to 19, White male children are at greatest risk for successful suicide, and, as age increases, the chance of using firearms as the method for suicide increases (Rosenberg et al., 1990). In addition, firearms are responsible for the increased number of homicides involving children and the increased number of unintentional firearm fatalities (Rivara, 1985). Childhood homicides and unintentional firearm injuries are 5 times greater among Black children than among White children (Rosenberg et al., 1990).

Etiology of Childhood Injury

Garbarino (1988) described the possible origins of childhood injuries. He began by noting that unintentional injuries lie on a continuum from "random accidents" to "fully preventable" circumstances. Where injuries are viewed on this continuum is subject to change, and is dependent on how much society knows about preventing injury and what kind of community standards exist to urge implementation of prevention efforts.

A minority of injuries do not have a clear, preventable causal agent. Such injuries appear to occur by "fate" or by circumstances that are beyond the control of the individuals involved. For example, if a child was walking carefully on the sidewalk and then was hit by a car which swerved to avoid another child and moved up onto the sidewalk, this would be an incident near the "random accident" end of the continuum. The circumstances appear to be beyond the control of the child. Barriers known to prevent pedestrian injury, such as fences, pedestrian lanes, and other barriers, cannot be erected

wherever children go. Even close supervision may not always keep a child from darting into the street. Sometimes vectors come together in ways that are both dangerous and difficult to predict.

In contrast, most injuries on the continuum are viewed as somewhat preventable. Preventable injuries occur when there are indications from researchers or from the community that one behavior can be implemented or another behavior avoided in order to decrease the chance for injury. It is worth noting that in order for injuries to be prevented, a barrier must not only be obtained but must be in place, or the parents and their children must be able to distinguish safe situations from dangerous situations in which injury is a possibility. Individuals must then be able to extract from the situation safe, versus risky, behavior. Often this discrimination must be made in situations where the threat of injury is not always obvious or where injury is a low baserate, unexpected occurrence (Peterson & Schick, 1993). Here, prevention becomes an issue of both learning and motivation.

At the upper end of the preventable continuum of injury noted by Garbarino (1988), lies another cause for injuries—negligence. That is, when parents or caregiving adults fail to take precautions that fall within the expectations of the community, injuries that occur are viewed as evidence of neglect. Like Garbarino, we argue that negligence is an expanding subtype of preventable accidents, dependent upon the leniency or strictness of community caregiving standards. Even when the caregiver is clearly not aware of the preventive measures that could have been taken to protect a child from injury, someone is at fault. In such a case, for example, the social and pediatric community did not fulfill their obligation to the child by educating the parent properly.

Within the continuum of injury etiologies, as described by Garbarino (1988), are specific origins of injury. He states that the sources of injury lie within the elements of situation risk for the child. First, environmental hazards are encountered by children daily. In order for the child to be safe, parents and children must differentiate between safe and hazardous situations and must know the appropriate preventive behavior to use (Peterson & Cook, 1993). Second, some injuries originate not with an environmental hazard but with dangerous child behavior. As will be described below, children participate in highly risky behavior as a part of their social and interpersonal development. Finally, as mentioned previously, inappropriate parenting contributes to childhood injury. Not only can parental neglect lead to injury, but those who use physical punishment increase their children's risk for injury as well.

Differential Diagnosis

As indicated previously, an injury is the result of tissue damage occurring due to extreme exposure to chemical or physical elements (Haddon & Baker, 1981). More specifically, we have defined an injury as "tissue damage with a specific time of onset, which left a visible mark for over an hour or which resulted in pain for over 15 minutes" (Peterson, Saldana, & Heiblum, 1996). Such tissue damage may be visible or may extend to internal organs, as in drowning or poisoning. This definition avoids labeling as an injury tissue damage due to repeated stresses and strains (e.g., forming a blister on a foot, making muscles sore by repeated lifting).

Actual injuries are diagnosed as a different type of occurrence from "near injuries." (Peterson, Farmer, & Mori, 1987). A near injury occurs in situations where an actual injury could take place but failed to, in the absence of any preventive behavior. There are four conditions that must be met to define an event as a near injury: the child is involved in a clearly risky situation, an event occurs that would have resulted in injury had the child contacted the injury vector, clear prevention efforts are not in place (e.g., the failure to fall down the stairs is not due to the presence of a child gate), and the child does not experience any tissue damage or pain lasting more than a few minutes (Peterson, Harbeck, & Moreno, 1993). Near injuries thus occur at a much higher rate than do actual injuries and, may in fact drive the continuation of risk taking behavior that eventually leads to injury because of the failure to contact negative consequences.

Prognosis if Left Untreated

Thus far, many statistics have been given indicating the number of children who are killed and who receive emergency treatment each year due to injuries. For every injury, there are direct costs such as immediate and long-term financial costs, as well as emotional distress and psychological adjustment costs (e.g., peer problems if mobility is impaired or disfigurement occurs). Even further, with every fatality are years of life lost (indirect costs). What can be expected if we as a society continue to fail to aim effective preventive endeavors at decreasing the number of unintentional injuries in children? This question can best be answered in a historical context. Financial costs for injury prevention, detection, and treatment are immense. Twenty years ago, $17.6 million were reportedly spent on childhood motor vehicle injuries alone (Hartunian, Smart, & Thompson, 1981). In 1982, an estimated $7.5 billion were spent on direct and indirect costs (Guyer & Ellers, 1990). More recently, $4,684,000,000 were spent annually on direct costs alone for injuries to children under 14 years of age (Rice, MacKenzie, et al., 1989).

Even more tragic than the monetary costs for childhood injuries are the indirect costs. Every injury is associated with a loss of productivity and a personal loss of a family member (Roberts & Brooks, 1987). Indirect costs represent not only the current losses due to the child injury, but include the future losses as well (Guyer & Ellers, 1990). The number of years annually lost due to injury-related fatalities is more than 3 million (Irwin et al., 1992). Thus, the annual number of life years lost as a result of injuries is greater than cancer (1.8 million years) or heart disease (1.6 million years) (Centers for Disease Control, 1984). Ironically, injuries rob our society of such a large number of life years because they occur disproportionately to children, who have the largest number of years of life ahead of them, prior to injury (Rivara & Mueller, 1987).

As long as preventable injuries continue to occur at such high rates, their direct and indirect costs will also increase. We cannot afford, as a social and medical community, to continue to sacrifice such large percentages of our children to unintentional injuries. The following sections will describe methods of assessing and identifying injuries, of analyzing the behaviors contributing to childhood injuries, of preventing injuries, and of evaluating the effectiveness of preventive endeavors.

Problem Identification

Assessment of Tissue Damage

There are a variety of dimensions of assessment that have been used to categorize or quantify injuries, to improve our ability to monitor injury occurrence, and to study the behavioral and environmental mechanisms by which injuries take place. The initial section of this chapter was organized by injury type and exemplifies the different structures used in classifying injuries. It is common to categorize injuries by both the source of the injury (e.g., automobile injuries, which might include burns, impact injuries, cuts) and the outcome (e.g., lacerations, asphyxiation, electrocution). This results in potentially overlapping categories, but allows preventionists the flexibility of considering interventions relevant to source or behavioral etiology and also aids in structuring interventions to improve trauma treatment following injury.

As noted earlier, injuries are also categorized as inflicted (child abuse, child homicide) or unintentional. Such categorization is anachronistic and ignores the reality that injury exists on a continuum. Many parents injure children by shaking their child, bathing their child in hot water, or striking a child who then falls and is injured. These injuries are both inflicted and unintentional, in the sense that the caregiver did not plan for or seek to create the outcome. In contrast, some children are injured while engaging in caregiver-prompted behavior that is dangerous and clearly developmentally inappropriate (e.g., sending a five-year-old alone across several lanes of traffic at twilight), but such injuries are not viewed as inflicted and thus are categorized as though parental behavior was not instrumental in their occurrence. Garbarino (1988) argued persuasively that the more we know about injury prevention, the more we are likely to criminally indict caregivers for failing to protect their children. This chapter focuses on the literature that examines non-inflicted injury, but we wish to once again remind the reader that the intentional/unintentional dichotomy may not be a sensible way to evaluate caregiver contributions to injury.

In addition to type and level of intentionally, injury severity forms an important dimension of study. As noted earlier, for epidemiologists to study injury, they must contact the injuries in some fashion. The bulk of what is known about injuries comes from hospital inpatient or emergency room records, with additional data coming from records obtained by state highway patrols and firefighters, police records, and medical examiners. Thus, most systems indexing injury severity consider only injury outcomes that are relatively severe.

The severity scales we will discuss are designed to index the amount of damage incurred by an injury. There are three indicators that are typically used when defining an injury: physiological and biochemical parameters, anatomical descriptors, and personal characteristics such as age and sex (MacKenzie, 1984). Some scales are intended for specific types of injuries (e.g., Glasgow Coma Scale; Teasdale & Jennett, 1974), and others are used as more global scales (e.g., Abbreviated Injury Scale; Petrucelli, 1981). The next section will focus on assessment measures that can be used to index a variety of injuries.

At this point it is important to note that no standardized instruments (interviews, measures, or treatments) exist to aid in protecting children from the types of injury that are presented in this chapter. There are a few measures in existence used to assess home safety hazards (e.g., Safe Home Checklist; Barone, Greene & Lutzker, 1986); however, most of the common home health hazards (e.g., electrical outlets without covers) are not the leading killers of children. Thus, the following section will describe the measures that do exist that assess the level of severity of injuries after they have occurred. Such scales could potentially be used to assess the dangers that various activities and environments present, by determining the level of injury severity that the activities or environments incur. The use of the current injury scales in such a manner remains to be determined by future research.

Major Severity Assessment Scales

The most common scale used in assessing injury severity is the Abbreviated Injury Scale (AIS; Petrucelli, 1981). The scale was originally developed to index injuries sustained from automobile crashes. Several years later, it was revised to include numerous classifications of injuries and has since been approved as an official assessment tool for all federally funded motor vehicle injury investigations (MacKenzie, 1984).

The AIS is a scale ranging from 1 to 6, of increasing anatomic injury (1 = minor; 2 = moderate; 3 = serious; 4 = severe; 5 = critical; 6 = maximum injury/unsurvivable). The AIS manual is divided into sections for head, neck, thorax, abdomen/pelvis, spine, extremities and bony pelvis. Although the scale primarily indexes anatomical injury, level of consciousness and neurological functioning are also used as considerations in indicating the severity of an injury. Injuries are categorized, using the AIS, by the anatomical region in which the injury was sustained (e.g., lung) and then by the type of injury (laceration). Common injuries that require medical attention, but are easily treated, are rated as a 1 on the AIS. Examples of injuries that are rated as a 1 are lacerations, hand fractures, and contusions. Slightly more serious injuries, rated as a 2, are hepatic contusions, concussions, and radius fractures. Injuries rated as a 3 include open bone fractures, skull fractures, and splenic lacerations (Manary & Hollifield, 1993).

The AIS was devised for and uses language appropriate for medical personnel. The primary source of information used to rate the injury is the hospital discharge records. Research on this method has indicated that raters have difficulty obtaining agreement on the type of injuries sustained simply by looking at medical charts; however, when injuries are agreed upon, there is acceptable interrater reliability regarding the level of severity of the injury (MacKenzie, Shapiro, & Eastham, 1985). In addition, test–retest reliability appears to be acceptable when the raters recognize the same injures during viewings of the same medical charts at time 1 and time 2 (K = .71–.89; MacKenzie et al., 1985).

Similar to the AIS, the Injury Severity Score (ISS; Baker, O'Neill, Haddon, & Long, 1974) was developed to index relatively serious injuries that require medical attention. Ratings are made using a 1–5 scale with an additional 6th rating for "unknown" outcomes. The ISS is simply a derivative of the AIS and can be calculated by taking the sum of squares of the three most severely rated AIS scores in different body regions (Manary & Hollifield, 1993). Ratings of 6 or greater on the AIS are rated as "unknown" on the ISS (Baker et al., 1974). The intention of the ISS is to rate the overall injury severity of an individual who may have sustained multiple injuries to different anatomical regions.

The AIS and ISS are appropriate severity scales for rating injuries that require medical attention. However, neither is useful for describing the majority of injuries experienced by children. A scale that allows quantification of minor severity is considered next.

Minor Severity Assessment Scale

Recently, we developed a measure to help in the identification of all injuries, especially minor injuries, that result in any tissue damage. The Minor Injury Severity Scale* (MISS; Peterson, Saldana, & Heiblum, 1996) was developed as a standardized method of rating injuries from low severity, such as paper cuts, increasing to pulled muscles, badly skinned knees, concussions, broken bones, and, ultimately, fatalities. Although the rating scales extend to permanent disability or death, the measure was designed to maintain its sensitivity in the spectrum of less severe injuries.

The MISS contains 22 separate empirically derived categories of injury types (e.g., animal scratch/bites, bump/bruises, burns, loss of consciousness, nosebleeds), created to rate injuries on a 0 to 7 scale (0 = no injury; 6 = severe damage resulting in disability; 7 = death). Ratings for each category are then distinct for a particular type of injury. We found such distinctions necessary due to the dissimilar nature (potential for pain, disabilities such as scarring, length of time to heal) of various types of injuries such as burns, cuts, and impact injuries. Within the same injury type, injury to different areas on the body of the same size, depth, and shape are rated differently. For example, equal amounts of swelling to the eye and to the shin do not equate as equally severe injuries because intense swelling to the eye is indicative of more severe damage than the same level of swelling to the shin.

The ratings of the MISS rely first on the selection of the appropriate category, then on observation of the parameters of the injury to assist in the measurement of the severity. Using such observations as the depth and width of the tissue damage, the color, and the amount of swelling produced by the injury, individuals with relatively little training can accurately rate the severity of an injury. Using

---

*Copies of the MISS can be obtained from the authors by writing to Department of Psychology, University of Missouri–Columbia, 210 McAlester Hall, Columbia, MO 65211.

self-reports of mothers and children who were trained to keep an ongoing report of injuries sustained, we found acceptable interrater reliability ($r = .71$) among undergraduate coders reading the reports. In addition, excellent test–retest reliability was obtained from reports from both mothers ($r = .99$) and children ($r = .98$) at two separate time periods. Furthermore, we were able to demonstrate discriminate and convergent validity for subjective variables such as the amount of fear and pain felt at the time of the injury in comparison with the amount of actual tissue damage sustained.

Etiology

A final way of categorizing injury is by the situation in which the injury occurred. Thus, a pedestrian injury (type of injury) that was severe (intensity rating) could come from deliberately crossing the street while returning home from school, from playing in the street, from accepting a dare to run across the street, or from being pushed into the street while roughhousing. Clearly, such information would be helpful to preventionists. For the most part, although some studies have differentiated broadly by etiology (e.g., bathtub drownings from swimming pool drownings), there has been little work describing the activity in which the child was engaged at the time of the injury.

In the last decade, there has been increasing emphasis on institutionalizing a molar rating for the etiology of injury. *The International Classification of Diseases, 9th Revision (ICD-9;* U.S. Department of Health and Human Services, 1989) includes a set of codes for environmental causes of tissue damage. These "E codes" provide a well-established system for indicating what situations precede injury. There are separate codes for each of the following injury causes: motor vehicle occupant—traffic, pedestrian—traffic, pedestrian—nontraffic, motorcyclist, bicyclist—MV involved, other motor vehicle, airplane crash, poison—solid/liquid, poison—gas/vapor, fall, house fire, drowning, aspiration—food, aspiration—other, suffocation, unintentional firearm, electric current, farm machinery, medical—surgical, other unintentional, suicide, homicide, and unknown (Department of Health and Human Services, 1992). Within each of these categories there are clear exceptions (e.g., transport accidents that involve vehicles which are regarded as industrial

equipment and used exclusively on industrial premises are coded as industrial rather than transport injuries) and specific subcategories (*ICD9-3R,* U.S. Department of Health and Human Services, 1989). It should be noted that E codes were devised to be used with adults' hospital records. Thus, the categories may not be entirely suitable for children's activities. In addition, E codes give only the most global information about the causal sequence of events leading to injury. In general, even after an E code is assigned, it often remains unclear as to how a given activity resulted in the actual injury event.

There have been a small number of studies recently, however, that have studied the behavioral mechanisms of injury. For example, Christoffel and her colleagues (1996) examined the sequence of events in pedestrian injuries and noted three variables that contributed to injury: the child's short stature, moving rapidly into traffic, and sudden appearance (e.g., coming out from between two automobiles). This work also explored the potential contributions of low levels of supervision, child behavior problems, and environmental risks (such as circular drives that do not allow the driver to see the road ahead).

Examination of minor injuries suggests that children more often sustain minor injuries while playing than while engaged in purposeful behavior, and are more likely to be injured in unstructured play than during structured games (Peterson, Brown, Bartelstone, & Kern, 1996). Approximately one in every three minor injuries reported occurred as a violation of family safety rules (Peterson & Saldana, 1996). These studies only begin the exploration of causal sequences resulting in injury. Although such research is extraordinarily labor intensive, it is crucial in the area of effective prevention interventions in the future.

In addition to attempting to classify etiology of an injury, studies that afford a functional analysis of injury risk behavior may offer scientists the links from environment and behavior to injury necessary for effective prevention. The next section considers such an approach.

Problem Analysis

Injuries have few positive consequences, with the exception of very rare secondary gain, and they are accompanied by multiple negative consequences. In contrast, injury risk behavior has frequent positive outcomes and only rarely actually results in injury. Every day, children around the nation engage in countless risk-taking behaviors. Every time a child crosses a street, climbs a tree, performs a gymnastics trick or plays with a pet, that child is at risk for injury (Roberts & Brooks, 1987). Fortunately, the most frequent sources of injuries, such as falls and sports-related injuries, are not often associated with fatal wounds (Zins et al., 1994). Nevertheless, the question remains as to why children place themselves in situations daily that could result in minor injury, serious injury, disabling injury, or death.

Competence

Children may engage in risk-taking as a way of gaining competence in a desired skill. If children never put themselves at risk of getting hit in the face with a ball, there would be no soccer goalies, no baseball catchers, no football players. Many of the activities that are valued by children in our society involve mild risk-taking behaviors. In order to become competent and not only succeed at an activity, but decrease one's chance for injury, one must first engage in what may be for a novice highly risky behavior. Furthermore, children value gaining competence and control over their environment.

Once competence is achieved, children may then feel relatively invulnerable to injuries. This concept that perceived competence increases risk is supported by data from our lab suggesting that children who rated themselves as having higher self-confidence in their bike riding skills also expected to have less pain and less serious injuries when encountering a simulated bicycle collision (Peterson, Brazeal, Oliver, & Bull, in press; Peterson, Gillies, et al., 1994). Additionally, boys, who are at greater risk for injury than girls (Matheny, 1987), are also more likely than girls to believe that they are resilient to injury. In our study regarding bicycle safety practices, males reported expecting less fear, less pain and less severe injuries than did females when shown a simulated collision. In addition, younger children at lower epidemiological risk were more likely to react fearfully than older children who are actually more likely to sustain injuries on a bicycle (Peterson, Gillies, et al., 1994). These re-

sults may be evidence that the feelings of accomplishment and gaining of skills increase the feeling of confidence and thus, increase the chance of future risk-taking behavior.

Excitement

As with gaining competence, there is excitement in risk-taking behavior. Physiologically, as the adrenaline flows, there is a feeling of pleasure and perhaps a little fear as well. When these feelings are associated with a behavior, they increase many children's desire to continue in risk-taking. For example, second-grade children, who are not as likely to sustain bicycle injuries as are older children, reported feeling more fear and less excitement than eighth graders when faced with simulated bicycle collisions (Peterson, Harbeck, et al., 1993). However, eighth-grade children, who are at the greatest risk for bicycle injury, reported feeling heightened exhilaration when faced with potentially hazardous situations while riding bicycles (Peterson, Gillies, et al., 1994).

Another study measured the level of exhilaration in fourth-grade children exposed to risk-taking situations (Cook, 1991). Children reported the degree to which they felt excitement or fear in a variety of injury risk situations. Later, they were observed in a situation which was perceived as being risky but actually was not (going off the diving board in a school-sponsored swim class). Children who reported higher exhilaration in general risky situations were more likely to respond on the board in a risky way (running or skipping on the board, bouncing on the board) and to leave the board in a risky way (flipping or diving), and were marginally less likely to engage in self-protective behavior such as wearing a life jacket, pausing on the board, and seeking instructor assistance. In contrast, children who had higher fear scores were much more likely to engage in protective behavior (Cook, 1991). These data suggest that children who feel the most excitement from risky situations are involved in the most risk-taking behavior.

Convenience

Some risk-taking behavior may simply be due to trying to minimize one's efforts. Cutting across a busy street may decrease the amount of time it takes to get home. So long as the child continues to make it home without injury from crossing the street, he or she is likely to continue to engage in the risky behavior. Many activities become more risky once shortcuts are taken to save time (e.g., riding bikes over curbs, mothers leaving young children alone in the tub in order to accomplish another task, cooking on the front burners instead of waiting for the back burners to become available). In most instances, so long as the child continues to succeed without being injured and without parental directives to do otherwise, he or she will continue to engage in the activity and his or her parent may become more accepting of the behaviors, even though each time the behavior occurs, the child is taking a chance for injury.

Peer Rewards

Finally, some risk taking may occur for the purpose of gaining peer rewards. Children, particularly boys, often engage in group activities that have an element of risk taking involved as a way of gaining social acceptance (Gärling & Valsiner, 1985). Children often encourage dangerous behavior with one another. Those who are willing to engage in highly risky behaviors, are also likely to be considered "cool" by their peers. For example, one of the most commonly cited reasons by children for not wearing bicycle helmets is that peers do not wear them and they are "uncool" (Gielen et al., 1994; Puczynski & Marshall, 1992). Furthermore, as with much risk-taking behavior, mothers of children who refuse to wear helmets due to peer influence fail to use effective discipline methods to ensure helmet use (Peterson, Saldana, & Schaeffer, 1997).

Consequences of Injury Risk Behavior

Why is it that children engage in injury risk behavior and that many children who are at greatest risk for injury are also those who are the least aware of injury risk? The most obvious reason may be that although injuries are the leading cause of death in children in our nation, injuries are also a relatively low baserate event (Rivara & Mueller, 1987). Thus, following the large majority of risk-taking occasions, children do not receive immediate negative consequences from their environment when they engage in highly risky behavior and they often do

receive positive consequences. For example, not only are children typically unlikely to receive negative consequences in the form of injury, but a study of mothers and their children indicated that even when children engaged in a risky behavior that did result in injury, mothers reported failing to follow through with an effective remediating consequence for the large majority of events (Peterson, Bartelstone, Kern, & Gillies, 1995). Specifically, mothers reported doing nothing following 80.1% of events and delivering a lecture 14.4% of the time. Their children reported receiving no consequences 96% of the time and recalled the mothers giving a lecture only 1.2% of the time. Thus, the few times that mothers actually lectured their children following risky behavior, children heard and/or remembered the lecture only a small fraction of the time. Furthermore, mothers reported using and children reported receiving other discipline methods such as restricting a privilege, grounding the child, or forming a family rule against the behavior less than 3% of the time.

Given that children receive only a small number of negative consequences either from an actual injury or from caregiver discipline, the law of probability indicates that a child can engage in risk-taking behavior a number of times without receiving any negative consequences. Thus, if a child experiences feelings of increased competence, or excitement, or enjoys convenience, or earns peer rewards by engaging in a risky behavior, and the child is able to do so with minimal risk for negative consequences from the external environment (i.e., sustaining injury or discipline), the probability of the behavior seems likely to increase. Said differently, when the assurity of positive reinforcement outweighs potential negative consequences, children are more likely to engage in injury risk behavior.

Plan Implementation

Intervention Conceptualization

Until the mid 1980s, the most prevalent method of conceptualizing the prevention of injuries was the host, agent, environment model (Gratz, 1979). In this model, the *host* indicated the victim of the injury (i.e., the child), the *agent,* the stimulus that caused the injury, and the *environment,* the continual temporal, physical and interpersonal setting in which the injury occurred. Although this model appears to be useful in conceptualizing where and when injuries occur (Rivara & Mueller, 1987), its success in directing thinking about how to prevent injuries is limited (Peterson & Mori, 1985). More recently, researchers in the areas of health psychology and public health have begun using a three-dimensional targets × methods × tactics conceptual model for prevention (Peterson & Mori, 1985).

Targets

Using Peterson and Mori's (1985) model, the *target* refers to the source at which the preventive intervention is aimed. For the prevention of childhood injury, the target is sometimes the manufacturer of the hazard, but is more typically the caregiver or the actual child. The decision whether to target the caregiver or the child is in part related to child development. The age of children greatly determines their ability to be reasonable targets for preventive measures. For example, a 2-year-old cannot reasonably be expected to know not to go out into the street. However, a child 8 years old can be expected to understand the dangers of playing in the street and be given some, but not total, responsibility for knowing not to do so. An adolescent of 14 is expected to be able to cross streets entirely independently. For the 2-year-old child, the appropriate target to prevent a child pedestrian injury is the caregiver. For a child of 8, both the parent and the child should be targeted. The influence of dares and alcohol on pedestrian safety might be the focus for adolescent targets.

The methods of intervention are typically either mandated (legislated) or educational (persuasive) (Peterson & Roberts, 1992). When preventive change occurs as a result of adherence to a law or a change in legal policy, the method of intervention is known as mandated. On the other hand, when change occurs as a result of a shift in knowledge or the successful use of persuasive techniques, the method of intervention is labeled educational persuasive.

Methods

National laws can be aimed at product safety, at caregivers (e.g., laws against corporal punishment), and at eliminating risky behaviors in chil-

dren (e.g., increased legal drinking age; Garbarino, 1988). Legislated or mandated interventions at the national level focused on the hazards themselves are among the most successful intervention strategies. For example, prior to the Poison Prevention Packaging Act, poisoning was an even stronger threat to children than it is currently. The act mandated child-resistant packaging and limiting the amount of a drug available in a single container to nonlethal dosages, reducing childhood poisoning by 50% (Walton, 1982). Another example of a population-wide intervention is the new design of automobiles. Air bags on the passenger side can greatly decrease child injuries. Recent changes in the design of cars now make it more likely that a child pedestrian who is struck by a car will be contacted by the wheels and the pavement, but will not be thrown up onto the car. Research predicts that this change will help reduce the number of serious pedestrian injuries by 30% (Rivara, 1990). Examples such as these give support for the continued federal effort that is necessary to fund injury prevention programs (Guyer & Ellers, 1990).

There are some mandated community-level efforts to help reduce childhood injuries, as well. For example, researchers have found the use of bicycle safety helmets decreases head injury risk by 85% and brain injury risk by as much as 88% (Rivara, 1985; Thompson, Rivara, & Thompson, 1989). Furthermore, in a five-year longitudinal study, it was shown that if all cyclists wore helmets, one death a day and one head injury every 4 minutes could be prevented (Sacks et al., 1991). Knowing that an increase in bicycle helmet use could prevent numerous childhood injuries, the city of Seattle, Washington, embarked on a city-wide campaign to increase the use of safety helmets in school-aged children. Parental awareness of the risk of injury when riding without a helmet was increased through personal contact with physicians, trade shows, and exposure to mass media such as newspapers, television, and radio. A successful effort was made to make helmets more available to the general population by not only decreasing the cost of helmets, but selling them at a general retail store as opposed to bicycle specialty shops. Furthermore, local professional sports figures promoted the theme that helmets are a necessary part of any "sports" uniform, school assemblies and bike rodeos were conducted to increase child awareness, and children were reinforced with free coupons (for french fries, etc.) for wearing helmets. Following the program, annual sales for safety helmets in the community rose from 1,500 in 1986 to 5,000 in 1987, to 20,000 in 1988, and to 30,000 during the first eight months of 1989 (Bergman, Rivara, Richards, & Rogers, 1990). Efforts such as these demonstrate that if campaigned properly, community interventions that combine passive (buying the helmet) and active (maintaining helmet use) efforts can greatly reduce childhood injury risk.

Despite the effectiveness of national and community interventions in reducing the number of fatalities and serious injuries, Matheny (1987) argued that although passive interventions at the national or community level are helpful in reducing the number of fatalities due to injury, they are not as helpful in reducing the large number of daily minor injuries that children sustain, nor will they avoid any types of fatal injuries that could have been prevented by parental supervision. He argued that preventionists should consider the child's world as the primary concern and thus, that intervention at the individual level cannot be ignored. Examples of individual interventions include educating parents to store dangerous materials such as poisons, guns, and knives in locked locations and to use barrier methods such as gates and fences around swimming pools (Wintemute, 1990). Additional individual intervention strategies will be considered later in the section "Parental Role in Reducing Childhood Injury."

Tactics: Active or Passive

Prevention exists on a continuum of action required from the child or caregiver to ensure safety. The literature has often dichotomized this continuum into passive and active methods. Passive methods at their extreme typically refer to one-time design changes that alter hazards so they are no longer dangerous. For example, requiring manufacturers to construct refrigerator doors so that they could not trap children inside removed the danger from this vector of asphyxiation for young children (Robertson, 1983). Other environmental barriers such as separating roadways from play and residential areas require no further action to protect children.

However, most forms of prevention do require some action from caregivers. Even environmentally based changes often require limited caregiver efforts. For example, there are one-time preventive actions, such as turning down water heater thermostats to prevent scalding burns, and installing smoke detectors. Other barrier methods require a single large-effort response such as purchasing a safety seat or installing a child gate, followed by a small-effort response such as fastening the infant into the car seat before each trip or unlatching and relatching the child gate every time one goes up the stairs. At one end of the preventive effort continuum are permanent changes to the injury vector, followed by barrier solutions, and at the other end are highly effortful responses such as supervising an infant in the bathtub or escorting small children across busy streets. The most effective prevention takes place in the center of this continuum of effort. Unfortunately, as this chapter documents, population- or community-level actions that produce permanent design changes are hard to institute; furthermore, most communities do not provide any guidelines or support for the high-effort prevention sometimes necessary to keep children safe (Peterson & Roberts, 1992).

A Focus on Behavioral Intervention

Most successful intervention methods at the national level have concentrated on passive intervention strategies (Peterson, Zink, & Downing, 1993). However, many injuries that occur in the home as a result of a caregiver's unsafe behavior will never be reduced by such methods. For instance, in one study, 31% of mothers reported drinking hot beverages with children aged 0–1 on their laps, 49.2% reported occasionally traveling in cars with their children on their laps, and 60.7% reported using electric appliances in the bathroom with 1–2-year-old children (Gofin & Palti, 1991). Keeping data such as these in mind and considering Matheny's (1987) argument that children are faced with daily minor injury risks, and Scheidt's (1988) and Peterson and Roberts' (1992) suggestions regarding the need for increased behavioral interventions to reduce serious and fatal injuries in children, this section will review behavioral interventions at the individual level that are focused on the caregiver targets. Both passive and active strategies will be considered as methods for preventing childhood injury.

Parental Role in Reducing Childhood Injury

There is a consensus among behavioral researchers that intervening to change parents' behavior is among the most promising modes of preventing childhood injury (Garbarino, 1988; Peterson & Roberts, 1992). However, one of the least researched areas in childhood injury prevention is the relationship between parental behaviors and childhood injury (Wortel & de Geus, 1993). Parents report that they influence their children's safety through teaching and family safety rules (Peterson, Farmer, & Kashani, 1990). In support of this report, we found a significant negative correlation ($r = -.48$) between the number of home safety rules that mothers reported advocating on an empirically derived list of Family Safety Rules and the number of childhood injuries sustained, suggesting that parents who have more safety rules in their homes also have children who sustain fewer injuries (Peterson & Saldana, 1996). Although these data are only correlational, they suggest that certain patterns of parenting may be associated with fewer injuries. In addition, parents who realize the threat of injuries to their children and who are willing to use preventive tactics to reduce the possibility of injury appear to have fewer hazards in their homes (Russell, 1991). Thus, it appears that, if parents are invested in reducing the number of injuries in their children, their preventive measures are often associated with lower injury rates.

However, it is difficult to maintain parental involvement and consistency in behavioral interventions such as safety enforcement. For instance, in the same study linking higher number of safety rules to fewer minor injuries, we also found that mothers inconsistently enforced family safety rules 26.82% of the time (Peterson & Saldana, 1996). Similarly, parents appear to believe that their efforts to maintain safety for their children do not necessitate an ongoing commitment. For example, early research from our lab indicated that parents believed that their 8- to 10-year-old children knew and understood their safety rules, and, thus, could be left unsupervised (Peterson, Mori, & Scissors, 1986). However, when the children were then interviewed, the family rules that they described disagreed with their parent's responses on the majority of serious rules (e.g., allow adult neighbor to enter home = 60% disagreement; if sees a fire should contact a parent = 100% disagreement; if power goes out, child can light candles = 91% disagreement; if child has a serious cut, wait for the parent to get home = 100% disagreement; Peterson et al., 1986). Thus, it appears that parents often believe that family safety rules can act as a passive rather than an active intervention strategy prior to their child's actual developmental readiness to be protected by rules in the absence of parental supervision.

Even more disturbing are findings that parents recognize risk-behavior changes that could be made, and yet they proceed to "gamble with the odds." Examples of this phenomenon are evident in the bicycle safety literature. One study indicated that 61% of all parents interviewed believed that bicycle helmets are effective in preventing head injuries and that these parents do worry that their children will be in a serious biking collision (Schneider, Ituarte, & Stokols, 1993). Yet, when asked why their children did not wear safety helmets, one-third of all parents asked had no specific reason to offer (Hu, Wesson, Parkin, Chipman, & Spence, 1994). When mothers of second- and eighth-grade children were asked how they would respond if their children continued to refuse to wear a helmet, mothers tended to let their older, more at-risk children get away with not wearing a helmet more often than they did younger children (Peterson, Saldana, & Schaeffer, 1997). Furthermore, another recent study indicated that most parents in one Alabama county had not even thought about purchasing a helmet for their child bicycle-riders, and that of those who had made the purchase, only 35% reported their child regularly wearing the helmet (Jones, King, Poteet-Johnson, & Wang, 1993).

How then can preventionists work with parents to consistently follow through with intervention strategies to decrease childhood injury? One study with mothers of infants and toddlers reported that 95% of mothers believed that the suggested childproofing techniques would make them feel like better parents, would not be inconvenient, and would increase the safety of their child (Gielen et al., 1994). Individual injury prevention many times requires that a parent engage in active prevention without any external reinforcement (Peterson & Oliver, 1994). Thus, elements of individual-directed intervention methods may be (1) to reinforce the internal belief system parents have that they will be better parents if they increase the safety of their children and (2) to increase self-reinforcement and family support for such efforts. Once parents become invested in their children's safety, educational methods can be used both to help parents recognize particularly risky behaviors that increase the chance of injury and to increase knowledge of the risks associated with differing developmental stages of childhood.

One instance of successful parental education was part of the Seattle bicycle helmet campaign (Bergman et al., 1990). As noted earlier, parents were educated through pediatricians, pamphlets, mass media, and the presentation of ongoing up-to-date statistics about bicycle injuries sustained in the area. Although it is not possible from this study to determine whether the parental education was the most important factor in increasing helmet usage in the Seattle area, it can be stated that such education strategies were a part of the successful campaign.

Another method for increasing child safety may be to help parents recognize the need to enforce safety in all areas of child behavior. In our naturalistic observation of children's injuries, mothers reported that their children received remediating consequences, on the average, no more than 36% of the time for injuries encountered in 24 different activity categories. Injuries sustained in certain categories (e.g., such as structured team play) received, on the average, almost no remediation (less than 4% of the events were followed by preventive interventions; Peterson et al., 1995). Although parents cannot change the rules of team sports activities, they can help by insisting that their children wear appropriate safety equipment and working closely with coaches and athletic directors to insure that safety precautions are taken on the field (Derksen & Strasburger, 1994). To completely protect a child, generalization of safety behaviors is necessary across settings, activities, and caregivers. In essence, injury prevention needs to be adopted as a lifestyle for children and all those who work with them (Peterson & Cook, 1993).

Most importantly, preventionists need to develop appropriate contingencies for parental safety behavior. This can be done in part by decreasing the cost of behavior change for parents (e.g., giving away smoke detectors) and by increasing the positive consequences received upon a behavior change (Peterson, Zink, & Downing, 1993). One way of increasing positive consequences that appears to re-

duce injury is helping parents recognize secondary gain from use of safety interventions (e.g., parents' use of car seats helps in the management of children's car behavior and makes the car ride more pleasant for the parent; Christopherson & Gyulay, 1981). Explicit incentives may also be used. In a different study of car safety seats, parents who failed to comply with using safety restraints simply because it was mandated by law, increased their use of restraints when lottery tickets were given to those parents who arrived at day care with their children in a safety restraint (Roberts & Turner, 1986). Similar attempts to develop positive reinforcements for parents are necessary to decrease the incidence of risky behavior.

Finally, injury prevention should focus on helping parents instill safety beliefs and rules in their children. Although parents are the primary socialization agents for safety in their children (Peterson et al., 1995), children are not always under the supervision of their parents (Rivara, Calonge, & Thompson, 1989). This is especially true for older children, who are often given more freedom and self-responsibility. However, to be safe, the process of relinquishing supervision and control over risky behavior is a gradual one. Parents must gradually transfer the responsibility of monitoring safe behavior from themselves to their children. They must be aware of when their child is developmentally capable of performing a safe behavior on his or her own. This can be tested by allowing a child to engage in a low- to moderate-risk activity while still under the supervision of the parent. As children reach three years of age, they begin to direct their own behaviors and to test their freedom, thereby requiring constant supervision to ensure that safety needs are met. As children increase in age, it is important for parents to maintain co-regulation with their children to balance freedom and supervision (Scheidt, 1988). As with parents, contingencies should be set up and followed through with children. Parents can establish positive consequences for children engaging in safe behavior (e.g., wearing bicycle helmets without being told) and enforce negative consequences for engaging in high-risk behavior (e.g., loss of bike privileges for not wearing a helmet).

Several successful research attempts to train children to increase their home safety skills can be implemented by parents. In a series of studies using the "Safe at Home" manual (Peterson, 1984), seven modules of safe behavior were taught to children. These modules included (1) safe after-school activities, (2) safe answering the telephone, (3) safe answering the door, (4) safe selection and preparation of food, (5) appropriate responses to a home fire, (6) effective intervention for a bad cut, and (7) safe practices when looking after a younger child. Specific criteria were included for each of the modules with the best responses, acceptable responses, and unacceptable responses provided (e.g., food preparation: best response is nutritious and is not likely to cause an injury, such as grapes; acceptable response is somewhat nutritious and is not likely to cause an injury, such as bologna; unacceptable response uses a can opener, stove top, or knife and is likely to cause an injury, such as frying an egg). When compared with a discussion-oriented "Prepared for Today" training manual, the more standardized "Safe at Home" manual showed greater improvement for child safety practices and safe responses to potentially hazardous situations (Peterson, 1984). Research indicates that the "Safe at Home" manual can be taught to either an individual child or to a group of children, by an untrained instructor and still show significant results in child safety behaviors (Peterson & Thiele, 1988), Furthermore, with slight changes to the protocol (e.g., reducing the number of steps to be remembered in a procedure), the standardized manual can be used with children as young as three years old and show significant improvements in safety responses for all modules (Mori & Peterson, 1986). Thus, the "Safe at Home" manual appears to be a potentially useful and inexpensive tool for parents to use with their children when training safety beliefs and rules about a variety of home safety domains.

Future Research

Although the intervention strategies just described are focused at the individual level with the caregiver target, future research should consider the combination of intervention strategies at the national, community, and individual levels. It may seem at times that this is an impossible task. The belief system described at the beginning of this chapter suggests that there will always be injuries, and there is no way to guard against such random events. However, this is simply not the case. Changes

at national, community, and family levels can result, and have resulted, in substantial decreases in injury in the past. Sweden, for example, has significantly reduced its rate of child fatalities over a period of 10 years by combining national efforts providing funds and motivation for the Child Accident Committee, with efforts of community organizations such as the Red Cross, the police, physicians, nurses, and teachers. In addition, efforts were directed toward caregivers who increased day care during high-risk seasons (such as harvesting) and became more educated about appropriate expectations of children at varying developmental stages. In 1959, Sweden's injury death rate for children under the age of 4 was greater than the death rate in the United States, and for children ages 5 to 14, fatalities were equivalent to those in the United States. In 1986, the rates were reduced to less than half of those incurred in the United States in both age groups (Bergman & Rivara, 1991). Sweden's changes provide compelling evidence for the utility of injury prevention initiatives in our own country. In order to protect children from injury, efforts must be made by federal, state, and local agencies (Guyer & Ellers, 1990). Although such intervention combinations are challenging, difficult, and expensive, the long-term gain in life and quality of life for tomorrow's children would be invaluable.

References

Agran, P., Castillo, D., & Winn, D. (1990). Childhood motor vehicle occupant injuries. *American Journal of Diseases of Children, 144*(6), 653–662.

Baker, S.P., & Waller, A.E. (1989). *Childhood injury: State by state mortality facts.* Baltimore: Johns Hopkins University, School of Public Health.

Baker, S.P., O'Neill, B., & Ginsberg, M.J. (1992). *The injury fact book* (2nd. ed.). New York: Oxford University Press.

Baker, S.P., O'Neill, B., Haddon, W., & Long, W.B. (1974). The Injury Severity Score: A method for describing patients with multiple injuries and evaluating emergency care. *Journal of Trauma, 14,* 187–196.

Barone, V.J., Greene, B.F., & Lutzker, J.R. (1986). Home safety with families being treated for child abuse and neglect. *Behavior Modification, 10,* 93–114.

Bergman, A.B., & Rivara, F.P. (1991). Sweden's experience in reducing childhood injuries. *Pediatrics, 88,* 69–74.

Bergman, A.B., Rivara, F.P., Richards, D.D., & Rogers, L.W. (1990). The Seattle children's bicycle helmet campaign. *American Journal of Diseases of Children, 144*(6) 727–731.

Centers for Disease Control. (1984). Potential years of life lost. *Morbidity and Mortality Weekly Report, 34,* 27.

Centers for Disease Control and Prevention. (1991). Child passenger restraint use and motor-vehicle-related fatalities among children—United States, 1982–1990. *Morbidity and Mortality Weekly Report, 40,* 600–602.

Christoffel, K.K., Donovan, M., Schofer, J., Wills, K., Lavigne, J., & The Kids 'n' Cars Team. (1996). Psychosocial factors in childhood pedestrian injury: A matched case-control study. *Pediatrics, 97,* 33–42.

Christopherson, E.R., & Gyulay, J. (1981). Parental compliance with car seat usage: A positive approach with long-term follow-up. *Journal of Pediatric Psychology, 6,* 301–312.

Cook, S.C. (1991). *The perception of physical risk by children and the fear/exhilaration response.* Unpublished master's thesis, University of Missouri, Columbia.

Consumer Product Safety Commission. (1989, August). Large buckets are drowning hazards for young children. *Safety News.* Washington, DC: Consumer Product Safety Commission.

Davidson. L.L. (1987). Hyperactivity, antisocial behavior, and childhood injury: A critical analysis of the literature. *Developmental and Behavioral Pediatrics, 8,* 335–340.

Department of Health and Human Services. (1992). *Standard definitions for childhood injury research.* Report of NICHD Conference, March, 1989. Rockville, MD: NICHD.

Derksen, D.J., & Strasburger, V.C. (1994). Children and the influence of the media. *Primary Care: Clinics in Office Practice, 21,* 747–758.

Division of Injury Control. (1990). Childhood injuries in the United States. *American Journal of Diseases of Children, 144*(6), 627–646.

Durkin, M.S., Davidson, L.L., Kuhn, L., O'Connor, P., & Barlow, B. (1994). Low-income neighborhoods and the risk of severe pediatric injury: A small-area analysis in northern Manhattan. *American Journal of Public Health, 84,* 587–592.

Freide, A., Azzara, C.V., Gallagher, S.S., & Guyer, B. (1985). Injuries to bicycle riders. In J.J. Alpert & B. Guyer (Eds.), *The pediatric clinics in North America: Injuries and injury prevention* (pp. 141–151). Philadelphia: Saunders.

Garbarino, J. (1988). Preventing childhood injury: Developmental and mental health issues. *American Journal of Orthopsychiatry, 58,* 5–45.

Gärling, T., & Valsiner, J. (Eds.). (1985). *Children within environments: Toward a psychology of accident prevention.* New York: Plenum.

Gielen, A.C., Joffe, A., Dannenberg, A.L., Wilson, M.E., Beilenson, P.L., & DeBoer, M. (1994). Psychosocial factors associated with the use of bicycle helmets among children in countries with and without helmet use laws. *Journal of Pediatrics, 124,* 204–210.

Gofin, R., & Palti, H. (1991). Injury prevention practices of mothers of 0 to 2 year olds: A developmental approach. *Early Child Development and Care, 71,* 117–126.

Gratz, R.R. (1979). Accidental injury in childhood: A literature review on pediatric trauma. *Journal of Trauma, 19,* 551–555.

Guyer, B., & Ellers, B. (1990). Childhood injuries in the United States. *American Journal of Diseases of Children, 144*(6), 649–652.

Haddon, W., Jr., & Baker, S.P. (1981). Injury control. In D. Clark & B. MacMahon (Eds.), *Preventive and community medicine* (pp. 109–140). Boston; Little, Brown.

Hartunian, N.S., Smart, C.N., & Thompson, M.S. (1981). *The incidence and economic costs of major health impairments.* Lexington, MA: Lexington Books.

Hazinkinski, M.F., Francescutti, L.H., Lapidus, G.D., Micik, S., & Rivara, F.P. (1993). Pediatric injury prevention. *Annals of Emergency Medicine, 22,* 456–467.

Hu, X., Wesson, D., Parkin, P.C., Chipman, M.L., & Spence, L.J. (1994). Current bicycle helmet ownership, use and related factors among school-aged children in metropolitan Toronto. *Canadian Journal of Public Health, 85,* 121–124.

Insurance Institute for Highway Safety. (1991). *Fatality facts, 1991 edition.* Arlington, VA: Author.

Irwin, C.E., Cataldo, M.F., Matheny, A.P., & Peterson, L. (1992). Health consequences of behaviors: Injury as a model. *Pediatrics, 90,* 798–807.

Jones, C.S., King, W., Poteet-Johnson, D., & Wang, M.Q. (1993). Prevention of bicycle-related injuries in childhood: Role of the caregiver. *Southern Medical Journal, 86,* 859–864.

Jones, N.E. (1992). Prevention of childhood injuries part II: Recreational injuries. *Pediatric Nursing, 18,* 619–621.

Koop, C.E., & Lundberg, G.D. (1992). Violence in America: A public health emergency: Time to bite the bullet back. *Journal of American Medical Association, 267,* 3075–3076.

Losh, D.P. (1994). Injury prevention in children. *Primary Care, 21,* 733–746.

MacKenzie, E.J. (1984). Injury severity scales; Overview and directions for future research. *American Journal of Emergency Medicine, 2*(6), 537–549.

MacKenzie, E.J., Shapiro, S., & Eastham, J.N. (1985). The Abbreviated Injury Scale and Injury Severity Score; Levels of inter- and intrarater reliability. *Medical Care, 23,* 823–835.

Manary, M.J., & Hollifield, W.C. (1993). Childhood sledding injuries in 1990–1991. *Pediatric Emergency Care, 9,* 155–158.

Martin, V., Langley, B., & Coffman, S. (1995). Patterns of injury in pediatric patients in one Florida community and implications for prevention programs. *Journal of Emergency Nursing, 21,* 12–16.

Matheny, A.P. (1987). Psychological characteristics of childhood accidents. *Journal of Social Issues, 43,* 45–60.

McLoughlin, E., & McGuire, A. (1990). The causes, cost, and prevention of childhood burn injuries. *American Journal of Diseases of Children. 144*(6), 677–683.

Mori, L., & Peterson, L. (1986). Training preschoolers in home safety skills to prevent inadvertent injury. *Journal of Clinical Child Psychology, 15*(2), 106–114.

National Committee for Injury Prevention and Control. (1989). *Injury prevention: Meeting the challenge.* New York: Oxford University Press.

Patterson, R.F. (Ed.). (1989). *Webster's Dictionary and Thesaurus.* Miami, FL: P.S.I.

Peterson, L. (1984). Teaching home safety and survival skills to latch-key children; A comparison of two manuals and methods. *Journal of Applied Behavior Analysis, 17*(3), 279–293.

Peterson, L., & Brown, D. (1994). Integrating child injury and abuse-neglect research: Common histories, etiologies, and solutions. *Psychological Bulletin, 116*(2), 293–315.

Peterson, L., & Cook, S. (1993). Preventing children's injuries. In R.O. Brinkman & L.L. Mullins (Eds.), *Problems in pediatric psychology* (pp. 304–313). New York: Springer.

Peterson, L., & Mori, L. (1985). Prevention of child injury: An overview of targets, methods, and tactics for psychologists. *Journal of Consulting and Clinical Psychology, 53,* 586–595.

Peterson, L., & Oliver, K. (1995). Prevention of injuries and diseases. In M.C. Roberts (Ed.), *Handbook of pediatric psychology* (pp. 185–199). New York: Guilford.

Peterson, L., & Roberts, M.C. (1992). Complacency, misdirection, and effective prevention of children's injuries. *American Psychologist, 47,* 1040–1044.

Peterson, L., & Saldana, L. (1996). Accelerating children's risk for injury: Mother's decisions regarding common safety rules. *Journal of Behavioral Medicine, 19*(4), 317–331.

Peterson, L., & Schick, B. (1993). Empirically derived injury prevention rules. *Journal of Applied Behavior Analysis, 26,* 451–460.

Peterson, L., & Thiele, C. (1988). Home safety at school. *Child and Family Behavior Therapy, 10*(1), 1–8.

Peterson, L., Mori, L., & Scissors, C. (1986). Mom or dad says I shouldn't: Supervised and unsupervised children's knowledge of their parents' rules for home safety. *Journal of Pediatric Psychology, 11,* 177–188.

Peterson, L., Farmer, J., & Mori, L. (1987). Process analysis of injury situations: A complement to epidemiological methods. *Journal of Social Issues, 43,* 33–44.

Peterson, L., Farmer, J., & Kashani, J.H. (1990). Parental injury prevention endeavors: A function of health beliefs? *Health Psychology, 9,* 177–191.

Peterson, L., Harbeck, C., & Moreno, A. (1993). Measures of children's injuries: Self-reported versus maternal-reported events with temporally proximal versus delayed reporting. *Journal of Pediatric Psychology, 18,* 133–147.

Peterson, L., Zink, M., & Downing, J. (1993). Childhood injury prevention. In D. Glenwick & L. Jason (Eds.), *Promoting health and mental health in children, youth, and families* (pp. 51–74). New York: Springer.

Peterson, L., Brazeal, T.J., Oliver, K.K., & Bull, C.A. (in press). Gender and developmental patterns of affect, belief, and behavior in stimulated injury events. *Journal of Applied Developmental Psychology.*

Peterson, L., Gillies, R., Cook, S.C., Schick, B., & Little, T. (1994). Developmental patterns of expected consequences for simulated bicycle injury events. *Health Psychology, 13,* 218–223.

Peterson, L., Bartelstone, J., Kern, T., & Gillies, R. (1995). Parent's socialization of children's injury prevention. *Child Development, 66,* 224–235.

Peterson, L., Brown, D., Bartelstone, J., & Kern, T. (1996). Methodological consideration in participant event monitoring of low baserate events in health psychology: Children's injuries as a model. *Health Psychology, 15,* 124–130.

Peterson, L., Saldana, L., & Heiblum, N. (1996). Quantifying tissue damage from childhood injury: The Minor Injury Severity Scale (MISS). *Journal of Pediatric Psychology, 21*(2), 251–267.

Peterson, L., Saldana, L., & Schaeffer, C. (1997). Maternal intervention strategies in effecting children's bicycle helmet use. *Journal of Health Psychology, 2*(2), 225–330.

Petrucelli, E. (1981). *The Abbreviated Injury Scale (AIS)—Ten years of progress* (Technical Publication No. 810212). Warrendale, PA: Society of Automotive Engineers.

Puczynski, M., & Marshall, D.A. (1992). Helmets! All the pros wear them. *Journal of Diseases of Children, 146,* 1465–1467.

Rice, D.P., MacKenzie, E.J., Jones, A.S., Kaufman, S.R., deLissovoy, G.V., Max, W., McLoughlin, E., Miller, T.R., Robertson, L.S., Salkever, D.S., & Smith, G.S. (1989). *Cost of injury in the United States: A report to congress.* San Francisco: Johns Hopkins University.

Rivara, F.P. (1985). Traumatic deaths of children in the United States: Currently available prevention strategies. *Pediatrics, 75,* 456–462.

Rivara, F.P. (1990). Child pedestrian injuries in the United States. *American Journal of Children, 144*(6), 692–696.

Rivara, F.P., & Mueller, B.A. (1987). The epidemiology and causes of childhood injuries. *Journal of Social Issues, 43,* 13–31.

Rivara, F.P., Bergman, A.B., LoGerfo, J., & Weiss, N.S. (1982). Epidemiology of childhood injuries: II. Sex differences in injury rates. *American Journal of Diseases of Children, 136,* 502–506.

Rivara, F.P., Calonge, N., & Thompson, R.S. (1989). Population-based study of intentional injury incidence and impact during childhood. *American Journal of Public Health, 79,* 990–994.

Roberts, M.C., & Brooks, P.H. (1987). Children's injuries: Issues in prevention and public policy. *Journal of Social Issues, 43,* 1–12.

Roberts, M.C., & Turner, D.S. (1986). Rewarding parents for their children's use of safety seats. *Journal of Pediatric Psychology, 11,* 25–36.

Robertson, L.S. (1983). *Injuries.* Lexington, MA: Lexington Books.

Rodriguez, J.G. (1990). Childhood injuries in the United States: A priority issue. *American Journal of Diseases of Children, 144*(6), 625–626.

Rosenberg, M.L., Rodriguez, J.G., & Chorba, T.L. (1990). Childhood injuries: Where we are. *Pediatrics* (Supplement) *86,* 1084–1091.

Russell, K.M. (1991). Development of an instrument to assess maternal childhood injury health beliefs and social influence. *Issues in Comprehensive Pediatric Nursing, 14,* 163–177.

Sacks, J.J., Holmgreen, P., Smith, S.M., & Sosin, D.M. (1991). Bicycle-associated head injuries and deaths in the United States from 1984 through 1988: How many are preventable? *Journal of the American Medical Association, 266,* 3016–3018.

Scheidt, P.C. (1988). Behavioral research toward prevention of childhood injury. *American Journal of Diseases of Children, 142,* 612–617.

Schneider, M.L., Ituarte, P., & Stokols, D. (1993). Evaluation of a community bicycle helmet promotion campaign; What works and why. *American Journal of Health and Promotion, 7,* 281–287.

Selbst, S.M., Baker, D., & Shames, M. (1990). Bunk bed injuries. *American Journal of Diseases of Children, 144*(6), 721–723.

Teasdale, G., & Jennett, B. (1974). Assessment of coma and impaired consciousness. *Lancet, 2,* 81–84.

Thompson, D.C., Thompson, R.S., & Rivara, F.P. (1990). Incidence of bicycle-related injuries in a defined population. *American Journal of Public Health, 80,* 1388–1390.

Thompson, R.S., Rivara, F.P., & Thompson, D.C. (1989). A case-control study of the effectiveness of bicycle safety helmets. *New England Journal of Medicine, 320,* 1361–1367.

U.S. Department of Health and Human Services, Health Care Financing Administration. (1989). *The International Classification of Diseases, 9th revision, clinical modification.* Washington, DC: U.S. Government Printing Office.

Walton, W.W. (1982). An evaluation of the Poison Prevention Packaging Act. *Pediatrics, 69,* 363–370.

Williams, A.F. (1976). Observed child restraint use in automobiles. *American Journal of Diseases of Children, 130,* 1311–1317.

Wintemute, G.J. (1990). Childhood drowning and near-drowning in the United States. *American Journal of Diseases of Children, 144*(6), 663–669.

Wortel, E., & de Geus, G.H. (1993). Prevention of home related injuries of pre-school children: Safety measures taken by mothers. *Health Education Research, 8,* 217–231.

Zavoski, R., Lapidus, G., Lerer, T., & Banco, L. (1995). Bicycle injury in Connecticut. *Connecticut Medicine, 59,* 3–9.

Zins, J.E., Garcia, V.F., Tuchfarber, B.S., Clark, K.M., & Laurence, S.C. (1994). Preventing injury in children and adolescents. In R.J. Simeonsson (Ed.), *Risk, resilience and prevevention: Promoting the well-being of all children* (pp. 183–201). Baltimore: Paul H. Brooks.

Bibliography

Baker, S.P., O'Neill, B., Ginsburg, M.J., & Li, G. (1992). *The injury fact book* (2nd ed.). New York: Oxford University Press.

Finney, J.W., Christophersen, E.R., Friman, P.C., Kalnins, I.V., Maddux, J.E, Peterson, L., Roberts, M.C., & Wolraich, M. (1993). Society of Pediatric Psychology Task Force report: Pediatric psychology and injury control. *Journal of Pediatric Psychology, 18,* 499–426.

Peterson, L., & Roberts, M.C. (1992). Complacency, misdirection, and effective prevention of children's injuries. *American Psychologist, 47,* 1040–1044.

Roberts, M.C., & Brooks, P.H. (1987). Children's injuries: Issues in prevention and public policy. *Journal of Social Issues, 43,* 1–12.

Wilson, M.H., Baker, S.P., Teret, S.P., Shock, S., & Garbarino, J. (Eds.). (1991). *Saving children.* New York: Oxford University Press.

13

Elimination Disorders in Children

PATRICK C. FRIMAN AND KEVIN M. JONES

General Introduction

This chapter will discuss enuresis and encopresis, the two most commonly occurring elimination disorders in children. Although the primary clinical features of both disorders are medical/organic, a fusion of medical, psychological, and behavioral literature supports biobehavioral methods of assessment and treatment as state of the art. For many years, the interpretation and treatment of both problems was governed primarily by a psychological perspective. This perspective shifted with respect to imputation of personal responsibility. Elimination disorders were initially perceived as volitional acts occurring as a function of character defect; thus, treatment tended to be highly punitive (Glicklich, 1951; Levine, 1982). Although a cultural residue of this early characterological perspective remains (i.e., children are still frequently punished for urinary and fecal accidents), toward the middle of this century the characterological position was superseded by a psychopathological perspective. This position lifted the emphasis on volition and personal responsibility and instead emphasized variables such as aberrant family dynamics and toilet training practices and their potentially maladaptive influence on subsequent psychic development (Sperling, 1982; Warson, Caldwell, Warinner, & Kirk, 1954). In the past two decades, the strictly psychopatho-

logical perspective has shifted to the aforementioned biobehavioral perspective (Friman, 1986, 1995; Friman & Chrisophersen, 1986; Houts, 1991; Levine, 1982; Mellon & Houts, 1995; Warzak & Friman, 1994). Our approach to assessment and treatment will be guided by that perspective.

This chapter will primarily address nocturnal enuresis and retentive encopresis, with less extensive discussions of diurnal or mixed enuresis and nonretentive encopresis. Primary topics are divided into the following sections: introduction, problem identification, problem analysis, plan implementation, and plan evaluation. Our intent is to inform potential treatment providers about the current literature on each of these topics, with optimal treatment planning as the overarching goal.

Nocturnal Enuresis

Introduction

Nocturnal enuresis is one of the most prevalent and persistent sleep disturbances in children. Despite extensive clinical research many enuretic children in the United States remain untreated, mistreated, or treated ineffectively (Foxman, Valdez, & Brook, 1986; Shelov, Gundy & Weiss, 1981). For example, surveys suggest many parents use punishment and/or fluid restriction to treat their children's enuresis (Shelov et al., 1981), while many primary care physicians recommend drug treatment or no treatment at all (Foxman et al., 1986). Effective behavioral alternatives are available but they are prescribed infrequently by physicians, who typically prefer drug treatments.

PATRICK C. FRIMAN • Father Flanagan's Boys' Home, Boys Town, Nebraska 68010; and Creighton University School of Medicine, Omaha, Nebraska 68178-0001.   KEVIN M. JONES • Father Flanagan's Boys' Home, Boys Town, Nebraska 68010.

Handbook of Child Behavior Therapy, edited by Watson and Gresham. Plenum Press, New York, 1998.

Defining Characteristics

Criteria for including children in enuretic study groups has varied widely in the past three decades. The current criteria for enuresis from *DSM-IV* (American Psychiatric Association, 1994) are (a) repeated urination into bed or clothing; (b) at least two occurrences per week for at least three months or a sufficient number of occurrences to cause clinically significant distress; (c) chronological age of five or, for children with developmental delays, a mental age of at least five; (d) not due exclusively to the direct effects of a substance (e.g., diuretics) or a general medical condition (e.g., diabetes).

There are three subtypes of enuresis: nocturnal only, diurnal only, and mixed nocturnal and diurnal. There are two courses: primary and secondary. The primary course includes children who have never established continence and the secondary course involves children who, after establishing continence for at least six months, resume having accidents.

Physiology of the Bladder and Continence Skills

The bladder (detrusor) is the central component in a complex set of physiological systems that govern urination. A comprehensive review of these systems is far beyond the scope of this chapter (for more thorough discussions see Muellner, 1951, 1960, 1961; Vincent, 1974). However, a rudimentary description of the systems is necessary to underscore the logic behind treatment approaches for enuresis. The bladder is an elastic hollow organ resembling an upside-down balloon with a long narrow neck; it has two primarily mechanical functions: storage and release of urine (Vincent, 1974). Extended storage and volitional release are the defining properties of urinary continence. The body of the bladder is composed of smooth muscle and its nerve supply is autonomic. Thus, it cannot be directly controlled by volitional maneuvers—that is, one cannot "will" the bladder to contract or relax.

Fortunately, there are components of the urogenital system (other than the bladder itself) that can be volitionally controlled to establish continence. These involve three large muscle groups: the thoracic diaphragm, the lower abdominal musculature, and the pubococcygeus (anterior end of the levator ani) (Muellner, 1951, 1960, 1961). Deliberate urination at all levels of bladder filling involves a coordination of these three groups resulting in intra-abdominal pressure directed to the bladder neck. This coordinated action lowers the bladder neck, and results in reflexive contractions of the bladder body, opening of the internal and external sphincters, and bladder emptying.

Urine retention generally involves an obverse of the process described above. That is, except during imminent or actual urination, pelvic floor muscles remain in a state of tonus, or involuntary partial contraction, which maintains the bladder neck in an elevated position and sphincter muscles closed (Vincent, 1974). Even after initiation of urination has begun, contraction of the pelvic floor muscles can abruptly raise the bladder neck and terminate urination, but this requires some training and concentrated effort. Thus, the voluntary components of the bladder system can be used to "trigger" the involuntary components to achieve urination or continence.

Establishing nocturnal continence involves a sequence of continence skills, including detection of the impulse to urinate concurrent with bladder filling, and inhibiting actual and impending urination while asleep. Mastery of continence skills requires abundant practice, especially for enuretic children.

Prevalence

Research from several countries suggests nocturnal enuresis is most prevalent in the United States (Gross & Dornbusch, 1983). The National Health Examination Survey reported as many as 25% of boys and 15% of girls were enuretic at age 6, with as many as 8% of boys and 4% of girls still enuretic at age 12 (Gross & Dornbusch, 1983; see also Foxman et al., 1986). Prevalence studies from outside the United States, although more conservative, indicate at least 7% of all 8-year-old children wet their beds, with an approximate two-to-one ratio of boys over girls (Verhulst et al., 1985; see reviews by De Jong, 1973; Mellon & Houts, 1995). Estimates of the percentage of children with nocturnal enuresis whose condition is primary range from 80% (Mellon & Houts, 1995) to 90% (Scharf & Jennings, 1988).

Etiology

Enuresis has a heterogenous clinical presentation, which makes establishing its etiology a complex affair. Not only are its initiating causes and maintaining variables also heterogenous and thus different from child to child, but they can actually differ within the same child at different points in time (D.M. Fielding & Doleys, 1988; MacKeith, 1968). The most prominent causal factors in the literature on etiology for nocturnal enuresis are family history, maturation, functional bladder capacity, sleep dynamics, physical pathology, psychopathology, and nocturnal polyuria.

Family History

Family history is the most consistently supported etiological variable. The research shows that the probability of enuresis increases as a function of closeness or number of blood relations with a positive history (Bakwin, 1971, 1973; Hallgren, 1957; Kaffman & Elizur, 1977). These findings suggest a genetic linkage which some theorists argue against, suggesting that families convey tolerant attitudes toward bed-wetting, not enuretic "genes" (Kanner, 1972). But, even in settings where family custom plays a minimal role in child development (such as the Israeli kibbutzim) a high correlation between family history and enuresis in children exists (Kaffman & Elizur, 1977).

Maturation

The possibility of a genetic connection suggests a biologic factor, the identity of which is still unclear, but the evidence points to maturational lag (Scharf & Jennings, 1988). For example, children with decreased developmental scores at the ages of one and three years are significantly more likely to develop enuresis than are children with higher scores (Fergusson, Horwood, & Sannon, 1986). There is also an inverse relationship between birth weight and enuresis at any age. Enuretic children tend to lag slightly behind their nonenuretic peers in Tanner sexual maturation scores, bone growth, and height (Gross & Dornbusch, 1983). The increased prevalence of enuresis in boys also suggests maturation lag because boys generally have a slower rate of development than girls throughout childhood and adolescence (Fergusson et al., 1986; Gross & Dornbusch, 1983; Verhulst et al., 1985). Finally, enuretic children exhibit a 15% annual spontaneous remission rate, which is consistent with the notion that

they are lagging behind in the acquisition of continence, a developmental milestone for all children (Forsythe & Redmond, 1974). Despite the apparent maturational lag in many (perhaps most) enuretic children, their scores on standardized intelligence tests are in the average range (Gross & Dornbusch, 1983). Thus, the maturational lag appears more anatomical and/or physiological than intellectual and its cardinal expression is reduced bladder control (Barbour, Borland, Boyd, Miller, & Oppe', 1963; Gross & Dornbusch, 1983; Muellner, 1960, 1961).

Functional Bladder Capacity (FBC)

FBC refers to voiding capacity as distinguished from true bladder capacity (TBC), which refers to bladder structure (Troup & Hodgson, 1971). FBC is established in various ways, examples of which include the higher volume in either of the first two voidings after ingestion of a specified water load (e.g., 30 ml/kg body weight) (Starfield, 1967; Zaleski, Gerrard, & Shokeir, 1973), the average of all voidings in 24 hours (Hauri, 1982), or the average of all voidings in one week (Zaleski et al., 1973). The research suggests that the FBC of enuretic children is generally lower than that of their nonenuretic siblings (Starfield, 1967) and peers (Muellner, 1961; Starfield, 1967; Troup & Hodgson, 1971; Zaleski et al., 1973) but their TBC is about the same (Troup & Hodgson, 1971). Overall, the research on FBC suggests that many enuretic children urinate more frequently with less volume than do their nonenuretic peers and siblings. Their urinary pattern can be compared to that found in infants and very young children (Muellner, 1960, 1961).

Sleep Dynamics

Enuresis is regarded as a parasomnia by most sleep researchers (Ferber, 1985, 1989; Hauri, 1982), as a manifestation of sleep disturbance by some sleep researchers (Broughton, 1968), and as an outcome of deep sleep by most parents (Shelov et al., 1981). Still, sleep dynamics have not been established as a cause of enuresis. Wetting episodes occur in all stages of nonrapid eye movement (NREM) sleep and the probability of their occurrence appears to be a function of the amount of time spent in each stage (Ferber, 1989; Mikkelson & Rapoport, 1980).

Enuretic episodes also rarely occur during REM sleep, therefore thematically related dreams (e.g., dreaming of urinating) may be a result rather than a cause of wetting (Hauri, 1982; Perlmutter, 1985).

A final issue pertaining to sleep involves whether enuretic children are more difficult to awaken than their nonenuretic peers. Generally, findings from early related studies were mixed (Bostock, 1958; Boyd, 1960; Finley & Wansley, 1977; G.C. Young & Morgan, 1973). In addition to equivocal findings, the early research is limited because it did not establish sleep depth at the time of attempted awakening. Recent research with 15 enuretic boys and 18 controls resolved this problem by employing sleep EEGs and auditory tones delivered via earphones. During 512 arousal attempts, enuretic children awoke 8.5% of the time compared to 39.6% of the time for controls (Gellis, 1994). Thus, the common parental complaint about bedwetting children who are difficult to awaken may have an empirical basis.

Pathophysiology

There are numerous well-known potential physiopathologic causes of enuresis. These include urinary tract infection, urinary tract anomaly, bladder instability, occult spina bifida, epilepsy, diabetes mellitus, and sleep apnea. Most of these causes can be ruled out by complete history, physical exam, and urinalysis. When unanswered questions remain, other, more elaborate, laboratory examinations such as voiding cystourethrogram or polysomnographic evaluation are available (Ferber, 1989; Gross & Dornbusch, 1983; Perlmutter, 1985).

Psychopathology

Although vestiges of the once prominent (if not dominant) position that enuresis was a function of underlying psychopathology remain (Mishne, 1993; Sperling, 1982), the majority position appears to be that psychopathology is not a causal variable for primary enuresis (Couchells, Bennet-Johnson, & Carter, 1981; Ferber, 1985, 1989; Fergusson et. al., 1986; Friman, 1986, 1991, 1995; Moffat, Kato, & Pless, 1987; Scharf & Jennings, 1988; Schmitt, 1984; Shaffer, 1973; Werry & Cohrssen, 1965). Although some studies suggest that enuretic children exhibit anxiety and/or problematic conduct

(Couchells et al., 1981; Shaffer, 1973), the research (Morgan & Young, 1975; Werry & Cohrssen, 1965) and the prevailing position in the literature is that these symptoms are more likely a result than a cause of enuresis (Ferber, 1985, 1989; Friman & Christophersen, 1986; Friman, 1986, 1995; Friman & Warzak, 1990; Schmitt, 1984). Moreover, recent longitudinal research showing that maturational variables were predictive of enuresis also showed that psychosocial variables such as emotional disposition were not predictive of enuresis (Fergusson et al., 1986). If the underlying cause of enuresis were psychopathology, then eliminating only the wetting would presumably give rise to other expressions of the pathology. Yet symptom substitution does not occur following successful nonpsychiatric treatment of enuresis (Werry & Cohrssen, 1965). In fact, enuretic children successfully treated with conditioning therapy actually exhibit improvement in psychological status (Moffat et al., 1987).

A possible exception to the preceding involves increased emotional problems in a subsection of children with secondary enuresis (Shaffer, 1973). First, as noted in the physiology section, continence involves skilled practice and necessary skills can be lost, regained, and even lost again. Thus, secondary enuresis, by itself, does not indicate presence of emotional problems. But life stressors (e.g., loss of parent, moving, academic failure) may result in various types of temporary skill loss, including loss of continence skills (Muellner, 1960). These stressors and their accompanying upsets do not necessarily lead to pathological dysfunction (Jarvelin, Moilanen, Vikevainen-Tervonen, & Huttunen, 1990). If enuresis is a side effect of serious psychopathology or if it is secondary to traumatic stress, it is unlikely to be subtle enough to elude a clinically astute therapist.

Nocturnal Polyuria

The presence of antidiuretic hormone (ADH), or arginine vasopression, causes the kidneys to increase the osmality (or concentration) of urine (by increasing reabsorption of free water in the renal-collecting duct). Theoretically, serum ADH levels increase at night and thereby protect sleep from urinary urgency and facilitate nocturnal continence. Recent research has shown that a subset of enuretic children do not exhibit the normal diurnal rhythm of ADH secretion and perhaps wet their beds as a result of increased urine production while sleeping (Norgaard, Pedersen, & Djurhuus, 1985; Rittig, Knudsen, Norgaard, Pedersen, & Djurhuus, 1989). Earlier (and subsequent) related research showed that desmopressin (DDAVP), an intranasally administered vasopressin analogue, reduced nocturnal enuretic episodes in children (e.g., Dimson, 1977; and see DDAVP in the treatment section). Whether the effectiveness of DDAVP is due to restoration of insufficient nocturnal ADH or is merely the result of decreased urine production and thus independent of a primary causal variable is not established (Houts, 1991; Key, Bloom, & Sanvordenker, 1992). Support for decreased nocturnal ADH as a primary causal variable is limited for several reasons. First, the sample sizes in related studies have been small (Norgaard et al., 1985; Rittig et al., 1989). Second, fewer than one quarter of treated children achieve short-term dryness (Moffat, Harlos, Kirshen, & Burd, 1993). Third, not all children with known urine concentrating problems wet the bed (e.g., only 50% of children with sickle cell anemia are enuretic). Finally, lower ADH is not linked in any empirical way to a reason for children's not awakening to full bladders. Furthermore, many persons (children and adults alike) sleep through the night when their bladders are full and still do not wet their beds. In conclusion, nocturnal enuresis is multiply determined and abnormality in nocturnal ADH secretion is only one of several possible causal possibilities.

Problem Identification

The initial stage of an enuresis evaluation should contain a "go no further" maxim. That is, once a history has been obtained and preliminary information about enuresis has been shared with the parents and child, the therapist should go no further with direct treatment until a medical examination has been obtained. As indicated in the etiology section, any of a number of pathophysiological variables can cause enuresis and, although these are rare, they are nonetheless a possibility and must be ruled out medically before a primary treatment plan is implemented (Cohen, 1975; D.M. Fielding & Doleys, 1988; Friman, 1986, 1995; Gross & Dornbusch, 1983; Mellon & Houts, 1995; Schmitt, 1984).

This emphasis on initial medical examination should not be construed as delimiting the role of the behavior therapist. The examination is but one of a constellation of therapeutic maneuvers necessary for effective management of enuresis, most of which are implemented by the therapist.

Treatment of enuresis is approached both directly and indirectly, and the go no further clause is pertinent only for direct treatment. Thus, the evaluation process is actually the first stage of treatment, albeit indirect. The parents and child will most likely have contended unsuccessfully with enuresis for some time and thus it is likely to seem beyond their control. In addition, because a residue of characterological and psychopathological interpretations of enuresis still exist in Western culture, it is possible that the parents and the child will have misinterpreted the problem. In the initial evaluation, the therapist can introduce optimism about management and disabuse parents and child of notions about enuresis leading to blaming or shaming the child (or a parent).

While taking the history, the therapist should include questions derived from the sections on defining characteristics (e.g., primary vs. secondary) and etiological factors mentioned previously (e.g., family history of enuresis, disease history, mental health history). Some screening for mental health problems should be included (e.g., behavior checklists, related inquiry). As indicated above, mental health problems do not appear to have a direct forward causal relationship with enuresis (i.e., they are much more likely to be caused by, rather than to cause, enuresis). However, if the patient presents with mental health problems, these should be addressed in the ultimate treatment plan.

Problem Analysis

After evaluating medical and psychological complications, the evaluation should address three important topics. First, the therapist should probe all aspects of the child's life to determine sources of punishment for wetting and take steps to eliminate them. This can be done directly, by warning parents away from punishment, and indirectly, by demonstrating logically that the problem is a skills deficit. Second, the therapist should assess the motivational level and the availability of social resources for the parents. If the parent is minimally motivated and/or has few social resources (e.g., single working parent), the number of treatment maneuvers they will be able to implement will likely be limited. Third, the therapist should assess the motivation of the child. As will be seen in the treatment section, optimal treatment plans include many components and require compliance from the child for completion of most steps. An unmotivated or noncompliant child would be difficult to treat with any method known to cure enuresis. Fortunately, enuresis itself contributes to the motivation of the child. As the quantity of pleasant experiences missed (e.g., sleepovers, camp) and unpleasant experiences encountered (e.g., social detection, embarassment) accumulate, motivation will likely increase as well. Therefore, if a child appears unmotivated and the case is medically and psychologically uncomplicated, the best approach may be to request that the parents return to clinic for reevaluation in three months.

Evaluation should include a period of 10 to 15 days during which bedwetting episodes are monitored. A convenient monitoring procedure utilizes a standard monthly calendar; each morning the parent marks a "D" if the bed is dry and a "W" if bedwetting occurred. These data may be used to establish baseline levels and to evaluate treatment effects.

Plan Implementation

The treatment of enuresis is even more heterogenous than are its clinical manifestations or its etiology. In fact, the range of treatments described in the literature is too extensive to review here. Instead, the following discussion focuses on the two major empirically derived approaches to treatment, medication and skills training, and the major subcomponents of each.

Medication

Surveys (Foxman et al., 1986) substantiate what much of the literature on enuresis suggests that physicians prescribe drug therapy for enuresis more frequently than any other treatment (Blackwell & Currah, 1973; Cohen, 1975; Fergusson et al., 1986; Friman, 1986, 1995; Friman & Chris-

tophersen, 1986; Rauber & Maroncelli, 1984). A broad spectrum of drugs have been prescribed for enuresis but two types comprise the majority of current prescriptions: antidepressants and antidiuretics.

Tricyclic Antidepressants

Historically, tricyclic antidepressants were the drugs of choice for treatment of enuresis and imipramine was the most frequently prescribed drug treatment (Blackwell & Currah, 1973; Foxman et al., 1986; Rauber & Maroncelli, 1984; Stephenson, 1979). The mechanism by which imipramine reduces bed-wetting is still, for the most part, unknown (Stephenson, 1979). Most experts now agree its antidepressant and sleep effects are not the significant mechanisms leading to a decrease in wetting. A review and synthesis of the research on mechanisms is beyond the scope of this paper. It is important to know, however, that imipramine somehow reduces premature contractions of the detrusor following partial filling of the bladder and thereby increases functional bladder capacity (Stephenson, 1979).

Imipramine, in doses between 25 and 75 mg given at bedtime, produces initial reductions in wetting in a majority of children, often within the first week of treatment (Blackwell & Currah, 1973). The primary therapeutic gain from imipramine, however, appears to be the respite from wetting obtained while the child is on the drug. Reviews of both short- and long-term studies show enuresis usually recurs when tricyclic therapeutic agents are withdrawn (Ambrosini, 1984). The permanent cure produced with imipramine is only 25% (ranging from 5% to 40%) (Blackwell & Currah, 1973; Houts, Berman, & Abramson, 1994). Subtracting the annual spontaneous remission rate of 15% (Forsythe & Redmond, 1974) leaves only about a 10% increment in cure rate using this medication. Thus, imipramine is superior to no treatment or to placebo, but not by much.

Furthermore, use of imipramine does not teach continence skills. In fact, by diminishing detrusor contractions it reduces opportunities for learning sensory awareness of those contractions and practice of needed responses. This reduced opportunity to learn may account for the high relapse rate following termination of the medication and for reports showing that drug regimens may impair subsequent continence skill training programs (Houts, Peterson, & Liebert, 1984). Finally, imipramine can cause several untoward side effects ranging in severity from excessive sweating, irritability, nausea, and vomiting to convulsions, collapse, coma, and death (Cohen, 1975; Friman & Christophersen, 1986; Friman, 1986; Friman & Warzak, 1990; Herson, Schmitt, & Rumack, 1979).

Given its low cure rate and high relapse rates, side effects, potential to diminish skill development, and potential toxicity, imipramine should not be used as a primary treatment for enuresis (Ferber, 1989; Friman & Christophersen, 1986; Friman, 1986, 1995; Friman & Warzak, 1990; Gross & Dornbusch, 1983; Herson et al., 1979; Scharf & Jennings, 1988). However, because its effects are seen so quickly (when they occur), it can be a valuable adjunct to treatment, especially when other methods are failing and a dry night is needed to heighten motivation, or when a child plans to attend camp or a sleepover (Friman, 1986, 1995; Friman & Christophersen, 1986; Friman & Warzak, 1990; Herson et al., 1979; Schmitt, 1984).

Antidiuretics

As described in the section on nocturnal polyuria, Norgaard and colleagues reported on a small number of enuretic children who had abnormal circadian patterns of plasma vasopressin concentration (Norgaard et al., 1985; Rittig et al., 1989). As a result of these reports and because of its known antidiuretic properties, DDAVP rapidly became a popular treatment for enuresis and it may now have displaced the tricyclics as the treatment most prescribed. DDAVP concentrates urine, thereby decreasing urine volume and intravesical pressure; this makes bladder neck descent and detrusor contraction less probable and nocturnal continence more probable. DDAVP also has fewer side effects than imipramine (Dimson, 1986; Ferrie, MacFarlane, & Glen, 1984; Norgaard et al., 1985; Novello & Novello, 1987; Pedersen, Hejl, & Kjoller, 1985; Post, Richman & Blackett, 1983). Recommended dosages are 10 to 20 μg taken at bedtime.

Research on DDAVP has yielded mixed results, with success in some studies (Dimson, 1986; Pederson et al., 1985; Post et al., 1983) but not in others (Ferrie et al., 1984; Scharf & Jennings,

1988). A recent review by Moffat and colleagues (1993) indicated that fewer than 25% of children become dry on the drug (a much larger percentage show some improvement) and, as with tricyclics, its effects appear to last only as long as the drug is taken and are less likely to occur in younger children or children who have frequent accidents (see also Houts et al., 1994; Pederson et al., 1985; Post et al., 1983). In addition, DDAVP is very expensive. Finally, because DDAVP reduces urine output, it also reduces opportunities to practice continence skills (similar to imipramine). Nonetheless, its treatment effects, when they occur, are as immediate as are those of imipramine but with fewer side effects. Thus, DDAVP may be preferable to imipramine as an adjunct to treatment.

Behavioral Treatment

Behavioral treatment requires more effort than drug treatment but it is safer, in terms of side effects, and more effective, in terms of higher cessation rates and lower relapse rates. Behavioral treatment is superior to drug treatment because the drugs used for enuresis cause changes in body chemistry and corresponding physiology that are impermanent—they last only as long as the drugs are in the system. Behavioral treatment, however, trains skills that are necessary for continence and these skills outlast the implementation of the methods employed to teach them in all children and are permanent in most. Initially, the provider should inform the child and parents that numerous other children, many probably in the child's neighborhood and school, also have enuresis. Then, with the child in attendance, the provider should tell the parents to avoid blaming or shaming the child for wetting. The provider should then enthusiastically solicit the child's cooperation in treatment and work with the child and family on a treatment plan. The following sections describe the most commonly used behavioral treatments for enuresis.

Urine Alarm

The alarm works using a moisture-sensitive switching system, the closing of which rings the alarm. Numerous safe, efficient, and effective alarms are available, many of which attach directly to the child's pajamas and thus increase the child's access to alarm feedback (Mountjoy, Ruben, & Bradford, 1984; Schmitt, 1984).

The mechanism of action in alarm treatment was initially described as classical conditioning, with the alarm as the unconditioned stimulus, bladder distension the conditioned stimulus, and waking as the conditioned response (Mowrer & Mowrer, 1938). More recent literature emphasizes a negative reinforcement or avoidance paradigm (Doleys, 1977; Perlmutter, 1985) in which the child awakens to the alarm, stops urinating and either completes urination in the toilet or holds urine until a more convenient time. Cures are obtained slowly, and during the first few weeks of alarm use the child often awakens only after voiding completely (Schmitt, 1984). The aversive properties of the alarm, however, inexorably strengthen the skills necessary to avoid it. These skills include sensory awareness of urinary need, waking to urinate, or exercising anatomical responses which offset urination.

Reports of controlled comparative trials show the alarm to be superior to imipramine (Wagner, Johnson, Walker, Carter, & Wittmer, 1982), DDAVP (Wille, 1986) and other skill-based methods (Fournier, Garfinkel, Bond, Beauchesne, & Shapiro, 1987). In fact, the literature has consistently described the urine alarm as the single most effective treatment for enuresis (Broughton, 1968; Cohen, 1975; Doleys, 1977; Ferber, 1985, 1989; Friman, 1986, 1995; Friman & Warzak, 1990; Gross & Dornbusch, 1983; Houts et al., 1994; Mikkelson & Rapoport, 1980; Novello & Novello, 1987; Perlmutter, 1985; Schmitt, 1984; Werry, 1966). Reviews of the literature show its success rate is higher (approximately 75%) and its relapse rate lower (approximately 41%) than any other drug or skill-based treatment (Doleys, 1977; Werry, 1966). Furthermore, when an intermittent alarm schedule is used (e.g., alarm rings after every other accident) the relapse rate can be as low as 17% (Doleys, 1977).

Retention Control Training (RCT)

The emergence of RCT followed the observation that many enuretic children had reduced functional bladder capacity (Muellner, 1960, 1961; Starfield, 1967). RCT expands functional bladder capacity by requiring children to drink extra fluids (e.g., 16 oz of water or juice) and delay urination as long as possible (Muellner, 1960, 1961; Starfield, 1967; Starfield & Mellits, 1968). In order to assess progress, an enuretic child's parents should set up a weekly game in which the child urinates in an appropriate container and tries to produce more urine than in previous weeks.

RCT is successful in as many as 50% of cases (Doleys, 1977; Starfield & Mellits, 1968) but it is not as effective as the urine alarm. This lesser effectiveness is not surprising, because RCT does not train nocturnal skills directly. It directly trains volume-control skills during the day and this indirectly affects nocturnal continence skills.

Kegel Exercises

Kegel exercises involve purposeful manipulation of the muscles necessary to prematurely terminate urination, or contraction of the muscles of the pelvic floor (Kegel, 1951; Muellner, 1960). Originally developed for stress incontinence in women (Kegel), a version of these exercises, stream interruption, has been used in enuresis treatment packages for years (Friman, 1986, 1995; Friman & Warzak, 1990; Scharf & Jennings, 1988; Schmitt, 1984). For children, stream interruption requires initiating and terminating urine flow during a urinary episode at least once a day. The use of stream interruption exercises in the treatment of enuresis is logical from a physiological perspective, because, as indicated in the physiology section, terminating an actual or impending urinary episode involves the same muscle systems. Thus, regular practice could increase a child's capacity to retain urine longer and could expedite attainment of continence. No evaluation of the effects of stream interruption has been reported. A recent study of Kegel exercises, however, showed their regular practice eliminated enuresis in 47 of 79 children with diurnal enuresis. Although stream interruption was used initially to train the appropriate muscle contractions, the exercises primarily consisted of dry contraction of pelvic musculature. Specifically, children were required to "hold" the contraction for 5 to 10 seconds, followed by a 5-second rest, at least 10 times on three separate occasions a day (Schneider, King, & Surwit, 1994). Of the 52 children who also wet at night, nocturnal episodes were eliminated in 18 and improved in 9 children. Thus, Kegel exercises may have a functional role in enuresis treatment.

Paired Association

Paired association involves pairing stream interruption (or Kegel exercises) with the urine alarm in a reinforcement paradigm. With stream interruption, the parent stands outside the bathroom door with the alarm while the child urinates. The parent sounds the alarm and the child practices stream interruption. With Kegel exercises the alarm could be used merely to cue the exercise. The parent praises and rewards accordingly. A more convenient version of this sequence involves making an audiotape of the alarm played intermittently; this would allow the child to practice alone with either stream interruption and/or Kegel exercises.

The paired association procedure has not yet been evaluated, but some basic literature supports its potential effectiveness. For example, sleeping persons can make discriminations between stimuli on the basis of meaningfulness and prior training (Oswald, Taylor, & Treisman, 1960) and the probability of a correct discrimination is significantly improved through contingent reinforcement (Zung & Wilson, 1961). Thus, reinforcing a relationship between stream interruption and the alarm while the child is awake may increase the probability that the child will interrupt urination in response to the alarm while asleep.

Waking Schedule

This treatment component involves waking the children and guiding them to the bathroom for urination. Results obtained are attributed to a change in arousal, increased access to the reinforcing properties of dry nights (Bollard & Nettlebeck, 1982), and urinary urge in lighter stages of sleep (Scharf & Jennings, 1988). In a representative study using a staggered waking schedule, four of nine children reduced their accidents to less than twice a week, suggesting a waking schedule may improve but is unlikely to cure enuresis (Creer & Davis, 1975). A less effortful schedule involves waking the children just before the parents go to bed and systematically

fading the schedule by waking them one-half hour earlier on nights following several successive dry nights (Bollard & Nettlebeck, 1982).

Visual Sequencing

This procedure involves mentally rehearsing nightime continence skills. Although its empirical support is still at the successful case-report stage, visual sequencing is often included in multicomponent treatment plans (Friman, 1995; Friman & Warzak, 1990; Scharf, 1986). The procedure involves visualization of either or both of the behavioral sequences leading to nocturnal continence. Both sequences include detection of urgency and contraction of the external urethral sphincter, with holding urine throughout the night in the first sequence and awakening to a dry bed in the second. The procedure can be taught in the office. The provider should ask the child to sit in a comfortable chair, take three to four deep breaths, close the eyes, and relax fully. The provider should then discuss each detail of what will happen during the night, while asking the child to focus on a mental picture of urge sensation, urge suppression, and waking up to a dry bed.

Reinforcement Systems

Reinforcement systems may not cure enuresis but they can sustain a child's motivation to participate in treatment, especially when the system reinforces success in small steps (Friman, 1986, 1995; Friman & Christophersen, 1986; Friman & Warzak, 1990). An example involves a dot-to-dot drawing and a grab bag (see Figure 1). The child identifies an affordable and desirable prize and the parent draws (or traces) a picture of it using a dot-to-dot format with every third or fourth dot bigger than the rest. The child then connects two dots for each dry night and when the line reaches a larger dot, they earn access to a grab bag with small rewards (e.g., small toys, edibles, money, privileges, special time with parents). When all the dots are connected, the child earns the prize (see Jenson & Sloane, 1979, for more details).

Responsibility Training

All of the skill-based components mentioned previously are designed to promote a mature void-

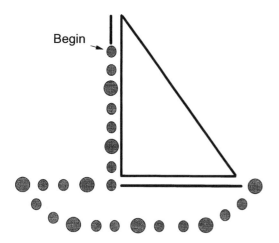

FIGURE 1. Sample Dot-to-Dot drawing of a toy sailboat for reinforcement-based training.

ing repertoire in the child. To be consistent with this design, the child should be treated in a way that promotes maturation (Ferber, 1985, 1989). For example, they should not be left in diapers at night. They should be assigned household responsibilities associated with their accidents. In younger children this may merely mean bringing their sheets to the laundry basket. In older children, however, it may mean actually laundering the sheets. These responsibilities should not be presented as a punishment but as a correlate of increased responsibility and a demonstration of the parent's confidence in and respect for their maturing child.

Plan Evaluation

Historically, the choice of treatment for enuresis was governed more by the desire to establish continence than by concern for the child's health and well-being. Fortunately, medical care for enuretic children has evolved substantially since that time. Nonetheless, the sustained reliance on drugs as a primary treatment, the abiding parental use of punishment, and the often excessive restriction on fluid intake still place the health and well-being of many enuretic children at risk. Treatments most likely to cure enuresis with minimal risk to child health are those which specifically teach continence skills. Because the probability for cure increases with the number of components included in the treatment plan (Bollard & Nettlebeck, 1982), it

is imperative that the therapist carefully address barriers to plan implementation.

Although the initial choice of components should be based on child maturation, child and parent willingness, and family resources, the components in the plan can be "titrated" over time in accord with family resources and motivation until cure is obtained. For example, a two-parent, one-wage-earner, middle-income family with a motivated 10-year-old bed-wetting child and at least one motivated parent could be given a waking schedule, a motivational system, and the alarm on the initial visit. Over the course of one or two additional visits, other skill-based treatment components could be added as needed, along with a small prescription of DDAVP or imipramine for sleepovers or camp-outs. Families with fewer resources and less motivation would be given fewer components. A single-parent, low-income family with a motivated 10-year-old child and a nonmotivated parent could be given urine retention and stream interruption. The chances for cure, other things being equal, are lower in the second case than in the first, but they are still higher than if no treatment were used. Furthermore, the active involvement of the child may lead to increased involvement by the parent, at which point the provider could add more components. Developing an effective skill-based treatment plan will require a substantial time investment for parents and child. The investment of that time, however, is more than offset by the substantial decrease in potential harm to the enuretic child and the increase in potential for eliminating the enuresis.

Diurnal Enuresis

Introduction

Diurnal enuresis is important for a number of reasons, one of which is psychological. In a survey of 20 potential fears completed by school children, "wetting pants in class" was third behind "losing a parent" and "going blind" (Ollendick, King, & Frary, 1989). The research on diurnal and mixed enuresis is much smaller (and the problems occur less frequently) and thus virtually all aspects of this problem are less understood. In fact, the *DSM-IV* criteria notwithstanding, no widely accepted definitional criteria exist for diurnal enuresis. Prevalence estimates for diurnal and mixed enuresis for both boys and girls at ages six and seven years range between 0.5% to 2% (Blomfield & Douglas, 1956; Hallgren, 1956a, b; see also Berk & Friman, 1990; D.M. Fielding & Doleys, 1988). Population figures on primary versus secondary diurnal enuresis are not established, but secondary diurnal enuresis is not rare (Van Gool & Jonge, 1989).

The pathophysiological etiology of diurnal enuresis can be grouped into bacteriuria (much more likely in girls), disease (e.g., diabetes), anatomical abnormalities (e.g., nephropathy), and functional abnormalities (e.g., unstable bladder). Although these conditions all may require behavioral interventions as part of a comprehensive treatment plan, the initial and primary management is medical. The class of diurnal enuresis for which primary management is behavioral (after all medical issues have been addressed or ruled out) has various labels (e.g., daytime dribbling; nonneuorgenic bladder) but the one we prefer to use is *urge incontinence* (Meadow, 1990; Van Gool & Jonge, 1989).

One of the key variables in the treatment of urge incontinence is similar to routine toilet training. It includes awareness of bladder distension and incipient or actual bladder neck descent (see section on physiology of bladder). This distension and/or descent gives rise to postural changes and limb movements suggestive of urinary urgency. The function of these movements appears to be maintenance of bladder neck ascent. For example, when children scissor their legs or compress their thighs the movements produce upward pressure in the perineal region that lifts the bladder neck and forestalls urination (D. Fielding, 1982; Muellner, 1960, 1961; Vincent, 1974). However, children are often unaware of these movements and their function. So, when parents advise their children to go the bathroom, based on observation of the movements, the children may appear unaware of the need to urinate. Routine aspects of parental teaching can be applied to help the child make the necessary connections, initially between body movements and need, and ultimately between bladder contraction and need, and thus enable the child to complete or forestall urination based on a plan.

A major factor inhibiting attainment of awareness and progress toward continence for these children is the limited capacity of their bladder to hold urine (D. Fielding, 1980, 1982; D.M. Fielding & Doleys, 1988). This limitation is primarily due to either functional capacity variables (as with nocturnal enuresis) or partial emptying. These children have poor control over their pelvic floor musculature and/or immature (oversensitive to filling) bladders. Behavior problems (e.g., noncompliance) may also have a role in the limited attainment of continence.

Little empirically derived information is available on behavioral treatment of diurnal enuresis, although recent studies have emerged. For example, two studies have employed the nocturnal urine alarm to heighten awareness of urge and thus treat daytime wetting (Friman & Vollmer, 1995; Halliday, Meadow, & Berg, 1987). Another recent study targeted increased control of pelvic floor musculature using Kegel exercises and eliminated daytime wetting for 44 of 79 children (Schneider et al., 1994).

Optimal Treatment Approach

The optimal approach to diurnal enuresis involves comprehensive assessment (medical and psychological). Medical conditions need to be ruled out initially and psychological complications (e.g., oppositional behavior) need to be addressed prior to behavioral intervention. Behavioral treatment should focus on training skills necessary for continence, including increased awareness and sufficient pelvic floor musculature. Reinforcement-based motivational systems such as the dot-to-dot game mentioned previously have rarely been investigated, but should be included to increase child motivation.

Functional Encopresis

Introduction

Functional encopresis is less prevalent than enuresis but, if untreated, is the more likely of the two conditions to lead to serious (and potentially life-threatening) medical sequelae and seriously impaired social acceptance, relations, and development. The reasons for the former will be described later. A primary reason for the latter is that soiling appears to evoke more revulsion and rejection by peers, parents, and important others. As recently as the late 19th century, influential medical experts recommended beatings for children with encopresis (Henoch, 1889). The professional approach to encopresis has evolved substantially since that time, but approaches by many laypersons are not keeping pace. The afflicted children are still frequently shamed, blamed, and punished for a condition over which they have little control (Levine, 1982; Pierce, 1985). For reasons that will become clear below, encopresis differs from enuresis in that physicians (especially pediatricians) are most likely to recommend an initial course of treatment that leads to cure (cf. Levine, 1982). The intention of this part of the chapter is to remedy that disparity for behavior therapists.

Defining Characteristics

Functional encopresis (encopresis) is a disorder without organic pathogenesis in which individuals either voluntarily or involuntarily pass feces into or onto an inappropriate location, usually their clothing (Wright, 1973). The current criteria from *DSM-IV* (American Psychiatric Association, 1994) are (a) inappropriate passage of feces at least once a month for at least three months; (b) chronological or developmentally equivalent age of four years; (c) not due exclusively to the direct physiological effects of a substance (e.g., laxatives) or a general medical condition except through a mechanism involving constipation. There are two subtypes: encopresis with and without constipation (and overflow incontinence).

Physiology of Bowel

The large intestine or colon is the distal end of the alimentary tract sequentially composed of the esophagus, stomach, biliary tract, and intestines, small and large. Although physiologically simpler than the bladder system, a thorough review of the colonic system is also beyond the scope of this chapter (for more thorough review see Whitehead & Schuster, 1985). Some rudimentary description of the system, however, is necessary to understand the logic of treatment. The colon is a tubular shaped organ that connects to the small intestine (via the ileum) from which it receives waste in liquid form. It is best understood in terms of its six components, the ascending, transverse, descending, and sigmoid colons, and the rectum and anus. It has three primary functions, fluid absorption, storage, and evacuation. Extended storage and planned evacuation are the defining features of fecal continence. Evacuation is achieved through a motor function called peristalsis, involving a wavelike motion of the colon walls. Retrograde peristalsis in the ascending colon keeps chyme in contact with the absorptive surface of the colon, turning liquid into semisolid waste which begins to move as it takes on mass. Movement occurs over an extended period and is potentiated by external events that instigate intracolonic dynamics. These events include motor activity (resulting in the orthocolonic reflex) and eating a meal (resulting in the gastrocolonic reflex).

Normally the rectum contains little or no feces, but when colonic movement causes contraction of the sigmoid colon, feces are propelled into the rectum and its distension stimulates sensory receptors in the rectal mucosa and in the muscles of the pelvic floor. This results in relaxation of the internal sphincter which allows bowel contents to contact more sensory receptors. The process is involuntary until rectal distension occurs, at which point the child can manipulate the external sphincter and use the same three muscle groups (diaphragm, abdominal musculature, levator ani) that instigate or forestall urination to instigate or forestall defecation. The push used to complete most bowel movements is called a Valsalva Maneuver, and it is physiologically and phenomenologically similar to the push needed to blow up a balloon or deliver a baby.

Prevalence

Estimates of the prevalence of encopresis vary from 1.5% to 5% of the pediatric population, depending on the source of the estimate. Encopresis comprised 1.5% of all pediatric referrals from an Israeli kibbutz (Lifshitz & Chovers, 1972) and 5% of all child psychiatric referrals from a Scandinavian province (Olatawuria, 1973). In a study of American pediatric patients, Levine (1975) found a 3% incidence of encopresis. Despite the higher incidence of encopresis found in psychiatric clinics, pediatricians probably encounter more encopretic children because of larger pediatric caseloads (Wright, Schaefer, & Solomons, 1979). Another factor that artificially lowers incidence statistics for the psychiatric and pediatric encopretic populations is parental reluctance to report, or parental ignorance of, the condition. Wright (1973) reported that most cases of encopresis are discovered during the assessment of other presenting problems. Therefore, encopresis may be a larger problem for pediatrics than the literature suggests.

Etiology

The literature is not clear on whether the causes of encopresis are more homogeneous than those of enuresis or simply that much less is known about the former. But between 80% and 95% of encopresis cases can be traced directly to stool retention (Levine, 1975; Wright et al., 1979). A smaller subset of encopretic children have either a true organic etiology (see pathophysiology section) or nonretentive encopresis. The latter group is composed of children with psychological complications (see psychopathology section).

Fecal retention and impaction. As indicated in the defining characteristics section, *DSM-IV* distinguishes between encopresis with and without constipation (retention). Although definitions for constipation vary, children who frequently go two or more days without a bowel movement are probably prone to constipation. A common complaint by parents of encopretic children is that their children deliberately soil their clothing (Wright et al., 1979) but this accusation is usually false (Levine, 1982). The primary cause of excess soiling is fecal retention, which in most cases is not the result of personality characteristics (e.g., stubbornness) but is the result of a constellation of factors, many of which are beyond a child's immediate control (Levine, 1982, 1983). These factors include a constitutional predisposition, diet, insufficient leverage for passage of hard stools, and occasional or frequent painful passage of hard stools (Christophersen, 1994). For some children, especially those with extreme constipation and/or treatment failure, there is an increased threshold of awareness of rectal distension, a possibly weak internal sphincter, and/or a tendency to contract the external sphincter during the act of defecation (Meunier, Marechal, & De Beaujeu, 1979; Loening-Baucke & Younoszai, 1982; Loening-Baucke & Cruikshank, 1986; Wald, Chandra, Chiponis, & Gabel, 1986). The combined effect of all these factors is a lowered probability of volun-

tary stool passage and a heightened probability of fecal retention.

Chronic fecal retention results in fecal impaction, which results in enlargement of the colon. Colon enlargement results in decreased motility of the bowel system and occasionally in involuntary passage of large stools and frequent soilings due to seepage of soft fecal matter. The seepage is often referred to as "paradoxical diarrhea" because the children retain large masses of stool and thus are functionally constipated, but their colon allows passage of soft stool around the mass, and this results in diarrhea (Christophersen, 1994; Levine, 1982).

That fecal impaction is related to encopresis has been established by several investigators, primary among whom are Davidson (1958), Levine (1975), and Wright (1973, 1975). All independently reported that 80% of their patients had fecal impaction accompanying fecal incontinence at the first clinic visit. Subsequent to his 1975 report, Levine and his colleagues developed a simple clinical procedure to identify fecal impactions from a KUB (x-ray of the lower abdomen including the kidneys, ureter, and bladder; Barr, Levine, Wilkinson, & Mulvihill, 1979). As a result of the improved diagnostic method, Levine revised his initial 80% estimate of fecal impaction's coexistence with fecal incontinence to 90% (Christophersen, 1994).

Pathophysiology. As with enuresis, there are known physiopathic causes of encopresis, although when differential defecation dynamics due to constipation are excluded, there are not as many. Various kinds of eccentric formations and locations of the anus can lead to encopresis, yet these are rare, readily detectable on physical exam, and require medical management (Hatch, 1988). The most likely differential diagnosis is Hirschsprung's disease, or congenital aganglionosis. Its incidence is approximately 1 in 25,000 and thus is rare. A comparison between encopresis and Hirschprung's disease across 16 different variables showed the two were distinct on all but one, prevalence of males (Levine, 1981). Thus, the clinical presentation itself should prevent the astute clinician from mistaking one for the other. The possible exception is "ultra short segment" Hirshsprung's disease, which has a more subtle clinical picture. However, the existence of this condition is controversial, and, even if it does exist, following the recommendations in the evaluation section should ensure that, in the unlikely event a behavior therapist encounters a case, appropriate workup and treatment do occur. There are several other pathophysiological conditions that involve encopresis (e.g., hypothyroidism, myelomeningocele) but their clinical presentations are well known and they are unlikely to be missed in routine medical workups.

Psychopathology. Historically, the role of behavioral and personality disturbance has been emphasized in the etiology and course of encopresis (cf. Wright et al., 1979). Yet three studies conducted in the late 1980s failed to confirm this position (Friman, Mathews, Finney, & Christophersen, 1988; Gabel, Hegedus, Wald, Chandra, & Chaponis, 1986; Loening-Bauke, Cruikshank, & Savage, 1987). Two studies found levels of behavioral problems higher than those of normal samples but still significantly lower than those of clinical samples (Gabel et al., 1986; Loening-Bauke et al., 1987) and one study found no difference between normal and encopretic samples (Friman et al., 1988). All three studies found clinically significant levels of behavior problems in a subsample of the children with encopresis ranging from 18% (Friman et al., 1988) to 21% (Loening-Bauke et al., 1987). Thus, as a group phenomenon, encopresis cannot be traced to psychopathological variables. In fact, similar to enuresis, the research on positive behavioral changes following successful treatment suggests that the increased behavior problems in many encopretic children may be more of a consequence than a cause of encopresis (Levine, Mazonson, & Bakow, 1980; M.H. Young, Brennen, Baker, & Baker, 1995). Yet there are several caveats to this conclusion.

For example, children with elevated behavior problems are also at risk for treatment failure (Levine & Bakow, 1976; L.J. Stark, Spirito, Lewis, & Hart, 1990). This risk may be related to treatment resistance, because a cardinal constituent of any set of child behavior problems is noncompliance. Children who sufficiently resist toilet training may cause stool retention; if they are predisposed to constipation, then their opposition to training could devolve delayed toilet training into chronic encopresis (Levine, 1982; Levine & Bakow, 1976).

Children with nonretentive encopresis appear to be the most likely children to resist and thus fail any form of direct treatment (Landman, Levine, &

Rappaport, 1983; Landman & Rappaport, 1985; Levine, 1981). Very little can be said about this subsample because of a distressing gap in the literature. According to known experts (Levine, Landman) and the *DSM-IV,* nonretentive encopresis appears to involve a distinct subsample, which is typically accompanied by elevated psychopathology and treatment resistance and/or failure. Although not considered idiopathic, the origins and course of nonretentive encopresis are not well understood.

Problem Identification

As with enuresis, the initial stage of encopresis contains a go no further maxim—following the history, or if possible, prior to the initial visit, the behavior therapist should refer the child to a physician (e.g., a pediatrician) for a medical examination. The encopresis exam should include a routine check of history and systems and abdominal palpation, rectal examination, and preferably a KUB (flat plate radiograph of the abdomen to determine the extent of fecal impaction). A barium enema is rarely necessary unless features of the exam suggest Hirschprung's disease. A thorough history should include questions similar to those regarding enuresis, including defining characteristics (primary vs. secondary) and etiological factors (e.g., family history of encopresis), and a screening for psychological problems (e.g., behavior checklists).

Problem Analysis

In addition to routine behavior and psychological assessments, the behavioral interview for encopresis should include questions that are pathognomonic (see Table 1). These include asking whether there is ever a long period between bowel movements, whether bowel movements are atypically large (stop up the toilet), whether fecal matter ever has an unusually foul odor, whether fecal matter is ever difficult or painful to pass, and whether the child ever complains of not being able to feel the movement or make it to the toilet on time. An additional question that pertains more to treatment history than to pathogenesis is whether the child ever hides soiled underwear. Affirmative answers to any or all of the pathognomonic questions is highly suggestive of retentive encopresis, and hiding underwear indicates a history that may include some form of punishment.

TABLE 1. Recommended Questions for Encopresis Interview

1. Is there ever a long period (2–3 days) between bowel movements?
2. Are the bowel movements often large? Do they ever stop up the toilet?
3. Does fecal matter have an unusually foul odor?
4. Is fecal matter difficult or painful to pass?
5. Does the child ever complain of not being able to feel the movement or make it to the toilet on time?
6. Does the child ever hide soiled underwear?

Similar to enuresis, the encopresis evaluation is the first step in treatment. Encopresis is not well understood outside of the medical community and the child's parents are likely to be under the influence of the characterological and psychopathological interpretations that are prevalent in Western culture. A parent's interpretation of the condition is also likely to influence how the children view their problem. Thus, the encopresis evaluation can actually begin treatment by providing accurate information to "demystify" the problem. The evaluation should also address three of the evaluation topics emphasized for enuresis: (a) punishment, (b) parent motivation, and (c) child motivation. Last, the evaluation should include questions about diet and timing of meals. Low-fiber diets and irregular meals can be contributing factors in encopresis.

Monitoring of bowel movements can be facilitated by using a chart (see Appendix). This chart allows the parent to monitor the number of bowel movements per day, the number of times the child soils his clothes, and a brief description of the stools. In order to assess the integrity of treatment components, this chart also includes categories for monitoring any dietary changes, medications, and rewards.

Plan Implementation

Retentive Encopresis

During the past 15 years, several descriptive and controlled experimental studies have supported a multicomponent approach to treatment of chronic retentive encopresis partly derived from the pioneering work of Davidson (1958), Christophersen and Rainey (1976), Levine (1975), and Wright (1975). As indicated previously, the first component can be addressed within the evaluation. Specifically, the entire elimination process including its disordered manifestations should be "demystified"

(Christophersen, 1994; Levine, 1982, 1983). The belief that bowel retention and bowel accidents are generally associated with personality development, and specifically with such characteristics as stubbornness, immaturity, or laziness, can result in parents shaming and blaming their children into the bathroom. But a disordered process of elimination such as encopresis should no more be a target for censure and blame than should a disordered process of respiration, digestion, or motor movement. The data-based literature does not support the association between behavioral profiles and bowel habits (Friman et al., 1988; Gabel et al., 1986; Loening-Baucke et al., 1987). On the contrary, this literature recommends that parents avoid blaming the child and suggests that they restructure toileting conditions in order to increase the likelihood of proper elimination (Levine, 1982). Second, if there is a fecal impaction it should be removed with enemas and/or laxatives (Christophersen, 1994; Levine, 1982; O'Brien, Ross, & Christophersen, 1986). Third, the child should sit on the toilet for about five minutes one or two times a day (O'Brien et al., 1986; Wright, 1975). Fourth, the parents should promote proper toileting with encouragement and not with coercion. In addition, they should not reserve all their praise and affection for proper elimination; a child should be praised initially for sitting on the toilet (Christophersen, 1994; Levine, 1982,1983; Wright, 1975). Fifth, a stool softener such as mineral oil (Davidson, 1958) or glycerin suppositories (O'Brien et al., 1986; Wright & Walker, 1977) should be used in order to ease the passage of hard stools. Sixth, dietary fiber should be increased in the child's diet (Houts, Mellon, & Whelan, 1988; O'Brien et al., 1986). L.J. Stark, Spirito, et al. (1990) recommend at least 20g of fiber per day, which can easily be consumed from fresh vegetables, whole grains, and fruit (popcorn and high-fiber snack bars for finicky children). Seventh, in order to increase and maintain motility in the child's colon, the child's activity levels and fluid intake should be increased (Levine, 1982, 1983). Eighth, during toileting episodes the child's feet should be on a flat surface. Foot placement is crucial to the "Valsalva maneuver" (grunting push necessary to produce a bowel movement; Levine, 1982, 1983; O'Brien et al., 1986). And ninth, the child should be rewarded for all bowel movements in the toilet (Christophersen & Rainey, 1976; Levine, 1982, 1983; O'Brien et al., 1986; Wright & Walker, 1977).

The literature on this approach (or variations thereof) has progressed sufficiently to lead to group trials. For example, in a study of 58 children with encopresis, 60% were completely continent after five months and those who did not achieve full continence averaged a 90% decrease in accidents (Lowery, Srour, Whitehead, & Schuster, 1985).

Nonretentive Encopresis

Treatment of nonretentive encopresis is not well established; thus, recommending an optimal course of treatment is premature. Perhaps the best approach would begin with a comprehensive psychological evaluation that includes behavioral assessment techniques. Virtually all investigators who have described this subsample of children report emotional and behavioral problems and treatment resistance (e.g., Landman & Rappaport, 1985; Landman et al., 1983) and it is possible that some of these children's soiling is related to modifiable aspects of their social ecology. Some investigators have employed versions of the approach outlined previously and have included supportive verbal therapy (Landman & Rappaport, 1985) or behavior management for the parents of these children (L.J. Stark, Spirito, et al., 1990). Clearly, the various problems, other than soiling, exhibited by this subsample require some form of treatment, but the soiling itself needs direct attention. It is a medical condition first and foremost and has the potential to devolve to a life-threatening status (McGuire, Rothenberg, & Tyler, 1983). Furthermore, public detection of accidents is likely to worsen the social, emotional, and behavioral aspects of the condition. Thus successful treatment, because it eliminates the possibility of public detection, should be pursued aggressively (Levine, 1981).

Plan Evaluation

Not all children succeed with these approaches, and for these children augmentive methods have been developed. For example, one study of 18- treatment-resistant children showed that using a group format for treatment delivery and teaching parents to use relevant behavior management strategies resulted in an 83% decrease in accidents, and these positive results were maintained or even improved at six months follow-up (Stark, Owens-Stively, Spirito, Lewis, & Guevremont, 1990).

Another augmentive method for treatment-resistant cases is biofeedback training (obviously, access to appropriately trained professionals, parent consent, and child assent are essential criteria). For those children with very limited awareness of rectal distension and/or with abnormal defecation dynamics (cf. Loening-Baucke & Younoszai, 1982; Loening-Baucke & Cruikshank, 1986; Wald et al., 1986), biofeedback has been successfully used to increase awareness and retrain bowel habits (e.g., Loening-Baucke, 1990; Wald, Chandra, Gabel, & Chiponis, 1987).

Thus, a variety of effective primary and augmentive treatment approaches are available for remediation of chronic retentive encopresis. It is also possible that aspects of these approaches could be used to prevent encopresis.

Prevention

Encopresis (retentive) more so than enuresis, can be a preventable condition. There are known risk factors and often a predictable developmental course. In his discussion of the causes of encopresis, Levine (1982) described three stages of its development. Such descriptions aid the identification of children who most likely would benefit from preventive interventions.

In stage I (infants and toddlers) the primary causal variables are simple constipation and parental overreaction. In this stage a provider (probably a pediatrician but possibly a psychologist) should use "demystification" to initiate a preventive intervention. The general "demystified" instructions for parents should emphasize consistent, nonaggressive, well-informed management of any or all bowel problems, especially constipation. Parents should also be encouraged to follow the readiness criteria established by Azrin and Foxx (1974) before setting up a bowel training program. In general, no reaction at all to a bowel problem is better than an overreaction (Levine, 1982, 1983).

During stage II (three to five years) the various stresses associated with toilet training are of paramount concern. Preventive efforts should include continued demystification, which at this stage involves gentle assistance with all toileting tasks, and encouragement to work on and to talk about toileting tasks. During stage II such aids as toilet seats and small stools for foot leverage may be helpful. Increased dietary fiber will loosen and moisten stools and help to prevent painful passage of hard stools. Most important is the avoidance of coercion, negative feedback, and inducements to rush the toileting process. The child should be encouraged to sit on the toilet at least once a day but for not longer than five minutes. The time for this toileting episode should be consistent across days. And the child should be praised for adherence to the schedule (Christophersen, 1994; Levine, 1983; Wright & Walker, 1977).

During stage III (early school years) scheduling toileting episodes becomes the primary concern. Toileting schedules at this stage are particularly critical for children whose risk of encopresis has increased because of problems during stages I and II. The psychosocial reactions to bowel movements at school, especially schools without doors on toilet stalls, can be a problem for the child at risk (Levine, 1982, 1983). For such children, a preventive effort should involve the regulation of bowel movements so that they occur in the children's home either before or after school. Perhaps the best method of increasing adherence to a home schedule is the use of suppositories (Christophersen, 1994). When the regulation of bowel movements becomes consistent as a result of using suppositories, the suppositories should be faded out of the toileting routine (Christophersen & Rainey, 1976). In addition to regulation of bowel movements, the preventive intervention for the school-aged child at risk should include increased dietary fiber, elevated activity levels, increased fluid intake, continued demystification, and praise for the absence of accidents (Levine, 1982, 1983).

The preventive intervention recommended here is, at its most burdensome point, a mild treatment procedure, and, at its least burdensome point, a mild

toilet training procedure. Thus, implementation may not require a great deal of extra effort from the parents or the provider. In fact, with the exception of those cases where suppositories are needed, prevention is equivalent to ordinary toilet training conducted at an appropriate age level. Therefore, the best preventive maneuver would be to provide this recommended intervention for all children. Bowel training is, after all, a human experience that is often fraught with complications (Levine, 1982). It is difficult to ascertain how the interventions used to ease those complications in children at risk for encopresis would cause problems when used with children whose risk is lower. Conversely, the procedure might simplify the entire bowel training process for everyone concerned. Thus, even in the absence of supportive data, our position is that informed providers can prevent at least some (perhaps a lot) of encopresis with timely health education.

Concluding Remarks

Incontinence in children involves primarily medical problems that require biobehavioral solutions. The antecedent emphasis on "bio" in the word biobehavioral should be matched by antecedent emphasis on medicine in assessment and treatment of these conditions. In other words, the children should be seen by medical practitioners first to rule out rare but nonetheless real pathophysiological variables. In addition, a medical workup can clarify the clinical picture for the child, family, and provider and can lead to optimal treatment planning.

There is a longstanding cultural bias against children with incontinence and it is perpetuated in adult and peer communities. This bias may have some roots in the contingencies of survival that influence humans as a species. That is, revulsion at human waste is a hygienic reaction that may have survival value. But the bias also has roots in widespread misinterpretations of incontinence involving characterological and psychopathological emphasis. The provider can begin treatment indirectly by responding to these interpretations as psychological pathogens (e.g., laziness is not a causal variable) and taking steps to eliminate or modify them so they are more consistent with known causes of incontinence. In addition, the presenting case is likely to have an extended history of failure with home remedies, and, thus, child and parents may have an inflated sense of the problem or a deflated sense of their own ability to resolve it. The provider can address both of these by instilling confidence about the expected success of treatment and in the potential of the child and parents as partners in its delivery. Enuresis and encopresis that are not pathophysiological (i.e., the vast majority) are medical conditions that require—and respond well to—behavioral treatment. Thus, behavioral treatment of childhood incontinence represents a crowning achievement of behavior therapy and should be a standard procedure in the clinical repertoire of any child-oriented behavioral practitioner. Despite this achievement, an abundance of cases remain unmanaged, mismanaged, and overmedicated. In addition to the question of how to expand delivery of appropriate treatment (e.g., in the medical community), there are many other questions across the spectrum of incontinence variables (e.g., sleep, hormone release, learning factors) that need further study. Behavior therapy has achieved much success with childhood incontinence; now is the time to energetically generate more.

APPENDIX: Bowel Movement Chart

Patient: _____

Month: _____

Days	# Bowel Movements	Size/ Consistency	Soilings	Diet change (if any)	Medication (if any)	Contingent Reward (if any)	Comments
1							
2							
3							
4							
5							
6							
7							
8							
9							
10							
11							
12							
13							
14							
15							
16							
17							
18							
19							
20							
21							
22							
23							
24							
25							
26							
27							
28							
29							
30							

Note: # Bowel Movements: In toilet; Size/consistency; Approximate no. of cups; H = Hard, S = Soft, D = Diarrhea

References

Ambrosini, P.J.(1984). A pharmacological paradigm for urinary continence and enuresis. *Journal of Clinical Psychopharmacology, 4,* 247–253.

American Psychiatric Association. (1994). *Diagnostic and statistical manual of mental disorders* (4th ed.). Washington, DC: Author.

Azrin, N.H., & Foxx, R.M. (1974). *Toilet training in less than a day.* New York: Simon & Schuster.

Bakwin, H. (1971). Enuresis in twins. *American Journal of Diseases in Children, 121,* 222–225.

Bakwin, H. (1973). The genetics of enuresis. In I. Kolvin, R.C. MacKeith, & S.R. Meadow (Eds.), *Bladder control and enuresis* (pp. 73–78). Philadelphia: Lippincott.

Barbour, R.F., Borland, E.M., Boyd, M.M., Miller, A., & Oppe', T.E. (1963). Enuresis as a disorder of development. *British Medical Journal, 2,* 787–790.

Barr, R.G., Levine, M.D., Wilkinson, R.H., & Mulvihill, D. (1979). Chronic and occult stool retention: A clinical tool for its evaluation in school aged children. *Clinical Pediatrics, 18,* 674–686.

Berk, L.B., & Friman, P.C. (1990). Epidemiologic aspects of toilet training. *Clinical Pediatrics, 29,* 278–282.

Blackwell, B., & Currah, J. (1973). The psychopharmacology of nocturnal enuresis. In I. Kolvin, R.C. MacKeith, & S.R. Meadow (Eds.), *Bladder control and enuresis* (pp. 231–257). Philadelphia: Lippincott.

Blomfield, J.M., & Douglas, J.W.B. (1956). Bed wetting: Prevalence among child aged four to seven years. *Lancet 1,* 850–852.

Bollard, J., & Nettlebeck, T. (1982). A component analysis of dry-bed training for treatment of bed wetting. *Behavior Research & Therapy, 20,* 383–390, 1982.

Bostock, J. (1958). Exterior gestation, primitive sleep, enuresis, and asthma: A study in aetiology. *Medical Journal of Australia, 2,* 185–192.

Boyd, M.M. (1960). The depth of sleep in enuretic school children and in non-enuretic controls. *Journal of Psychological Research, 4,* 274–281.

Broughton, R.J. (1968). Sleep disorders: Disorders of arousal. *Science, 159,* 1070–1078.

Christophersen, E.R. (1994). *Pediatric compliance.* New York: Plenum.

Christophersen, E.R., & Rainey, S. (1976). Management of encopresis through a pediatric outpatient clinic. *Journal of Pediatric Psychology, 1,* 38–41.

Christophersen, E.R., Finney, J.W., & Friman, P.C. (Eds.). (1986). Prevention in primary care [Special issue]. *Pediatric Clinics of North America, 33.*

Cohen, M.W. (1975). Enuresis. *Pediatric Clinics of North America, 22,* 545–560.

Couchells, S.M., Bennet-Johnson, S., & Carter, R. (1981). Behavioral and environmental characteristics of treated and untreated enuretic children and match nonenuretic controls. *Journal of Pediatrics, 99,* 812–816.

Creer, T.L., & Davis, M.H. (1975). Using a staggered waking procedure with enuretic children in an institutional setting. *Journal of Behavior Therapy & Experimental Psychiatry, 6,* 23–25.

Davidson, M. (1958). Constipation and fecal incontinence. *Pediatric Clinics of North America, 5,* 749–757.

De Jong, G.A. (1973). Epidemiology of enuresis: A survey of the literature. In I. Kolvin, R.C. MacKeith, & S.R. Meadow (Eds.), *Bladder control and enuresis* (pp.39–46). London: Heinemann.

Dimson, S.B. (1977). Desmopressin as a treatment for enuresis. *Lancet, 1,* 1260.

Dimson, S.B. (1986). DDAVP and urine osmolality in refractory enuresis. *Archives of Diseases in Children, 61,* 1104–1107.

Doleys, D.M. (1977). Behavioral treatments for nocturnal enuresis in children: A review of the recent literature. *Psychological Bulletin, 84,* 30–54.

Ferber, R. (1985). *Solve your child's sleep problems.* New York: Simon & Schuster.

Ferber, R. (1989). Sleep-associated enuresis in the child. In M.H. Kryger, T. Roth, & W.C. Dement (Eds.), *Principles and practice of sleep medicine* (pp. 643–647). Philadelphia: Saunders.

Fergusson, D.M., Horwood, L.J., & Sannon, F.T. (1986). Factors related to the age of attainment of nocturnal bladder control: An 8-year longitudinal study. *Pediatrics, 78,* 884–890.

Ferrie, B.G., MacFarlane, J., & Glen, E.S. (1984). DDAVP in young enuretic patients: A double-blind trial. *British Journal of Urology, 56,* 376–378.

Fielding, D. (1980). The response of day and night wetting children and children who wet only at night to retention control training and the enuresis alarm. *Behavior Research and Therapy, 18,* 305–317.

Fielding, D. (1982). An analysis of the behavior of day- and night-wetting children: Towards a model of micturition control. *Behavior Research and Therapy, 49,* 49–60.

Fielding, D.M., & Doleys, D.M. (1988). Elimination problems: Enuresis and encopresis. In E.J. Mash & L.G. Terdal (Eds.), *Behavioral assessment of childhood disorders* (pp. 586–623). New York: Guilford.

Finley, W.W., & Wansley, R.A. (1977). Auditory intensity as a variable in the conditioning treatment of enuresis nocturia. *Behavior Research and Therapy, 15,* 181–185.

Forsythe, W., & Redmond, A. (1974). Enuresis and spontaneous cure rate study of 1129 enuretics. *Archives of Diseases in Children, 49,* 259–269.

Fournier, J.P., Garfinkel, B.D., Bond, A., Beauchesne, H., & Shapiro, S.K. (1987). Pharmacological and behavioral management of enuresis. *Journal of the American Academy of Child and Adolescent Psychiatry, 26,* 849–853.

Foxman, B., Valdez, R.B., & Brook, R.H. (1986). Childhood enuresis: Prevalence, perceived impact, and prescribed treatments. *Pediatrics, 77,* 482–487.

Friman, P.C. (1986). A preventive context for enuresis. *Pediatric Clinics of North America, 33,* 871–886.

Friman, P.C. (1991, March). *Enuresis and clinically significant behavior problems.* Paper presented at the annual Teaching Family Association Conference, Omaha, NE.

Friman, P.C. (1995). Nocturnal enuresis in the child. In R. Ferber & M.H. Kryger (Eds.), *Principles and practice of sleep medicine in the child* (pp. 107–114). Philadelphia: Saunders.

Friman, P.C., & Christophersen, E.R. (1986). Biobehavioral prevention in primary care. In N. Krasnegor, J.D. Arasteh, & M.F. Cataldo (Eds.), *Child health behavior: A behavioral pediatrics perspective* (pp. 254–280). New York: Wiley.

Friman, P.C., & Vollmer, D. (1995). Successful use of the nocturnal urine alarm for diurnal enuresis. *Journal of Applied Behavior Analysis, 28,* 89–90.

Friman, P.C., Warzak, W.J. (1990). Nocturnal enuresis: A prevalent, persistent, yet curable parasomnia. *Pediatrician, 17,* 38–45.

Friman, P.C., Mathews, J.R., Finney, J.W., & Christophersen, E.R. (1988). Do children with encopresis have clinically significant behavior problems? *Pediatrics, 82,* 407–409.

Gabel, S., Hegedus, A.M., Wald, A., Chandra, R., & Chaponis, D. (1986). Prevalence of behavior problems and mental health utilization among encopretic children. *Journal of Developmental and Behavioral Pediatrics, 7,* 293–297.

Gellis, S.S. (1994). Are enuretics truly hard to arouse? *Pediatric Notes, 18,* 113.

Glicklich, L.B. (1951). An historical account of enuresis. *Pediatrics, 8,* 859–876.

Gross, R.T., & Dornbusch, S.M. (1983). Enuresis. In M.D. Levine, W.B. Carey, A.C. Crocker, & R.T. Gross (Eds.), *Developmental–behavioral pediatrics* (pp. 575–586). Philadelphia: Saunders.

Hallgren, B. (1956a). Enuresis: I. A study with reference to the morbidity risk and symptomatology. *ACTA Psychiatrica et Neurologica Scandinavica, 31,* 379–404.

Hallgren, B. (1956b). Enuresis: II. A study with reference to certain physical, mental and social factors possibly associated with enuresis. *ACTA Psychiatrica et Neurological Scandinavica, 31,* 405–436.

Hallgren, B. (1957). Enuresis: A clinical and genetic study. *ACTA Psychiatrica et Neurologica Scandinavica, 32* (Suppl. 114), 73–90.

Halliday, S., Meadow, S.R., & Berg, I. (1987). Successful management of daytime enuresis using alarm procedures: A randomly controlled trial. *Archives of Diseases in Children, 62,* 132–137.

Hatch, T.F. (1981) 1988 IN TEXT. Encopresis and constipation in children. *Pediatric Clinics of North America, 35,* 257–281.

Hauri, P. (1982). *The sleep disorders: Current concepts.* Kalamazoo, MI: Upjohn.

Henoch, E.H. (1889). *Lectures on children's diseases* (Vol. 2, J. Thompson, Trans.). London: New Syndenham Society.

Herson, V.C., Schmitt, B.D., & Rumack, B.H. (1979). Magical thinking and imipramine poisoning in two school-aged children. *Journal of the American Medical Association, 241,* 1926–1927.

Houts, A.C. (1991). Nocturnal enuresis as a biobehavioral problem. *Behavior Therapy, 22,* 133–151.

Houts, A.C., Peterson, J.K., & Liebert, R.M. (1984). The effects of prior imipramine treatment on the results of conditioning therapy with enuresis. *Journal of Pediatric Psychology, 9,* 505–508.

Houts, A.C., Mellon, M.W., & Whelan, J.P. (1988). Use of dietary fiber and stimulus control to treat retentive encopresis: A multiple baseline investigation. *Journal of Pediatric Psychology, 13,* 435–445.

Houts, A.C., Berman, J.S., & Abramson, H. (1994). Effectiveness of psychological and pharmacological treatments for nocturnal enuresis. *Journal of Consulting and Clinical Psychology, 62,* 737–745.

Jarvelin, M.R., Moilanen, I., Vikevainen-Tervonen, L., & Huttunen, N. (1990). Life changes and protective capacities in enuretic and non-enuretic children. *Journal of Child Psychology and Psychiatry, 31,* 763–774.

Jenson, W.R., & Sloane, H.N. (1979). Chart moves and grab bags: A simple contingency management. *Journal of Applied Behavior Analysis, 12,* 334.

Kaffman, M., & Elizur, E. (1977). Infants who become enuretics: A longitudinal study of 161 Kibbutz children. *Monographs of the Society for Research on Child Development, 42,* 2–12.

Kanner, L. (1972). *Child psychiatry.* Springfield, IL: Thomas.

Kegel, A.H. (1951). Physiologic therapy for urinary stress incontinence. *Journal of the American Medical Association, 146,* 915–917.

Key, D.W., Bloom, D.A., & Sanvordenker, J. (1992). Low-dose DDAVP in nocturnal enuresis. *Clinical Pediatrics, 32,* 299–301.

Landman, G.B., & Rappaport, L. (1985). Pediatric management of severe treatment-resistant encopresis. *Development and Behavioral Pediatrics, 6,* 349–351.

Landman, G.B., Levine, D., & Rappaport, L. (1983). A study of treatment resistance among children referred for encopresis. *Clinical Pediatrics, 23,* 449–452.

Levine, M.D. (1975). Children with encopresis: A descriptive analysis. *Pediatrics, 56,* 407–409.

Levine, M.D. (1981). The schoolchild with encopresis. *Pediatrics in Review, 2,* 285–291.

Levine, M.D. (1982). Encopresis: Its potentiation, evaluation, and alleviation. *Pediatric Clinics of North America, 29,* 315–330.

Levine, M.D. (1983). Encopresis. In M.D. Levine, W.B. Carey, A.C. Crocker, & R.T. Gross (Eds.), *Developmental–behavioral pediatrics* (pp. 586–595). Philadelphia: Saunders.

Levine, M.D., & Bakow, H. (1976). Children with encopresis: A study of treatment outcome. *Pediatrics, 58,* 845–852.

Levine, M.D., Mazonson, P., & Bakow, H. (1980). Behavioral symptom substitution in children cured of encopresis. *American Journal of Diseases in Childhood, 134,* 663–667.

Lifschitz, M., & Chovers, A. (1972). Encopresis among Israeli kibbutz children. *Israel Annals of Psychiatry and Related Disciplines, 4,* 326–340.

Loening-Baucke, V.A. (1990). Modulation of abnormal defecation dynamics by biofeedback treatment in chronically constipated children with encopresis. *Journal of Pediatrics, 116,* 214–221.

Loening-Baucke, V.A., & Cruikshank, B. (1986). Abnormal defecation dynamics in chronically constipated children with encopresis. *Journal of Pediatrics, 108,* 562–588.

Loening-Baucke, V.A., & Younoszai, M.K. (1982). Abnormal anal sphincter response in chronically constipated children. *Journal of Pediatrics, 100,* 213–218.

Loening-Baucke, V.A., Cruikshank, B., & Savage, C. (1987). Defecation dynamics and behavior profiles in encopretic children. *Pediatrics, 80,* 672–679.

Lowery, S., Srour, J., Whitehead, W.E., & Schuster, M.M. (1985). Habit training as treatment of encopresis secondary to chronic constipation. *Journal of Pediatric Gastroenterology and Nutrition, 4,* 397–401.

MacKeith, R. (1968). A frequent factor in the origins of primary nocturnal enuresis: Anxiety in the third year of life. *Developmental Medicine and Child Neurology, 10,* 465–470.

McGuire, T., Rothenberg, M., & Tyler, D. (1983). Profound shock following interventions for chronic untreated stool retention. *Clinical Pediatrics, 23,* 459–461.

Meadow, S.R. (1990). Day wetting. *Pediatric Nephrology, 4,* 178–184.

Mellon, M.W., and Houts, A.C. (1995). Elimination disorders. In R.T. Ammerman and M. Hersen (Eds.), *Handbook of Child Behavior Therapy in the Psychiatric Setting* (pp. 341–366). New York: Wiley.

Meunier, P., Marechal, J.M., & De Beaujeu, M.J. (1979). Rectoanal pressures and rectal sensitivity in chronic childhood constipation. *Gastroenterology, 77,* 330–336.

Mikkelson, E.J., & Rapoport, J.L. (1980). Enuresis: Psychopathology, sleep stage, and drug response. *Urological Clinics of North America, 7,* 361–377.

Mishne, J.M. (1993). Primary nocturnal enuresis: A psychodynamic clinical perspective. *Child and Adolescent Social Work Journal, 10,* 469–495.

Moffatt, M.E.K., Kato, C., & Pless, I.B. (1987). Improvements in self-concept after treatment of nocturnal enuresis: Randomized controlled trial. *Journal of Pediatrics, 110,* 647–652.

Moffatt, M.E.K., Harlos, S., Kirshen, A.J., & Burd, L. (1993). Desmopressin acetate and nocturnal enuresis: How much do we know? *Pediatrics, 92,* 420–425.

Morgan, R.T., & Young, G.C. (1975). Parental attitudes and the conditioning of childhood enuresis. *Behavior Research Therapy, 13,* 197–199.

Mountjoy, P.T., Ruben, D.H., & Bradford, T.S. (1984). Recent technological advancements in the treatment of enuresis. *Behavior Modification, 8,* 291–315.

Mowrer, O.H., & Mowrer, W.M. (1938). Enuresis: A method for its study and treatment. *American Journal of Orthopsychiatry, 8,* 436–459.

Muellner, S.R. (1951). The physiology of micturition. *The Journal of Urology, 65,* 805–813.

Muellner, R.S. (1960). Development of urinary control in children. *Journal of the American Medical Association, 172,* 1256–1261.

Muellner, R.S. (1961). Obstacles to the successful treatment of primary enuresis. *Journal of the American Medical Association, 178,* 147–148.

Norgaard, J.P., Pedersen, E.B., & Djurhuus, J.C. (1985). Diurnal antidiuretic hormone levels in enuretics. *Journal of Urology, 134,* 1029–31.

Novello, A.C., & Novello, R. (1987). Enuresis. *Pediatric Clinics of North America, 34,* 719–733.

O'Brien, S., Ross, L.V., & Christophersen, E.R. (1986). Primary encopresis: Evaluation and treatment. *Journal of Applied Behavior Analysis, 19,* 137–145.

Olatawuria, M.O. (1973). Encopresis: A review of 32 cases. *Acta Paediatrica Scandinavica, 62,* 358–364.

Ollendick, T.H., King, N.J., & Frary, R. (1989). Fears in children and adolescents: Reliability and generalizability across gender, age, and nationality. *Behavior Research and Therapy, 27,* 19–26.

Oswald, K., Taylor, A.M., & Treisman, M. (1960). Discriminative responses to stimulation during human sleep. *Brain, 83,* 440–445.

Pedersen, P.S., Hejl, M., & Kjoller, S.S. (1985). Desamino-D-Arginine Vasopressin in childhood nocturnal enuresis. *Journal of Urology, 133,* 65–66.

Perlmutter, A.D. (1985). Enuresis. In P.P. Kelalis, L.R. King, & A.B. Belman (Eds.), *Clinical Pediatric Urology* (2nd ed., pp. 311–325). Philadelphia: Saunders.

Pierce, C.M. (1985). Encopresis. In H.I. Kaplan & B.J. Sadock (Eds.), *Comprehensive handbook of psychiatry* (4th ed., pp. 1487–1489). Baltimore: Williams & Wilkins.

Post, E.M., Richman, R.A., & Blackett, P.R. (1983). Desmopressin response of enuretic children. *American Journal of Diseases in Children, 137,* 962–963.

Rauber A., & Maroncelli, R. (1984). Prescribing practices and knowledge of tricyclic antidepressants among physicians caring for children. *Pediatrics, 73,* 107–109.

Rittig, S., Knudsen, U.B., Norgaard, J.P., Pedersen, E.B., & Djurhuus, J.C. (1989). Abnormal diurnal rhythm of plasma vasopressin and urinary output in patients with enuresis. *American Journal of Physiology, 252,* F664-F671.

Scharf, M. (1986). *Waking up dry.* Cincinnati: Writer's Digest Books.

Scharf, M.B., & Jennings, S.W. (1988). Childhood enuresis: Relationship to sleep, etiology, evaluation, and treatment. *Annals of Behavioral Medicine, 10,* 113–120.

Schmitt, B.D. (1984). Nocturnal enuresis. *Primary Care, 11,* 485–495.

Schneider, M.S., King, L.R., & Surwitt, R.S. (1994). Kegel exercises and childhood incontinence: A new role for an old treatment. *Journal of Pediatrics, 124,* 91–92.

Shaffer, D. (1973). The association between enuresis and emotional disorder: A review of the literature. In I. Kolvin, R.C. MacKeith, & S.R. Meadow (Eds.), *Bladder control and enuresis* (pp. 118–136). Philadelphia: Lippincott.

Shelov, S.P., Gundy J., & Weiss, J.C. (1981). Enuresis: A contrast of attitudes of parents and physicians. *Pediatrics, 67,* 707–710.

Sperling, M. (1982). *The major neuroses and behavior disorders in children.* New York: Jason Aronson.

Starfield, B. (1967). Functional bladder capacity in enuretic and nonenuretic children. *Journal of Pediatrics, 70,* 777–782.

Starfield, B., & Mellits, E.D. (1968). Increases in functional bladder capacity and improvements in enuresis. *Journal of Pediatrics, 72,* 483–487.

Stark, L., Owens-Stively, J., Spirito, A., Lewis, A., & Guevremont, D. (1990). Group behavioral treatment of retentive encopresis. *Journal of Pediatric Psychology, 15,* 659–671.

Stark, L.J., Spirito, A., Lewis, A.V., & Hart, K.J. (1990). Encopresis: Behavioral parameters associated with children who fail medical management. *Child Psychiatry and Human Development, 20,* 169–179.

Stephenson, J.D. (1979). Physiological and pharmacological basis for the chemotherapy of enuresis. *Psychological Medicine, 9,* 249–263.

Troup, C.W., & Hodgson, N.B. (1971). Nocturnal functional bladder capacity in enuretic children. *Journal of Urology, 105,* 129–132.

Van Gool, J.D., & Jonge, G.A. (1989). Urge syndrome and urge incontinence. *Archives of Diseases of Childhood, 64,* 1629–1634.

Verhulst, F.C., van der Lee, J.H., Akkeruis, G.W., Sanders-Woudstra, J.A.R., Timmer, F.C., & Donkhorst, I.D. (1985). The prevalence of nocturnal enuresis: Do DSM III criteria need to be changed? A brief research report. *Journal of Child Psychology and Psychiatry, 26,* 989–993.

Vincent, S.A. (1974). Mechanical, electrical and other aspects of enuresis. In J.H. Johnston & W. Goodwin (Eds.), *Reviews in Pediatric Urology* (pp. 280–313). New York: Elsevier.

Wagner, W., Johnson, S.B., Walker, D., Carter, R., & Wittmer, J. (1982). A controlled comparison of two treatments for nocturnal enuresis. *Journal of Pediatrics, 101,* 302–307.

Wald, A., Chandra, R., Chiponis, D., & Gabel, S. (1986). Anorectal function and continence mechanisms in childhood encopresis. *Journal of Pediatric Gastroenterology and Nutrition, 5,* 346–351.

Wald, A., Chandra, R., Gabel, S., & Chiponis, D. (1987). Evaluation of biofeedback in childhood encopresis. *Journal of Pediatric Gastroenterology and Nutrition, 5,* 346–351.

Warson, S.R., Caldwell, M.R., Warinner, A., & Kirk, A.J. (1954). The dynamics of encopresis. *American Journal of Orthopsychiatry, 24,* 402–415.

Warzak, W.J., Friman, P.C. (1994). Current concepts in pediatric primary nocturnal enuresis. *Child and Adolescent Social Work Journal, 11,* 507–523.

Werry, J. (1966). The conditioning treatment of enuresis. *American Journal of Psychiatry, 123,* 226–229.

Werry, J.S., & Cohrssen, J. (1965). Enuresis: An etiologic and therapeutic study. *Journal of Pediatrics, 67,* 423–430.

Whitehead, W.E., & Schuster, M.M. (1985). *Gastrointestinal disorders: Behavioral and physiological basis for treatment.* New York: Academic.

Wille, S. (1986). Comparison of desmopressin and enuresis alarm for nocturnal enuresis. *Archives of Diseases in Children, 61,* 30–33.

Wright, L. (1973). Handling the encopretic child. *Professional Psychology, 3,* 137–144.

Wright, L. (1975). Outcome of a standardized program for treating psychogenic encopresis. *Professional Psychology, 6,* 453–456.

Wright, L., & Walker, E. (1977). Treatment of the child with psychogenic encopresis. *Clinical Pediatrics, 16,* 1042–1045.

Wright, L., Schaefer, A.B., & Solomons, G. (1979). *Encyclopedia of pediatric psychology.* Baltimore: University Park Press.

Young, G.C., & Morgan, R.T.C. (1973). Conditioning treatment of enuresis: Auditory intensity. *Behavior Research and Therapy, 11,* 411–416.

Young, M.H., Brennen, L.C., Baker, R.D., & Baker, S.S. (1995). Functional encopresis: Symptom reduction and behavioral improvement. *Developmental and Behavioral Pediatrics, 16,* 226–232.

Zaleski, A., Gerrard, J.W., & Shokeir, H.K. (1973). Nocturnal enuresis: The importance of a small bladder capacity. In I. Kolvin, R.C. MacKeith, & S.R. Meadow (Eds.), *Bladder control and enuresis* (pp. 95–101). Philadelphia: Lippincott.

Zung, W.W., & Wilson, W.P. (1961). Responses to auditory stimulation during sleep. *Archives of General Psychiatry, 4,* 548–552.

IV

Medical/Pediatric Problems

The problems in this section are those that are typically first recognized and/or diagnosed through consultation with medical professionals. That does not mean, however, that treatment will necessarily occur in the medical setting. In fact, many of the behavioral sequelae associated with a particular problem are treated in the home or in school environments. Managing chronic pain, for example, often requires parents to change their pain supporting behaviors as well as requiring children to learn relaxation skills (Chapter 14, by Allen and Matthews). The types of problems discussed in Chapter 15 (e.g., seizures, TBI, postconcussive syndrome) pose a different, and sometimes difficult, challenge for the behavior analyst in that many of the behaviors are the result of neurological insult that affects the effectiveness of certain behavioral procedures.

Chronic illnesses often evoke behavioral changes in children as well as changes in how parents interact with their children. In addition, medical regimens for chronic illnesses are often aversive or time-consuming, making treatment compliance a central issue in disease management. Chapter 16 (McMahon, Lambros, & Sylva), recommends a two-pronged approach for treating behaviors associated with chronic illness: hypothesis testing and keystone behaviors.

Problems associated with eating (i.e., anorexia, bulimia) are some of the most troublesome and difficult to treat problems, as many variables (e.g., social, family, individual, biological) contribute to their development and maintenance. Williamson, Womble, and Zucker (Chapter 17) present a case formulation approach for assessing and treating eating disorders and compare the effectiveness of different types of treatments (behavior therapy, cognitive therapy, cognitive–behavior therapy, and pharmacotherapy). Somewhat related to the eating disorders chapter is Chapter 18, by Linscheid, on feeding disorders. Noting that problems related to feeding may arise from normal developmental processes or medical complications, Linscheid describes the most effective procedures for assessing and treating many different types of feeding problems that occur in young children.

14

Behavior Management of Recurrent Pain in Children

KEITH D. ALLEN AND JUDITH R. MATTHEWS

Introduction

Recurrent pain represents a clinically significant health problem for many children and adolescents. Recurrent pain is characterized by repeated painful episodes experienced across several months that occur in the absence of well-defined organic pathology. The most common types of recurrent pain involve headaches and recurrent abdominal pain (RAP), and those most affected are typically school-aged children and adolescents who are usually healthy and pain-free between episodes.

The most common headaches in children are tension headaches (characterized by dull, mild to moderate diffuse pain) and common migraine headaches (characterized by sharp, throbbing, moderate to severe pain). Although prevalence rates vary, recurrent headaches appear in about 2–3% of all children under 10, and 4–15% of all adolescents (Bille, 1962; Linet, Stewart, Celentano, Ziegler, & Sprecher, 1989; Newacheck & Taylor, 1992; Sillanpaa, 1983). Overall, however, evidence suggests that the typical onset is around 6–7 years of age, with recurrent headaches typically becoming more prevalent with age and with adolescent girls experiencing more headaches than do adolescent boys (P.A. McGrath, 1990).

Recurrent abdominal pain (RAP) is characterized by pain that is periumbilical and/or epigastric and is usually described in vague terms (Farrell, 1984). Prevalence estimates range from 6% to 30% (Apley & Naish, 1958; Oster, 1972; Apley, 1975; Parcel, Nader, & Meyer, 1977; P.A. McGrath, 1990). The best estimate is that about 10–15% of school-aged children experience RAP at some point. Combined, recurrent pain syndromes can occur in as many as 30% of all children (P.A. McGrath, 1990), representing a major health problem for school-aged children.

Clinical evidence does suggest some spontaneous remission of recurrent pain syndromes with age, but there are no clear indicators of who may become pain-free and who will continue to suffer. It is clear, however, that the longer children endure relative unpredictable episodes of pain the more likely they are to develop other emotional/behavioral difficulties, particularly without access to age-appropriate coping strategies. For example, acute pain experiences generally are associated with increases in anxiety as pain intensity increases. Typically, the anxiety decreases as the source of the acute pain is controlled. In recurrent pain, however, the anxiety associated with painful episodes may persist and in some cases evolve into depression, particularly as the health care system fails in repeated attempts to identify and remediate organic pathology that does not exist. Yet efforts to identify common emotional/behavioral characteristics of children with recurrent pain have proven equivocal (Cooper, Bawden, Camfield, & Camfield, 1987;

KEITH D. ALLEN AND JUDITH R. MATTHEWS • Division of Pediatric Psychology, Munroe-Meyer Institute for Genetics and Rehabilitation, and University of Nebraska Medical Center, Omaha, Nebraska 68198–5450.

Handbook of Child Behavior Therapy, edited by Watson and Gresham. Plenum Press, New York, 1998.

Andrasik et al., 1988; Guidetti et al., 1987; Hodges, Kline, Barbero, & Flanery, 1985; Hodges, Kline, Barbero, & Woodruff, 1985; P.J. McGrath, Goodman, Firestone, Shipman, & Peters, 1983). Childrens' emotional/behavioral responses to recurrent pain are likely to be unique to the context in which they occur, and, even in children where collateral responses such as increased anxiety or depression are identified, these conditions are a result rather than a cause of the recurrent pain episodes (Cunningham et al., 1987).

The most important differential diagnosis in identifying recurrent pain is to rule out organic pathology or disease (tumors, allergies, etc.). Given the prominence of the biomedical or disease model, most children will have been taken repeatedly by their parents to a variety of physicians (e.g., pediatrician, gastroenterologist, ENT, neurologist) who will seek to identify and treat an underlying pathological condition with the expectation that the symptoms will then disappear. If organic pathology exists, this treatment is relatively efficient and effective in eliminating the child's pain. Indeed, treating recurrent pain from a behavioral perspective when organic pathology exists and has not been identified can place the psychologist at ethical and legal risk and the child at considerable physical and emotional risk. This is not to imply that behavioral approaches are contraindicated where organic pathology exists, but rather that they should be seen as ancillary to medical interventions. In this chapter, however, we address only those disorders with no known pathology.

Note that once organic pathology has been ruled out, the pain is often called psychogenic. The call for psychological intervention is then generally based on the same disease model perspective as that identified above; that there must be some underlying pathology (now psychological in nature) that needs to be treated in order for the pain to cease (Fordyce & Steger, 1979). This etiological model is inadequate, as it is now generally recognized that the pain experienced in recurrent pain syndromes is multidimensional in nature and that the sensory system involved in episodes of recurrent pain is complex. Episodes of pain can be affected by external and internal factors alike, many of which can be modified to alter the experience of pain. Indeed, it is clear that recurrent pain is not simply a prolonga-

tion of the same mechanisms induced by acute pain; recurrent pain activates different mechanisms (Wall, 1984). Although there have been a variety of alternative etiological models offered to account for recurrent pain (e.g., Barr, 1983; Levine & Rappaport, 1984; Routh, Ernst, & Harper, 1988), we have not found a satisfactory biobehavioral model. For example, not all models acknowledge operant features of pain behavior and some suggest that recurrent pain can be conceptualized almost exclusively as a sign of psychopathology. Operant models, on the other hand, have focused almost exclusively on chronic pain (Fordyce & Steger, 1979; Rachlin, 1985) in which no organic etiology exists. A biobehavioral model of the etiology of recurrent pain in children requires attention to both organic and operant variables.

Organic (Organismic) Variables

By definition, recurrent pain is not a symptom of an underlying organic disease that requires medical treatment. However, the absence of organic disease does not mean the absence of organic etiology. There is increasing evidence that individuals with recurrent pain syndromes have different predispositions or thresholds of responsiveness to environmental stress that activates a poorly regulated nervous system. Environmental stress can be any stimuli that disturb the organism's homeostasis. Given a different threshold of responsiveness, it is neither the stressful stimulus or the organism's reactivity that results in pain, but the combination of the two that can precipitate or trigger painful episodes. For example, migraine headaches appear to be related to an inherited basic defect resulting in neurovasomotor instability (Barlow, 1984). Common stimuli that then elicit reactivity and subsequent headache pain include exercise, caffeine, alcohol, academic demands, and emotional distress. Similarly, recurrent abdominal pain appears to be related in part to gastrointestinal susceptibility or enhanced sensitivity (Gaffney & Gaffney, 1987; Kopel, Kim, & Barbers, 1967). Common stimuli that elicit reactivity and subsequent abdominal pain might include lactose, low-fiber diets, academic demands, and emotional distress (Levine & Rappaport, 1984). Note that unusual autonomic reactivity or abnormal physiological responses to stress have not been identified in all children with recurrent pain syndromes (e.g., Apley, Haslam, & Tulloch, 1971; Feuerstein, Barr, Francoeur, Houle, & Rafman, 1982). However, because individuals may have unique responses to stress, it is possible that efforts to identify reliable autonomic reactivity have failed to monitor relevant response systems (Schwartz, 1995) . In sum, both the child's individual physiological responsiveness and the stimuli that elicit that responsiveness are relevant in understanding at least part of the etiology of recurrent pain (Zeltzer, Barr, McGrath, & Schechter, 1992).

Operant (Contingencies of Reinforcement) Variables

The importance of learning factors in understanding pain has now been well established (Fordyce, 1976; Fordyce & Steger, 1979; Rachlin, 1985). Individuals can display a range of pain behaviors that are a function of reinforcement contingencies. Unfortunately, these operant factors are often oversimplified as "secondary gain," suggesting that pain behavior is strengthened by escape from demands or unpleasant experiences (such as school) or access to preferred activities (such as watching TV with a parent). While these are certainly important factors to consider, the pain relief produced by pain behavior should not be underestimated. That is, pain behaviors (e.g., lying down, taking medication, body posturing, staying home from school) may be reinforced because they result in pain reduction. In addition, maintenance of pain behavior may be enhanced through imitation or modeling effects (Apley, 1975; Oster, 1972; Christensen & Mortensen, 1975; Fordyce & Steger, 1979) and through the nonreinforcement of well behavior (Allen & McKeen, 1991). Of course, even in situations in which a close operant relationship is persuasive, the problem can be the result of some organic etiology (Fordyce, 1976), and certainly not all recurrent pain in children is operant (Turk & Flor, 1987). Still, the importance of reinforcement contingencies in the maintenance of recurrent pain in children cannot be overemphasized. It is perhaps this fact more than any other, that response to pain can be changed by environmental factors, that has lead to the growing interest in behavioral methods of intervention.

Problem Identification

The most important initial step in identifying recurrent pain problems is the differential diagnosis. Diagnosis can be particularly helpful in three important ways. First, the diagnosis should initially assist the clinician in determining whether behavioral intervention should be pursued at all. Second, the diagnosis can assist the clinician in determining a priori what critical questions may need to be covered during the assessment. Finally, the diagnosis should assist the clinician in selecting the most appropriate treatment strategy. Once an appropriate diagnosis has been made, a behavioral assessment can then be conducted.

Differential Diagnosis of Recurrent Pain Conditions

Rule Out Pathology

Any disorder with a potential organic pathology, as in any case of recurrent pain, should be and usually will have been evaluated initially by a physician to rule out disease processes (i.e., tumors, infections, etc.). If the child has not been to a physician for a recurrent pain condition, it is prudent to refer that child to the family physician for a medical evaluation before continuing further. For recurrent headaches, the most common organic causes include recent infections, increased intracranial pressure from excessive fluid or swelling, solid tumors, diseases such as hypertension, or dental problems (P.J. McGrath & Unruh, 1987). The most common organic etiologies of RAP are gastrointestinal (e.g., chronic constipation) and genitourinary (e.g., urinary tract infections and dysmenorrhea) (Dimson, 1971; P.J. McGrath & Unruh, 1987). Other less common causes are intake-related (e.g., lactose intolerance) or related to trauma or infection. However, even if a client has been to a physician and organic pathology has been ruled out, professionals working with children with recurrent pain syndromes should be aware of symptoms or "red flags" that might indicate a more serious condition suggesting a need to refer back to a physician. Table 1 presents red flag symptoms that may be identified during differential diagnosis of headaches or RAP and that may be

TABLE 1. Red Flag Symptoms Indicative of Organic Pathology

Headaches*	Recurrent abdominal pain**
Worsening pain	Pain away from umbilicus
Nausea/vomiting without migraine symptoms	Weight loss or growth failure
Constant pain	Fever
Intellectual decline	Anemia
Personality change	Bloody stools or vomit
Pain in face	Changes in symptoms or functioning
Waking at night with pain	Waking at night with pain
Motor or perceptual difficulties during pain free episodes	Difficulty or painful urination

* Based in part on McGrath & Unruh, 1987.
** Farrell, 1985; Levine & Rappaport, 1984.

indicative of pathology suggesting the need for a medical referral.

Type of Recurrent Pain

Although distinguishing between headaches and stomachaches appears relatively straightforward, it is not always so. There can be some overlap, the symptoms can covary, and in some cases RAP may actually be a symptom of a headache condition (i.e., abdominal migraine).

Headache. The two most common types of headaches in children are common migraine and tension headaches. Although a combination of these two headaches are occasionally seen in children, they are typically coded as being one of these two primary types. "Common migraine" is the most common type of headache in children. Characteristics of common migraine include pain lasting anywhere from 4 to 72 hours that is unilateral in location, pulsating in quality, moderate or severe in intensity, aggravated by routine physical activity, and associated with nausea, photo- and phonophobia. Common characteristics of tension headaches typically include pain lasting minutes to days that is pressing/tightening in quality, mild or moderate in intensity, bilateral in location, and does not worsen with routine physical activity. Nausea is absent, but photophobia or phonophobia may be present. These criteria were developed with adult study populations and complete diagnostic criteria can be found in the International Headache Society

diagnostic criteria (International Headache Society, 1988).

In our clinical experience with children, the intensity and the quality are the best indicators of type of headache, whereas location and associated features overlap too much to be reliable diagnostic criteria. Interestingly, this supports the notion that these two types of headaches may fall on the same etiological continuum. Whether the differential diagnosis is important is unclear. Although both may involve autonomic reactivity, migraine and tension headaches may involve different response systems, vasomotor and muscular, respectively. As a result, treatments for migraine have typically included thermal biofeedback to control vasomotor instability, whereas treatment for tension headache has typically included electromyographic biofeedback to reduce muscle tension. To our knowledge, the importance of this distinction to treatment outcome remains unaddressed in children. Until it has been shown to be irrelevant for treatment, differential diagnosis of headache type should be pursued.

Recurrent Abdominal Pain. Recurrent abdominal pain typically involves at least three episodes of pain over at least three months, sufficient to interfere with daily activities and with no known organic cause (Apley, 1975). Usually, the diagnosis is made by elimination of organic difficulties, such as gastrointestinal dysfunctions (e.g. constipation), intake-related pain (e.g., lactose intolerance), acquired noninflammatory impairments (e.g., peptic ulcer), chronic infections (e.g., Crohn's disease), metabolic diseases (e.g., diabetes mellitus), delayed effects of congenital anomalies (e.g., Hirschprung's disease), neurologic disorders (e.g., abdominal epilepsy), late complications of trauma (e.g., adhesions), and genitourinary disorders (dysmenorrhea, urinary tract infection, Levine & Rappaport, 1984). Onset is rarely before the age of 5 and tends to peak at 9–10 years of age (Apley, 1975). Although not necessary for diagnosis, there are a number of common symptoms (Rappaport & Leichtner, 1993). Pain location is usually periumbilical (around the umbilicus) and is generally described as diffuse and aching (Farrell, 1984), although on occasion we have seen children with pain symptoms severe enough to result in a trip to the hospital emergency room. In fact, one child was incorrectly diagnosed with acute appendicitis and underwent unnecessary surgery. Duration of the pain symptoms is usually short (less than 3 hours) and is usually during waking hours (wakening from sleep with abdominal pain is typically considered an indicator of organic pathology). Associated autonomic symptoms include nausea and vomiting, flushing, perspiration, and palpitations. Pain is rarely alleviated through medication. Finally, school absence is high in children with RAP (Walker, Garber, Van Slyke, & Greene, 1995).

Problem Assessment

During the assessment process, there are several concerns that arise that are endemic to the assessment of pain in general and recurrent pain in particular. First, as with any private event, pain can only be assessed indirectly, often through self-report. The difficulty lies in that self-reports of private events are established by the child's verbal community which does not have access to the private event. The verbal community can (and does) resort to public accompaniments of the private event (pain behavior), but "this method of circumventing the privacy of the individual is not foolproof because the public and private events may not be perfectly correlated (Skinner, 1957).

Second, observed pain behaviors (including self-report, facial and postural expression, and activity change) are subject to contingencies of reinforcement (sometimes subtle, sometimes not), making it difficult to interpret discrepancies in pain

behavior. For example, those who adhere to the oversimplified dichotomy of pain being either "organic" or "psychogenic" often assume that pain without pathology is "in the child's head" (Rappaport & Leichtner, 1993). If this message has been conveyed by the medical community prior to referral, there may be an extinction burst, in which pain behaviors increase in response to a decrease in reinforcement (i.e., lost credibility, lost attention), or there may actually be a decrease in pain behavior in response to punitive references to psychopathology. Consequently, it is important to determine whether the child and family have the impression that the pain is "in the child's head" and to educate them regarding this inaccuracy.

A third problem in assessing recurrent pain in particular is its episodic nature. The precipitating event is rarely directly observable and the occurrence of the pain is often unpredictable. With recurrent pain, a psychologist must settle for proxy measures such as self-report. And, as with all self-monitoring, the ongoing process of rating pain intensity may actually alter the reports of pain. In some cases, unobtrusive measures by the parents may be appropriate.

Pain Assessment Guidelines

When assessing pain in children, the child's skill and developmental level should be taken into consideration (Zeltzer et al., 1992). For instance, the child's language development and learning history will determine who answers the interview questions, how pain intensity is reported, and which intervention is most appropriate. The components of a thorough assessment will vary somewhat across conditions, but general knowledge of pain assessment strategies, as well as knowledge of the particular pain condition, should ensure adequate assessment of any pain disorder. Although the focus here is on headaches and recurrent abdominal pain, the following assessment procedures can be adapted easily to other recurrent pain disorders. The critical components of any good assessment should cover four areas:

1. *Historical/contextual variables:* A review of significant medical history, family history of recurrent pain, time and circumstances of pain onset, previous treatment attempts (medical and behav-

ioral/psychological), and any comorbidity (e.g., depression, anxiety, parent–child conflict, or marital conflict).

2. *Pain variables:* Assessment of pain location, frequency, intensity, duration, quality, associated features (e.g., nausea, vomiting, light/sound sensitivity, other pain), and pain behavior (e.g., grimacing, moaning, postural guarding).

3. *Organic variables:* Physiological setting events (e.g., fatigue, hunger, hyperarousal) and antecedents (e.g., academic demands, food, physical activity, emotion, and weather) as well as psychophysiological hyperarousal and delayed recovery.

4. *Operant variables:* Specific discriminative stimuli that may evoke pain behaviors and consequences that may reinforce, punish, or extinguish pain behaviors.

There are three primary methods for assessing each of these components. Most clinicians use a combination of methods to enhance the reliability of individual measures.

Self- or Parent-Report

Client and Parent Interview. The interview is the primary means of obtaining information regarding the historical and contextual variables just listed. It also provides a means of assessing both client and parent perceptions and/or awareness of pain, organic and operant variables. Although a standard interview form is not necessary, it can assist the interviewer by prompting for certain types of information. For example, a standard interview form for assessing headaches has been developed by P.A. McGrath (1990). It prompts specific inquiries about common headache precipitants (e.g., foods with caffeine, yeast, MSG, or nitrates; fatigue; emotional stress; academic demands or difficult school situations) and some common consequences (e.g., leaving school, elimination of responsibilities, special treatment). In addition, a parent rating scale has been developed for identifying common environmental variables associated with headache (Budd, Workman, Lemsky, & Quick, 1994). Note, however, that although it may be helpful to know some common antecedents and consequences to headaches, the assessment should not be constrained or limited to lists provided in standard interviews or rating forms.

There do not appear to be any published standard interview forms for RAP. Specific components of the interview should include diet (fiber content) and toileting history to rule out chronic constipation, and corollary physical effects such as nausea, vomiting, and headaches. Although there are fewer known triggers for RAP than for headaches, stress related to family, peers, and school appears to be high in many children with RAP (P.A. McGrath, 1990). Although not the case for the majority of children with RAP, school avoidance can be an integral part of RAP (P.J. McGrath & Unruh, 1987). If the child has excessive school absences, special attention should be given to school-related antecedents and consequences. The clinician should assess the child's morning routine, academic performance, peer relations, and any events at school that might be aversive for the child. In addition, activities occurring at home if school is missed should be documented to determine whether they might be reinforcing.

Daily Monitoring. Although the interview provides a historical review, monitoring provides a more direct assessment of pain, organic and operant variables. Visual analogue scales (VAS), in which the length of a line is adjusted to match the strength of a perception, are often used with children to enable them to rate pain intensity. Having them rate intensity on a daily basis throughout the day also provides frequency and duration measures. Studies have found that the VAS is a reliable and valid measure of perceptions of pain in persons over the age of five, regardless of age, gender, and health status (e.g., P.A. McGrath, 1987; P.A. McGrath & deVerber, 1986). Other pain intensity rating techniques include pain thermometers in which the amount of red (mercury) is adjusted to match the strength of a perception, poker chips, and Likert-type scales using numbers on a 0–10 or 1–100 scale (indicating increasing pain intensity) or faces depicting differing amounts of comfort (P.A. McGrath, 1990). The ratings are typically behaviorally anchored. Daily monitoring should also include reports of the impact of pain on activity and medication taken.

As with interview forms, there are numerous monitoring forms that have been used with children (e.g., P.J. McGrath, Cunningham, Lascelles, and Humphreys, 1990). Form 14.1 presents a form used in our clinic that is appropriate for children

FORM 14.1. Sample Pain Monitoring Form

Name_____**Age**_____**Sex:** Male / Female

INTENSITY - <u>Four</u> times each day, please update the pain graph according to the following scale.

I N T E N S I T Y
(0) NO PAIN
(1)
(2) SLIGHTLY PAINFUL - I only notice my pain when I focus my attention on it.
(3)
(4) MILDLY PAINFUL - I can ignore my pain most of the time.
(5)
(6) PAINFUL - It is painful, but I can continue what I am doing.
(7)
(8) VERY PAINFUL - My pain makes concentration difficult, but I can perform undemanding tasks.
(9)
(10) EXTREMELY PAINFUL - I can't do anything when I have such pain.

MEDICATION - Each time you take medication for pain, please indicate the type and amount of medication.

MONDAY (Date_____)

INTENSITY — graph, vertical axis 0–10, horizontal axis 6 AM, 8, 10, 12 PM, 2, 4, 6, 8, 10, 12

MEDICATION (type and amount)
_____
_____
School Missed?   Yes   No
Classes Missed:
_____
Activities Missed:

TUESDAY (Date_____)

INTENSITY — graph, vertical axis 0–10, horizontal axis 6 AM, 8, 10, 12 PM, 2, 4, 6, 8, 10, 12

MEDICATION (type and amount)
_____
_____
School Missed?   Yes   No
Classes Missed:
_____
Activities Missed:

WEDNESDAY (Date_____)

INTENSITY — graph, vertical axis 0–10, horizontal axis 6 AM, 8, 10, 12 PM, 2, 4, 6, 8, 10, 12

MEDICATION (type and amount)
_____
_____
School Missed?   Yes   No
Classes Missed:
_____
Activities Missed:

OVER

(continued)

FORM 14.1 (*Continued*)

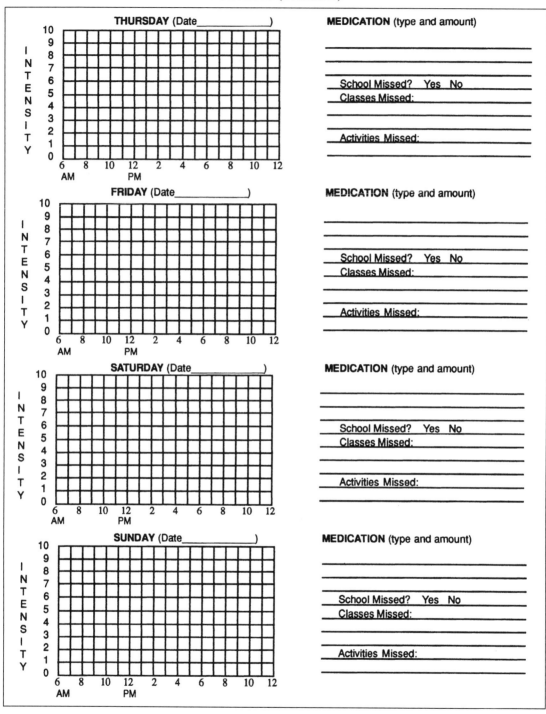

THURSDAY (Date_____)

INTENSITY

MEDICATION (type and amount)

_____

_____

School Missed?   Yes   No
Classes Missed:
_____

Activities Missed:
_____

FRIDAY (Date_____)

INTENSITY

MEDICATION (type and amount)

_____

_____

School Missed?   Yes   No
Classes Missed:
_____

Activities Missed:
_____

SATURDAY (Date_____)

INTENSITY

MEDICATION (type and amount)

_____

_____

School Missed?   Yes   No
Classes Missed:
_____

Activities Missed:
_____

SUNDAY (Date_____)

INTENSITY

MEDICATION (type and amount)

_____

_____

School Missed?   Yes   No
Classes Missed:
_____

Activities Missed:
_____

age seven and older. Common features of pain records include an intensity rating that is behaviorally anchored, time of the day, and specific consequences (e.g., medication, taken, activities missed). Some forms (e.g. P.A. McGrath, 1990) also include other symptoms, possible causes, and coping strategies. Although monitoring of actual headache and abdominal pain are likely to be quite similar, the assessment of RAP may also include monitoring of dietary fiber and bowel habits (including frequency, size and consistency of bowel movements) to continuing assessing for constipation that may be associated with RAP.

Monitoring should also involve a descriptive functional assessment in which the antecedents and consequences to pain are reported by the child and/or parents. The purpose should be to identify the circumstances under which the pain occurs and to look for patterns that suggest that pain is reinforced (either positively or negatively) or punished. It may be useful to have the child attempt to record data on specific antecedents and consequences associated with specific episodes of pain. For this purpose, a daily recording form similar to the one depicted in Form 14.2 may be used. This type of detailed record keeping can be important because the patient or family may not be aware of the significance of the events correlated with pain behavior

FORM 14.2. Sample Daily Monitoring of Pain, Pain Antecedents, and Pain Consequences

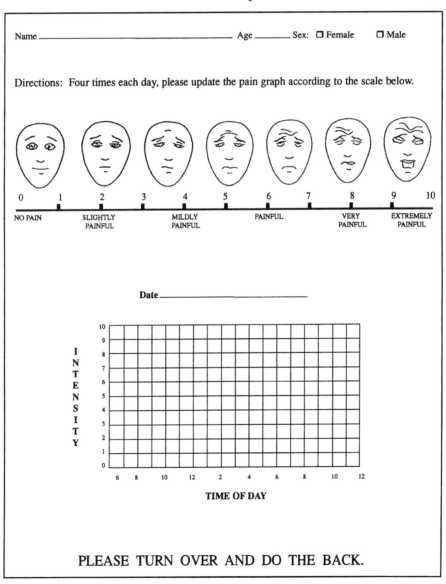

Adapted using Bieri, Reeve, Champion, Addicoat, & Zeigler (1990).   (*continued*)

FORM 14.2 (*Continued*)

Please put a check mark in front of each thing that happened before your headache,
and each thing that happened after headache occurred.

What Happened Before Headache

☐ Ate something
    specify what _____

_____

☐ Drank something
    specify what _____

_____

☐ Glare or bright light
☐ Weather or temperature change
☐ Too much sleep
☐ Strong odors, fumes
☐ Game or competition
☐ Worried about something
☐ Sad/unhappy
☐ Difficult school work or test
☐ Angry about something
☐ Problem/fight with parents
☐ Problem/fight with friends
☐ Concentrated hard on something
☐ Something embarassing happened
☐ Too much physical activity
☐ Other (please specify) _____

_____

What Happened During/After Headache

☐ Took medication (indicate type and how much) _____

_____

☐ Missed school
☐ Missed one or more classes
    Specify which class(es) _____

_____

☐ Did not complete homework
☐ Could not get out of bed in morning
☐ Chose a quiet activity to manage the pain
☐ Did not complete chores
    Specify which chores missed _____

_____

☐ Missed practice/appointment/lesson
    Specify which practice/appointment(s) _____

_____

☐ Asked parent for help
☐ Asked parent for medication
☐ Tried to ignore headache
☐ Slept
☐ Rested
☐ Turned off lights, shut blinds, shades, or shutters
☐ Turned off sounds (T.V. , music)
☐ Ate or drank something
☐ Put cloth on head/neck
☐ Massaged head/neck
☐ Got a massage from someone else
☐ Started exercise or other recreation
☐ Cried
☐ Tried to distract yourself (listen to music, watch T.V.)
☐ Practiced relaxation
☐ Tried to remain active
☐ Did normal activity/routine
☐ Talked to parent/friend about pain
☐ Other (please specify) _____

(Rachlin, 1985). Note that listing likely antecedents and consequences on a recording form may bias responses.

Direct Observation. Because recurrent pain is intermittent, it is uncommon to have repeated op-portunities to directly observe pain behavior. Clinicians can, however, look for common pain behaviors such as postural guarding, grimacing, crying, squinting, withdrawal, changes in temperament (irritability), kneading or holding part of the body (head or abdomen), verbal complaints of pain, gagging or vomiting, and pallor. Clients should be asked to rate their pain during each clinic visit to look for correlations between pain ratings and pain behavior. Direct observation may also involve psychophysiological monitoring. This typically involves recording one or a number of physiological modalities (e.g., heart rate, hand temperature, electromyography, respiration, electrodermal responses) under a number of different stressful or relaxing conditions. Psychophysiological assessment is not always practical or necessary; however, it can be useful for several reasons. First, psychophysiological assessment can facilitate the education of patients about their own physiology and psychophysiological activity, reactivity, and recovery from stress. Second, it can permit pre- and posttreatment comparisons, thus documenting progress for clinical research and/or for insurance purposes. Finally, both reactivity to stress and rate of recovery from stress can help in identifying critical behaviors for targeting in intervention (Haynes, et al., 1991). For example, delayed poststress recovery should alert the therapist that the child does not have the ability to regulate physiological reactivity (Schwartz, 1995). Impaired poststress recovery may suggest unhealthy functioning of homeostatic control of the autonomic nervous system.

A typical psychophysiological assessment might involve some combination of an adaptation or habituation period (during which the client rests quietly), and then periods of relaxation, or stress (e.g., oral reading, silent math [serial 7's], personal imagery of a stressful event) followed by poststress or postrelaxation phases. Stressors are individualized based on the intake interview. A complete assessment protocol is beyond the scope of this chapter and the reader is referred to Schwartz (1995) for more detailed information.

Permanent Product Measures. Permanent product measures involve sources of data that can be recorded independent of self-report. Efforts to assess the number of days of school missed, the number and type of activities missed both at home and at school, the number of emergency room visits, and the amount of medication taken (both prescription and nonprescription) are critical when assessing recurrent pain syndromes. While these do not measure actual pain, they do measure the impact of pain on daily living. Note that in most cases,

these data are collected through self-report, in the daily monitoring by either the client or the parent.

Problem Analysis

The analysis of the data obtained during the assessment involves careful consideration of both organismic and operant variables that may be involved in the maintenance of the recurrent pain. Those variables identified during the analysis then permit development of an appropriately individualized treatment plan. Because the nature of pain makes it impossible to measure the private experience of pain, function is determined primarily in terms of the effect of pain behavior on the environment. In addition, because recurrent pain is typically episodic, function is based primarily on data obtained from self-monitoring of pain parameters as well as self and parent report rather than from direct observation of pain episodes and corresponding contextual events.

The determination of when sufficient data have been collected to conduct a meaningful analysis depends primarily on the characteristic parameters of the pain. For example, pain that is very frequent (i.e., several episodes per week) may require less time for assessment in order for meaningful relations to emerge. One week may be sufficient to observe temporal patterns of significance or to identify clear situational antecedents to pain episodes. On the other hand, less frequent pain (one episode per week) may require a longer period of monitoring for patterns to emerge, in some cases up to four weeks of recording. In general, it is difficult to imagine a situation in which less than one week of self-monitoring would be sufficient. Clinicians should attempt to obtain self-monitoring of at least three separate pain episodes to establish any trends. Two weeks of self-monitoring is often sufficient to obtain this amount of data and seems reasonable in most cases of recurrent pain. Information obtained during interviews and psychophysiological assessment can usually be obtained during a single clinic visit.

Analysis of Organic Variables

Data from all sources provide an assessment in which patterns in pain episodes may be identified, revealing reliable organic variables. Identification of organic variables, however, provides no real assessment of function. That is, in situations where reliable antecedents, or pain triggers, are identified, it is unclear whether the resulting pain behaviors are a result of contingencies of survival (respondents) or contingencies of reinforcement (operants). Most antecedents seem to serve an eliciting function, and, the longer children experience recurrent pain, the larger the number of conditioned pain "triggers" likely to be present (Zeltzer, et al., 1992). Similarly, in situations where stressors are identified that elicit significant autonomic reactivity and/or delayed poststress recovery, pain behavior can be only hypothesized to be escape motivated (i.e., strengthened through reduction in arousal and escape from or reduction in pain). Regardless of such considerations, the analysis of pain triggers may suggest opportunities for intervention in terms of eliminating or avoiding some antecedents. In addition, an analysis of the psychophysiological data may show autonomic reactivity that suggests interventions involving the development of alternative means of reducing arousal or speeding poststress recovery.

Analysis of Operant Variables

Data from the assessment will also provide a descriptive functional assessment in terms of consequences maintaining pain behavior. Pain elicited via organismic variables is likely to acquire discriminative properties; that is, the pain may set the occasion for pain behavior. The descriptive assessment data may show that subsequent pain behavior is then strengthened in one of three ways. First, pain behavior may be strengthened and maintained because even intermittently, it results in a reduction in or an escape from pain experienced. Typical pain behaviors strengthened through this relation include reductions in activity level (e.g., lying in bed, missing school, missing activities), increases in medication ingestion, and increases in palliative techniques (e.g., massaging part of the body, trying to relax). Note that while these behaviors often do result in reduction in immediate pain *intensity,* they rarely produce significant reductions in long-term pain *frequency.*

Second, pain behavior may be strengthened because it results in a reduction in or an escape from aversive experiences other than pain. Many of the same behaviors listed previously (e.g., reduction in activity level) can also result in avoidance of stressful demands at school or at home, escape from nonpreferred activities (e.g., chores), or escape or avoidance of family conflict. In our opinion, however, the most important experience to look for during the assessment is avoidance or escape from the responsibility for independent management of the recurrent pain. Children with recurrent pain can often avoid the responsibility of being good observers of their own behavior because their parents will do it for them. One result is that the children are not good at identifying reliable triggers of pain. Similarly, they avoid the demands of learning helpful pain management techniques because their parents will provide medications, take them to the doctor, and let them stay in bed when the pain is bad. Thus, the assessment may reveal a child who engages in little independent pain management behavior.

Third, pain behavior may also be strengthened through an increase in access to desirable or preferred activities. The assessment may show pain behavior resulting in a greater proportion of time spent with mom or dad or special attention from family and relatives who ask about and are interested in the child's pain. Even in cases where little attention is regularly provided in response to recurrent pain episodes, the assessment may show that on intermittent occasions during which the pain intensity increases, there is a change in the response of those around the child (i.e., more serious pain results in more serious response).

Decisions about how to proceed with treatment are based on the assessment data and the subsequent analysis. Treatment decisions are based in part on answers to the following questions:

1. Are there any reliable antecedents/triggers that can reasonably be removed that will allow prevention of at least some pain episodes? These may involve changes in lifestyle (changing dietary habits, moderating exercise, normalizing sleep patterns). They may also involve attempts to eliminate prominent emotional/academic stressors or to resolve difficult school or family situations.

2. Are there self-regulation skills that can be taught to the patient that will allow the child to manage potential autonomic reactivity in response to stress and/or pain?

3. Are there specific responses to pain that parents should be eliminating to discourage pain behavior or adding to encourage well behavior?

Plan Implementation

Since the answers to each of the three questions from the previous section are likely to be affirmative, treatment is likely to include features of responses to all three. But because pain and the treatment of pain can often seem mysterious and is often poorly understood by parents and children, an initial effort to demystify the treatment process may improve compliance with the treatment protocol and, ultimately, treatment outcome.

Demystification and Validation

Pain behavior has typically demanded a social response of some kind. Society generally gives each child the right to claim to be in pain regardless of evidence to the contrary (Rachlin, 1985). This has especially been true with acute pain, but with recurrent pain, the absence of well-defined organic pathology has led to questions about the authenticity of the pain. There is no reason, however, to question the veracity of pain reports. Although one should not rely exclusively on self-reports of pain intensity (Turk & Flor, 1987), treatment should always begin with a verbal intervention that involves the demystification of the recurrent pain process and an acknowledgement of the validity of the pain report. The following is a presentation of a sample demystification and validation that can be presented to children and parents:

> "Now that we've talked with you and your parents and have had you keep track of your pain for a while, we think that your pain partly comes from having a body that is particularly sensitive to things around you, like stress and other things in the environment. The fact that your body reacts is not unusual at all. What your body does that is different is that it reacts sooner and does not recover or calm down as quickly as others. Over time, this continuing reactivity can result in pain. Understand that it is not stress that causes your pain, nor is it your

body's reactivity that causes pain, it is the combination of the two that can trigger painful episodes. Your body's reactivity is very real and so is the pain you experience."

Control of Organic Variables

Precipitants

In cases in which clear pain precipitants or triggers are identified during the problem assessment and analysis, attempts to eliminate or control these triggers may prove valuable. Unfortunately, eliminating or controlling triggers often involves a change in lifestyle (i.e., diet, exercise, sleep habits) and there is little research on this area as an intervention for recurrent pain. The lack of research on eliminating triggers as an intervention probably reflects the fact that there is little evidence that triggers account for a significant number of headaches or stomachaches. Certainly, there is some evidence of a few common triggers of recurrent pain, such as chocolate leading to headaches and constipation (or slow gut motility) and lactose intolerance leading to stomachaches (Egger, Carter, Wilson, Turner, & Soothill, 1983; Barr, Levine & Watkins, 1979). And there is evidence, for example, that some children with RAP can be treated with increased dietary fiber (Barr et al, 1979; Edwards, Finney, Bonner, 1991; Feldman, McGrath, Hodgson, Ritter, & Shipman, 1985). But there are few other studies supporting lifestyle changes as an intervention, and many of those that have been done have utilized treatment packages (Finney, Lemanek, Cataldo, Katz, & Fuqua, 1989; P.J. McGrath et al., 1992; Sanders, Shepherd, Cleghorn, & Woolford, 1994). In addition, the complexity of changing the lifestyle of child and family appears to make it a relatively inefficient intervention, except perhaps in cases where strong evidence of reliable precipitants is clearly determined in the assessment.

Self-Regulation

Learning to control autonomic reactivity in response to pain precipitants appears to be one of the most effective interventions available. Indeed, this is one of the most researched areas of intervention in managing recurrent pain in children.

Self-regulation training for children typically involves biofeedback (thermal or electromyographic) or progressive muscle relaxation or some combination of the two, and these treatments have been found to be quite effective (see Duckro & Cantwell-Simmons, 1989, for a review; Grazzi, Leone, Frediani, & Bussone, 1990; Labbe, 1995; Larsson, Melin, & Doberi, 1990; P.J. McGrath et al., 1992). More recently, researchers have extended clinic-based success into the home and found that reducing clinical contact and increasing home practice has resulted in equally significant improvements (Allen & McKeen, 1991; Burke & Andrasik, 1989; Guarnieri & Blanchard, 1990). There are other self-regulation strategies that can be used with children, such as visual imagery, diaphragmatic breathing, and autogenics; however, none of these strategies has the research support that biofeedback and relaxation do. Part of the success of biofeedback may be the immediacy of the feedback. That is, biofeedback may succeed because the immediacy of the feedback provides reinforcement of intermediary behaviors until pain reduction can be achieved. This is important because the temporary pain relief achieved by maladaptive pain behaviors is so immediate that it interferes with acquisition of more adaptive behaviors. Biofeedback is also attractive because, in this technological age, it holds particular appeal for children. In fact, self-regulation training can be considered an important component of treatment, regardless of the outcome of the assessment, because (a) the research support is substantial, (b) the absence of observed autonomic reactivity does not mean it does not exist, only that it was undetected, and (c) parents who will be asked to comply with operant pain behavior management recommendations may resist in the absence of evidence that their children are being given strategies for managing (responding to) pain themselves.

Thermal biofeedback is the most extensively researched method for treatment of recurrent pain in children, is extremely easy to learn and to teach, and can be portable and easily used within a variety of settings, including the classroom. An introduction to thermal biofeedback treatment can be presented following the demystification and could include the following information:

"Now there are several things *you* can do to deal with your body's reactivity. First, some things are more likely to produce a reaction by your body than others, and you can try to eliminate obvious stressors or triggers. But you will never be able to eliminate them all. Second, you can try to find medications that will eliminate your pain. But the medications do not solve the problem of your body's reactivity. As soon as you stop the medication, the pain will likely return. Finally, you can learn to control your body's reactivity. The skills for learning to control reactivity are easy and once you learn them, you will have them to use whenever you need them. You are going to learn to control your reactivity using thermal biofeedback. In biofeedback, bio refers to 'body' and feedback refers to 'information.' Biofeedback, then, is simply a means of giving you information about what your body is doing so that you can learn to control it better. You are going to learn to control your body by using information about your hand temperature. The computer will tell you how warm or cold your hands are and then assist you in learning to warm your hands. Children who learn to warm their hands using biofeedback can reduce the reactivity of the body that is associated with pain and in many cases can reduce the frequency of their pain."

It is important to emphasize changes in pain frequency as the likely outcome of learning and using biofeedback. Research has shown that frequency is the most consistently modified pain parameter (Duckro & Cantwell-Simmons, 1989), and it supports the importance of regular practice of the biofeedback skills. That is, biofeedback has proven to be better in prevention of recurrent pain episodes than in reduction of intensity once the pain has occurred. This finding is consistent with the conceptualized autonomic reactivity; frequent use of biofeedback may reduce reactivity and thereby prevent the onset of painful episodes.

The actual course of treatment can vary widely depending upon how quickly the child learns the skills, the cognitive capabilities of the child, and resources available. Clinic-based treatment has typically involved 8–12 sessions over 6–10 weeks. A home-based protocol, however, is more efficient and accessible to more children. A typical treatment might involve 4 clinic visits across 8 weeks, with most learning occurring during daily home practice. The initial clinic visit usually involves 10–15 minutes of equipment hookup and habituation and then 10 minutes of therapist-directed strategies for handwarming (imagery and/or diaphragmatic breathing). The therapist-guided imagery might go as follows:

"You can begin the process of warming your hands by closing your eyes and then taking a long, slow, deep breath in through your nose, and, when you are ready, out through your nose as slowly as possible. When you breathe in, feel your belly-button push out, and, as you breathe out, feel yourself go loose and limp, warm and heavy. Now we are going to think of a place or situation that would be pleasant and warm, like lying on a beach, taking a hot bath, or snuggling up next to a fire. Imagine that you are walking out on a beach with white sand as far as you can see. There is a blue sky with a scattering of white fluffy clouds. The sun is warm and the water is sparkling. You lie down on your back in the sand to enjoy the warmth and you notice, as you settle in the sand, the warmth from the sand on the back of your legs, arms, back, and shoulders. You can also feel the rays of the sun soaking into the front of your body; your legs . . . your arms . . . your chest . . . your face . . . your cheeks. As the heat from the sun and sand soak into your body, you can feel that warmth drain slowly into your fingers. As the warmth slowly moves into your hands and fingers, you notice that they feel surrounded, enveloped by warmth. Your fingers, hands and arms may feel heavy and limp, like they are sinking into the sand, or they may feel light and tingly, like they could lift right off the sand."

Guided imagery usually involves helping the child create pictures and experience sensations that are pleasant and warm, although there is no imagery that reliably works for all children. It is best to tell the children that they will need to be "scientists" and experiment with different images during bio-feedback to see what works best. The child can then engage in 10–15 minutes of independent biofeedback practice. The child can also be instructed to practice at least once a day at home for 10–15 minutes. Research has shown that there is a relation between amount of home practice and improvement in pain (Allen & McKeen, 1991), so emphasis should be on home practice at least once a day. For school-aged children, it appears that most of these skills can be learned primarily at home with home temperature trainers. These temperature trainers can be as simple as a 25-cent alcohol thermometer or as sophisticated as a digital trainer with threshold capabilities ($40–60), most of which are available from biomedical supply houses (e.g., Biomedical Instruments, Warren, MI; Stens Corporation, San Francisco).

To help insure that home practice occurs and that the quality of that practice is adequate, any one of several strategies should be used. Asking the client to complete a daily practice log (See Form 14.3), detailing frequency, length and quality of practice (amount of temperature change) may serve as a prompt to practice, and also as a means of identifying and solving problems in the practice routine. In addition, during each clinic visit, the client can be asked to practice in front of the therapist and to attempt handwarming without feedback. Plans for generalization should include the use of increasing distraction during practice in the clinic and at home (e.g., open doors, static noise, or TV), practicing in less relaxing situations (e.g., sitting up rather than lying down, kitchen rather than bedroom), increasing the frequency of practices without feedback, and initiation of practice in situations where pain may be likely to occur (e.g., in the classroom). Although many practitioners use audiotapes to enhance relaxation, they are not necessary for successful intervention. In addition, there may be some concern that reliance on audiotapes to achieve relaxation may diminish generalization. There do not appear to be published data, however, to specifically support or discourage use of tapes.

Management of Operant Variables: Pain Behavior Management

Pain behavior management strategies are designed to discourage maladaptive pain behavior by

FORM 14.3. Thermal Biofeedback Home Practice Log

NAME _____

WEEK 1 2 3 4 5 6 7 8 9 10 11 12

NOT RELAXED	0 1 2 3 4 5 6 7 8 9	VERY RELAXED
	RELAXATION SCALE	

	BEGIN				END			
DATE	Temp	Time	Relax #		Temp	Time	Relax #	COMMENT
MONDAY 1								
2								
TUESDAY 1								
2								
WEDNESDAY 1								
2								
THURSDAY 1								
2								
FRIDAY 1								
2								
SATURDAY 1								
2								
SUNDAY 1								
2								

removing any reinforcement that may be supporting the maintenance of that behavior. These strategies are also designed to differentially reinforce more adaptive behaviors that are incompatible with pain behaviors. The assessment may have identified obvious reinforcers for pain that will need to be addressed, or the assessment may have demonstrated a distinct lack of support for more adaptive behavior. However, as in the situation with self-regulation training, even if reinforcing consequences are remote, obscure, or few in number, recommendations for strategies to strengthen well behavior and discourage pain behavior are still applicable. That is, the absence of obvious reinforcing consequences does not mean they do not exist or that they might not emerge in the near future.

Not surprisingly, research has shown that the consequences of recurrent pain are closely related to the level of disability created by pain in children and adolescents (Holden, Gladstein, Trulsen, &

Wall, 1994), and that the modification of consequences in response to recurrent pain is an important part of treatment (Allen & McKeen, 1991; P.J. McGrath & Feldman, 1986; McMahon, Harper, & Cruikshank, 1990; Sanders et al., 1989). The parents' introduction to pain behavior management guidelines may be as follows:

"Now that your child has begun to learn the skills that are important for controlling [his/ her] own pain (i.e., knowledge of triggers, problem-solving skills, control over their reactivity), it is important to create an environment in which independent use of these skills is encouraged. You need to be aware, however, that a child's natural reaction to pain is to wait for a parent or a doctor to alleviate the pain. And a parent's natural reaction is to do just that: fix it or take them to a doctor who can. This is adaptive with acute pain or injury-related pain episodes. But this approach is not adaptive with recurrent pain. Your child can and should become more independent in managing pain, because your child is the only one who can. In a practical sense this means doing less for your child in terms of solving [his/her] pain problem and doing more for [him/her] in terms of en-

couraging adaptive coping. Here are specific recommendations for how you can do this."

Recommendations should direct parents to pay less attention to pain behaviors, pay more attention to adaptive coping, and to insist upon continuation of normal activities, chores, and responsibilities (See Table 2). Anecdotal clinical experience suggests that parents are more likely to follow through with these recommendations if they can see that their child is learning skills that will enable him or her to manage the pain. Thus, introduction of the parents to pain behavior management should be prefaced with evidence that the child is developing self-regulation strategies (e.g., is capable of producing hand temperature increases with and without feedback). Parents who follow these guidelines have been found to have children who exhibit more adaptive coping, regardless of how much they practice other coping strategies, whereas parents who do not follow through with these recommendations have children who exhibit less adaptive coping, regardless of how much they practice the coping strategies (Allen & McKeen, 1991; Kuhn & Allen, 1993).

Although these pain management techniques have been developed and researched in traditional clinical settings, there is no reason to believe they

TABLE 2. Operant Pain Behavior Management Guidelines

1. *Eliminate status checks:*
   No questions about pain intensity, frequency, duration, location.

2. *Reduce response to pain behavior:*
   No effort should be made to assist the child in coping (other than to issue a single prompt to practice self-regulation skills). Do not offer assistance or suggesttions for coping. Do not offer medication.

3. *Reduce pharmacological dependence:*
   No not offer over-the-counter or abortive medication. If medication is requested, deliver only as prescribed and not PRN (i.e., follow directed time table).

4. *Encourage normal activity:*
   Insist upon attendance at school, maintenance of daily chores and responsibilities, participation in regular activities (lessons, practices, clubs).

5. *Encourage independent management of pain:*
   Praise and publicly acknowledge independent practice of self-regulation skills during pain-free episodes. If pain is reported, issue a single prompt to practice self-regulation skills. Praise and reward compliance with #4 when report of pain has been made.

6. *Recruit others to follow rules 1–5:*
   School personnel should not send child home, child should be encouraged and permitted to practice self-regulation skills in the classroom, workload should not be modified.

7. *Treat pain requiring a reduction in activity as illness:*
   If school, activities, chores, or responsibilities are missed, the child should be treated as ill and sent to bed for the remainder of the day, even if pain is resolved. Do not permit watching television, playing games (video) or special treatment.

could not be implemented easily in any environment. Because recurrent pain syndromes can be responsible for missed classes and prolonged absences, specific recommendations have been advanced for management of some recurrent pain conditions in the school environment (McMahon, et al., 1990). Indeed, it makes sense that school psychologists, counselors, and school nurses should be aware of fundamental assessment and intervention strategies. At the most basic level, an interview and daily pain diary maintained for two weeks should identify significant school-based precipitants that may be modifiable. An intervention may then involve introduction of a simple self-regulation strategy and appropriate operant recommendations to the family, including regular school attendance. Similar strategies have been implemented in a primary care setting for treatment of another recurrent pediatric paroxysmal disorder (Kuhn, Allen, & Shriver, 1995), with excellent outcome. While many primary care physicians may not have the time to implement the assessment and treatment themselves, psychologists who have established collaborative relationships with pediatricians and have shown that behavioral technology can be efficiently integrated into a primary care practice will likely be recruited by primary care providers to handle many child health behavior problems (Allen, Barone, & Kuhn, 1993), including recurrent pain.

Plan Evaluation

Deciding whether treatment efforts have been successful depends upon outcome in a number of areas. Reduction in pain parameters is a critical variable. A 50% reduction in pain has often been used in recurrent pain research as an indication of clinically significant change (Duckro & Cantwell-Simmons, 1989). This can be applied to any one or all of the pain parameters, but is often applied to some composite measure of pain. A pain "index" is a typical composite score, in which repeated daily measures of pain intensity, are averaged, producing a score that reflects frequency, intensity, and duration. Producing changes in pain parameters, however, is inadequate as a sole measure of treatment outcome. Since these measures are dependent on verbal reports, clinicians must be careful to avoid simply teaching children to reduce reports of pain,

a practice that may not be in the child's best interest (P.J. McGrath & Feldman, 1986). Changes in pain parameters are best supported by permanent product measures that corroborate verbal reports. The clinician should see changes in measures of adaptive behavior, such as increases in the number of days in school, reductions in medication usage, and fewer missed activities. Clinicians and/or parents may also observe changes in directly observed pain behaviors during reported episodes.

The determination of when sufficient data have been collected to evaluate success is quite similar to the determination of when there is sufficient assessment data to conduct a meaningful analysis. Frequent episodes of pain may require less time to evaluate improvement than does less frequent pain. Clinicians should be aware, however, that because some of the features of the operant guidelines involve extinction of pain behavior, there may initially be an increase in reported and observed pain behavior. Children and parents must be encouraged to maintain compliance with the program.

Determining what to do when the intervention is ineffective depends in part on determining why it has been ineffective. Ongoing assessment should assist in that process. In general, the reasons for treatment failure can generally fall into four categories (see Table 3).

Motivational Deficits

Children with low-frequency pain may exhibit poor motivation to practice and learn new skills that are infrequently needed (Allen & McKeen, 1991). In addition, few children are motivated to practice self-regulation skills or remain active when they are in the midst of pain. A supplemental incentive program for changing diet, avoiding precipitants, practicing self-regulation, and/or remaining active could be implemented if motivation appears to be a problem. However, the development of a motivational program risks placing the onus of responsibility for management of pain upon the parent. A strategy more consistent with the treatment objectives would be to insure that the parents are enforcing the operant guidelines, demanding continued activity and leaving no alternative for managing pain other than the strategies that were offered. Research has suggested that even in situations in which poorly motivated children take little initiative to practice

TABLE 3. Problem-Solving Treatment Failures

Problem	Possible solution
Motivational deficit (see page 280)	1. Supplemental motivational program 2. Referral back for medical evaluation 3. Emphasize operant recommendations
Skills deficit (page 281)	1. Increase frequency of practice 2. Enhance the biofeedback sensitivity or resolution 3. Enhance relative performance feedback 4. Introduce alternative relaxation strategy
Assessment error (page 281)	1. Conduct new A-B-C assessment 2. Review assessment and need to resolve family factors (e.g., marital conflict, general parent–child conflict) 3. Review assessment and need to resolve child factors (e.g., depression, anxiety) 4. Referral back for further medical evaluation
Inadequate planning for generalization and maintenance (page 282)	1. Train more exemplars or arrange for more common stimuli across settings, people, stimuli, and time 2. Booster sessions for skill maintenance

self-regulation or manage precipitants, parents who have adhered to operant guidelines have had children who used less medication and engaged in more adaptive functioning (Allen & McKeen, 1991; Kuhn & Allen, 1993).

In situations in which parents are not compliant with operant guidelines or other recommendations for lifestyle changes, the alternatives are fewer. Children can still be taught to manage their own pain, and many are successful, even without the support of their parents. Some parents, however, may not have explored all the alternative medical evaluations that were available prior to their referral, and they may not be willing to comply until their concerns about potential medical problems or their hopes for medical solutions have been addressed.

Skill Deficits

In situations in which children are having a difficult time learning self-regulation skills, several alternatives are available. Changing or enhancing the feedback may improve outcome. For example, enhancing the sensitivity (or resolution) of the equipment will lead to more dramatic changes in feedback in response to actual changes in hand temperature. Providing feedback showing performance in relation to other (anonymous) children who are doing more poorly has also been found to be an effective way to enhance feedback for some children (Allen & Shriver, 1997). In addition, the child may require more learning repetitions, and increasing the number of practices may help (Allen & McKeen, 1991; Allen & Shriver, 1997). Finally, biofeedback may prove too overwhelming for some children, especially younger children, and a less complex self-regulation strategy may be employed, such as visual imagery, regulated deep-breathing, or diaphragmatic breathing. Some have suggested that altered breathing patterns may actually mediate some of the positive effects of relaxation and biofeedback through autonomic nervous system changes (Janis, Defares, & Grossman, 1983).

Assessment Error

Treatment failures may also occur because the descriptive assessment was incomplete or because a critical variable went unnoticed. Assessment error could involve missing a reliable precipitant that could be eliminated or modified (e.g, diet change), not identifying remote but powerful consequences for pain behavior (e.g., pain behavior that helps maintain family homeostasis), or targeting a less reactive response mode (e.g., handwarming instead of EMG). Because these types of errors are always a possibility, and because new variables (e.g., new triggers, new functions) can develop even in the midst of treatment, assessment should be an ongoing process that continues throughout treatment and follow-up.

Poor Generalization or Maintenance of Skills

Even if children and parents are motivated to learn and implement recommended behavior changes, some children may experience treatment failure because their knowledge and skills fail to generalize from the clinic. Good intervention, of course, includes systematic planning for generalization (Stokes & Baer, 1977). However, even the most thorough clinician may fail to train sufficient exemplars or to program enough common stimuli across settings. In addition, parents and children may reduce the frequency with which they use the skills learned in clinic as they begin to experience reductions in pain. A subsequent relapse often renews the vigor with which parents once again pursue medical interventions. The skills learned in clinic may be forgotten or ignored. Booster sessions may be needed to encourage maintenance of the skills learned, even as pain reduction occurs. Booster sessions should be a part of good long-term follow-up.

The manner in which contact with the therapist is faded and follow-up is conducted depends in large part on the individual client and family and their response to treatment. Clients and families who have been highly motivated and have adhered closely to recommendations may be able to maintain improvements with decreasing contact after only two to three clinic sessions. Follow-up at 6 and 12 months would be appropriate. Clients and families, however, who have had more difficulty learning techniques or who have shown some motivational deficits may require contact with the clinician for a longer period to insure treatment integrity and adjust the program as needed to response to changing client motivation and skills. In this case, follow-ups may also be conducted more frequently (e.g., every 3 months) until stability is established.

Summary and Directions for Research

Recurrent pain episodes, the most common of which are headaches and abdominal pain, represent a clinically significant health problem for many children and adolescents. Recurrent pain can occur in as many as 30% of all children and can, left untreated, lead to significant impairment of daily emotional and behavioral functioning. Although the causes of recurrent pain problems remain uncertain, there is increasing evidence that both organic and operant factors play an important role in understanding and treating recurrent pain in children. While organic features such as autonomic overresponsiveness have often been ignored, operant factors have often been oversimplified as "secondary gain." The temporary relief from pain is an immediate and powerful reinforcer for pain behaviors that has little impact on the long-term frequency of recurrent pain episodes and often results in increasing functional limitations.

Although there are inherent problems in assessing pain (e.g., it is private, episodic, and inextricable from pain behavior), assessment techniques that include self-report, direct observation, and permanent product measures have proven reliable in assessing pain in children. The resulting analyses of organic and operant variables have led to the development of relatively effective treatment strategies and refinements that are increasingly cost-effective. Treatment typically involves efforts to identify and eliminate reliable precipitants, regulate and control autonomic arousal as a precursor or in response to pain, and management of the home and school environments in such a way that they are supportive of adaptive coping and discouraging of maladaptive pain behavior. It appears that the treatments could easily be implemented in a variety of environments, including school or primary care setting, and there is some evidence suggesting that long-term follow-up can be beneficial.

Although there is research supporting each of these strategies in some fashion in the management of recurrent pain, there is a paucity of well-controlled outcome studies exploring these techniques across recurrent pain conditions. For example, support for biofeedback has come primarily from studies treating children with migraines, whereas there is little research exploring biofeedback as a part of treatment for children with tension headaches or recurrent abdominal pain. Support for operant strategies has come primarily from the adult literature and somewhat from research on children with recurrent abdominal pain, whereas outcome studies investigating the treatment of headaches in children have rarely addressed operant features of pain. In addition, the volume of discussions and opinions published on recurrent abdominal pain belies the actual number of controlled outcome studies on treatment of RAP. Additional areas of research that warrant investigation include the application of home-based methods to RAP, the exploration of typical psychophysiological responses to stress in children with recurrent pain syndromes and the changes in those responses as a result of treatment, and a closer look at the management of recurrent pain in school and primary care settings. In the meantime, research evidence to date suggests that clinicians who rule out organic pathology, then perform a reasonable descriptive functional assessment and analysis, and then develop and implement an intervention based on the strategies that have been described, are likely to be successful in the behavioral management of recurrent pain in children.

ACKNOWLEDGMENTS

This manuscript was supported in part by grant MCJ 319152 from the Maternal and Child Health Bureau, Health Resources Services Administration, and by grant 90 DD 032402 of the Administration on Developmental Disabilities.

References

Allen, K.D., & McKeen, L. (1991). Home-based multicomponent treatment of pediatric migraine. *Headache, 31,* 467–472.

Allen, K.D., & Shriver, M.D. (1997). Enhanced performance feedback to strengthen biofeedback treatment outcome with childhood migraine. *Headache, 37,* 169–173.

Allen, K.D., Barone, V.J., & Kuhn, B.R. (1993). A behavioral prescription for promoting applied behavior analysis within pediatrics. *Journal of Applied Behavior Analysis, 26,* 493–502.

Andrasik, F., Kabela, E., Quinn, S., Attanasio, V., Blanchard, E., & Rosenblum, E.L. (1988). Psychological functioning of children who have recurrent migraine. *Pain, 34,* 43–52.

Apley, J. (1975). *The child with abdominal pain* (2nd ed). Oxford, England: Blackwell.

Apley, J., & Naish, N. (1958). Recurrent abdominal pains: A field survey of 1,000 school children. *Archives of Disease in Children, 33,* 165–170.

Apley, J., Haslam, D.R., & Tulloch, G. (1971). Pupillary reaction in children with recurrent pain. *Archives of Diseases in Children, 46,* 337.

Barlow, C.F. (1984). *Headaches and migraine in childhood.* Philadelphia: Lippincott.

Barr, R.G. (1983). Recurrent abdominal pain. In M.D. Levine, W.B. Carey, A.C. Crocker, & R.T. Gross (Eds.), *Developmental behavioral pediatrics* (pp. 521–528). Philadelphia: Saunders.

Barr, R.G., Levine, M.D., & Watkins, J.B. (1979). Recurrent abdominal pain of childhood due to lactose intolerance, *New England Journal of Medicine, 300,* 1449–1452.

Bieri, D., Reeve, R.A., Champion, G.D., Addicoat, L., & Zeigler, J.B. (1990). The faces pain scale for the self-assessment of the severity of pain experienced by children: Developmental, initial validation, and preliminary investigation for ratio scale properties. *Pain, 41,* 139–1250.

Bille, B. (1962). Migraine in schoolchildren. *Acta Paediatrica Scandinavica, 51,* 1–151.

Budd, K.S., Workman, D.E., Lemsky, C.M., & Quick, D.M. (1994). The Children's Headache Assessment Scale (CHAS): Factor structure and psychometric properties. *Headache, 17,* 159–179.

Burke, E., & Andrasik, F. (1989). Home vs clinic-based biofeedback treatment for pediatric migraine: Results of treatment through one-year follow-up. *Headache, 29,* 434–440.

Christensen, M.F., & Mortensen, O. (1975). Long-term prognosis in children with recurrent abdominal pain. *Archives of Disease in Children, 50,* 110–114.

Cooper, P., Bawden, H., Camfield, P., & Camfield, C. (1987). Anxiety and life events in childhood migraine. *Pediatrics, 79,* 999–1104.

Cunningham, S.J., McGrath, P.J., Ferguson, H.B., Humphreys, P., D'Astous, J., Latter, J., Goodman, J., & Firestone, P. (1987). Personality and behavioral characteristics in pediatric migraine. *Headache, 27,* 16–20.

Dimson, S.B. (1971). Transit time related to clinical findings in children with recurrent abdominal pain. *Pediatrics, 47,* 666–674.

Duckro, P.N., & Cantwell-Simmons, E. (1989). A review of studies evaluating biofeedback and relaxation training in the management of pediatric headache. *Headache, 29,* 428–433.

Edwards, M.C., Finney, J.W., & Bonner, M. (1991). Matching treatment with recurrent abdominal pain symptoms: An evaluation of dietary fiber and relaxation treatments. *Behavior Therapy, 22,* 257–267.

Egger, J., Carter, C.M., Wilson, J., Turner, M.W., & Soothill, J.F. (1983). Is migraine food allergy? A double-blind controlled trial of oligoantigenic diet treatment. *Lancet, 2,* 865–869.

Farrell, M.K. (1984). Abdominal pain. *Pediatrics, 74*(Suppl.), 955–957.

Feldman, W., McGrath, P.J., Hodgson, C., Riter, H., & Shipman, R.T. (1985). The use of dietary fibre in the management of simple childhood idiopathic recurrent abdominal pain: Results in a prospective double blind randomized controlled trial. *American Journal of Disease in Children, 139,* 1216–1218.

Feuerstein, M., Barr, R.G., Francoeur, T.E., Houle, M., & Rafman, S. (1982). Potential biobehavioral mechanisms of recurrent abdominal pain in children. *Pain, 13,* 287–298.

Finney, J.W., Lemanek, K.L., Cataldo, M.F., Katz, H.P., & Fuqua, R.W. (1989). Pediatric psychology in primary health care: Brief targeted therapy for recurrent abdominal pain. *Behavior Therapy, 20,* 283–291.

Fordyce, W.E. (1976). *Behavioral methods for chronic pain and illness.* St. Louis: Mosby.

Fordyce, W.E., & Steger, J.C. (1979). Chronic pain. In O.F. Pomerleau & J.P. Brady (Eds.). *Behavioral medicine: Theory and practice* (125–153). Baltimore: Williams & Wilkins.

Gaffney, A., & Gaffney, P.R. (1987). Recurrent abdominal pain in children and the endogenous opiates: A brief hypothesis. *Pain, 30,* 217–219.

Grazzi, L., Leone, M., Frediani, F., & Bussone, G. (1990). A therapeutic alternative for tension headache in children: Treatment and 1-year follow-up results. *Biofeedback and Self-Regulation, 15*(1), 1–6.

Guarnieri, P., & Blanchard, E.B. (1990). Evaluation of home-based thermal biofeedback treatment of pediatric migraine headache. *Biofeedback and Self-Regulation, 15,* 179–184.

Guidetti, V., Fornara, R., Ottaviano, S., Petrilli, A., Seri, S., & Cortesi, F. (1987). Personality inventory for children and childhood migraine. *Cephalalgia, 7,* 225–230.

Haynes, S.N., Gannon, L.R., Orimoto, L., O'Brien, W.H., & Brandt, M. (1991). Psychophysiological assessment of post-stress recovery. *Psychological Assessment, 3,* 356–365.

Hodges, K., Kline, J.J., Barbero, G., & Flanery, R. (1985). Depressive symptoms in children with recurrent abdominal pain and in their families. *Journal of Pediatrics, 107,* 622–626.

Hodges, K., Kline, J.J., Barbero, G., & Woodruff, C. (1985). Anxiety in children with recurrent abdominal pain and their parents. *Psychosomatics, 26,* 859–866.

Holden, E.W., Gladstein, J., Trulsen, M., & Wall, B. (1994). Chronic daily headache in children and adolescents. *Headache, 34,* 508–514.

International Headache Society. (1988). Classification and diagnostic criteria for headache disorders, cranial neuralgias and facial pain. *Cephalalgia, 8,* 19–28

Janis, I., Defares, P., & Grossman, P. (1983). Hypervigilant reactions to threat. In H. Selye (Ed.), *Selye guide to stress research* (Vol. 3). New York: Scientific and Academic Editions.

Kopel, F.B., Kim, I.C., & Barbers, G.J. (1967). Comparison of rectosigmoid motility in normal children, children with recurrent abdominal pain and children with ulcerative colitis. *Pediatrics, 64,* 539–545.

Kuhn, B.R., & Allen, K.D. (1993, November). Long-term follow-up of home-based treatment of pediatric migraine. Paper presented at the annual convention of Association for Advancement of Behavior Therapy, Atlanta, GA.

Kuhn, B.R., Allen, K.D., & Shriver, M.D. (1995). Behavioral management of children's seizure activity: Intervention guidelines for primary care providers. *Clinical Pediatrics, 34,* 570–575.

Labbe, E. (1995). Treatment of childhood migraine with autogenic and skin temperature biofeedback: A component analysis. *Headache, 35,* 10–13.

Larsson, B., Melin, L., & Doberi, A. (1990). Recurrent tension headache in adolescents treated with self-help relaxation training and muscle relaxant drug. *Headache, 30,* 665–671.

Levine, M.D., & Rappaport, L.A. (1984). Recurrent abdominal pain in school children: The loneliness of the long distance physician. *Pediatric Clinics of North America, 31,* 969–991.

Linet, M.S., Stewart, W.F., Celentano, D.D., Ziegler, D., Sprecher, M. (1989). An epidemiological study of headache among adolescents and young adults. *Journal of American Medical Association, 261*(15), 2211–2216.

McGrath, P.A. (1987). The multidimensional assessment and management of recurrent pain syndromes in children and adolescents. *Behavior Research and Therapy, 25,* 251–262.

McGrath, P.A. (1990). *Pain in children: Nature, assessment and treatment.* New York: Guilford.

McGrath, P.A., & deVerber, L.L. (1986). The management of acute pain evoked by medical procedures in children with cancer. *Journal of Pain and Symptom Management, 1,* 145–150.

McGrath, P.J., & Feldman, W. (1986). Clinical approach to recurrent abdominal pain in children. *Developmental and Behavioral Pediatrics, 7,* 56–63.

McGrath, P.J., & Unruh, A.M. (1987). *Pain in children and adolescents.* New York: Elsevier.

McGrath, P.J., Goodman, J.T., Firestone, P., Shipman, R., Peters, S. (1983). Recurrent abdominal pain: A psychogenic disorder? *Archives of Disease in Childhood, 58,* 888–890.

McGrath, P.J., Cunningham, S.J., Lascelles, M.A., & Humphreys, P. (1990). *Help yourself: A treatment for migraine headaches* [Patient manual and audiotape]. Ottawa, Ontario, Canada: University of Ottawa Press.

McGrath, P.J., Humphreys, P., Keene, D., Goodman, J., Lascelles, M., Cunningham, J., & Firestone, P. (1992). The efficacy and efficiency of a self-administered treatment for adolescent migraine. *Pain, 49,* 321–324.

McMahon, C., Harper, D.C., & Cruikshank, B. (1990). Assessment and treatment of recurrent abdominal pain: Guidelines for the school psychologist. *School Psychology Review, 19*(2), 212–222.

Newacheck, P.W., & Taylor, W. (1992). Childhood chronic illness: Prevalence, severity, and impact. *American Journal of Public Health, 82,* 364–371.

Oster, J. (1972). Recurrent abdominal pain, headache and limb pains in children and adolescents. *Pediatrics, 50,* 429–436.

Parcel, G.S., Nader, P.R., & Meyer, M.P. (1977). Adolescent health concerns, problems, and patterns of utilization in a true ethnic urban population. *Pediatrics, 60,* 157.

Rachlin, H. (1985). Pain and behavior. *Behavioral and Brain Sciences, 8*(1), 43–83.

Rappaport, L.A., & Leichnter, A.M. (1993). Recurrent abdominal pain. In N.L. Schechter, C.B. Berde, & M. Yaster (Eds.), *Pain in infants, children, and adolescents* (pp. 561–569). Philadelphia: Williams & Wilkins.

Routh, D.K., Ernst, A.R., & Harper, D.C. (1988). Recurrent abdominal pain in children and somatization disorder. In D.K. Routh (Ed.), *Handbook of pediatric psychology* (pp. 492–504). New York: Guilford.

Sanders, M.R., Rebgetz, M., Morrison, M., Bor, W., Gordon, A., Dadds, M., & Sheperd, R. (1989). Cognitive–behavioral treatment of recurrent nonspecific abdominal pain in children: An analysis of generalization, maintenance, and side-effects. *Journal of Consulting and Clinical Psychology, 57,* 294–300.

Sanders, M.R., Shepherd, R.W., Cleghorn, G., & Woolford, H. (1994). The treatment of recurrent abdominal pain in children: A controlled comparison of cognitive–behavioral family intervention and standard pediatric care. *Journal of Consulting and Clinical Psychology, 62,* 306–314.

Schwartz, M.S. (1995). Baselines. In M.S. Schwartz (Ed.), *Biofeedback: A practitioners guide.* (2nd ed.). New York: Guilford.

Sillanpaa, M. (1983). Changes in the prevalence of migraine and other headaches during the first seven school years. *Headache, 23,* 15–19.

Skinner, B.F. (1957). *Science and human behavior.* New York: Macmillan.

Stokes, T.F., & Baer, D.M. (1977). An implicit technology of generalization. *Journal of Applied Behavior Analysis, 10,* 349–367.

Turk, D.C., & Flor, H. (1987). Pain>pain behaviors: The utility and limitations of the pain behavior construct. *Pain, 31,* 277–295.

Walker, L.S., Garber, J., Van Slyke, D.A., & Greene, J.W. (1995). Long-term health outcomes in patients with recurrent abdominal pain. *Journal of Pediatric Psychology 20,* 233–245.

Wall, P.D. (1984). Mechanisms of acute and chronic pain. In L. Kruger & J.C. Liebeskind (Eds.), *Advances in pain research and therapy* (Vol. 9, pp. 575–587). New York: Raven.

Zeltzer, L.K., Barr, R.G., McGrath, P.A., & Schechter, N.L. (1992). Pediatric pain: Interacting behavioral and physical factors. *Pediatrics, 90*(5), 816–821.

Bibliography

Barlow, C.F. (1984). *Headaches and migraine in childhood.* Philadelphia: J.B. Lippincott.

Barr, R.G. (1983). Recurrent abdominal pain. In M.D. Levine, W.B. Carey, A.C. Crocker, & R.T. Gross (Eds.), *Developmental behavioral pediatrics* (pp. 521–528). Philadelphia: Saunders.

Fordyce, W.E. (1976). *Behavioral methods for chronic pain and illness.* St. Louis: Mosby.

Levine, M.D., & Rappaport, L.A. (1984). Recurrent abdominal pain in school children: The loneliness of the long distance physician. *Pediatric Clinics of North America, 31,* 969–991.

Rachlin, H. (1985). Pain and behavior. *Behavioral and Brain Sciences, 8*(1), 43–83.

Schwartz, M.S. (Ed.). (1995). *Biofeedback: A practitioners guide* (2nd ed.). New York: Guilford.

Zeltzer, L.K., Barr, R.G., McGrath, P.A., & Schechter, N.L. (1992). Pediatric pain: Interacting behavioral and physical factors. *Pediatrics, 90*(5), 816–821.

15

Central Nervous System Dysfunction

Brain Injury, Postconcussive Syndrome, and Seizure Disorder

WILLIAM J. WARZAK, JOAN MAYFIELD, AND JANICE McALLISTER

Introduction

Central Nervous System (CNS) dysfunction, whether the result of acquired injury, congenital defect, or developmental events, can have significant consequences for a child's psychosocial functioning and classroom performance. The long-term sequelae of CNS insult may impair performance on many levels, with the severity of a student's limitations being associated with the severity of the neurological insult. This chapter will focus on three types of CNS dysfunction and their implications for the student, school staff and school psychologist. We will provide the reader with a general understanding of the most common consequences of pediatric traumatic brain injury (TBI), postconcussion syndrome, and seizure disorders. Relevant medical management and rehabilitation issues will be presented across all conditions. Pharmacological issues, especially as they pertain to seizures, will be presented

because performance in the classroom may be affected by these medications. Behavioral interventions will receive special emphasis. Indeed, behavioral approaches to address CNS dysfunction have become increasingly important and commonplace (see for example, Dahl, 1992; Dahl, Brorson, & Melin, 1992; Fenwick, 1991; Horton & Miller, 1985; Horton & Sautter, 1986; Kuhn, Allen, & Shriver, 1995; Warzak & Kilburn, 1990).

Bringing effective behavior change procedures to bear upon CNS dysfunction as it presents in school settings enhances classroom behavior, academic performance, and activities of daily living, tasks important to the overall habilitation of these students (Chelune & Moehle, 1986; Cynkin, 1979; Heaton & Pendleton, 1981). Although different sorts of CNS dysfunction may require different strategies to address neurological and behavioral deficits, behavioral principles have been demonstrated to have wide generality (cf. Honig & Staddon, 1977; Leitenberg, 1976), and there is no reason to believe that these principles will vary from student to student as a function of particular injuries. Behavioral procedures, however, will vary as a function of neurological insult and the factors that influence the behavioral expression of the insult. This will be reflected in the behaviors selected for remediation, the selection and delivery of reinforcers, the development of discriminative stimuli, and the individual

WILLIAM J. WARZAK • Department of Psychology, Munroe-Meyer Institute for Genetics and Rehabilitation, and University of Nebraska Medical Center, Omaha, Nebraska 68198–5450.   JOAN MAYFIELD • Division of Pediatric Psychology, Munroe-Meyer Institute for Genetics and Rehabilitation, and University of Nebraska Medical Center, Omaha, Nebraska 68198–5450.   JANICE McALLISTER • Division of Pediatric Neurology, University of Nebraska Medical Center, Omaha, Nebraska 68198-2165.

Handbook of Child Behavior Therapy, edited by Watson and Gresham. Plenum Press, New York, 1998.

protocols developed for each child in need of intervention (Warzak & Kilburn, 1990).

Problem Identification

Traumatic Brain Injury

Types, Prevalence, Etiology, and Consequences

Traumatic brain injuries (TBI) are of two types: penetrating and closed head. Penetrating injuries involve perforation of the skull and laceration of brain tissue (e.g., gunshot wound) and tend to result in more focal and localized deficits. Closed head injuries tend to be more diffuse, caused primarily by blunt trauma and the associated acceleration–deceleration forces to the head and brain, such as that sustained in motor vehicle accidents (Lezak, 1995). Mild injuries that result in minimal cerebral bruising, swelling, or tissue strain may lead to only temporary impairment and loss of function. Permanent impairment may result from more significant injuries, which in turn may interrupt normal neurological development of brain structure and result in deficits not immediately apparent at the time of injury (Rutter, Chadwick, & Shaffer, 1983).

Pediatric patients account for approximately 40% of the 500,000 to 1.5 million Americans who sustain traumatic brain injuries annually (Brandstater, Bontke, Cobble, & Horn, 1991; Crouchman, 1990). The majority of these injuries occur to youth between the ages of 15 and 19 years old (Farmer & Peterson, 1995). One of every 25 students will experience some form of head trauma by the time they graduate from high school; as many as 20% of all special education students are believed to have sustained TBI prior to their eligibility for special services (Savage, 1991). Approximately 50% of children with TBI will need educational support during the first year following their injury (Donders, 1994).

There are many factors that influence the sequelae of traumatic brain injury in children. Among these are the nature of the injury, such as closed head versus penetrating wound, and the location and severity of the wound. Patient characteristics that affect outcome include genetics, premorbid development, age at time of onset or injury, and pre-existing medical, behavioral, and affective status. Students with above average intelligence, academic skills, and social skills tend to have a better prognosis (D. Harrington, 1990). Students who are premorbidly impaired are likely to continue to evidence those deficits and may experience an exacerbation of them. Sociocultural and psychosocial factors (e.g., family beliefs and responses to disability, SES) also may influence outcome (Dean, 1985).

Another potential differentiating factor, perhaps most relevant in young children, is the brain's apparent ability to compensate for some injuries by reorganizing neural function (i.e., the concept of plasticity). The exact nature of plasticity and the potential for reorganization of brain function postinjury is controversial. Nevertheless, evidence supports the occurrence of denervation supersensitivity (i.e., an increase in postsynaptic responsiveness to neurotransmitters following a neurological insult) and reactive synaptogenesis (i.e., axonal collateral sprouting). Whether these mechanisms account for observed sparing or recovery of function postinjury is unclear (Almli & Finger, 1992; Laurence & Stein, 1978). It may be that functional recovery postinjury is not the result of structural change, but rather, is due to other factors such as resolution of edema (i.e., swelling) or the use of alternative behavioral compensatory strategies (Rutter et al., 1983).

There are data to suggest that the effects of plasticity may occur during critical periods of brain development that coincide with critical periods for the acquisition of certain neuropsychological skills. Particularly during the preschool years, the brain appears to have some reorganizational capacity for the initiation or resumption of function that might be expected to be impaired as a result of brain insult (Chelune & Edwards, 1981; Dean, 1985). The data in this regard are perhaps most supportive of the reassignment (or preservation) of language functioning, which appears to be subsumed by the right hemisphere if the left hemisphere is compromised at an early age in right dominant children (Rutter et al., 1983).

However, it has been suggested that injury to the brain at an early age may impair future brain development, thereby limiting the potential for cognitive and neuropsychological development (Reitan & Wolfson, 1992). In fact, neural regrowth or reorganization may lead to interference in function (e.g., delayed posttraumatic epilepsy) (Almli & Finger, 1992; Rutter et al., 1983). There is considerable evidence to suggest that individuals who sustain significant brain injury at an early (preschool) age recover considerable academic function but never attain the level of performance of their unimpaired peers (Jaffe, Polissar, Fay, & Liao, 1995; Koskiniemi, Kyykka, Nybo, & Jarho, 1995; Reitan & Wolfson, 1992). Therefore, recovery is often a function of the severity of brain injury.

Brain Injury Severity

Depth and duration of coma and duration of posttraumatic amnesia (PTA) are considered to be the most useful indices of the severity of brain injury and are among the critical factors in determining its sequelae (Alexander, 1984; Levin, Benton, & Grossman, 1982; McGuire & Rothenberg, 1986). Presence and depth of coma are estimated with various measures, including the Glasgow Coma Scale (GCS; Teasdale & Jennett, 1974), duration of loss of consciousness (LOC), and time elapsed since injury before the patient obeys commands (i.e., time to obey commands [TOC]). The GCS is a 15-point scale computed as the sum of a patient's best-rated response (from 0 to 5) in eye movements, motor movements, and verbal functioning (Heiden, Small, Caton, Weiss, & Kurze, 1983; Teasdale & Jennett, 1974). The GCS is of limited utility with younger children because many of the responses require mature levels of neurodevelopment (Simpson & Reilly, 1982), but alternative measures for use with comatose pediatric patients have been developed (see, for example, Gordon, Fois, Jacobi, Minns, & Seshia, 1983; Seshia, Seshia, & Sachdeva, 1977; Simpson & Reilly, 1982; Yager, Johnston, & Seshia, 1990).

The severity of TBI has commonly been translated into three levels: mild, moderate, and severe. *Severe brain injury* has been defined as a GCS score immediately after injury of 3 to 8 (e.g., absence of eye opening, inability to obey commands, failure to utter recognizable words) and posttraumatic amnesia of at least 10 days (Teasdale & Jennett, 1974). Students who have experienced severe injuries will require an array of special services and are unlikely to return to a traditional classroom setting without considerable support. Recovery of academic skills tends to be seen primarily within the first year postinjury, with subsequent plateau (Chadwick, 1985; Chadwick, Rutter, Brown, Shaffer, & Traub, 1981). Residual impairment ranges from extended coma with little apparent response to sensory stimulation, to chronic speech and language impairment, and deficits in attention and concentration, memory, sensation and perception, reasoning, and impulse control. General cognitive disorganization, motor retardation, and behavioral and affective disturbance are also common (Mitiguy, Thompson, & Wasco, 1990).

Moderate brain injury (GCS of 9–12 with responses such as eyes open, normal flexor response, intelligible speech but no sustained conversation) also often results in significant residual impairment. PTA of one to seven days is not uncommon (Van Zomeren & Van Den Burg, 1985). Even patients who make a relatively good recovery from a moderate injury frequently complain of persistent headaches, memory deficits, and difficulties with activities of daily living, including interacting with friends and family (Rimel, Giordani, Barth, & Jane, 1982). Students with this level of injury often resume traditional classroom activities but may require special education services and extra consideration in terms of programming, scheduling, and so on.

Moderate and severely injured children often experience chronic neuropsychological deficits that affect academic performance. Over the first year postinjury, moderately and severely injured children may display dramatic progress and reacquire many previously learned skills. Continued follow-up suggests that adaptive living skills continue to improve while intellectual, neurocognitive, and academic skills plateau, with performance levels remaining substantially below those of uninjured peers after the first year (Jaffe et al., 1995). However, while the injured student attempts to regain lost function, his or her peers continue in their general social, cognitive, and academic development. Therefore, the task for these children is not simply to recover lost function, but to reestablish parity with peers who have continued to acquire new skills during the injured child's rehabilitation (Jaffe et al., 1995).

Mild brain injury (i.e., a GCS of 13–15 which reflects little or no impairment of verbal functioning or of eye/motor movement) may occur in patients who have experienced brief LOC or no LOC, with no known structural damage to the brain (Binder, 1986; Rimel, Giordani, Barth, Boll, & Jane, 1981). Approximately 80% of all closed head injuries fall into this category (Kraus et al., 1984). Students who experience mild injury often make a very good academic recovery but may experience fatigue and deficits in sustained attention and memory for new information for varying lengths of time. Deficits following mild injury are often subtle but may have considerable impact on social, familial, academic, and occupational functioning (Eisenberg, 1989; Levin et al., 1982; Rosenthal, 1983). Indeed, brain injury has been termed the "silent epidemic" because its frequency and disabling effects are often unrecognized (Conboy, Barth, & Boll, 1986). Clusters of symptoms in affective, cognitive, somatic, and sensory areas often persist following mild head injury. These are often associated with postconcussion syndrome (Cicerone & Kalmar, 1995).

Postconcussive Syndrome

There is no universally accepted definition of concussion (Cantu, 1992a), but several features of the phenomenon are commonly cited in the literature. The hallmark of concussion is immediate and transient impairment of neural function commonly characterized by amnesia and confusion. These alterations in function are the consequence of mechanical trauma to the brain. These alterations in mental status can occur without loss of consciousness. One does not have to lose consciousness to be concussed (Fick, 1995; D.E. Harrington, Malec, Cicerone, & Katz, 1993; J.P. Kelly et al., 1991).

Mild head trauma, with potential for concussive effects, occurs with some regularity among youth involved in collision sports. For example, it has been estimated that as many as 20% of varsity high school football players sustain a concussion annually (Gerberich, Priest, Boen, Straub, & Maxwell, 1983), with as many as 250,000 concussions a year occurring in contact sports such as gymnastics, football, hockey, and wrestling (Cantu, 1988; Le-Blanc, 1994). These latter sports have the highest risk of head or neck injury per 100,000 participants (Mueller & Cantu, 1990). For those who have sustained a concussion, the odds of sustaining additional concussive injuries is greatly increased (Gerberich et al., 1983).

The severity of postconcussive symptoms is related to a number of factors including the student's history of prior head injury. This is a critical factor in assessing the danger posed to an individual student by any given concussive event. Repeated concussions may result in cortical atrophy and cumulative impairment in neuropsychological functioning (Gronwall & Wrightson, 1975; Jordan & Zimmerman, 1990; Unterharnscheidt, 1970). Because symptoms may be delayed or not initially apparent, and because students themselves are often unable to report their condition, students may not be evaluated properly or may be returned to athletic competition too soon (Fick, 1995; Hugenholtz & Richard, 1982; J.P. Kelly et al., 1991). In rare cases this can lead to second-impact syndrome.

Second-impact syndrome is seen in individuals who continue to be symptomatic from a previous mild head injury and then sustain another ostensibly mild injury. This second injury triggers a series of pathophysiological events that lead to vascular engorgement, brain swelling, herniation, and death (Cantu, 1992a,b; J.P. Kelly et al., 1991; Leblanc, 1994). For these reasons it is essential that school staff be familiar with concussive injuries and their sequelae. In particular, knowing when to withhold a student from competition or when to refer for further evaluation is critical if catastrophic outcomes are to be avoided (Genuardi & King, 1995; J.P. Kelly et al., 1991).

Perhaps the most important single factor in protecting youth who sustain mild head injuries is providing an adequate amount of recovery time before returning to activity that places them at risk for additional insult (Cantu, 1988; Hugenholtz & Richard, 1982; Wilberger, 1993). Several efforts have been made to classify concussions and establish decision-making rules for returning athletes to competition (see for example, Cantu, 1992a; Fick, 1995; Leblanc, 1994). Of more relevance in the present context are the symptoms of concussion that should trigger further evaluation.

Staff present at the moment of injury should try to ascertain whether the student has experienced a loss of consciousness. Simple questions related to orientation are helpful (e.g., "Where are you?" "What were you doing?" "What quarter is it?"). Memory for events immediately preceding a concussive event is often impaired (i.e., retrograde amnesia). Memory for events following an injury (anterograde amnesia) is suggestive of more significant injury (Fick, 1995).

Students who have sustained a concussion should be evaluated by medical personnel. If the concussion occurs during an athletic contest, questions regarding whether a student athlete should return to a competition should be deferred to the judgement of medical staff. The relevant issues are whether or not the student is currently symptom free, and the number and recency of previously sustained concussions. Several researchers believe that students who experience an initial concussion should be withheld from athletic competition until they have been completely symptom free for at least one week, with further restrictions imposed upon those who have sustained more frequent or severe injuries. Certainly any student with any residual symptoms whatsoever should not be allowed to compete in an athletic contest that puts them at risk for further injury (Cantu, 1988, 1992a; Fick, 1995, Leblanc, 1994; Wilberger, 1993).

Although not all concussions or mild head injuries result in postconcussive syndrome, up to 50% of patients who sustain mild head injuries report symptoms three or more months postinjury (Rimel et al., 1981; Rutherford, 1989). Headache, memory deficits, dizziness, and fatigue are among the most common symptoms (Edna & Cappelen, 1987). Postconcussive deficits tend to remit spontaneously over time but this is not universally so, with up to 20% of patients continuing to experience headaches and 4% reporting impaired memory at one year postinjury (Evans, Evans, & Sharp, 1994; Wilberger, 1993).

In the classroom, students with a history of recent concussion may experience deficits in attention, concentration, and memory. This may be misinterpreted by school staff as lack of motivation, noncompliance, or defiance. Compounding the problem is the fact that there are often no physical findings to support subjective complaints although school performance and day-to-day functioning may be impaired. Because of this, even some professional staff may be uncomfortable with the diagnosis of postconcussive syndrome (Cicerone, & Kalmar, 1995; D.E. Harrington et al., 1993); this results in students and school staff who remain uninformed about this syndrome. This greatly hampers students who attempt to return to school in the face of subtle but real symptoms (Cicerone, 1991).

Seizure Disorders

Seizure disorders are among the most common neurologic illnesses seen in childhood, with an annual incidence rate of 0.56 per 1,000 through the first 20 years of life (Berg & Shinnar, 1994).

Seizures are "the clinical manifestation of an abnormal and excessive discharge of a set of neurons of the brain" (Hauser, Annegers, & Kurland, 1993, p. 453). There are many seizure presentations and a variety of etiologies, including head injury, central nervous system infections, metabolic imbalances, withdrawal from addictive substances, exposure to certain toxins, and, for some children, simply a febrile illness.

Some seizures are provoked by external factors such as trauma, and they resolve once the underlying factors are treated. These may be treated prophylactically with anticonvulsants; however, these may not prevent seizure activity and may have undesirable side effects such as cognitive slowing or depression (Gaultieri & Cox, 1991). Other seizures are unprovoked and have no clear precipitant. They appear to result from an organic tendency for abnormal and excessive electrical discharge from cortical neurons. Still other seizures may be affected by physiological, psychological, and behavioral variables, with particular sensory stimuli and mental activity precipitating seizure activity in some individuals (Brown & Fenwick, 1989; Fenwick & Brown, 1989). The name given to recurrent, unprovoked seizures is epilepsy. An overview of the most common types of childhood epileptic seizures and syndromes follows.

Generalized Seizures

Generalized seizures show clinical signs of bilateral cerebral hemispheric involvement. Generalized tonic-clonic seizures (grand mal seizures) are perhaps the most commonly known. This seizure begins without warning. The student suddenly loses consciousness and falls to the ground with the muscles tonically contracted, making the body rigid. Breathing is shallow and irregular, frequently resulting in poor oxygenation (i.e., cyanosis) often first manifested by the child's lips turning blue. Incontinence may occur and the tongue may be bitten. Following the tonic contraction phase, clonic activity (repetitive jerking movements) is seen in the extremities. Finally, the person relaxes, breathes more deeply and regularly, and awakens. Afterward, patients are usually in a postictal state of varying duration, during which they are sleepy and perhaps confused. The child may have a feeling of muscle soreness, generalized stiffness and headache.

Should such an episode occur in the classroom, school staff should document what the child was doing prior to, during, and after the seizure. Information pertaining to fever or other symptoms of illness is of particular importance.

Myoclonic Seizures. The hallmark of myoclonic seizures is the myoclonic jerk defined as a sudden, brief, shocklike contraction of an individual muscle or group of muscles (Commission on Classification and Terminology of the International League Against Epilepsy, 1981). Because the onset is sudden and large muscle groups are often involved, these seizures are often associated with falls which may cause additional head injury. Myoclonic seizures are often associated with developmental delays (Aicardi, 1994) or neurodegenerative syndromes but may occur in children with normal intellect.

Atonic Seizures. A similar seizure type often associated with myoclonic seizures is the atonic seizure. Atonic seizures are characterized by the sudden loss of postural tone with brief, if any, loss of consciousness (Commission on Classification and Terminology of the International League Against Epilepsy, 1981). These seizures also are frequently associated with falls and ensuing injury to the face and head. As a whole, atonic seizures are difficult to control with medication, often necessitating the use of protective helmets in affected children. Children with atonic seizures also are often developmentally delayed.

Absence Seizures. Absence seizures are usually first observed in school-age children and are often first identified by teachers (Olsson, 1988). During an absence seizure, the child suddenly stops whatever activity he or she was engaged in and has a blank, staring facial expression. The child may have minor facial movements (e.g., blinking) during an episode, but does not have tonic-clonic activity and does not lose postural tone. The child then awakens, usually unaware of the lapse of consciousness, and resumes prior activities.

These seizures last less than 20 seconds and occur multiple times each day. Because these children repeatedly miss bits of instructional time, they often will have increasing difficulty with schoolwork (Aicardi, 1994; Menkes & Sankar, 1995). Approximately half of those children with absence seizures will develop other seizure types (most commonly generalized tonic-clonic seizures) and should be closely monitored for seizure activity. Absence seizures are usually controlled by medication.

Absence seizures must be differentiated from simple daydreaming (Berkovic, Andermann, Andermann, & Gloor, 1987). An inattentive child may have a blank expression and be unaware of classroom activities, but, ordinarily, will respond when his or her name is called and will know that their thoughts have drifted off classroom work. Daydreaming also responds more readily to contingency management procedures than do seizures, although behavioral contributions to seizure management can be considerable for some children.

Partial Seizures

The second major group of epileptic seizures is partial (focal) seizures. Symptoms of a partial seizure are defined by the area of the brain affected. For example, if the motor area is affected, then the seizure is clinically manifested as jerking, trembling or other abnormal movement of a part of the body. The primary sensory cortex or special sensory systems may be involved, yielding symptoms such as an abnormal sensation or the appearance of a flashing light. Partial seizures begin with abnormal electrical activity in one area of the brain and do not initially affect both cerebral hemispheres (Commission on Classification and Terminology of the International League against Epilepsy, 1981).

Simple Partial Seizures. Simple partial seizures begin focally and never spread to involve both brain hemispheres. Consciousness is not lost or impaired and the child remains alert and retains memory for the seizure (Devinsky, Kelley, Porter, & Theodore, 1988). Seizure activity may spread to affect other parts of the body (e.g., moving from the leg to the arm and then to the face). Following a simple partial seizure, the child does not have post-seizure (i.e., postictal) confusion or sleepiness but may have a weakness of one side or part of the body known as Todd's paralysis. This weakness may last several hours or for one or more days (Aicardi, 1994; Menkes & Sankar, 1995).

Complex Partial Seizures. Complex partial seizures begin focally in the brain and are associated with an impairment of consciousness. These seizures have commonly been referred to as psychomotor epilepsy or temporal lobe epilepsy because many of these seizures begin in the temporal lobe of the brain, although they may begin in the frontal or the occipital lobes as well.

The complex partial seizure often begins with an unusual or unpleasant sensation (an aura), such as the feeling of "rising" in the abdomen, or smelling a foul odor, or other vaguely noxious special sensory symptoms. A feeling of inappropriate familiarity (déjà vu) or inappropriate strangeness (jamais vu) may also occur. As the seizure progresses, the child stares or has a blank facial expression. There may be automatisms or stereotyped behavior sequences such as movements resembling waving, pulling at clothing, shouting, laughing, crying, lip smacking, or chewing. The child may move about without apparent awareness of the surroundings or may say a few stereotyped phrases while appearing to look at someone. If approached during this phase of automatisms, the child may push or strike at the person (Adams & Victor, 1993). Following the seizure, he or she will have no memory of the event and may be sleepy or somewhat confused. Complex partial seizures are generally brief, usually lasting only a few minutes. If the complex partial seizure lasts a few seconds and is manifest only as a staring facial appearance, it may be confused with absence seizures. The two seizure types are then differentiated by the electroencephalographic (brain wave) appearance of the seizures.

Seizure Syndromes

Seizure syndromes are epileptic disorders grouped by seizure type(s) and associated symptoms. The following exemplify the most common syndromes that affect school-age children.

Febrile Seizures. Simple febrile seizures are perhaps the most common provoked seizures seen in childhood. Two to five percent of children in the United States and Europe will have at least one simple febrile seizure (Forsgren, Sidenvall, Bloomquist, & Heijbel, 1990; Van Den Berg & Yerushalmy, 1969; Verity, Butler, & Golding, 1985). These seizures are usually generalized tonic-clonic in type (but may be partial), and they occur in febrile children between the ages of 6 months and 6 years. The seizures are benign, are not associated with intellectual deterioration, and they are not recurrent in 60% of children who experience them (Ellenberg & Nelson, 1978; Nelson & Ellenberg, 1976). If a child has a febrile seizure while at school, the student should be treated as a child with a generalized tonic-clonic seizure. Evaluation by a physician is warranted to rule out a serious central nervous system infection.

Lennox-Gastaut Syndrome. This syndrome, encountered most frequently in early intervention programs, is characterized by frequent seizures of multiple types, an identifiable EEG pattern, and developmental delay (Livingston, 1988). This syndrome comprises approximately 1% to 2% of all childhood epilepsy cases, with an estimated prevalence of 0.13 per 1,000 children aged 0 to 9 years (Cowan, Bodensteiner, Leviton, & Doherty, 1989; Hauser et al., 1993). The cause of Lennox-Gastaut Syndrome is thought to be early brain injury or brain malformation. Children presenting with Lennox-Gastaut Syndrome are typically 2 to 5 years old. Of children with this syndrome, 20% to 60% evidence developmental delays at onset, with 75% to 90% diagnosed with developmental delay within five years post onset, obviating the ability of most individuals to live independently as adults (Chevrie & Aicardi, 1972; Aicardi, 1994).

Infantile Spasms. Infantile spasms (or West Syndrome) is the name given to an epileptic syndrome which has typical onset between 3 and 12 months of age. With a prevalence rate of 0.19 per 1,000 children between the ages of birth to 10 years, this is an epileptic syndrome commonly seen by neurologists (Cowan et al.,1989). These children have neurological problems that affect their school performance and may require early intervention services from school staff. During an Infantile Spasm, multiple myoclonic jerks affecting the extremities and neck muscles are observed. The baby rapidly folds his or her arms over the chest, raises the knees to the abdomen, and drops the head downward, in a movement that has been likened to the act of closing a jackknife. Some infants will throw the head back and jerk the arms and legs in an outward movement. Jackknife Seizures or Salaam Seizures (referring to the bowing head movement) are common names for these seizures.

The myoclonic jerks usually occur in clusters that last up to several minutes and may be followed by a tonic-clonic seizure. Most of these children eventually stop having spasms but are usually developmentally delayed and frequently develop other types of seizures (Glaze, Hrachovy, Frost, Kellaway, & Zion, 1988; Riikonen, 1981).

Landau-Kleffner Syndrome. Landau-Kleffner Syndrome, also known as acquired epileptiform aphasia, is a rare syndrome that has generated a great deal of recent interest (Deonna, 1991). Children with this syndrome are without apparent deficit prior to the onset of aphasia between the ages of 18 months and 13 years (the majority are 4 to 7 years at the onset of the illness). A variety of seizure types are present in most, but not all, of these children; all of the children have an abnormal EEG. Treatment with anticonvulsant drugs has had little effect on the aphasia or EEG abnormalities but some success has been achieved with corticosteroids (Paquier, Van Dangen, & Loonen, 1992).

Pseudoseizures. Pseudoseizures (also known as psychogenic seizures) are seizurelike events which are not associated with abnormal electrical cortical discharges. They may occur in grade-school-aged children but are more frequent in adolescents and are more common in females (Finlayson & Lucas, 1979, Wyllie et al., 1970; Lancman, Asconape, Graves, & Gibson, 1994). Pseudoseizures usually mimic generalized tonic-clonic or complex partial seizures but may consist only of staring. They may be preceded by auras and in some cases may be followed by a postictal-like state of sleepiness. Urinary incontinence and tongue biting are rare. Suggestive statements made by a health care professional may precipitate a pseudoseizure or may end an event, unlike true epileptic seizures, which are not brought on or stopped by suggestive statements alone. As a whole, adolescents and children are unlikely to have severe psychopathology as the cause of their pseudoseizures (Wyllie et al., 1991) but stress may be contributory (Lancman et al., 1994; Silver, 1982).

Problem Analysis

Our analysis of school-related issues common to children with CNS dysfunction will focus primarily on those children who have experienced TBI. Children who present with postconcussion syndrome and seizure disorder may benefit from temporary curricular changes and classroom modification, allowances by school staff, and careful monitoring. They are unlikely, however, to require evaluation and planning to the same extent as children with TBI. They may not require special programming unless their postconcussion syndrome or seizure disorder coexists with other conditions (such as developmental delay and associated behavioral and cognitive deficits) that require adaptive curricular changes.

Children with brain injury may present with a variety of dysfunctions resulting in academic, social, and behavioral issues. Evaluation of these children may require neuropsychological and behavioral assessment to determine basic brain-behavior integrity, identify behaviors to be shaped and maintained by the social environment, and determine the conditions under which target behaviors appear. These analyses take time, and parents may express frustration and feel a sense of urgency to complete a plan and commence therapy or resume school activities. They may see assessment procedures as obstacles to progress and may need help to understand the assessment process (Szekers & Neserve, 1994).

From a classroom perspective, several issues need to be addressed. A primary concern is the student's ability to cope with the classroom environment, ranging from the level of stimulation in the classroom to the pace of academic instruction. If a child returns to the classroom too soon after a neurological event they may be disoriented, disinhibited, or otherwise unprepared to deal with the traditional expectations of the classroom (Ylvisaker, Hartwick, & Stevens, 1991). The rate at which they work, process information, acquire new learning (and the sort of learning), and their ability to work independently must be ascertained. Students also should be evaluated to ensure they have a functional classroom repertoire including the ability to:

—tolerate general classroom stimulation
—attend to task
—follow simple directions
—function within a group
—communicate effectively
—evidence learning potential (Cohen, 1991)

Neuropsychological Assessment Strategies

Two assessment strategies contribute greatly to this evaluation. First, students with recently acquired brain injuries may benefit from a comprehensive *neuropsychological evaluation.* Neuropsychological assessment examines brain–behavior relationships through tests that assess specific domains of brain functioning, especially those sensitive to impairment as a function of brain damage. With the exception of the Luria-Nebraska and the Halstead-Reitan test batteries, there are very few test batteries that have been developed for children with traumatic brain injury and even fewer that have been standardized using brain-injured children as subjects (Batchelor, Sowles, Gean, & Fischer, 1991; D. Harrington, 1990). Among those areas evaluated by the latter batteries are attention and concentration, various aspects of memory and learning, perceptual–motor skills, speech and language skills, problem solving, and abstract reasoning (Farmer & Peterson, 1995). Results of testing procedures are used to generate specific recommendations concerning curriculum and instructional tactics, class scheduling, and general systemic changes important to reintegration into the school setting.

Neuropsychological findings may also have significant implications for classroom behavior in a way that traditional psychoeducational assessment does not. For example, frontal lobe syndrome may present as behavioral excesses that are maintained not only by current defective contingencies of reinforcement but also are exacerbated by defective monitoring and self-regulation and by an inability to respond quickly to changing environmental contingencies (i.e., difficulty learning from trial-by-trial feedback) (Rosenthal, 1983). Older students, in particular, are likely to manifest changes in behavior as a function of frontal lobe injuries. Young children may not exhibit the effects of a frontal injury until they are older and their cortex has matured, thereby presenting with behavioral, affective, and cognitive consequences far removed in time from the original injury. Knowing a student's history of brain trauma as well as understanding frontal lobe syndrome may affect how this student is subsequently evaluated and how initial contingencies are structured.

Understanding a student's current problem behavior may be facilitated by knowing whether it is consistent with premorbid behavior or is newly developed postinjury. School disciplinary reports and information obtained from previous school teachers can provide data regarding the premorbid behavioral and affective aspects of a student. Brain injuries often exaggerate premorbid behavioral features, but injuries also change an individual's behavior in ways not previously seen, making it difficult to understand the contingencies controlling current behavior without a formal analysis.

Another example is to be found in the difficulty students with right hemisphere injury may have in reading social cues and in changing their behavior as a function of feedback from the social environment. Because it is the right hemisphere that analyzes the paralinguistic features of the voice, difficulty in recognizing verbal nuances that influence much of daily behavior is impaired (Rhawn, 1990). An inability to alter one's behavior as a function of social cues is likely to result in behavior that is inappropriate and aversive to others, thus discouraging future social interaction. This deficiency may manifest itself as a social skill deficit that is not a deficit of socially skilled behavior, per se, but is rather a function of defective stimulus control, the result of faulty perception of facial, postural, vocal, and other cues to the affective status of others. Intervention directed toward the acquisition of appropriate behavior instead of assessing the ability of relevant stimuli to evoke relevant aspects of the current repertoire may be insufficient.

On a more instructional level, right hemisphere injury may also result in a defect in attending to the left hemi-attentional field (i.e., inattention or neglect) (Heilman, Watson, & Valenstein, 1993). This phenomenon, if undetected, might result in a variety of ineffective rehabilitation and educational strategies, and raises concerns about general school and playground safety. If information is presented to the wrong visual field of a student (e.g., presenting a block design task in the left visual field of a right dominant individual) with a right hemisphere injury, the result may be impaired performance unrelated to the student's ability to perform the task. At the most basic level, such an oversight will create difficulties in teaching situations. The extent to which these difficulties are aversive to the student increases the probability of inappropriate affective responses that disrupt ongoing task performance (Skinner, 1953).

Applied Behavior Analysis

The second evaluative strategy, and the one that ultimately can determine the circumstances under which appropriate and inappropriate behavior are most probable, is the use of applied behavior analysis (Baer, Wolf, & Risley, 1968). Often associated with the evaluation of problem behaviors, applied behavior analysis can assist in identifying the circumstances under which any behavior occurs and in identifying the optimal conditions under which adaptive behavior occurs. This strategy has particular relevance to children who have sustained TBI and, in some cases, to children with seizure disorders.

Applied behavior analysis has long been used in the rehabilitation of children with CNS dysfunction (Cicerone, 1989; Cicerone & Wood, 1987). Inherent in this approach is the blend of assessment, treatment, and evaluation into a seamless strategy to determine the controlling variables under which behavior occurs. The development and maintenance of a functional repertoire begins with a task analysis of the student's goals and dissecting each goal into component behavioral objectives. The behavior required to meet each objective is operationally defined to permit accurate measurement of student performance and to facilitate the delivery of appropriate consequences contingent upon the student's behavior. Target behaviors are frequently measured and the functional relationships between behavior and consequences ascertained. The identification of discriminative stimuli that reliably evoke seizures, disruptive behavior, or other instances of maladaptive behavior, is equally important and well served by this approach.

An essential initial step is to determine which consequences function as reinforcers and under what conditions. Reinforcers may be identified through discussion with the student, staff, and family members, completion of reinforcer survey schedules (e.g., Cautela & Kastenbaum, 1967; Clement & Richard, 1976) or by observing a student's daily preferred activities. Participation in activities that the student frequently engages in may be used to reinforce other, less probable behavior (Premack, 1959). New reinforcers may be developed by having students sample activities that have been found to be effective in reinforcing the behavior of other students (Ayllon & Azrin, 1968). In

some cases a structured reinforcer assessment may be required (Pace, Ivancic, Edwards, Iwata, & Page, 1985) to ensure that consequences intended to increase behavior will actually do so. It cannot be assumed that consequences that generally serve to increase or decrease the behavior of students in general will be effective with any particular student (e.g., Solnick, Rincover, & Peterson, 1977; Warzak, Kewman, Stefans, & Johnson, 1987). Nor can it be assumed that a particular reinforcer will always be effective, due to the nature of setting events (Wahler, 1983) and establishing operations (Michael, 1982, 1993) that may influence the proximal effectiveness of any given stimulus as either discriminative or reinforcing. Finally, patient compliance with, and affective response to, task demands should be monitored. These responses may themselves become the focus of intervention (Cicerone, 1989; Jain, 1982).

Plan Implementation

Preparation

Recommendations for placement, curriculum planning, and specialized services are often deferred until behavioral targets have been identified by neuropsychological and behavioral assessment. Neuropsychological findings may identify areas of deficiency that cannot be adddressed directly but which may be susceptible to compensatory strategies. Aphasic students, for example, may benefit from phonemic cueing; students with right hemisphere dysfunction and resulting social skills deficits may benefit from strategies to prompt social repertoires in response to various social contexts. A functional analysis will identify the controlling variables for each of these repertoires, whether they result from behavioral excess or deficiency, and provide a means of evaluating student progress.

During this process, parents need to be informed of their child's rights regarding educational placement and services, special education categories, and the nature and significance of the IEP, including how special services are provided within their specific school district (Ylvisaker et al., 1991). Their child's limitations and strategies for intervention should be made clear. We provide examples of strategies relevant to most common classroom situations below.

Peer Relationships

The activities of many students with brain injuries are restricted because of concerns about additional injury, as well as because of physical, cognitive, or social limitations. These limitations reduce a student's functional repertoire, decrease opportunities for maintaining old friendships, and limit opportunities to develop new ones. Even minor injuries may result in poor self-monitoring and difficulty responding appropriately to social cues, thereby contributing to defective social behavior (Alexander, 1984; Goethe & Levin, 1984; Hopewell, Burke, Weslowski, & Zawlocki, 1990). Behavior that once served to reinforce the social behavior of peers now may be lacking or simply unavailable; new behavior may appear that is maladaptive or may be aversive to others, thus discouraging peer social interaction.

For an adolescent at a time of increasing independence, being unable to participate effectively in activities such as driving or dating may functionally isolate the student. A return to premorbid activities, to the extent possible, is crucial to maintaining social and peer interactions and preventing social isolation (Warzak, Allan, Ford, & Stefans, 1995). Reduced or modified participation in a service club, athletic function, or other school-related activity may be a critical element in supporting a student's return to school.

The success of these efforts often depends on the nature of the student's current social repertoire. Some students may require both social skills and contingency management strategies to facilitate an appropriate repertoire. Social skills may be acquired through a combination of procedures such as modeling, behavioral rehearsal, feedback, and reinforcement. (cf. J.A. Kelly, 1982). Social skills ranging from conversational skills (Brotherton, Thomas, Wisotzek, & Milan, 1988) to refusal skills for unwanted sexual activity (Warzak & Page, 1990) have been taught successfully to students with CNS dysfunction. Other students may not need skills training per se but may benefit from a structured program to assist them in reading social cues correctly and to facilitate the appearance of appropriate social behavior under appropriate stimulus conditions. Contingency management procedures which incorporate information obtained from task analyses and a functional analysis are appropriate for this purpose.

The generalization of social skills training to the extra-therapeutic environment has long been particularly difficult. Indeed, issues related to generalization are important considerations whenever behavior change is an issue. Several strategies have been identified to facilitate generalization (Stokes & Baer, 1977). Training that employs exemplars that closely approximate real-world conditions is crucial. Key individuals, situations, and verbal and contextual cues should be incorporated into training (e.g., Cicerone & Wood, 1987; Warzak & Page, 1990). In vivo training should always be considered as a terminal training procedure when possible. Transporting discriminative stimuli from the therapeutic environment, be it the counselor's office, an after-school training setting, or the home, into the actual environment where target behaviors are to occur also may be helpful (e.g., Ayllon, Kuhlman, & Warzak, 1982).

Staff Preparedness

School personnel play an important role in the reentry process of a student who has sustained a brain injury. Few staff members have experience in working with these children (Blosser & DePompei, 1991; Cooley & Singer, 1991) and it may be disconcerting to some to have a child in the classroom with newly acquired cognitive and behavioral deficits. Concerns might be addressed both by providing information about a student's current functioning and by providing the behavioral tools to the staff to assist them in solving day-to-day concerns.

For example, children who must adjust to CNS dysfunction are more likely to experience emotional and behavioral problems that compromise school functioning than are their unimpaired peers (Dean, 1986). The core of behavioral symptoms typically associated with childhood neurologic disorders involves deficits in attention and concentration, poor impulse control, and emotional lability (Nassbaum & Bigler, 1990), consistent with findings that many injuries to young children result in more generalized, rather than specific, patterns of deficits (Boll, 1974). Deficits in organizing, initiating, and sustaining effort until task completion also are common.

This behavior pattern may be interpreted by staff as noncompliance or as a lack of motivation when it may be that the child is unable, because of his or her injury, to complete these tasks successfully without considerable assistance (Hopewell, et al., 1990; Lezak, 1988). Learning-to-learn strategies (e.g., how to perform a task analysis, how to take notes, study skills) may need to be incorporated into didactic contexts which, in turn, have been modified for the student's benefit. Slowing the pace of instruction, ensuring that material is presented in consideration of identified deficits, developing compensatory strategies that address specific deficits, providing active learning tasks, teaching the process of an activity, and shaping students to become more independent, are examples of staff modifications to assist the impaired student (Cohen, 1991). Classroom structure and consistent routine with minimal disruption to educational activities are especially important (D. Harrington, 1990). If these cannot be provided within the regular classroom or resource room, additional intervention may be required.

More importantly, school personnel require skills of their own to address the behavioral needs of the impaired student. These might include training in the essentials of (a) behavioral assessment, (b) the acquisition and maintenance of behavior, and (c) strategies to promote the generalization of target behaviors to relevant contexts. These latter skills may be important even in the treatment of ostensibly medical problems such as seizures and, especially, pseudoseizures.

Seizure activity in students presents a particularly vexing problem for school staff, and an awareness of common interventions for seizure activity, including the effects of medication, deserves special mention here. In the case of pseudoseizures, providers must be careful not to alienate the child or family by suggesting that the seizure activity results from operant factors alone. It may be more productive to identify operant factors as among potential precipitating events (Dahl, 1992). Coping strategies such as relaxation and imagery may be effective in forestalling seizures with competing response training when seizures appear imminent (Brown & Fenwick, 1989). These strategies also provide significant others an opportunity to reinforce adaptive behavior that competes with seizure activity. In addition, an emphasis upon differential reinforcment

for adaptive behavior throughout the day, such as school attendance and performance, shifts the schedule of reinforcement from one that is closely tied to seizure activity to one that is contingent upon adaptive behavior (Kuhn et al., 1995; Zlutnick, Mayville, & Moffatt, 1975).

The presence of seizures with a medical etiology requires more specific staff preparation. A student experiencing a tonic-clonic seizure should be laid on the floor (never held upright) with the head turned to one side. This allows the tongue to fall away from the airway and allows saliva or vomitus to flow out of the mouth rather than pooling in the throat, causing choking and potential aspiration into the lung. No attempt should be made to put any object (such as a pencil or spoon) into the child's mouth to try to prevent the tongue from blocking the airway. It is far more likely that teeth will be chipped or mouth structures will be injured than that the child will choke on or bite through the tongue. Upon awakening, the child will likely be confused or sleepy and should be observed until fully awake. If a generalized tonic-clonic seizure lasts longer than five to ten minutes, the child should be taken to a hospital for treatment. Seizures lasting longer than thirty minutes are a serious cause of concern and may result in brain damage (Aicardi, 1994). These latter seizures may need long-term medication to control excessive neuronal activity.

Anti-Epileptic Medications

Although behavioral procedures may be the primary treatment modality for pseudoseizures (Kuhn et al., 1995) and a useful adjunct even in cases of refractory seizures (Dahl, 1992; Dahl, Brorson, & Melin, 1992; Fenwick, 1991; Zlutnick et al., 1975), pharmacological intervention is the primary treatment modality for these conditions. Anticonvulsant medication controls seizures in many children, but some children are only poorly responsive to medicine, and undesirable side effects such as cognitive slowing are not uncommon (Gaultieri & Cox, 1991). Antiepileptic medication also may be sedating, or cause speech dysfluency or dizziness. These and other factors affect a child's cognitive and social functioning, thus having a major impact on the child's classroom performance.

The mechanisms of action specific to each medication are beyond the scope of this chapter (the interested reader is directed to Coulter, Huguenard, & Prince, 1989; Macdonald & Kelly, 1995). In general, these medications work by decreasing rapid-fire electrical potentials in neurons, thereby limiting unregulated neuronal activity expressed as seizures. All seizure medications have side effects which should be known to school staff. The most common medications are reviewed below and are summarized in Table 1.

Phenobarbital is a drug that has been commonly used for treatment of generalized tonic-clonic seizures, partial seizures, and simple febrile seizures. Phenobarbital is an effective and inexpensive medication which, unfortunately, can have significant effects on behavior and cognition. Toddlers taking phenobarbital have been found to have sleep disturbances and irritability (Camfield et al., 1979). Phenobarbital also has been shown to impair children's performance on intelligence tests (Farwell et al., 1990). The cognitive slowing seen in some individuals can be quite remarkable, characterized by long latencies between presenting questions or instructions and the student's response. School staff who interact with these children should be aware of these manifestations and inform the student's parents should they first be observed in the school set-

TABLE 1. Common Seizure Types and Treatment

Seizure Type	Seizure Description	Treatment*
Generalized tonic-clonic	• Child loses consciousness • Falls down if standing • Shaking of arms and legs, alternating with stiffened arms and legs • Sleepy or confused afterward	Carbamazepine Phenobarbital Phenytoin Valproic acid
Myoclonic	• Sudden contraction of a group of muscles which may cause child to fall or to have head-bobbing movement	Valproic acid Vigabatrin
Atonic	• Sudden loss of postural tone which may cuase child to fall	Valproic acid
Absence	• Sudden, brief episodes of staring lasting less than 30 seconds • Child resumes activities after the seizure without sleepiness or confusion	Ethosuximide Valproic acid
Simple partial	• May have jerking of one part of the body or have a repetitive sensory symptom such as seeing a flashing light	Carbamazepine Phenytoin Lamotrigine Gabapentin
Complex partial	• Simple partial seizure which spreads to cause child to lose awareness of the environment	Carbamazepine Phenytoin Lamotrigine Gabapentin
Simple febrile seizures	• Seizures brought on simply by a rise in fever in a child under the age of six.	Reduce fever May use oral or rectal Diazepam
Lennox-Gastaut syndrome	• Multiple type of seizures • Mental retardation common	Carbamazepine Felbamate Valproic acid
Infantile spasms	• Clusters of myoclonic seizures found in children with early brain injury • Children often are mentally retarded	Valproic acid Vigabatrin
Landau-Kleffner syndrome	• Onset of aphasia between 18 months and 13 years • Multiple seizure types • Abnormal EEG	Poorly responsive to most anticonvulsants Corticosteroids have been tried
Pseudo-seizures	• Seizure-like events with normal EEG • Often brought on by stress	Behavioral management

*This is a partial listing of medications which might be used for each type of seizure. Medication regimens vary widely.

ting. *Primidone* (Mysoline) is an anticonvulsant which has phenobarbital as an active metabolite. Its mechanism of action and side-effect profile are similar to that of phenobarbital.

Phenytoin (Dilantin) is used to treat generalized tonic-clonic seizures, partial seizures, and, secondarily, generalizing seizures. This drug has multiple side effects in some patients, including abnormal hair growth (hirsutism), gum hypertrophy, and coarsening of facial features, as well as nystagmus and ataxia. Phenytoin is very effective and has few cognitive effects but the aforementioned side effects preclude its use in many cases (Aman, Werry, Paxton, & Turbot, 1994).

Carbamazepine (Tegretol) was originally used for partial seizures but is now commonly used for generalized tonic-clonic seizures as well. It is also prescribed prophylactically to individuals at risk for seizure activity. When carbamazepine is first taken, the patient will often experience nausea and sedation as side effects. With prolonged use of carbamazepine, however, the sedation and nausea usually abate. An effect on bone marrow production of white and red blood cells can be seen with carbamazepine use, but only rarely does a serious anemia result. Because carbamazepine is very effective and also has fewer cognitive side effects than other medications, it is now a first-line anticonvulsant medicine.

Valproic acid (Depakote or Depakene) is a medication used to treat myoclonic seizures (including infantile spasms), absence seizures, and generalized tonic-clonic seizures. When first taken, Valproate will cause nausea, but this effect usually diminishes with long-term use. Long-term effects, however, may include weight gain and tremulous hand movements. Rarely, Valproate has been associated with serious liver damage. Valproate does not commonly cause long-term cognitive effects.

Ethosuximide is a drug used only to treat absence seizures, which it does very effectively. Nausea is a common complaint when ethosuximide is first started, but this lessens with prolonged use. Cognitive side effects are not prominent.

Felbamate (Felbatol), *Gabapentin* (Neurontin), and *Lamotrigine* (Lamictal) are newly released anticonvulsants. The mechanism of action for these drugs is not as yet fully understood. Felbamate has been used to treat Lennox-Gastaut syndrome in children and partial seizures in adults (Leppik,

1995). Unfortunately, Felbamate has been associated with bone marrow failure (aplastic anemia) and with liver dysfunction, making it now seldom used. Gabapentin and Lamotrigine have been used for partial seizures in adults and teenagers (Messenheimer et al., 1994). Lamotrigine also has shown some effect in children with Lennox-Gastaut syndrome, absence epilepsy, and generalized epilepsy (Schulmberger et al., 1994). Gabapentin may cause sedation, dizziness, and ataxia (McLean, 1995). Rash, headache, and dizziness have been seen with Lamotrigine use (Richlens, 1994).

Vigabatrin is an anticonvulsant now used in Europe to treat partial seizures as well as infantile spasms. Side effects of Vigabatrin, include fatigue and dizziness, and, less commonly, impaired concentration, confusion, and abnormal thinking (Ben-Menacham, 1995).

Systemic Factors

Students who have missed school for any length of time may find themselves far behind their peers academically. This is especially true for students in high school, who have a far more daunting task of academic catch-up than students in elementary school. Upon return to school, high school students may pursue a class load that is inconsistent with their current abilities. Some students may catch up with their peers by increasing their class load, going to summer school, or taking correspondence courses, but others may be unable to pursue this level of activity because fatigue is a significant factor in cases ranging from postconcussive syndrome to severe brain injury (Cohen, 1991; Warzak et al., 1995). Issues related to falling behind classmates, not graduating with one's class, and missing class activities (e.g., senior field trips, proms) need to be addressed with students and their parents. Students who are close to completing their required coursework might be allowed to attend graduation with their class even if they themselves do not graduate until the following fall or spring.

The practical day-to-day issues that arise when accommodating students who have sustained neurological insult are numerous. Educational support materials such as computers, calculators, tape recorders, writing aids, positioning equipment, or augmentative communication devices may be essential equipment in providing an appropriate educational environment and should be considered within the IEP. Consideration of such classroom aids should be made before a student returns to the classroom following neurological insult and should be made with the consultation of relevant professionals such as speech, occupational, and physical therapists.

Limited mobility may result not only from physical limitations, such as use of a wheel chair, cane, or crutches, but also from cognitive deficits that hinder independent navigation of busy school hallways. Classes may need to be in close proximity to each other with extra time provided for traveling between classes, perhaps at a time when the school halls contain fewer students. Students who experience difficulty moving from class to class may find a "buddy" helpful in assisting their movement between classes.

Excessive stimulation may pose a problem for some students, with difficulties occurring in settings ranging from placement in the classroom to cafeteria seating. In the classroom, for example, a student may need to be placed at the front of the class to better see and hear instruction from school staff but also to minimize noise and distraction from the rest of the classroom. For other children, excessive stimulation may be present in social settings, such as the halls between classes, the cafeteria, and other assembly points. For children who are hypersensitive to noise, even activities that are supposed to be relaxing, such as lunch, may be stressful (Begali, 1992) due to noise or general activity level. Modifications that limit stimulation may be helpful. For example, eating with a few friends in a separate area or playing board games with a few friends instead of participating in large group activities may reduce stress.

Vocational Considerations

Significant CNS dysfunction will require careful examination of academic and vocational goals. For example, a vocational school, community college or deferring college altogether may be more consistent with a student's current cognitive abilities than attending a four-year university away from home. Students with significant CNS dysfunction should seek vocational counseling early in high school. The more severe the student's dysfunction

or the more assistance a student requires to function within his or her environment, the earlier vocational evaluation and counseling should begin. Too often students with long-standing injuries put off vocational considerations until they are juniors or seniors in high school. At that late date, many programs may be precluded because of inadequate student preparation or insufficient lead time to enroll in programs. Partial placement in the community, perhaps with a job coach (Jacobs, 1988), may provide an assessment of work potential while providing a framework for an adaptive work repertoire for the older student. Finally, vocational assessment may be helpful for high school students and result in a better match between the student's interests, abilities, and academic programming.

Family Support

The needs of a child who has acute deficits may be quite different from those of a child who has been long identified as a special needs student because of a chronic disability. Accommodations must quickly be made by the child, family members, and school staff. Rapid changes in family life, school programming, and academic and vocational aspirations may place considerable stress on the student and family members. Children and adolescents typically have limited coping skills to respond to deficits in behavioral and emotional functioning. These frustrations can lead to anxiety and depression (Crowley & Miles, 1991). Students with mild injuries are often aware of deficits and tend to overestimate their limitations, whereas more severely injured students often underestimate the extent of their deficits (Cicerone, 1991). In both cases, assistance is needed to facilitate adjustment. Individual counseling, group therapy programs, and peer support groups are an important means of supporting the student (D. Harrington, 1990).

Parents of children with significant brain injury must learn to adapt to a child who is different from the person they knew premorbidly, perhaps with significant cognitive and behavioral limitations, a different social repertoire, and affective and behavioral deficits (Bond, 1976; Brooks & Aughton, 1979; Cooley & Singer, 1991; Oddy, Humphrey, & Uttley, 1978; Warzak, Evans, & Ford, 1992; Warzak, et al., 1995). It is common for parents to become overloaded with the responsibilities of their roles as caregivers, planners, and nurturers. They may find themselves overextended without sufficient energy to function in any role successfully (Leaf, 1993). Siblings must adapt to changes in routine and status; the need for this adaptation often causes resentment of the impaired sibling, a finding not uncommon among siblings of children with chronic illness (Michaelis, Warzak, Stanek, & Van Riper, 1992; Warzak, Ayllon, Milan, Majors, & Delcher, 1993).

The degree of stress differs from family to family depending on premorbid cohesiveness, family attitudes about illness, and financial and social support (Lezak, 1988; Leaf, 1993). The most common family system problems tend to be financial difficulties, behavioral problems with siblings, and marital tension (Wade, Drotar, Taylor, & Stancin, 1995). These factors may dictate long-term therapeutic support for all family members. Because of the complexity of issues involved in the care of children with CNS dysfunction, it is recommended that therapeutic support be provided by professionals who have experience working with these children.

Familiarizing family members with the student's pattern of abilities and teaching family members behavioral strategies is an important component of treatment. Informing parents of the availability of support groups and respite care also may be helpful. Unfortunately, most school staff have little or no experience in working with students with CNS dysfunction and are not acquainted with community resources. Nevertheless, useful classroom (and home) strategies are most commonly developed from within a framework of traditional task analysis and contingency management.

Plan Evaluation

The effectiveness of a given intervention must be empirically determined. Many academic skills can be evaluated using standard psychoeducational testing, but much important classroom behavior occurs beyond the purview of traditional ability and achievement testing and requires a different assessment approach. For these occasions, small n research designs provide perhaps the best tool to evaluate the effects of environmental factors on specific behaviors of interest. This analysis owes much to the tradition of intensively studying individual subjects and using subjects as their own controls (Ferster & Skinner, 1957; Sidman, 1960).

These designs require operational definitions of target behaviors, reliable and frequent observation of them, and a careful tracking of the occurrence of these behaviors as a function of different interventions across time. The designs provide early identification of problems in learning or of plateaus in progress, and permit experimental evaluation of school and classroom intervention. Several designs typical to education and rehabilitation settings are illustrated in Chapter 2, this volume.

The application of these evaluative procedures is consistent with strategies used to initially evaluate target behavior. Indeed, behavioral strategies of assessment, treatment, and evaluation create a seamless pattern for working with students whether or not they have special needs. Considerations for promoting the acquisition and maintenance of an adaptive school and classroom repertoire may be found in Table 2.

Summary and Directions for Future Research

CNS dysfunction is a low-incidence problem with significant ramifications for the children who experience neurological impairment and the school and classroom staff who assist them. Children with CNS dysfunction will generally present in the classroom in one of three ways. First, children who have a chronic history of dysfunction will have been identified at an earlier time in their lives and receive services to address their limitations. Second, children will return to the classroom following a brain injury or neurological insult which is known to school staff. The sequelae of these events will vary as a function of the many factors that affect postinjury outcome and will have implications for the child's general behavior and academic performance. Third, the child will present with behavior in the classroom that is unanticipated and is associated with poorly understood contingencies or conditions. These children may manifest behavior from which neurological impairment or insult may be inferred.

Students with TBI often present with difficult problems for school staff and they will need comprehensive planning and a detailed IEP. Concus-

TABLE 2. Considerations for Developing a Behaviorally Based Program for Students with CNS Dysfunction[1]

1. A student who has experienced significant CNS insult should undergo a comprehensive assessment prior to the development of an IEP. Psychoeducational, neuropsychological, and behavioral evaluations may all be needed to clarify student strengths and weaknesses. Psychoeducational evaluation will not suffice to identify ability patterns or the variables that control day-to-day behavior.

2. A task analysis may be required before developing a program to shape and maintain multicomponent target behaviors. Each behavior of interest needs to be operationally defined and measured reliably and frequently. Repeated measurement permits early identification of plateaus or obstacles to progress and provides detection of subtle changes in behavior which might be missed by intermittent data collection procedures.

3. A reinforcer assessment should demonstrate that "reinforcers" actually influence the probability of behavior occurring. Reinforcers found in the student's natural environment are preferred over reinforcers unobtainable without extraordinary effort or expense.

4. Reinforcers should be readily available contingent on patient performance. Reinforcers that are to be delivered at a time removed from the actual occurrence of the target behavior need to be supported with token systems that bridge the gap between the target behavior and the actual occurrence of reinforcement.

5. Reinforcement should follow every success early in skill acquisition or in rebuilding a previous adaptive repertoire. A more variable (and less frequent) schedule of reinforcement should be implemented over time to facilitate generalization to extra-therapeutic settings.

6. Stimuli that are expected to evoke behavior in vivo must be available and salient in the training setting. Neuropsychological functioning must be considered in this regard. Different stimuli will be salient for different students as a function of locus of injury, nature of injury, and so on. The same stimuli, events, or conditions that functioned to evoke or reinforce behavior premorbidly may no longer be functional because of physical or cognitive limitations.

7. Generalization strategies should be considered from the outset of any treatment plan. Strategies to promote transfer of training include using a variety of examples, staff, students, and contexts to broaden stimulus control to the extra-therapeutic environment; thinning the schedule of reinforcement; and ensuring that trained behaviors are likely to be maintained by the student's everyday environment.

8. The student's behavioral program should be clearly understood by all staff members and no changes in the program should be made without a consensus of relevant staff and parents, as appropriate. Key issues should include clearly specifying which stimuli, events, or conditions are to be used as reinforcers or aversive consequences, who will provide them, under what circumstances they will be delivered or withdrawn, and according to what schedule.

9. Small n designs should be used to identify variables that affect the occurrence of target behaviors and to evaluate the effectiveness of treatment for individual students. These designs simultaneously incorporate repeated measurement of target behaviors with the imposition of the different contingencies that comprise intervention.

10. Staff considerations are important when imposing interventions that will draw on staff time over and above typical staffing requirements. Particularly in cases where extensive data collection or changes in staff routines may be required, motivation for compliance may be low. Providing reinforcing consequences for school staff can greatly influence the success or failure of any student's program.

[1] Adapted from Warzak & Kilburn, 1990.

sions occasionally occur on the playground, and students who have sustained concussions through sports activities may present with symptoms in the classroom or on the athletic field that require attention. They may not require an IEP, but planning their return to the classroom, with monitoring, is important. Seizure disorders may occur without any known prior neurological insult or other CNS dysfunction. Classroom and curricular modifications are more often dictated by associated comorbidity, such as developmental delay, than by the seizures themselves.

In spite of the complicated picture presented by children with CNS dysfunction, research has led to an increased understanding of the cognitive, behavioral, and psychosocial implications of these conditions (e.g., Barry & O'Leary, 1989; Lezak, 1988; Warzak et al., 1993). Day-to-day obstacles that confront pediatric patients and family members, at home and in the classroom, have been empirically identified; this knowledge has furthered our understanding of children's brain injuries and their sequelae (Asarnow, Satz, Light, Lewis, & Neuman, 1991; Warzak et al., 1995). This information is especially relevant to school staff in view of recent federal mandates to provide special education services to children with brain injuries (Individuals with Disabilities Education Act, 1990). These mandates have arisen in recognition of the fact that children with brain injuries require assistance if they are to maximize their potential and that academic settings may require modification to accommodate the special needs of these children (Begali, 1992; Mira, Tucker, & Tyler, 1992; Sherrets, 1984).

Although the federal government has recognized the need to provide special education services to individuals who have sustained traumatic brain injury, practical guidelines for providing these services are often lacking. School staff are frequently unfamiliar with this group of students and find it difficult to recognize and address their special needs effectively. Even school psychologists, who are often called upon as primary providers of services to children with central nervous system dysfunction, are frequently unprepared to work effectively with this population (Mayfield, Warzak, Ford, & Poler, 1996; Warzak, Ford, & Grow, 1992). To the extent that the problems targeted for evaluation and treatment are not congruent with the problems students and their families actually experience, student and family needs will remain ineffectively addressed. Greater staff awareness of obstacles to teaching and interacting with these students is needed to best match educational and follow-up services with the needs of individual students.

Often overlooked is the emotional impact of disability on the student and other family members. School psychologists can better support students, family members, and school staff through the emotional turmoil which results from CNS dysfunction and its sequelae if they themselves have sufficient understanding of the nature of CNS dysfunction and have the tools to address the emotional and behavioral ramifications experienced by their students at home and in the classroom (Warzak et al., 1995).

In recent years there has been an explosion of neuropsychological and behavioral research with children who experience CNS impairment and many of the findings relevant to school and classroom functioning are reported here. What is often lacking is a practical link between these two sources of data and practical ideas regarding how these data are to be integrated for the benefit of the student (Warzak, Mayfield, & McAllister, 1996). Children will be best served if and when both neuropsychological and behavioral findings are clearly understood by staff, are integrated into the IEP, and are implemented in the classroom. Improvement in cur-

rent educational strategies for these children will require further collaborative work between these two distinct but intertwined technologies.

ACKNOWLEDGMENTS

The editorial comments of Crystal Grow, Ph.D., and Christine T. Majors, M.S., University of Nebraska Medical Center, are gratefully acknowledged in the preparation of this manuscript.

References

Adams, R.D. & Victor, M. (1993). *Principles of neurology* (5th ed). New York: McGraw Hill.

Aicardi, J. (1994). *Epilepsy in children* (2nd. ed.). New York: Raven.

Alexander, M.P. (1984). Neurobehavioral consequences of closed head injury. *Neurology and Neurosurgery: Update series, 5*(20), 2–7.

Almli, C.R. & Finger, S. (1992). Brain injury and recovery of function: Theories and mechanisms of functional reorganization. *Journal of Head Trauma Rehabilitation, 7,* 70–77.

Aman, M.G., Werry, J.S., Paxton, J.W., & Turbot, S.H. (1994). Effects of phenytoin on cognitive–motor performance in children as a function of drug concentration, seizure type, and time of medication. *Epilepsia, 35,* 172–180.

Asarnow, R.F., Satz, P., Light, R., Lewis, R., & Neuman, E. (1991). Behavior problems and adaptive functioning in children with mild and severe closed head injury. *Pediatric Psychology, 16,* 543–555.

Ayllon, T.A, & Azrin, N.H. (1968). *The token economy: A motivational system for therapy and rehabilitation.* New York: Appleton-Century-Crofts.

Ayllon, T., Kuhlman, C., & Warzak, W.J. (1982). Programming resource room generalization using lucky charms. *Child Behavior Therapy, 4,* 61–67.

Baer, D.M., Wolf, M.M., & Risley, T.R. (1968). Some current dimensions of applied behavior analysis. *Journal of Applied Behavior Analysis, 1,* 91–97.

Barry, P., & O'Leary, J. (1989). Roles of the psychologist on a traumatic brain injury rehabilitation team. *Rehabilitation Psychology, 34*(2), 83–90.

Batchelor, E.S., Sowles, G., Gean, R.S., & Fischer, W. (1991). Construct validity of the Halstead-Reitan Neuropsychological Battery for children with learning disorders. *Journal of Psychoeduacational Assessment, 9,* 16–31.

Begali, V. (1992). *Head injury in children and adolescents: A resource and review for school and allied professionals* (2nd ed.). Brandon, VT: Clinical Psychology Publishing Company.

Ben-Menachem, E. (1995). Vigabatrin. *Epilepsia, 36*(Suppl. 2), S95–S104.

Berg, A.T., & Shinnar, S. (1994). The contributions of epidemiology to the understanding of childhood seizures and epilepsy. *Journal of Child Neurology, 9*(Suppl.), 2S19–2S26.

Berkovic, S.F., Andermann, F., Andermann, E., & Gloor, P. (1987). Concepts of absence epilepsies: Discrete syndromes or biological continuum? *Neurology, 37*, 993–1000.

Binder, L.M. (1986). Persisting symptoms after mild head injury: A review of the postconcussive syndrome. *Journal of Clinical and Experimental Neuropsychology, 8*(4), 323–346.

Blosser, J.L., & DePompei, R. (1991). Preparing education professional for meeting the needs of students with traumatic brain injury. *Journal of Head Trauma Rehabilitation, 6*(1), 73–82.

Boll, T.J. (1974). Behavioral correlates of cerebral damage in children aged 9 through 14. In R.M. Reitan & L.A. Davison (Eds.), *Clinical neuropsychology: Current status and applications.* Washington, DC: Winston.

Bond, M.R. (1976). Assessment of the psychosocial outcome after severe head injury. *Acta Neurochirurgica* (Vienna), *34*, 57–70.

Brandstater, M.E., Bontke, C.F., Cobble, N.D., & Horn, L.J. (1991). Rehabilitation in brain disorders: Specific disorders. *Archives of Physical Medicine and Rehabilitation, 72*, S332–S340.

Brooks, D.N., & Aughton, M.E. (1979). Psychological consequences of blunt head injury. *International Journal of Rehabilitation Medicine, 1*, 160–165.

Brotherton, F.A., Thomas, M.S., Wisotzek, M., & Milan, M.A. (1988). Social skills training in the rehabilitation of patients with traumatic closed head injury. *Archives of Physical Medicine and Rehabilitation, 69*, 827–832.

Brown, S.W., & Fenwick, P.B.C. (1989). Evoked and psychogenic seizures: II. Inhibition. *Acta Neurologica Scandinavia, 80*, 541–547.

Camfield, C.S., Chaplin, S., Doyle, A.B., Shapiro, S.H., Cummings, C., & Camfield, P.R. (1979). Side effects of phenobarbital in toddlers: Behavioral and cognitive aspects. *Journal of Pediatrics, 95*, 361–365.

Cantu, R.C. (1988). When to return to contact sports after a cerebral concussion. *Sport Medicine Digest, 10*, 1–2.

Cantu, R.C. (1992a). Cerebral concussion in sport: Management and prevention. *Sports Medicine, 14*, 64–74.

Cantu, R.C. (1992b). Second impact syndrome: Immediate management. *Physician Sports Medicine, 20*, 55–58.

Cautela, J.R., & Kastenbaum, R. (1967). A reinforcement survey schedule for use in therapy, training, and research. *Psychological Reports, 20*, 1115–1130.

Chadwick, O. (1985). Psychological seqelae of head injury in children. *Developmental Medicine and Child Neurology, 27*, 69–79.

Chadwick, O., Rutter, M., Brown, G., Shaffer, D., & Traub, M. (1981). A prospective study of children with head injuries: II. cognitive sequelae. *Psychological Medicine, 11*, 49–61.

Chelune, G.J., & Edwards, P. (1981). Early brain lesions: Ontogenic–environmental considerations. *Journal of Consulting and Clinical Psychology, 49*, 777–790.

Chelune, G.J., & Moehle, K.A. (1986). Neuropsychological assessment and everyday functioning. In D. Wedding, A.M. Horton, Jr., & J. Webster (Eds.), *The neuropsychology handbook.* New York: Springer.

Chevrie, J.J., & Aicadi, J. (1972). Childhood epileptic encephalopathy with slow spike-wave. A statistical study of 80 cases. *Epilepsia, 36* (Suppl. 2), S34–S45.

Cicerone, K.D. (1989). Psychotherapeutic interventions with traumatically brain-injured patients. *Rehabilitation Psychology, 34*(2), 105–114.

Cicerone, K.D. (1991). Psychotherapy after mild traumatic brain injury: Relation to the nature and severity of subjective complaints. *Journal of Head Trauma Rehabilitation, 6*, 30–43.

Cicerone, K.D., & Kalmar, K. (1995). Persistent postconcussion syndrome: The structure of subjective complaints after mild brain injury. *Journal of Head Trauma Rehabilitation, 10*, 1–17.

Cicerone, K.D., & Wood, J. (1987). Planning disorder after closed head injury: A case study. *Archives of Physical Medicine and Rehabilitation, 68*, 111–115.

Clement, P.W., & Richard, R.C. (1976). Identifying reinforcers for children: A children's reinforcement survey. In E.J. Mas & L.G. Terdal (Eds.) *Behavior therapy assessment: Diagnosis, design, and evaluation.* New York: Springer.

Cohen, S.B. (1991). Adapting educational programs for students with head injuries. *Journal of Head Trauma Rehabilitation, 6*(1), 47–55.

Commission on Classification and Terminology of the International League Against Epilepsy. (1981). Proposal for revised clinical and electroencephalographic classification of epileptic seizures. *Epilepsia, 22*, 489–501.

Conboy, T.J., Barth, J., & Boll, T.J. (1986). Treatment and rehabilitation of mild and moderate head trauma. *Rehabilitation Psychology, 31*, 203–216.

Cooley, E., & Singer, G. (1991). On serving students with head injuries: Are we reinventing a wheel that doesn't roll? *Journal of Head Trauma Rehabilitation, 6*(1), 47–55.

Coulter, D.A., Huguenard, J.R., Prince, D.A. (1989). Characterization of ethosuximide reduction of low-threshhold calcium current in thalamic neurons. *Annals of Neurology, 25*, 582–593.

Cowan, L.D., Bodensteiner, J.B., Leviton, A., & Doherty, L. (1989). Prevalence of the epilepsies in children and adolesents. *Epilepsia, 30*, 94–106.

Crouchman, M. (1990). Head injury: How community pediatricians can help. *Archives of Diseases in Children, 65*, 1286–1287.

Crowley, J.A., & Miles, M.A. (1991). Cognitive remediation in pediatric head injury: A case study. *Journal of Pediatric Psychology, 16*(5), 611–627.

Cynkin, S. (1979). *Occupational therapy: Toward health through activities.* Boston: Little, Brown.

Dahl, J. (1992). *Epilepsy: A behavior management approach to assessment and treatment in children.* Seattle, WA: Hogrefe & Huber.

Dahl, J., Brorson, L., & Melin, L. (1992). Effects of a broad spectrum behavioral medicine treatment program on children with refractory epileptic seizures: An eight-year follow-up. *Epilepsia, 33*, 98–102.

Dean, R.S. (1985). Foundation and rationale for neuropsychological bases of individual differences. In L. Hartledge & K. Telzrow (Eds.), *Neuropsychology of individual differences* (pp. 7–39). New York: Plenum.

Dean, R.S. (1986). Neuropsychological aspects of psychiatric disorders. In J.E. Obrzut & G.W. Hynd (Eds.), *Child neuropsychology: Clinical practice* (Vol. 2, pp. 83–112). London: Academic.

Deonna, T.W. (1991). Acquired epileptiform aphasia in children (Landau-Kleffner Syndrome). *Journal of Clinical Neurophysiology, 8,* 288–298.

Devinsky, O., Kelley, K., Porter, R.J., & Theodore, W.H. (1988). Clinical and electroencephalographic features of simple partial seizures. *Neurology, 38,* 1347–1352.

Donders, J. (1994). Academic placement after traumatic brain injury. *Journal of School Psychology, 32,* 53–65.

Edna, T.H., & Cappelen, J. (1987). Late post-concussional symptoms in traumatic head injury. An analysis of frequency and risk factors. *Acta Neurochirurgica, 86,* 12–17.

Eisenberg, M.G. (1989). Introduction: Special issue on traumatic brain injury rehabilitation. *Rehabilitation Psychology, 34*(2), 67.

Ellenberg, J.H., & Nelson, K.B. (1978). Febrile seizures and later intellectual performance. *Archives of Neurology, 35,* 17–21.

Evans, R.W., Evans, R.I., & Sharp, M.J. (1994). The physician survey on post-concussion and whiplash syndromes. *Headache, 34,* 268–274.

Farmer, J.E., & Peterson, L. (1995). Pediatric traumatic brain injury: Promoting successful school reentry. *School Psychology Review, 24*(2), 230–243.

Farwell, J.R., Lee, Y.J., Hirtz, D.G., Sulzabacher, S.I., Ellenberg, J.H., & Nelson, K.B. (1990). Phenobarbital for febrile seizures—effects on intelligence and on seizure frequency. *New England Journal of Medicine, 322,* 364–369.

Fenwick, P. (1991). Evocation and inhibition of seizures: Behavioral treatment. *Advances in Neurology, 55,* 163–183.

Fenwick, P., & Brown, P.B.C. (1989). Evoked and psychogenic seizures. 1. Precipitation. *Acta Neurologica Scandinavica, 80,* 541–547.

Ferster, C.B., & Skinner, B.F. (1957). *Schedules of reinforcement.* Englewood Cliffs, NJ: Prentice-Hall.

Fick, D.S. (1995). Management of concussion in collision sports. *Postgraduate Medicine, 97,* 53–60.

Finlayson, R.E., & Lucas, A.R. (1979). Pseudoepilyptic seizures in children and adolescents. *Mayo Clinic Proceedings, 54,* 83–87.

Forsgren, L., Sidenvall, R., Bloomquist, H.K., & Heizbel, T. (1990). A prospective incidence study of febrile convulsions. *Acta Paediatrica Scandinavia, 79,* 550–557.

Gaultieri, T., & Cox, D. (1991). The delayed neurobehavioral sequelae of traumatic brain injury. *Brain Injury, 5,* 219–232.

Genuardi, F.J., & King, W.D. (1995). Inappropriate discharge instructions for youth athletes hospitalized for concussion. *Pediatrics, 95,* 216–218.

Gerberich, S.G., Priest, J.D., Boen, J.R., Straub, C.P., & Maxwell, R.E. (1983). Concussion incidences and severity in secondary school varsity football players. *American Journal of Public Health, 73,* 1370–1375.

Glaze, D.G., Hrachovy, R.A., Frost, J.D., Kellaway, P., & Zion, T.E. (1988). Prospective study of outcome of infants with infantile spasms treated during controlled studies of ACTH and predisone. *Journal of Pediatrics, 112,* 389–396.

Goethe, K.E., & Levin, H.S. (1984). Behavioral manifestations during the early and long term stages of recovery after closed head injury. *Psychiatric Annals, 14,* 540–546.

Gordon, N.S., Fois, A., Jacobi, G., Minns, R.A., & Seshia, S.S. (1983). Consensus statement: The management of the comatose child. *Neuropediatrics, 14,* 3–5.

Gronwall, D., & Wrightson, P. (1975). Cumulative effect of concussion. *Lancet, 2,* 995–997.

Harrington, D. (1990). Educational strategies. In M. Rosenthal, E. Griffith, M. Bond, & J.E. Miller (Eds.), *Rehabilitation of the adult and child with traumatic brain injury* (2nd ed., pp. 476–492). Philadelphia: Davis.

Harrington, D.E., Malec, J., Cicerone, K., & Katz, H.T. (1993). Current perceptions of rehabilitation professionals towards mild traumatic brain injury. *Archives of Physical Medicine and Rehabilitation, 74,* 579–586.

Hauser, W.A., Annegers, J.F., & Kurland, L.T. (1993). Incidence of epilepsy and unprovoked seizures in Rochester, MN 1935–1984. *Epilepsia, 34,* 453–468.

Heaton, R.K., & Pendleton, M.G. (1981). Use of neuropsychological tests to predict adult patients' everyday functioning. *Journal of Consulting and Clinical Psychology, 49,* 807–821.

Heiden, J.S., Small, R., Caton, W., Weiss, M., & Kurze, T. (1983). Severe head injury: Clinical assessment and outcome. *Physical Therapy, 12,* 1946–1951.

Heilman, K.M., Watson, R.T., & Valenstein, E. (1993). Neglect and related disorders. In K.M. Heilman & E. Valenstein (Eds.),. *Clinical neuropsychology* (pp. 279–336). New York: Oxford University Press.

Honig, W.K., & Staddon, J.E.R. (1977). *Handbook of operant behavior.* Englewood Cliffs, NJ: Prentice-Hall.

Hopewell, C.A., Burke, W.H., Weslowski, M., & Zawlocki, R. (1990). Behavioral learning therapies for the traumatically brain-injured patient. In R.L. Wood & I. Fussey (Eds.), *Brain damage behavior & cognition: Cognitive rehabilitation in perspective* (pp. 229–245). New York: Taylor & Francis.

Horton, A.M., Jr., & Miller, W.G. (1985). Neuropsychology and behavior therapy. In M. Hersen, R.M. Eisler, & P.M. Miller (Eds.), *Progress in behavior modification* (Vol. 19, pp. 1–55), New York: Academic.

Horton, A.M., Jr., & Sautter, S.W. (1986). Behavioral neuropsychology: Behavioral treatment for the brain injured. In D. Wedding, A.M. Horton, Jr., & J. Webster (Eds.), *The neuropsychology handbook: Behavioral and clinical perspective.* New York: Springer.

Hugenholtz, H., & Richard, M.T. (1982). Return to athletic competition following concussion. *Canadian Medical Association Journal, 127,* 827–829.

Jacobs, H. (1988). The Los Angeles head injury survey: Procedures and initial findings. *Archives of Physical Medicine and Rehabilitation, 69,* 425–431.

Jaffe, K.M., Polissar, N.L., Fay, G.C., Liao, S. (1995). Recovery trends over three years following pediatric traumatic brain injury. *Archives of Physical Medicine and Rehabilitation, 76,* 17–26.

Jain, S. (1982). Operant conditioning for management of a non-compliant rehabilitation case after stroke. *Archives of Physical Medicine and Rehabilitation, 63,* 374–376.

Jordan, B.D., & Zimmerman, R.D. (1990). Computed tomography and magnetic resonance imaging comparisons in boxers. *Journal of the American Medical Association, 263,* 1670–1674.

Kelly, J.A. (1982). *Social skills training.* New York: Springer.

Kelly, J.P., Nichols, J.S., Filley, C.M., Lillehei, K.O., Rubinstein, D., & Kleinschmidt-Masters, B.K. (1991). Concussion in sports: Guidelines for the prevention of catastrophic outcome. *Journal of the American Medical Association, 266,* 2867–2869.

Koskiniemi, M., Kyykka, T., Nybo, T., & Jarho, L. (1995). Long-term outcome after severe brain injury in preschoolers is worse than expected. *Archives of Pediatric and Adolescent Medicine, 149,* 249–254.

Kraus, J.F., Black, M.A., Hessol, N., Ley, P., Rokaw, W., Sullivan, C., Bowers, S., Knowlton, S., & Marsghall, L. (1984). The incidence of acute brain injury and serious impairment in a defined population. *American Journal of Epidemiology, 119,* 186–201.

Kuhn, B.R., Allen, K.D., & Shriver, M.D. (1995). Behavioral management of children's seizure activity. *Clinical Pediatrics, 34*(11), 570–575.

Lancman, M.E., Asconpe, J.J., Graves, S., & Gibson, P.A. (1994). Psychogenic seizures in children: Long term analysis of 43 cases. *Journal of Child Neurology, 9,* 404–407.

Laurence, S., & Stein, D.G. (1978). Recovery after brain damage and the concept of localization of function. In S. Finger (Ed.). *Recovery from brain damage* (pp. 369–409). New York: Plenum.

Leaf, L.E. (1993). Traumatic brain injury: Affecting family recovery. *Brain Injury, 7*(6), 543–546.

LeBlanc, K.E. (1994). Concussions in sports: Guidelines for return to competition. *American Family Physician, 50,* 801–806.

Leitenberg, H. (1976). *Handbook of behavior modification and behavior therapy.* Englewood Cliffs, NJ: Prentice-Hall.

Leppik, I.O. (1995). Felbomate. *Epilepsia, 36*(Suppl. 2), S66–S72.

Levin, M.D., Benton, A.L., & Grossman, R.G. (1982). *Neurobehavioral consequences of closed head injury.* New York: Oxford University Press.

Lezak, M.D. (1988). Brain damage is a family affair. *Journal of Clinical and Experimental Neuropsychology, 10,* 111–123.

Lezak, M.D. (1995). *Neuropsychological assessment* (3rd ed.). New York: Oxford University Press.

Livingston, J.H. (1988). The Lennox-Gastaut Syndrome. *Developmental Medicine and Child Neurology, 30,* 536–549.

Macdonald, R.L., & Kelly, K.M. (1995). Antiepileptic drug mechanisms of action. *Epilepsia, 36*(Suppl. 2), S2–S12.

Mayfield, J.W., Warzak, W.J., Ford, & Poler, M. (1996, August). *Trends in neuropsychology training opportunities for school psychologists.* Paper presented at the 104th annual convention of the American Psychological Association. Toronto, Ontario, Canada.

McGuire, T.L., & Rothenberg, M.B. (1986). Behavioral and psychosocial sequelae of pediatric head injury. *Journal of Head Trauma Rehabilitation, 1*(4), 1–6.

McLean, M.J. (1995). Gabapentin. *Epilepsia, 36*(Suppl. 2), S73–S86.

Menkes, J.H., Sankar, R. (1995). Paroxysmal disorders. In J.H. Menkes (Ed.), *Textbook of child neurology* (pp. 725–814). Baltimore: Williams & Wilkins.

Messenheimer, J., Ramsay, R.E., Willmore, L.J., Leroy, R.F., Zielinski, J.J., Mattson, R., Pellock, J.M., Valakas, A.M., Womble, G., & Risner, M. (1994). Lamotrigine therapy for partial seizures: A multi-center, placebo-controlled, double-blind, cross-over trial. *Epilepsia, 35,* 113–121.

Michael, J. (1982). Distinguishing between discriminative and motivational functions of stimuli. *Journal of the Experimental Analysis of Behavior, 37,* 149–155.

Michael, J. (1993). Establishing operations. *Behavior Analyst, 16,* 191–206.

Michaelis, C., Warzak, W.J., Stanek, K., & Van Riper, C.L. (1992). Parental and professional perceptions of problems associated with long-term pediatric home tube feeding. *Journal of the American Dietetic Association, 92,* 1235–1238.

Mira, M.P., Tucker, B.F., & Tyler, J.S. (1992). *Traumatic brain injury in children and adolescents.* Austin, TX: Pro-Ed.

Mitiguy, J.S., Thompson, G., & Wasco, J. (1990). *Understanding brain injury: Acute hospitalization.* Lynn, MA: New Medico.

Mueller, F.O., & Cantu, R.C. (1990). Catastrophic injuries and fatalities in highschool and college sports, fall 1982–spring 1988. *Medicine and Science in Sports and Exercise, 22,* 737–741.

Nassbaum, N.L., & Bigler, E.D. (1990). *Identification and treatment of attention deficit disorder.* Austin, TX: Pro-Ed.

Nelson, K.B., & Ellenberg, J.H. (1976). Predictors of epilepsy in children who have experienced febrile seizures. *New England Journal of Medicine, 295,* 1029–1033.

Oddy, M., Humphrey, M., & Uttley, D. (1978). Stresses upon the relatives of head injured patients. *British Journal of Psychiatry, 133,* 307–313.

Olsson, I. (1988). Epidemiology of absence epilepsy. *Acta Paediatrica Scandinavia, 77,* 860–866.

Pace, G.M., Ivancic, M.T., Edwards, G.L., Iwata, B.A., & Page, T.J. (1985). Assessment of stimulus preference and reinforcer value with profoundly retarded individuals. *Journal of Applied Behavior Analysis, 18,* 249–255.

Paquier, P.F., Van Dangen, H.R., & Loonen, C.B. (1992). The Landau-Kleffner syndrome or "acquired aphasia with convulsive disorder"; long-term follow-up of six children and a review of the recent literature. *Archives of Neurology, 49,* 354–359.

Premack, D. (1959) Toward empirical behavior laws: I. Positive reinforcement. *Psychological Review, 66,* 219–233.

Reitan, R.M., & Wolfson, D. (1992). *Neuropsychological evaluation of older children.* Tucson, AZ: Neuropsychology Press.

Rhawn, J. (1990). *Neuropsychology, neuropsychiatry, and behavioral neurology.* New York: Plenum.

Richlens, A. (1994). Safety of lamotrigine. *Epilepsia, 35*(Suppl. 5), S37–S40.

Riikonen, R. (1981). A long-term follow-up study of 214 children with the syndrome of infantile spasms. *Neuropediatrics, 13,* 14–23.

Rimel, R.W., Giordani, B., Barth, J.T., Boll, T.J., & Jane, J.A. (1981). Disability caused by minor head injury. *Neurosurgery, 9,* 221–228.

Rimel, R.W., Giordani, B., Barth, J.T., & Jane, J.A. (1982). Moderate head injury: Completing the clinical spectrum of brain trauma. *Neurosurgery, 11,* 344–351.

Rosenthal, M. (1983). Behavioral sequelae. In M. Rosenthal, E.R. Griffith, M.R. Bond, & J.D. Miller (Eds.), *Rehabilitation of the head injured adult* (pp. 197–208). Philadelphia: Davis.

Rutherford, W.H. (1989). In H.S. Levin, H.M. Eisenberg, & A.L. Benton (Eds.), *Mild head injury.* New York: Oxford University Press.

Rutter, M., Chadwick, O., Shaffer, D. (1983). Head injury. In M. Rutter (Ed.), *Developmental neuropsychiatry* (pp. 83–111), New York: Guilford.

Savage, R.C. (1991). Identification, classification, and placement issues for students with traumatic brain injuries. *Journal of Head Trauma Rehabilitation, 6*(1), 1–9.

Schlumberger, E., Chavea, F., Palacios, L., Rey, E., Pajot, N., & Dulac, O. (1994). Lamotrigine in treatment of 120 children with epilepsy. *Epilepsia, 35,* 359–367.

Seshia, S.S., Seshia, M.M.K., & Sachdeva, R.K. (1977). Coma in childhood. *Developmental Medical Child Neurology, 19,* 614–628.

Sherretts, S.D. (1984). Neuropsychology and behavior disorders in youth. In C. Golden & P. Vicente (Eds.), *Foundations of clinical neuropsychology* (pp. 341–368). New York: Plenum.

Sidman, M. (1960). *Tactics of scientific research.* New York: Scientific Press.

Silver, L.B. (1982). Conversion disorder with pseudoseizures in adolescence: A stress reaction to unrecognized and untreated learning disabilities. (Case report). *Journal of American Academy of Child Psychiatry, 21,* 508–512.

Simpson, D., & Reilly, P. (1982). Pediatric coma scale. *Lancet, 9,* 450.

Skinner, B.F. (1953). *Science and human behavior.* New York: Free Press.

Solnick, J.V., Rincover, A., & Peterson, C.R. (1977). Some determinants of the reinforcing and punishing effects of time-out. *Journal of Applied Behavior Analysis, 10,* 415–424.

Stokes, T.F., & Baer, D.M. (1977). An implicit technology of generalization. *Journal of Applied Behavior Analysis, 10,* 349–367.

Szekers, S.F., & Neserve, N.F. (1994, November). Collaborative intervention in schools after traumatic brain injury. *Topics in Language Disorders, 15*(1), 21–36.

Teasdale, G., & Jennett, B. (1974). Assessment of coma and impaired consciousness: A practical scale. *Lancet, 2,* 81–84.

Unterharnscheidt, F. (1970). About boxing: Review of historical and medical aspects. *Texas Report of Biological Medicine, 28,* 421–495. Cited in J.P. Kelly, J.S. Nichols, C.M. Filley, K.O. Lillehei, D. Rubinstein, & B.K. Kleinschmidt-DeMasters. (1991). Concussion in sports: Guideline for prevention of catastrophic outcome. *Journal of the American Medical Association, 266,* 2867–2869.

Van Den Berg, B.J., & Yerushalmy, J. (1969). Studies on convulsive disorders in young children: I. Incidence of febrile and nonfebrile convulsions by age and other factors. *Pediatric Research, 3,* 298–304.

Van Zomeren, A.H., & Van Den Burg, W. (1985). Residual complaints of patients two years after severe head injury. *Journal of Neurological and Neurosurgical Psychiatry, 48,* 21–28.

Verity, C.M., Butler, N.R., & Golding, J. (1985). Febrile convulsions in a national cohort followed up from birth: I. Prevalence and recurrence in the first five years of life. *British Medical Journal, 290,* 1307–1310.

Wade, S., Drotar, D., Taylor, H.G., & Stancin, T. (1995). Assessing the effects of traumatic brain injury on family functioning: Conceptual and methodological issues. *Journal of Pediatric Psychology, 20*(6), 737–752.

Wahler, R.G. (1983). Setting events in social networks: Ally or enemy in child behavior therapy. *Behavior Therapy, 14,* 19–36.

Warzak, W.J., & Kilburn, J. (1990). Behavioral approaches to activities of daily living. In D.E. Tupper & K.D. Cicerone (Eds.), *The neuropsychology of everyday life. Vol. 1: Assessment and basic competencies* (pp. 285–305). New York: Martinus Nijhoff.

Warzak, W.J., & Page, T. (1990). Teaching refusal skills to sexually active adolescents. *Journal of Behavior Therapy and Experimental Psychiatry, 21,* 133–140 .

Warzak, W.J., Kewman, D.G., Stefans, V., & Johnson, E. (1987). Behavioral rehabilitation of functional alexia. *Journal of Behavior Therapy and Experimental Psychiatry, 18,* 171–177.

Warzak, W.J., Evans, J., & Ford, L. (1992). Working with the traumatically brain injured patient: Implications for rehabilitation. *Journal of Comprehensive Mental Health Care, 2,* 115–130.

Warzak, W.J., Ford, L., & Grow, C. (1992, August). *Are we prepared to provide school psychology services to students with TBI?* Paper presented at the 100th annual convention of the American Psychological Association, Washington, DC.

Warzak, W.J., Ayllon, T., Milan, M.A., Majors, C.T., & Delcher, H.K. (1993). Parental versus professional perceptions of obstacles to pediatric diabetes care. *Diabetes Educator, 19*(2), 121–124.

Warzak, W.J., Allan, T.M., Ford, L.A., & Stefans, V. (1995). Common obstacles to the daily functioning of pediatric traumatically brain injured patients: Perceptions of caregivers and psychologists. *Children's Health Care, 24*(2), 133–141.

Warzak, W.J., Mayfield, J.W., & McAllister, J.L. (1996, November). *Integrating neuropsychological and behavioral data to develop comprehensive assessment strategies in brain injured individuals.* Paper presented at the 30th annual convention of the Association for Advancement of Behavior Therapy, New York.

Wilberger, J.E. (1993). Minor head injuries in American football: Prevention of long term sequelae. *Sports Medicine, 15,* 338–343.

Wyllie, E., Friedman, D., Rothner, A.D., Luders, H., Dinner, D., Morris, H., Cruse, R., Erenberg, G., & Kotagal, P. (1970). Psychogenic seizures in children and adolescents: Outcome after diagnosis by ictal video and electroencephalographic recording. *Pediatrics, 85,* 480–484.

Wyllie, E., Friedman, D., Luders, H., Morris, H., Rothner, A.D., & Turnbull, J. (1991). Outcome of psychogenic seizures in children and adolescents compared with adults. *Neurology, 41,* 742–744.

Yager, J.Y., Johnston, B., & Seshia, S.S. (1990). Coma scales in pediatric practice. *American Journal of Diseases in Children, 144,* 1088–1091.

Ylvisaker, M., Hartwick, P., & Stevens, M. (1991). School reentry following head injury: Managing the transition from hospital to school. *Journal of Head Trauma Rehabilitation, 6*(1), 10–22.

Zlutnick, S., Mayville, W.J., & Moffatt, S. (1975). Modification of seizure disorders: The interruption of behavioral chains. *Journal of Applied Behavior Analysis, 8,* 1–12.

Bibliography

Aicardi, J. (1994). *Epilepsy in children* (2nd ed.). New York: Raven.

Almli, C.R. & Finger, S. (1992). Brain injury and recovery of function: Theories and mechanisms of functional reorganization. *Journal of Head Trauma Rehabilitation, 7,* 70–77.

Cantu, R.C. (1992). Cerebral concussion in sport: Management and prevention. *Sports Medicine, 14,* 64–74.

Chelune, G.J., & Edwards, P. (1981). Early brain lesions: Ontogenic–environmental considerations. *Journal of Consulting and Clinical Psychology, 49,* 777–790.

Dahl, J. (1992). *Epilepsy: A behavior management approach to assessment and treatment in children.* Seattle, WA: Hogrefe & Huber.

Jaffe, K.M., Polissar, N.L., Faye, G.C., Liao, S. (1995). Recovery trends over three years following pediatric traumatic brain injury. *Archives of Physical Medicine and Rehabilitation, 76,* 17–26.

Koskiniemi, M., Kyykka, T., Nybo, T., & Jarho, L. (1995). Long-term outcome after severe brain injury in preschoolers is worse than expected. *Archives of Pediatric and Adolescent Medicine, 149,* 249–254.

Levin, M.D., Benton, A.L., & Grossman, R.G. (1982). *Neurobehavioral consequences of closed head injury.* New York: Oxford University Press.

Menkes, J.H., Sankar, R. (1995). Paroxysmal disorders. In J.H. Menkes, (Ed.), *Textbook of child neurology* (pp. 725–814). Baltimore: Williams & Wilkins.

Rimmel, R.W., Giordani, B., Barth, J.T., Boll, T.J., & Jane, J.A. (1981). Disability caused by minor head injury. *Neurosurgery, 9,* 221–228.

Rimmel, R. Giordani, B., Barth, J.T., & Jane, J.A. (1982). Moderate head injury: Completing the clinical spectrum of brain trauma. *Neurosurgery, 11,* 344–351.

Savage, R.C. (1991). Identification, classification, and placement issues for students with traumatic brain injuries. *Journal of Head Trauma Rehabilitation, 6*(1), 1–9.

Ylvisaker, M., Hartwick, P., & Stevens, M. (1991). School reentry following head injury: Managing the transition from hospital to school. *Journal of Head Trauma Rehabilitation, 6*(1), 10–22.

16

Chronic Illness in Childhood

A Hypothesis-Testing Approach

COLLEEN M. McMAHON, KATINA M. LAMBROS,
AND JUDITH A. SYLVA

Introduction

The term *chronic illness* encompasses a variety of specific medical disorders and disease processes and their corresponding medical treatments and prognoses (Sexson & Swain, 1995; Varni & Wallander, 1988). A review of the pediatric research literature reveals that specific chronic illnesses share several common findings across disease processes. First, advancements in medical treatments have increased the survival rates for most pediatric conditions. Second, many childhood chronic illnesses can be cured or managed to the extent that children live to normal expected age ranges. Third, increased survival rates have afforded researchers the opportunity to study the psychosocial variables that influence the disease process in a variety of chronic illnesses. Fourth, psychosocial variables have been found to affect physical health and disease management. Finally, although much more is known about the relationship between psychosocial variables and chronic illness, research directly related to the efficacy of psychological interventions with chronically ill child populations remains limited (Drotar, 1993; LaGreca & Varni, 1993; Stehbens, 1988).

Definition and Background Information

It is estimated that 20% of the school-age population suffers from a chronic illness, and the percentage of children with chronic illnesses increases as early childhood and infant populations are included (Sexson & Swain, 1995). Given that this estimate is derived from the combined figures of more than a dozen disease processes, the likelihood that most educators and psychologists will have exposure to children with all of these illnesses is not very high. Therefore we have provided a general summary of the most common chronic illnesses of childhood and the typical course of treatment in Table 1. As can be seen from Table 1, childhood chronic illness encompasses a very diverse set of illnesses, with very different types of medical treatments. Prognostic indications also vary. For example, juvenile rheumatoid arthritis (JRA) is a chronic illness that is not considered life-threatening, while pediatric AIDS remains an illness that has resulted in death in almost all cases. Most chronic illnesses (e.g., hemophilia and sickle cell disease) are considered low-incidence problems; however, some illnesses, such as asthma, occur at a much higher rate, particularly in urban areas (Creer, Harm, & Marion, 1988). Some illnesses require frequent hospitalizations and school absences (e.g., cancer), while other illnesses may result in very few medical visits to manage the disease (e.g., congenital heart disease).

COLLEEN M. McMAHON, KATINA M. LAMBROS, AND JUDITH A. SYLVA • School of Education, University of California–Riverside, Riverside, California 92521-0102.

Handbook of Child Behavior Therapy, edited by Watson and Gresham. Plenum Press, New York, 1998.

TABLE 1. Diagnostic and Treatment Information for Common Chronic Illnesses of Childhood

Chronic illness	Prevalence	Age at diagnosis	Frequent hospitalizations/school absences	Course of medical treatment
Asthma	4.3% <18	<10 years	No	—Drug therapy (theo-phylline, corticosteroid) —Self-management/self-recording —Prevention/manage-ment of attacks
Cystic fibrosis	1 in 2,500 live births	40%—infancy; 60%—by 12 months	Variable	—Drug therapy
Juvenile diabetes (IDDM)	1 in 600 children under 18 years	5–6 years 11–13	Variable. If frequent, due to poor meta-bolic control	—Frequent monitoring of levels —Self-administration of insulin —Diet and exercise
Hemophilia	1 in 10,000 male births	Typically, <1 year	Limited	—Blood factor replace-ment therapy —Pain management —Therapeutic exercise
HIV/AIDS	8,000 cases AIDS—unknown HIV	Variable: >1 year–<19 years	Yes, during the end-stage of the disease	—Antiretroval drugs —Frequent monitoring of t-cell counts, general health
Juvenile rheumatoid arthritis	1 in 1,000	<16 years	Variable	—Nonsteroidal anti-inflammatory, cortico-steroid drugs —Therapuetic exercise —Pain management
Cancer: leukemia	All cancers: 1 in 600	<15 years	Yes	—Chemotherapy/radia-tion therapy —Bone marrow aspira-tions —Bone marrow trans-plant surgery —Frequent medical visits —Frequent invasive procedures during acture stage
Cancer: solid tumors	Same as above, except more boys than girls	<10 years for most tumors	Yes	—Chemotherapy/radiation —Surgery
Congenital heart disease	8 in 1,000 live births	Birth to early child-hood	Variable	—Surgery (e.g., open heart, pacemaker placement) —Drug therapy
Sickle cell disease	1 in 400 (Blacks)	<10 years	Variable	—Transfusions —Pain management
Seizure disorder	4 to 8 in 1,000	<2 years 11–13 years	Variable to none	—Antiepileptic medication

The psychological and behavioral sequelae dif-fer across and within disorders as well. Table 2 de-scribes the relationship between specific chronic illness and corresponding educational, psychologi-cal and behavioral problems. A review of the rele-vant educational, affective or behavioral problems

TABLE 2. Common Psychological and Behavioral Sequalae of Pediatric Chronic Illness

Chronic illness	Educational implications	Somatic complaints	Internalizing behavior problems	Externalizing behavior problems
Asthma	40% experience reading problems	No	Specific fears Anxiety/panic	Noncompliance
Cystic fibrosis	Frequent school absences	No	Specific fears Anxiety/panic	Noncompliance
Juvenile diabetes (IDDM)	Cognitive deficits, associated with attention and planning skills	Frequent	Depression Social anxiety School or social avoidance	Noncompliance Oppositional behavior
Hemophilia	Frequent school absences	Frequent	Depression Anxiety	Oppositional behavior High-risk behaviors
HIV/AIDS	Cognitive deficits, associated with end-stage disease	Frequent	Depression Anxiety	Noncompliance high-risk behaviors
Juvenile rheumatoid arthritis	Frequent school absences	Frequent	Depression Social anxiety School or social avoidance	None reported
Cancer: leukemia	Cognitive deficits associated radiation therapy	Frequent during acute phases; absent in remission	Depression Specific fears Social anxiety School or social avoidance	Aggression with siblings and peers Oppositional behavior/ noncompliance
Cancer: solid tumors	Frequent school absences during acute therapy with radiation	Frequent during acute phase; absent in remission	Depression Specific fears Social anxiety School or social avoidance	Aggression with siblings and peers Oppositional behavior/ noncompliance
Congenital heart disease	Frequent school absences	Infrequent	Generalized anxiety about the future	Noncompliance with diet, treatment
Sickle cell disease	Cognitive and motor deficits if associated strokes occur	Frequent	Depression Specific fears Social anxiety School or social avoidance	Noncompliance with treatment
Seizure disorder	Cognitive deficits, associated with location, severity, and treatment	Variable	School or social avoidance Social anxiety	Aggression Violent outbursts

for each disorder revealed considerable diversity in reporting these outcomes, even within disease processes. Therefore, Table 2 includes only those problems that were reported in the literature by empirical investigations, across years, and by multiple sources. The diagnostic categories in Table 2 are necessarily general, yet even with the general classifications used, variability across type of illness is noted. In addition, Table 2 provides some general information as to the expected occurrence of so-

matic complaints, typically chronic pain, experienced by the child. Chronic pain or other somatic complaints typically has been linked to either the disease process or the treatment (e.g., chemotherapy); however, in many cases frequent somatic complaints may be associated as often, or more often, with affective or psychosocial variables (McGrath, 1990).

The prevalence and outcome data regarding childhood chronic illness is so varied that it may be helpful to discuss assessment and treatment approaches with chronic illness in the context of specific disease processes. Two chronic illnesses, juvenile onset, Insulin Dependent Diabetes Mellitus (IDDM) and Acute Lymphocytic Leukemia (ALL), will be reviewed briefly in the following section. Examples of IDDM and ALL will also be provided throughout the problem identification, problem analysis, plan implementation, and plan evaluation sections. IDDM and ALL were selected as examples for several reasons. First, they represent extreme ends of the chronic illness continuum, with one disease process (IDDM) characterized as more chronic than life-threatening, requiring lifelong management to maintain health. Conversely, ALL is by definition an acute disease process that requires intensive treatment over a shorter time (1–5 years). Despite advances in medical treatment, ALL continues to result in death for approximately 30% to 40% of affected children. Once remission has been achieved, however, management of ALL is minimal, requiring only follow-up visits to the oncologist. Second, both ALL and IDDM typically have substantial social and emotional implications for afflicted children as well as increasing stressors within families. Finally, recent research with these illnesses demonstrates that educational impairments can result not only from missed school, but from changes in cognitive functioning due to either treatment or diagnostic factors.

Diabetes Mellitus

Diabetes mellitus is characterized by insufficient insulin production by the pancreas and is the most common endocrine or metabolic disorder of childhood (Holmes, O'Brien, & Greer, 1995; Johnson, 1988). In insulin dependent diabetes mellitus (IDDM), complete pancreatic failure occurs and insulin replacement by daily injection is necessary for survival. The onset of IDDM typically occurs in childhood and preadolescence, with the diagnosis of IDDM typically being made during either of two age periods, 5–6 years and 11–13 years of age. Disease onset may, however, occur at any time from infancy to young adulthood, striking males and females with equal frequency. The etiology of IDDM is unknown. Treatment of IDDM requires an extensive illness management regimen for the child

and parents. This typically involves self-injection of insulin, frequent monitoring of blood sugar levels, regulating food intake, and engaging in regular exercise (Johnson, 1988, 1995). Management of IDDM requires the child or adolescent to make ongoing decisions with regard to diet, insulin, and exercise to prevent episodes of hyper- and hypoglycemia. Adherence to the regimen has been shown to have a direct link to diabetic control in many children (Johnson, 1988; Weist, Finney, Barrinard, Davis, & Ollendick, 1993). Parent–child arguments over adherence to the regimen is often cited as a source of increasing family conflict. If metabolic control is established and maintained, children with IDDM may lead long and productive lives. For many children with IDDM and their families, maintaining metabolic control is difficult and clearly affected by the number and severity of psychosocial stressors (Holmes, 1990; Johnson, 1995). While the impact of psychosocial variables on the metabolic control of children with IDDM is well documented, the selection of treatment targets and effective interventions is less well known and is complicated by the sheer number of psychosocial variables that impact family and child functioning (Weist et al., 1993).

In addition to conflict over disease management, families of children with IDDM experience many stressors associated with the diagnosis and management of the disease, including differential treatment of the child with IDDM as compared with siblings, behavioral management issues, encouraging independence of the child with IDDM, and dealing with their fears about the child's future. Children and adolescents with IDDM often experience frequent school absences, social interaction problems with peers and siblings, and adjustment problems, including anxiety or depression about their future (Johnson, 1995). Also, children with IDDM often experience educational difficulties in academic content areas. It was previously thought that the reason for these academic problems was the children's frequent school absences. More recent research, however, has controlled for school absences in the investigation of academic and cognitive problems and has indicated that children with IDDM experience problems with memory, attention, and impulsivity well beyond those of healthy peers with comparable attendance records (Holmes et al., 1995).

Acute Lymphocytic Leukemia (ALL)

ALL is the most common form of cancer in children. Most children are between the ages of two and eight when diagnosed. Acute lymphocytic leukemia, also referred to as acute lymphoblastic leukemia, is a form of cancer in which bone marrow produces malignant cells that, in turn, reduce the number of normal blood cells and increase the white blood cell count. The etiology of ALL is unknown. Treatment is designed to destroy the cells, or blasts, prevent their recurrence, and restore the patient to a normal hematological (blood) status. ALL occurs slightly more frequently in boys than in girls and in Caucasians than in African Americans (National Cancer Institute, 1988). Once the diagnosis of ALL is made, children are categorized as being at either high, low, or medium risk. This classification is made based on the age at diagnosis, blood values, and initial symptomalogy (Powers, Vannatta, Noll, Cool, & Stehbens, 1995; Stehbens, 1988).

Survival rates for ALL have risen to above 80% according to some estimates—an increase from just 55% in 1976 (Granowetter, 1994; National Cancer Institute, 1988). Treatment for ALL usually requires chemotherapy and cranial radiation therapy, with remission (reduction of blasts) occurring following a one- or two-month course of treatment. In cases where remission appears stable, a course of two to three more years of chemotherapy is recommended. The side effects of such treatments are numerous and include frequent nausea and vomiting, loss of hair, lethargy, dental problems, and changes in brain structure or function typically associated with cognitive deficits and learning problems (Armstrong & Holmes, 1995; Moore, Copeland, Reid & Levy, 1992; Stehbens, 1988).

In addition to learning problems, children with ALL often suffer from chronic somatic complaints and affective disorders such as anxiety or depression. Social anxiety is often a problem for children with ALL, who may experience embarrassment about hair or weight loss associated with their treatments. Specific fears also develop as a result of the treatment for ALL. Children often develop anticipatory vomiting prior to receiving chemotherapy, or experience panic reactions to needles following invasive medical procedures such as bone marrow aspirations (BMA), in which a syringe is used to extract bone marrow for the purposes of monitoring disease progression. In addition, children with ALL may experience anxiety or hopelessness regarding their future, peer relation problems, delays in social development if the disease is diagnosed during the preschool or early childhood age, and delays in adaptive skills when relatives may limit the demands placed on the child with cancer. Even within ALL, however, affective, social, and behavioral outcomes are mixed, with some researchers finding no differences between children with cancer and their physically healthy peers in this domain and other researchers discovering large differences between groups (Noll, Bukowski, Davies, Koontz, & Kulkarni, 1993; Spirito, Stark, Cobiella, Dugan, Andiokites, & Hewett, 1990).

Families of children with ALL experience increased stress associated with this life-threatening illness, especially in the management of the intensive daily treatment process, marital distress, and the financial costs of treatment (Dahlquist, Czyzeski, Copeland, Jones, Taub, & Vaughan, 1993). Marital distress and parent coping style have been linked to child affective status and have been demonstrated to occur more frequently in families with a child with ALL than in families with physically healthy children (Dahlquist et al., 1993).

This brief description of two disease processes, IDDM and ALL, reveals the complexity involved in the assessment of and intervention with a child with either of these chronic illnesses. The sheer number of physical, psychological, behavioral, and familial factors to consider in the assessment or treatment of either of these illnesses appears overwhelming, particularly when the relevant literature reveals relationships between broad psychosocial variables and group characteristics. To date, there is minimal information in the pediatric literature as to (a) appropriate behaviors to target for intervention, (b) effective interventions for a variety of child behavior problems within these populations, and (c) the best approaches for the assessment and/or monitoring of critical psychosocial variables that influence and are influenced by the disease process (LaGreca & Varni, 1993).

Problem Identification

The assessment and treatment of a child with a chronic illness who experiences behavioral, cognitive, affective, or emotional problems is a difficult endeavor, complicated by the number of factors to consider and the interactive, reciprocal nature between factors. Figure 1 is a graphic illustration of the variables and potential combination of variables that may result in a child being referred for therapy services. As can be seen from Figure 1, any combination or any sequence of variables, such as family environment, cognitive/academic functioning, and adherence to medical regimen, may be related to the child's experiencing problems severe enough to warrant referral to a school psychologist, pediatric psychologist, or family therapist. In an effort to increase our knowledge regarding the relationship between psychosocial and physical health, several authors (Johnson, 1984; Weist, Ollendick, & Finney, 1991) have recommended that an empirical validation approach be used to identify appropriate psychological, familial, and behavioral targets for treatment. According to Weist et al., (1991), an empirical validation follows this sequence: (a) review of the relevant literature to identify potential variables of importance, (b) exploration of empirical validation through group studies, and (c) numerous treatment outcome studies, both group and idiographic approaches, to validate effective treatments. The empirical validation approach appears to be useful for identifying general variables for treatment and for exploring relationships between physical and psychological variables for a particular chronic illness.

With IDDM, for instance, psychosocial factors have been documented to affect a child's metabolic control and adjustment to the disease. The difficulty arises regarding the criteria for determining which psychosocial factor(s) to target for intervention. Typically, interventions for children and adolescents with IDDM are developed with the understanding that children need to manage their own disease, so noncompliance with the treatment regimen has been a frequent target for intervention. Compliance, rather than metabolic control, has been used as the standard for intervention success, with the assumption that better compliance leads to better metabolic control (Johnson, 1988). In an effort to select treatment targets based on empirical validation, Weist et al. (1993) used template matching to identify children with optimal control of diabetes, and compared them on psychosocial measures with children in nonoptimal diabetic control to identify variables empirically associated with optimal control. They found that optimally controlled children were not more compliant with the medical regimen than were children in the poorly controlled group. However, the groups did differ on measures of family, environment, and the child's health locus of control. Controlling family environments, decreased emphasis on independence, increased control rules, and monitoring enforced by the parents was associated with better metabolic control.

The findings of the Weist et al. (1993) study are important for several reasons. First, they demonstrate how little we know about the interactive or reciprocal nature between psychosocial variables, adherence to a medical regimen, and health status. Although their findings have yet to be replicated, it is interesting to note the possibility that compliance to a regimen may not be the critical variable to target for intervention, or, at least, that the presence or absence of factors may alter the importance of strict adherence to a regimen. For example, other researchers (e.g., Allen, Tenner, McGrade, Affleck, & Ratzan, 1983; Anderson, Auslander, Jung, Miller, & Santiago, 1990) have found that family disagreements regarding who should take responsibility for diabetes management are associated with poorly controlled children. Second, the findings support previous research with chronic illness that points to the family environment as a critical factor for optimal physical and psychological health for the child (e.g., Roberts & Wallander, 1992). Finally, these findings support an approach to assessment and treatment that rules out or rules in target variables in a systematic, empirical manner.

An empirical validation approach appears to be useful for identifying general variables to assess and target (e.g., Weist et al., 1993), particularly if future research in chronic illness is guided by this approach. The lack of current research addressing the empirical validation of treatment targets and the emphasis on nomothetic (e.g., group trait) characteristics limits the usefulness of the empirical validation approach as the sole index for selecting targets for assessment and treatment. In contrast, we propose a *hypothesis-testing approach* in conjunction with an ecological assessment and treatment approach for application with children with chronic illness. A hypothesis-testing approach

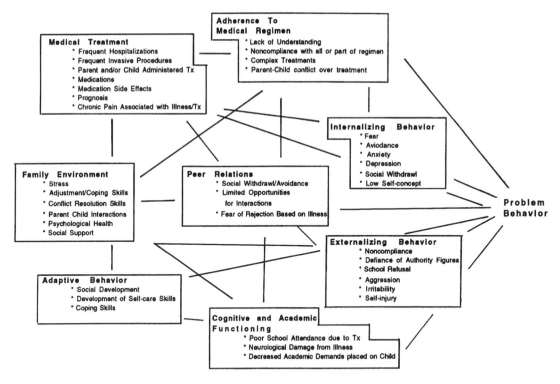

FIGURE 1. Contextual factors and influences related to chronic illness in childhood.

involves five steps: (a) hypothesis formulation, (b) descriptive functional analysis, (c) hypothesis refinement, (d) functional assessment and experimental functional analysis, and (e) hypothesis confirmation for intervention development.

The purpose of the hypothesis-testing approach is to develop a systematic method for the identification and analysis of child behavior problems. In this approach, each level serves to refine and reduce the variables to be targeted for intervention and monitoring, moving from very broad to very specific targets for identification, assessment, and treatment. Several fundamental principles of behavioral assessment are inherent in the hypothesis-testing approach. First, although assessment and intervention are separate activities, they are invariably linked as an ongoing process, because the assessment data lead directly to treatment and the intervention data may provide evidence that further assessment is warranted (Nelson & Hayes, 1986). Second, this approach is *ecological* because it provides a method by which to assess and treat broad as well as specific variables and to evaluate the im-

pact of multiple systems (or ecologies) on behavior and the impact of behavioral change on these systems (e.g., family, medical) (Martens & Witt, 1988). Finally, a *keystone behavior approach* is incorporated into a hypothesis-testing approach in which one or two responses are demonstrated to be emprically related to other responses (Hayes, Nelson, & Jarrett, 1987). Rather than treating all behaviors or responses, the keystone behavior approach identifies the keystone, or critical, behavior which, when changed in frequency or intensity, will result in changes for other, nontreated behaviors. Changes in the keystone behavior may produce concurrent changes (collateral effects) in a class of responses (Sulzer-Azaroff & Mayer, 1991). This approach is particularly useful in the examination of secondary and tertiary influences of behavior.

The first two steps in the hypothesis-testing approach, (a) hypothesis formulation and (b) descriptive assessment, are discussed in this section. The remaining steps with be discussed in the problem analysis section of this chapter.

Hypothesis Formulation

The purpose of hypothesis formulation is to generate initial hypotheses regarding the problem of interest and its maintaining variables. Data collection at this stage primarily involves (a) a review of the relevant literature and (b) informal interviews with parents, health care professionals, teachers, and the child. Even if the psychologist is familiar with the particular chronic illness of the referred child, a review of the current literature is necessary to ensure adequate assessment and treatment. Treatments thought to be positive and proactive can still result in unwanted side effects, and an adequate review of the literature may decrease the likelihood that inappropriate treatments will be recommended.

Informal interviews serve the purpose of gaining information regarding some of the variables depicted in Figure 1, such as disease status, behavioral history, medical problems, and medication use for the referred child and his family. In general, informal interviews should gather information that may serve to clarify or expand upon the referral information. Informal interviews should be structured to the extent that the interviewer gathers information relative to the eight domains in Figure 1: diagnosis/course of treatment, adherence to medical regimen, family environment, peer relations, adaptive behavior, cognitive/academic behavior, internalizing behaviors, and externalizing behaviors. With traditional medical or psychiatric approaches, these activities fall in the category of case formulation from which a treatment is prescribed that confirms or disconfirms the case formulation. In the hypothesis-testing approach, however, several competing hypotheses should emerge from completion of the activities. These hypotheses are be considered preliminary and should be operationalized for further analysis. At this step it should be possible to develop methods for either ruling in or ruling out each hypothesis formulated as the result of a review of the literature and the informal interviews. For example, in the case of a 13-year-old child with diabetes, we might hypothesize that poor adherence to a medical regimen is due to parent–child conflict, child anger regarding the responsibility of the disease management, or a lack of correspondence between adherence to regimen and good physcial health. These competing hypotheses could be ex-cluded or maintained depending on the data obtained during the descriptive functional analysis.

Descriptive Functional Analysis

An adequate analysis of a referral problem requires that the problem be operationalized in a quantifiable, reliable manner and that the analysis results in information that directly impacts intervention development. Functional analysis and assessment procedures have been used extensively with child behavior problems and have been shown to provide information critical to treatment selection and implementation (Carr, 1994; Gresham, 1991). Functional assessment methodology includes a wide range of strategies that are used to discover the functional, causal relationships between a problem behavior and environmental events which occasion or maintain the problem behavior. Functional assessment is not restricted in range or depth to mere descriptions of stimulus events occurring in close temporal proximity to a target behavior, but must also include data-based assessment of environmental ecologies, setting events, establishing operations, and so on, that may well be removed from a behavior but that reveal a functional relationship to it (Gresham, 1991). Functional analysis is subsumed in this assessment process, but involves a more systematic and scientific approach to data collection and behavioral observation that follows the S-O-R-C-K model for problem behavior analysis. The S-O-R-C-K model involves the assessment of critical individual child and environmental variables and includes developmental, physical, and psychological information about the child (O = Organism variables), antecedent stimuli or cues (S = Stimuli), target response(s) (R = Response), and the type and scheduling of consequences following the problem behavior (C = Consequences; K = Contingencies). The assessment process should yield information that can be interpreted and tested via a S-O-R-C-K model. To be consistent with both the ecological perspective and the keystone behavior approach, S-O-R-C-K information should be obtained across settings, situations, and behaviors.

The specific environments to be addressed and considered throughout the functional analysis include those variables depicted in Figure 1, including the child's (a) medical environment, (b) family and home life, (c) school setting, and (d) adaptive and social life. During this step in the identification and assessment process, broadly defined variables (e.g., depression, family stress) remain the focus. Assessment measures will include (a) structured interviews, (b) self-report scales, (c) rating scales, and (d) informal observations of the child. Perhaps the best place to begin is to conduct a structured interview with one to three key persons (i.e., parent, teacher, nurse) regarding the behaviors of interest, the contexts in which they occur, and the specific environmental events which precede and follow these behaviors. Although other suggestions for a functional analysis interview may be found elsewhere in this text (see Chapter 1, this volume), we have provided an adapted version of the Functional Analysis Interview Form (O'Neill, Horner, Albin, Sprague, Storey, & Newton, 1997) for use in the descriptive functional analysis with chronic illness. This assessment tool is conducted via a semistructured interview and may be administered to any person involved with the child. The Functional Analysis Interview Form was adapted for several reasons. First, the assessment of children with chronic illness involves more variables than would be expected with physically healthy children and more change in variables across time than may be experienced by the children and adolescents with developmental delays for whom the form was developed. Second, some of the adapted items reflect the use of the keystone behavior strategy in the identification of targets for treatment. Finally, many of the adapted items provide information specific to the child's medical treatment, medical regimen, and pain experiences as perceived by parents, teachers and nurses. Form 16.1 provides an example of the Adapted Functional Analysis Interview Form (AFA). The AFA should be administered initially to those persons from the environment in which the behaviors of concern have been reported (i.e., reported at home: the child's parents, caretakers, or siblings). Based on this information, supplementary and additional AFA interviews should be conducted with doctors, nurses, and, if applicable, teachers or psychologists.

Self-report and rating scales frequently have been used with pediatric populations. Both types of measures may be useful during the descriptive functional analysis step in both ruling in and ruling out variables for further assessment. A vast variety of child behavior rating scales exist, but many deal specifically with behaviors covered elsewhere in this book. These include rating scales for social skills (see Chapter 24), depression (see Chapter 20), anxiety (see Chapter 19), academic problems (see Chapter 4), and hyperactivity, aggression, and antisocial behavior (see Chapters 6 and 23). Table 3 provides a list of rating scales and self-report measures that have been used extensively or specifically with pediatric populations and their families.

Rating scales can be important in clarifying the role of those variables depicted in Figure 1 in the development and maintenance of the referral problem. Rating scales can also play an important role within a keystone behavior approach, not only in the identification of behavior for treatment, but in the identification of variables that are not necessarily amenable for treatment, but that can affect child and family functioning. For example, although cognitive variables such as parent and child health beliefs, parent causal attributions, and parent and child locus of control have been demonstrated to affect treatment implementation and success, cognitive variables themselves have not been demonstrated to be effective targets for change. Reimers and Wacker (1988) used the Behavioral Attribution Measure (BAM; Reimers, 1985) to assess the impact on treatment compliance of parental causal attribution for their child's behavioral problem to either a medical or behavioral cause. Reimers and his colleagues (1995) found that parental attributions for their child's behavior problem affected treatment compliance with carrying out behavioral interventions at home. However, their attributions changed when the behavioral intervention was effective. Cognitive variables such as parental causal attribution may be useful to assess and monitor, even if direct treatment is not possible.

Self-report scales should include pain reports, even if pain is not a primary target for intervention. Chronic pain and other somatic complaints are common for a variety of chronic illnesses and may be directly or indirectly related to referral problems such as school or social avoidance, depression, and anxiety. Form 16.2 includes a sample pain self-report form excerpted from McGrath (1990). Pain interview and self-report scales should be age-appropriate and provide multiple response opportunities, particularly for the child to indicate

FORM 16.1. Functional Analysis Interview Form

A. *Describe the behaviors(s)*

What are the behaviors of concern? For each, define the topography (how it is performed), frequency (how often it occurs per day, week, or month), duration (how long it lasts when it occurs), and intensity (what is the magnitude of the behaviors flow, medium, high? Does it cause harm?).

Behavior	Topography	Frequency	Duration	Intensity
1.				
2.				
3.				

B. *Define potential ecological events that may affect the behavior(s)*
   1. What medications is the person taking (if any) and how do you believe these may affect his/her behavior?
   2. Describe the sleep cycles of the individual and the extent to which these cycles may affect behavior.
   3. Describe the eating routines and diet of the person and the extent to which these routines affect behavior?
   4. Briefly list below the person's typical daily schedule of activities.

   6:00AM _____   3:00 _____

   9:00 _____   6:00 _____

   12:00 _____   9:00 _____

   5. About how often does the person get to make choices about activities, reinforcers? In what areas does that person get to make choices (e.g., food, clothing, leisure)?

C. *Define events and situations that predict occurrences of the behavior(s)*
   1. Time of day: When are the behaviors most likely? Least likely?
   2. Setting: Where are the behaviors most likely? Least likely?
   3. Social control: With whom are the behaviors most likely? Least likely?
   4. Activity: What activity is most likely to produce the behavior? Least likely?
   5. Are there particular situations that are not listed above that "set off" the behaviors that cause concern (particular demands, interruptions, transitions, delays, being ignored, etc.)?
   6. What would be the one thing you could do that would most likely make the undesirable behavior occur?

D. *Identify the "function" of the undesirable behavior(s). What consequences maintain the behavior(s)?*
   1. Think of each of the behaviors listed in Section A, and define the function(s) you believe the behavior serves for the person (i.e., what does he/she get and/or avoid by doing the behavior?

Behavior	What does he/she get	What does he/she avoid?
1.		
2.		

Describe the person's most typical response to the following situations.
   a. Are the above behaviors more likely, less likely, or unaffected if you present him/her with a difficult task?
   b. Are the above behaviors more likely, less likely, or unaffected if you interrupt a desired event (e.g., TV)?
   c. Are the above behaviors more likely, less likely, or unaffected if you deliver a "stem" request, reprimand?
   d. Are the above behaviors more likely, less likely, or unaffected if you are present but do not interact with (ignore) the person for 15 minutes?
   e. Are the above behaviors more likely, less likely, or unaffected by changes in routine?
   f. Are the above behaviors more likely, less likely, or unaffected if something the person wants is present but he/she can't get it (visible but out of reach)?
   g. Are the above behaviors more likely, less likely, or unaffected if he/she is alone (no one else present)?

E. *Define the efficiency of the undesirable behavior(s).*
   1. What amount of physical effort is involved in the behaviors (intense tantrum or simple verbal outbursts)?
   2. Does engaging in the behaviors result in a "payoff '(attention, avoiding work) every time? Once in a while?
   3. How much of a delay is there between the time a person engages in a behavior and gets the "payoff"? Is it immediate, a few seconds, longer?

F. *Define the primary method(s) used by the person to communicate*
   1. What are the general expressive communication strategies used by or available to the person (vocal speech, signs/gestures, communication books/boards, electronic devices)? How constantly are the strategies used?

FORM 16.1. (*Continued*)

2. With regard to receptive communication ability:
   a. Does the person follow verbal requests or instructions? If so, how many? List if only a few.

   _____

   _____

   b. Is the person able to imitate physical models for various tasks or activities?

   _____

   _____

G. *What events, actions, and objects are perceived zas positive by the person?*
   1. What are the events, activities, objects, people that appear to be reinforcing to the person? List them.

H. *What "functional alternative" behaviors are known by the person?*
   1. What socially appropriate behaviors/skills does the person perform that may be ways of achieving the same function(s) as the behaviors of concern?
   2. What things can you do to improve the likelihood that a teaching session will occur smoothly?
   3. What things can you do that would interfere or disrupt a teaching session?

I. *Provide a history of the undesirable behaviors and the programs that have been attempted*

   Behavior   How long has this been a problem?   Programs   Effect
   1. _____
   2. _____
   3. _____

Adapted from O'Neill, Horner, Albin, Sprague, Storey, & Newton (1997).

TABLE 3. Rating Scales Used with Pediatric Populations

Rating scale	Author/publisher	Target area	Respondent
Child Behavior Checklist (CBCL)	Achenbach & Edelbroch	Internalizing behaviors Externalizing behaviors Social competence	Parent Teacher Child
Pediatric Behavior Scale (PBS)	Lindgren		Parent
Treatment Acceptability Rating Form–Revised (TARF–R)	Reimers	Acceptability and understanding of behavioral interventions	Parent
Behavior Attribution Measure (BAM)	Reimers et al.	Parental beliefs regarding cause of child's behavioral problems	Parent
Parenting Stress Index (PSI)	Abidin	Parent rating of perceived stress in a variety of parenting situations	Parent
Family Environment Scale (FES)	Moos & Moos	Supportive environment Controlling environment Conflicted environment	Parent
Multidimensional Health Locus of Control	Thompson, Butcher, & Berenson	Internal locus of control Powerful others	Child
KIDCOPE	Spirito, Stark, & Williams	Use of cognitive and behavioral coping strategies	Child

FORM 16.2. Pain Self-Report Form

Children's Subjective Pain Experience

Average frequency of headaches _____   Range _____

Average length of headaches _____   Range _____

Notable changes in frequency or intensity _____

Current frequency _____   Current length _____

Why did you see Dr. _____ at this time? _____

Describe one of your usual headaches. (Note child's description of the following: where headache occurred; severity; accompanying symptoms; who intervened; duration; probable cause.)

_____

_____

Describe one of your worst headaches. (Note child's description of the following: where headache occurred; severity; accompanying symptoms; who intervened; duration; probable cause.)

_____

_____

Do you usually have any warning that you are going to get a headache?

        Yes _____   No _____   Sometimes _____

Verbatim response:_____

_____

When you have a headache, what else is happening to your body? (Note: After child answers, specifically ask about nausea, dizziness, weakness, aura.)

_____

_____

Where is your pain located? Tell me and then show me on these drawings. (Note: Verify by asking child to show on his/her head.)

_____

_____

Does your pain spread?   Yes _____   No_____   Where _____

What words describe your pain? _____

    (Prompt, after response:)

    Sharp _____   Aching _____   Stinging _____   Hammering _____   Dull _____

    Throbbing _____   Burning _____   Pounding _____   Cutting _____

When you have a headache, is your pain

    steady (the same)?   usually   always   sometimes   never

    up and down?   usually,   always   sometimes   never

    increasing (getting bigger)?   usually   always   sometimes   never

When you have a headache, is there a time in the day or night when it hurts worse?
(Inquire, after response, about waking up, morning, afternoon, bedtime, and meals.)

_____

_____

_____

FORM 16.2. (*Continued*)

Generally discuss natural temporal variations in frequency or intensity with child (weekdays vs. weekends, sports, school, TV).

_____

_____

_____

How much does your head ache? How strong is your pain usually? What words can you use to describe how much your head

hurts? _____

_____

_____

Now mark the line to show how strong that is.

I ——————————————————————————————————— I

How sad or depressed do you feel because of your pain?

I ——————————————————————————————————— I

Why does it make you sad? _____

Why do you think you have headaches? _____

What do your parents think causes them? _____

What do your friends think causes them? _____

How strong is your pain when it hurts the least? _____

Now mark the line to show how strong that is.

I ——————————————————————————————————— I

Which face on the face sheet looks the way you feel down inside when your pain hurts the most?

(Face sheet color: _____)

How unpleasant is your pain when it hurts the most?

I ——————————————————————————————————— I

What do you do to reduce the pain when you have a headache?

Method	Efficacy
At school _____	_____
_____	_____
_____	_____
At home _____	_____
_____	_____
_____	_____

Which works best? _____

(Prompt after response, to verify reliance on medication, sleep/rest, withdrawal from mental or physical activity.)

How well does it work? _____

_____

_____

_____

Excerpted from P. A. McGrath (1990), *Pain in Children: Nature, Assessment, and Treatment.*

information related to pain localization, pain intensity, and self-directed methods of controlling or decreasing pain. Such information is critical to developing effective pain management. For example, localized pain is typically associated with concurrent physical problems and may reflect a change in the child's medical status. Pain that is not localized is typically symptomatic of affective problems, including anxiety and depression.

Direct observation of child behavior under a variety of conditions is necessary in the process of ruling in or ruling out initial hypotheses about the referral problem. The application of common observational techniques to chronic illness is described briefly in this section. Functional assessment utilizes interviews and direct observations with the Antecedent-Behavior-Consequence (A-B-C) model to assess the function of the occurrence of a problem behavior through interactions within the environmental context (Sulzer-Azaroff & Mayer, 1991).

Problem identification is a complex process that involves the refinement of broad or general variables into quantifiable, objective units for further analysis. Hypothesis formulation through literature and record reviews; and a descriptive functional analysis through structured interviews, rating scale, and self-report completion, and direct observation of the child, should provide clarity as to the problem to be addressed and its positive, adaptive alternative. Understanding the relationship between the problem and the physical and psychosocial variables that are functionally related to the problem is developed through the problem analysis.

Problem Analysis

Problem behavior can serve many functions, typically involving attention, escape, sensory reinforcement, and tangible factors, and can appear in many forms, including externalizing behaviors (e.g., aggression, conduct problems, refusal behaviors) and internalizing problems (e.g., depression, anxiety, fear of invasive procedures) (Carr, 1994; Wallander & Thompson, 1995). Describing the form (topography) is necessary yet insufficient for developing effective interventions. It is crucial to determine the function of these problem behaviors so that they can be controlled, altered, or replaced

with more functionally appropriate or adaptive behaviors. To accomplish this, the description of the form or topography and the description of contextual factors related to the referral problem must be systematically investigated. Figure 2 provides a graphic chronology and description of the problem identification and analysis process. The context in which the behavior or behaviors of interest occur and the monitoring of related behaviors is critical. The actual analysis involves more specific variables (e.g., negative self-statements vs. low self-esteem; sleeping duration and recording of food intake vs. depression) under operationally defined contexts (e.g., bone marrow aspiration with mother present and supportive vs. medical visit). In problem analysis, the keystone behavior approach replaces a consideration of comorbidity so that the emphasis shifts from an interest in broad diagnostic variables in the beginning of the problem identification phase to a narrower analysis of the specific behaviors that are most problematic for the referred child and their relationship to other behaviors. That is, information related to a diagnosis of depression and anxiety disorder for a child with cancer is less important (or useful) than is information regarding child sleeping patterns improving along with decreases in reporting of specific fears associated with frequent bone marrow aspirations (BMA) are observed.

The problem analysis phase involves three steps that lead directly to the development of the intervention. These steps—hypothesis refinement, functional assessment, and experimental functional analysis—as well as hypothesis confirmation, are described below.

Hypothesis Refinement

Following the descriptive assessment stage, all collected data (interview, observational, and behavioral ratings/checklists) must be reviewed, graphed, scored, or coded. If the data confirm the initial hypothesis, the function of the behavior has been established via descriptive and correlational methods, and can be more stringently tested under a variety of conditions, which are systematically manipulated in a functional assessment. If the data are not consistent with the initial hypothesis, it will be necessary to refine or change the hypotheses about the function of the behavior based on the data collected.

Molar

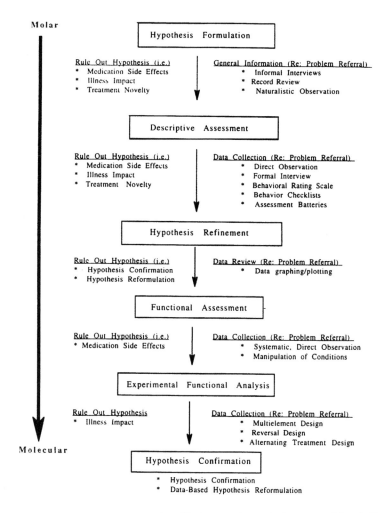

FIGURE 2. General problem identification, problem analysis process of chronic illness.

Functional Assessment and Experimental Functional Analysis

This level of assessment is largely represented by the single-case design methodology, which empirically examines the variables of interest on an individual level of analysis. The individual level analysis requires (a) the analysis of behavior–environment and behavior–behavior relationships with varying levels of experimental control to account for alternative explanations for behavior occurrence and (b) systematic measurement, typically observation of problem, alternative, and related (collateral) behaviors.

Single-Case Design Methodology

The use of single-case experimental design methodology for plan evaluation is described more completely in Chapter 2. However, in this section we provide a brief discussion regarding the application of these designs to assessment. Initially, baseline or pretreatment data are collected to assess the current functioning levels, and this process is followed by data collection both during and after a specific condition is implemented. Although several research designs exist, a reversal or withdrawal design or an alternating treatments design are typically utilized for functional assessment/experimental functional analysis purposes (Holmes et al., 1995; Sulzer-Azaroff, 1991). Although both designs effectively control against common threats to internal validity, the reversal design provides much stronger evidence for the identification of functional relationships between referral or problem behaviors and environmental events. In situations in which reversal designs are appropriate, an experimental functional analysis may be conducted whereby direct, causal information about the relationship between variables can be verified.

Some contextual variables, including medical and family variables, can safely be withdrawn to analyze the relationship with the referral and alternative behaviors. Examples of these include removing parental prompts to adolescents for diabetes management to evaluate the effect on metabolic control and removing tangible reinforcement for not crying and kicking during a BMA for a young child with ALL. In many other examples, however, the variables of interest cannot be withdrawn for either pragmatic or ethical reasons. Some medications may exacerbate behavioral problems, but cannot be withdrawn without adversely affecting the disease process. Another example involves the impractical removal of medications which require lengthy intake before physical affects can be observed, or that require some to be adequately removed from the body even after the child has stopped taking the medication. For certain forms of behaviors, such as internalizing behaviors, an experimental functional analysis of behavior is not practical because behaviors of interest involve withdrawal, avoidance, low appetite, and so on, which are less amenable than are high-frequency externalizing behaviors to an analysis under several changing conditions.

Alternating treatments (or alternating conditions) or multielement designs, however, provide a more practical, albeit less stringent, method for discovering behavior–environment relationships (Barlow & Hersen, 1985; Hains & Baer, 1989). When these designs are used without a withdrawal component, they can serve as a method for a functional assessment of the problem behavior. In this manner, behaviors of interest may be measured, typically over a longer period of time, for differential responding across conditions.

Although single-case methodology typically utilizes direct observation (see above sections or Chapter 2, this volume), self-recording and perma-

nent product analysis are often useful additions or substitutions for direct observation of behavior. Although this is true for most applications of behavioral analysis, it appears even more critical for accurate assessment with chronically ill children. For example, changes in blood glucose levels for a child with IDDM is a crucial measure of health. Obviously, monitoring glucose levels requires permanent product analysis (i.e., copy of lab report for results of blood analysis). Children's pain experiences can only be understood fully in the context of the individual child's perception of the intensity, frequency, and localization of the pain. For example, children with ALL preparing for bone marrow transplantation are confronted with frequent invasive procedures such as lumbar punctures and bone marrow aspirations. To fully assess their pain experiences before, during, and following the procedure, a self-monitoring method would need to be in place. In fact, when pain and a child's reaction to pain are the variables of interest, self-reporting mechanisms such as self-monitoring may be the most accurate measures available (McGrath, 1990).

Plan Implementation

The heterogeneity of the chronic illnesses in childhood makes it impossible to match particular treatments with particular disorders based on diagnostic information alone. We are therefore proposing a prescriptive model based on hypothesis-driven functional assessment data described in the preceding sections. Although a prescriptive model of treatment is, by definition, individualized, implementation of procedural steps should be done in a systematic, standardized fashion. Prescriptive procedural steps, such as target behavior selection, social validity assessment, and so on, are described in the following sections.

Selection of Target Behaviors, Alternative Behaviors, and Collateral Behaviors

The identification of appropriate targets for intervention is a relatively straightforward process following a hypothesis-driven functional assessment as described in the preceding section. The use of a keystone behavior approach may be new to many researchers and practitioners who are accustomed to targeting one problem behavior and one alternative behavior in a behavioral intervention. Although the procedures in the problem analysis step may still lead the clinician to treating two behaviors, it is much more likely that response relationships will be identified for intervention. For example, a traditional assessment may yield information relative to the antecedent cues and consequent events that maintain noncompliance with a four-year-old child with ALL who exhibits physical and verbal aggression with nurses during office visits. A behavioral intervention that stops there could miss other behaviors of concern, including aggression toward peers and adults in the preschool setting when novel activities are introduced.

When a keystone behavioral approach is used, more responses are analyzed, even if they do not appear to be similar to the referral behavior. The keystone behavioral approach could yield information relative to determining the relationship between the responses and could assist in developing one intervention to address multiple responses rather than implementing several interventions to aid in the reduction or increase of isolated behaviors. In the case example, the results of the keystone behavior-problem analysis is that the child's aggressive responding is maintained by social attention and avoidance of new, potentially painful, tasks and activities. In each setting, an adult (e.g., nurse, teacher) provides a one-to-one explanation of the day's schedule of activities, including who will be involved. Following the explanation, relaxation training and contingency management procedures are implemented to decrease the maladaptive responding of aggression and increase adaptive coping responses.

Beyond documenting the occurrence and severity of behaviors for intervention, it is important to identify more adaptive, alternative behaviors to replace the problematic behaviors. Alternative behaviors should be functional for the individual, that is, they should lead to meaningful social outcomes, be likely to be valued (or reinforced) in the natural environment following the intervention, and be important to the individual himself.

Social Validity Assessment

It is during the plan implementation phase that the social validity of the behaviors targeted for intervention are addressed. Social validity refers to the

process of asking the significant persons (e.g., parents, siblings, nurses, teachers) in the child's environment, as well as the individual child, to judge the importance of the behavior change to be targeted prior to the intervention and to assess their satisfaction with the results of the intervention (Hawkins, 1991). A measure of social validity may be obtained through semistructured interviews that focus on (a) social significance of the goals, (b) the social acceptability of the procedures, and (c) social importance of effects (Gresham & Lopez, 1996). Many authors discuss the importance of assessing social validity judgments following the implementation of the treatment (Wolf, 1978). Some authors (Gresham and Lopez, 1996), however, have argued that the true measure of social validity can be evaluated based not just on judgments, but rather, whether the intervention was implemented as prescribed and resulted in positive changes for child behavior.

We suggest that social validity assessments should be conducted throughout the assessment and intervention process. These assessments should include social validity judgments regarding the target behaviors to best ensure the promotion of functional, adaptive behaviors in the intervention. For example, a psychologist may recommend a self-management intervention for a preadolescent child with IDDM in an effort to enhance metabolic control. Suppose, however, the child experiences anxiety regarding self-management and states a desire for more parental support in disease management. Suppose also that teachers and parents report that the child demonstrates adequate self-management in other areas, such as academic performance. If increased child independence is not a generalized problem and anxiety and if parent–child conflict may be the antecedent for poor metabolic control, then increased parent involvement with enhanced supportive behaviors may be a more effective intervention. When assessment data as well as social validity data are considered, however, the intervention may be altered to reflect the values of the child and the family and better predict what will be reinforced in the natural community following the introduction of the intervention.

Selection of the Intervention

In most instances, the variety of successful intervention techniques that have been used with chronically ill populations have also been found to be successful with physically healthy children for a variety of psychosocial problems. As can be seen from Table 2, children with chronic illnesses often experience emotional or behavioral disorders that may be functionally related to the chronic illness. In addition, behavioral problems may be less related to the illness or to an emotional disorder than to the parental reaction to normative developmental behavior changes, as evidenced with preadolescent or adolescent children (Harris & Ferrari, 1989).

Common Psychosocial and Behavioral Treatment Targets in Chronic Illness

Despite the heterogeneity of chronic illnesses and their concomitant somatic, familial, and behavioral problems, some commonality across disorders exists in the identification of both treatments and targeted behaviors for intervention. In this section, we briefly review these common targets, which include (a) avoidance of aversive stimuli and (b) parent–child problems, for the two examples of IDDM and ALL.

Avoidance of Aversive Stimuli

During the acute phase of their medical treatments, children with ALL often experience painful invasive procedures. As previously described, bone marrow aspirations (BMA) and chemotherapy doses are two of the procedures that are most difficult for patients of all ages. It is not uncommon for a child to be referred for refusing to cooperate during these procedures, particularly with the BMA, or for a child to develop anticipatory vomiting up to one or two days before scheduled chemotherapy (Powers et al., 1995). Following an adequate problem analysis, environmental variables may be rearranged to decrease the avoidance behaviors and replace them with more adaptive coping strategies. With anticipatory vomiting, for example, relaxation training, visual imagery, and maternal distraction procedures have demonstrated the greatest efficacy for reducing incidences of vomiting and reported feelings of nausea and distress (Gonzales, Routh, & Armstrong, 1993; Shaw & Routh, 1993). Even with this information on treatment efficacy with anticipatory vomiting, data from the problem analysis phase must guide the selection of the intervention

because of the developmental and individual differences in response to treatment. While maternal distraction during aversive procedures is more effective than maternal reassurance with school-age children, the inverse is true for young children. Thus, treatments or conditions such as type of maternal responding might be used in the functional assessment phase to confirm an optimal match between child behavior and maternal responding. Once identified, the choice of the type of maternal responding to be implemented in an intervention plan is a relatively straightforward process.

In diabetes management, self-injections of insulin are often identified as aversive stimuli that the child or adolescent may seek to avoid. Again, this hypothesis is framed in a manner that can be tested and compared with other hypotheses, such as type of parental prompt for self-injection and presence or absence of peers during scheduled management times. As with ALL, successful treatment of avoidance behavior for children and adolescents with IDDM typically includes an approach that utilizes the differential reinforcement of incompatible (DRI) behavior by replacing the avoidant/maladaptive responding with more adaptive coping strategies. Such strategies include relaxation training, stress management training, and stress inoculation techniques (Johnson, 1995; Weist et al., 1993).

Parent–Child Problems

As previously discussed, the management of IDDM is a complex process that involves parents, children and health care providers. Family conflict surrounding the management issues is a common referral problem for pediatric, clinical, and school psychologists (Wallander & Thompson, 1995). In general, a family-based intervention is recommended for diabetes management that includes the following: (a) bolstering and maintaining parental monitoring of the child's regimen adherence and adjustment to diabetes through adolescence, (b) assisting parents and children in negotiating transfers in diabetes management, (c) assisting the child/ adolescent in accepting and feeling comfortable with the fact that competent adults (e.g., parents, nurses, physicians) (Weist et al., 1993) must make many decisions that affect their physical health.

Data regarding family functioning in general, and parent–child interactions specifically, should be obtained in the problem identification and problem analysis phases. Functional analyses of family problem behaviors have often been excluded from more traditional behavioral analysis approaches because of the assumed linear, rather than reciprocal, nature of the parent–child behaviors (Sanders & Dadds, 1993). Such information, however, is critical to individualizing and contextualizing behavioral family interventions to meet the specific needs of individual children and their families. Once critical interactional variables are identified, behavioral family interventions such as training parents in more positive interactional and child management skills or training parents as incidental teachers for more adaptive coping skills with their child are indicated (Sanders & Dadds, 1993; Wallander & Thompson, 1995).

Treatment Integrity

In a seminal article, Gresham (1989) discussed the importance of assessing treatment integrity in behavioral interventions. Treatment integrity is defined as the degree to which the intervention is implemented as intended. Factors related to treatment integrity in schools are (a) complexity of treatments, (b) time required to implement interventions, (c) materials and/or resources required, (d) number of treatment agents required, (e) perceived and actual effectiveness, and (f) motivation of treatment agents. All of these elements should be taken into account when choosing potential interventions.

Assessing the treatment integrity with which interventions are applied requires consideration of three technical issues: (a) specification of treatment components (i.e., define components in specific behavioral terms), (b) how much deviation from the intervention plan will still account for behavioral change, and (c) the reliable and valid measurement of treatment integrity. The first of these issues can be addressed by breaking down the intervention into a task analysis and defining each component in behavioral terms. The second technical issue has no concrete answer, but should be taken into consideration especially when the intervention is fairly complex. The reliability and validity of measurement will depend largely on how well the treatment components were operationally defined and on the approach used to evaluate treatment integrity.

The most commonly used measure of treatment integrity is direct observation (Gresham,

1989). Three steps are involved in using direct observation to evaluate treatment integrity: (a) the components of the intervention must be defined in operational terms, (b) both the occurrence and nonoccurrence of the treatment components must be recorded, and (c) the percentage of treatment components implemented must be calculated to assess the level of integrity. Gresham suggests that if the level of treatment integrity is calculated over time, it can be compared to the rate of behavior change over time to show a functional relationship between treatment integrity and treatment effectiveness. Indirect methods of assessing treatment integrity are rating scales, self-monitoring, self-report, and behavioral interviews. During the evaluation of treatment integrity, feedback to the consultee and additional training in the intervention components should be provided if necessary.

Planning for Generalization

Generalization has traditionally been defined as changes in untreated behaviors or occurrence of the treated behavior in nontraining situations (Stokes & Baer, 1977). Types of generalization include generalization across responses, settings, trainers or therapists, or materials. Generalization across time is typically referred to as maintenance. Behavioral interventions that exploit or incorporate naturally occurring stimuli and contingencies tend to demonstrate the best generalization outcomes (Scruggs & Mastropieri, 1994). In general, generalization in some form is desired as a result of a successful intervention. Even with hospital-based treatments, generalizations across stimuli (e.g., medical procedure, nurses, physicians) is desired.

Several generalization training strategies have been developed to assist clinicians with extending treatment effects across behaviors, time, settings, and situations. Some generalization training strategies may be more useful with chronically ill populations than with developmental or behavioral disorders and will be discussed briefly here. Stokes and Baer (1977) first delineated nine strategies to extend training effects over time and situations. These nine strategies fall into several categories, two of which are particularly useful with children with medical problems. The first category of generalization training strategies relies on the incorporation of naturally occurring antecedent and consequent events into the training, or treatment, session. By exploiting naturally occurring events and contingencies, interventionists program for generalization from the treatment to the generalization situations.

Even seemingly small events can increase the proximity between the treatment and the generalization situations. For instance, in a relaxation training intervention with a nine-year-old with ALL to reduce anticipatory vomiting prior to chemotherapy, the training session should be conducted in the same, or similar, setting, with the same materials and a similar chronology of events that precede and follow the chemotherapy and the child's target response. This child's response to the same materials may be too intense at the beginning of treatment to take place during the procedure, so toy needles and medical equipment may be used in the initial analogue treatment session. Treatment cannot end, however, until the child is able to demonstrate the adaptive responding (in place of the anticipatory vomiting) with the same materials that are used in chemotherapy. In addition, if a variety of nurses and technicians are responsible for administering the chemotherapy, then a variety of trainers should be used in the relaxation training so that child's adaptive responding is not hindered by limited exposure to the variety of antecedent cues present in the generalization situations. To program for generalization across situations, some relaxation training may need to occur in analogue conditions approximating aversive medical procedures, such as bone marrow aspirations and lumbar punctures.

Another category of generalization training strategies is mediated generalization. Mediated generalization refers to the practice of training children to regulate responding through various self-control procedures including self-monitoring, self-management, self-instructions, and visualization and relaxation training. Mediated generalization is particularly useful for the target behavior of pain management. Even very small children can be trained in these strategies for the purposes of cueing, or controlling, their own adaptive responding.

Mediated generalization and exploiting naturally occurring antecedent and consequent events are not mutually exclusive strategies and may need to be employed concurrently, or in a sequential fashion, for optimal effects. For many children, generalization training that exploits natural contingencies may need to come before the introduction of media-

tional strategies. Unlike developmentally or behaviorally disordered children, however, a great many children with chronic illness may require only mediational training to reduce maladaptive responding and increase coping skills. Progress monitoring throughout training and across situations will determine the efficacy of either or both of these generalization training strategies with a particular child.

Plan Evaluation

In the evaluation of ongoing interventions, one must address two empirical questions involving (a) the outcome of the intervention and (b) whether the intervention was responsible for the change in behavior. Outcome data are usually obtained through direct observation of behavior, as well as by examining recording forms kept by parents, teachers, and child and by evaluating permanent products where possible. Assessing the outcome of the intervention is relatively straightforward and is usually done by continuously tracking the target behavior during intervention and comparing it with pretreatment data. If positive changes have occurred in the target behavior, then the program must be faded so that the behavior is controlled by environmental variables that are less intrusive or "foreign" In other words, it is desirable that the target behavior be maintained by naturally occurring variables in the environment. Stimulus control procedures are most conducive to achieving this goal in that naturally occurring stimuli can be programmed to evoke the target behavior.

If one were only concerned with assessing outcome, a simple A-B design would be sufficient. However, answering the second question requires a more elaborate design (see Chapter 2, this volume). The difficulty in establishing functional relationships between changes in target behaviors and specific treatment components in cases of chronic illness is that reversals or withdrawals of treatment conditions, for example, may have life-threatening or serious health implications. Figure 3 illustrates the complex, dynamic relationship between the assessment, treatment, and evaluation process. Thus, a behavioral clinician must work closely with medical professionals to insure that the welfare of the individual is never compromised when using more complicated single-subject designs to demonstrate functional relationships.

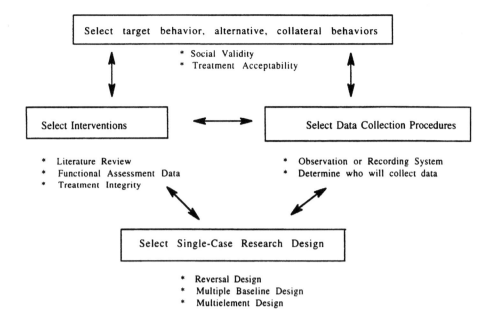

FIGURE 3. General plan evaluation procedures.

Summary and Directions for Future Research

Assessment and treatment with children who experience chronic illnesses are complex enterprises. In this chapter, we have attempted to delineate an empirically based approach to both assessment and treatment with these populations. Several important factors should be evident from this chapter. First, working with children with chronic illness and their families requires an adequate knowledge of the particular disease process, prognosis, and medical treatment protocol. The sheer variety of diseases makes it impossible for general clinicians and researchers to have this requisite knowledge, so a review of the recent medical and psychological literature is a critical first step. Second, successful treatment for children with chronic illness and their families depends on an adequate assessment of the child, the family, the disease, and the contextual factors that relate to the behaviors of concern, and testing the subsequent hypotheses in a systematic manner. The final intervention selected may have very little to do with the specific disease process and more to do with school functioning. The intervention has a greater chance of being effective if it is selected based on a hypothesis-testing approach which looks at multiple responding in a contextualized, socially valid manner. That is, although disease process information is necessary in an assessment with a chronically ill child, in the final analysis disease-specific (or medical treatment-specific) hypotheses may be ruled out in the earlier steps in the problem identification and analysis. Finally, chronic illnesses and their concomitant medical treatments can alter substantially in a short amount of time. Such quick and often drastic changes can impact the child, the family, and health professionals in various ways. Monitoring intervention effects and treatment integrity are the only methods to adequately understand and promote positive child and family outcomes.

References

Allen, D.A., Tenner, H., McGrade, B.J., Affleck, G., & Ratzan, S. (1983). Parent and child perceptions of the management of diabetes. *Journal of Pediatric Psychology, 8,* 129–141.

Anderson, B., Auslander, W., Jung, K., Miller, P., & Santiago, J. (1990). Assessing family sharing of diabetes responsibility. *Journal of Pediatric Psychology, 15,* 477–492.

Armstrong, F.D., & Holmes, M. (1995). Educational issues in childhood cancer. *School Psychology Quarterly, 10,* 292–304.

Barlow, D.H., & Hersen, M. (1985). *Single-case experimental designs: Strategies for studying behavior change* (2nd ed.). New York: Pergamon.

Carr, E.G. (1994). Emerging themes in the functional analysis of problem behavior. *Journal of Applied Behavior Analysis, 27,* 393–400.

Creer, T.L., Harm, D.L., & Marion, R.J. (1988). Childhood asthma. In D.K. Routh (Ed.), *Handbook of pediatric psychology* (pp. 162–189). New York: Guilford.

Dahlquist, L.M., Czyzewski, D.I., Copeland, K.G., Jones, C.L., Taub, E., & Vaughan, J.K. (1993). Parents of children newly diagnosed with cancer: Anxiety, coping and marital distress. *Journal of Pediatric Psychology, 18,* 365–376.

Drotar, D. (1993). Psychological perspectives in chronic childhood illness. In M.C. Roberts, G.P. Koocher, D.K. Routh, & D.J. Willis (Eds.), *Readings in pediatric psychology* (pp. 95–114). New York: Plenum.

Gonzalez, J.C., Routh, D.K., & Armstrong, F.D. (1993). Effects of maternal distraction versus reassurance on children's reactions to injections. *Journal of Pediatric Psychology, 18,* 593–604.

Granowetter, L. (1994). Pediatric oncology: A medical overview. In D.J. Bearison, & R.K. Mulhern (Eds.), *Pediatric psychoncology: Psychological perspectives on kids with cancer* (pp. 9–34). New York: Oxford.

Gresham, F.M. (1989). Assessment of treatment integrity in school consultation and prereferral intervention. *School Psychology Review, 18,* 37–50.

Gresham, F.M. (1991). What ever happened to the functional analysis in behavioral consultation. *Journal of Educational and Psychological Consultation, 2,* 387–392.

Gresham, F.M., & Lopez, M.F. (1996). Social validation: A unifying concept for school-based consultation research and practice. *School Psychology Quarterly, 11,* 273–284.

Hains, A.H., & Baer, D.M. (1989). Interaction effects in multielement designs: Inevitable, desirable, and ignorable. *Journal of Applied Behavior Analysis, 22,* 57–69.

Harris, S.L., & Ferrari, M. (1989). Developmental factors in child behavior therapy. In J.C. Witt, S.N. Elliott, & F.M. Gresham (Eds.), *Handbook of behavior therapy in education* (pp. 151–170). New York: Plenum.

Hawkins, R.P. (1991). Is social validity what we are interested in? Arguments for a functional approach. Special issue: Social validity: Multiple perspectives. *Journal of Applied Behavior Analysis, 24,* 205–212.

Hayes, S.C., Nelson, R.O., & Jarrett, R.B. (1987). Treatment utility of assessment: A functional approach to assessing quality. *American Psychologist, 42,* 963–974.

Holmes, C. (1990). Neuropsychological sequelae of acute and chronic blood glucose disruption in adults with insulin-dependent diabetes. In C. Holmes (Ed.), *Neuropsychological and behavior aspects of diabetes* (pp. 123–154). New York: Springer-Verlag.

Holmes, C.S., O'Brien, B., & Greer, T. (1995). Cognitive functioning and academic achievement in children with Insulin-Dependent Diabetes Mellitus (IDDM). *School Psychology Quarterly, 10,* 329–344.

Johnson, S.B. (1984). Knowledge, attitudes, and behavior: Correlates of health with childhood diabetes. *Clinical Psychology Review, 4,* 503–524.

Johnson, S.B. (1988). Diabetes mellitus in childhood. In D.K. Routh (Ed.), *Handbook of pediatric psychology* (pp. 9–31). New York: Guilford.

Johnson, S.B. (1995). Insulin-dependent diabetes mellitus in childhood. In M.C. Roberts (Ed.), *Handbook of pediatric psychology* (2nd ed., pp.263–285). New York: Guilford.

LaGreca, A.M., & Varni, J.W. (1993). Interventions in pediatric psychology: A look toward the future. *Journal of Pediatric Psychology, 18,* 667–680.

Martens, B.K., & Witt, J.C. (1988). On the ecological validity of behavior modification. In J.C. Witt, S.N. Elliot, & F.M. Gresham (Eds.), *Handbook of behavior therapy in education* (pp. 325–342). New York: Plenum.

McGrath, P.A. (1990). *Pain in children: Nature, assessment, and treatment.* New York: Guilford Press.

Moore, B.D., Copeland, D.R., Reid, H., & Levy, B. (1992). Neuropsychological basis of cognitive deficits in long-term survivors of childhood cancer. *Archives of Neurology, 49,* 809–817.

National Cancer Institute (1988). *Childhood cancer.* Bethesda, MD: National Institute of Health.

Nelson, R.O., & Hayes, S.C. (1986). The nature of behavioral assessment. In R.O. Nelson & S.C. Hayes (Eds.), *Conceptual foundations of behavioral assessment* (pp. 3–41). New York: Guilford.

Noll, R.B., Bukowski, W.M., Davies, W.H., Koontz, K. & Kulkarni, R. (1993). Adjustment in the peer system of adolescents with cancer: A two year study. *Journal of Pediatric Psychology, 18,* 351–364.

O'Neill, R.E., Horner, R.H., Albin, R.W., Sprague, J.R., Storey, K., & Newton, J.S. (1997). *Functional assessment and program development for problem behavior: A practical handbook,* (2nd ed.). Pacific Grove, CA: Brooks/Cole.

Powers, S.W., Vannatta, K., Noll, R.B., Cool, V.A., & Stehbens, J.A. (1995). Leukemia and other childhood cancers. In M.C. Roberts (Ed.), *Handbook of pediatric psychology* (2nd ed., pp. 310–326). New York: Guilford.

Reimers, T.M. (1985). Behavioral Attribution Measure (BAM). Unpublished scale.

Reimers, T.M., & Wacker, D.P. (1988). Parents' ratings of acceptability of behavioral treatment recommendations made in an outpatient clinic: A preliminary analysis of treatment effectiveness. *Behavioral Disorders, 14,* 7–15.

Reimers, T.M., Wacker, D.P., Derby, M., & Cooper, L. (1995). Relations between parent attributions and acceptability of behavioral treatment for their child's behavior problems. *Behavior Disorders, 20,* 171–178.

Roberts, M.C., & Wallander, J. (1992). *Family issues in pediatric psychology.* Hillsdale, NJ: Lawrence Erlbaum.

Sanders, M.R., & Dadds, M.R. (1993). *Behavioral family intervention.* Boston: Allyn & Bacon.

Scruggs, T.E., & Mastropieri, M.A. (1994). The effectiveness of generalization training: A quantitative synthesis of single-subject research. In T.E. Scruggs, & M.A. Mastropieri (Eds.), *Advances in learning and behavioral disabilities, Volume 8,* (pp. 259–280). Greenwich, CT: JAI Press.

Sexson, S., & Swain, A.M. (1995). The chronically ill child in the school. *School Psychology Quarterly, 10,* 359–368.

Shaw, E. G., & Routh, D.K. (1993). Effect of mother presence on children's reaction to aversive procedures. In M.C. Roberts, G.P. Koocher, D.K. Routh, & D.J. Willis (Eds.), *Readings in pediatric psychology* (pp. 237–246). New York: Plenum.

Spirito, A., Stark, L.J., Cobiella, C., Dugan, R., Andiokites, T., & Hewett, R. (1990). Social adjustment of children successfully treated for cancer. *Journal of Pediatric Psychology, 15,* 359–371.

Stehbens, J.A. (1988). Childhood cancer. In D.K. Routh (Ed.), *Handbook of pediatric psychology* (pp. 135–161). New York: Guilford.

Stokes, T.F., & Baer, D.M. (1977). An implicit technology of generalization. *Journal of Applied Behavior Analysis, 10,* 349–367.

Sulzer-Azaroff, B., & Mayer, G.R. (1991). *Behavior analysis for lasting change.* Fort Worth, TX: Holt, Rinehart, and Winston.

Varni, J.W., & Wallander, J.L. (1988). Pediatric chronic disabilities: Hemophilia and spina bifida as examples. In D.K. Routh (Ed.), *Handbook of pediatric psychology* (pp. 190–221). New York: Guilford.

Wallander, J.L., & Thompson, R.J. (1995). Psychosocial adjustment of children with chronic physical conditions. In M.C. Roberts (Ed.), *Handbook of pediatric psychology* (2nd ed., pp.124–143). New York: Guilford.

Weist, M.D., Ollendick, T.H., & Finney, J.W. (1991). Toward the empirical validation of treatment targets in children. *Clinical Psychology Review, 11,* 515–538.

Weist, M.D., Finney, J.W., Barrinard, M.U., Davis, C., & Ollendick, T.H. (1993). Empirical selection of psychosocial treatment targets for children and adolescents with diabetes. *Journal of Pediatric Psychology, 18,* 11–28.

Wolf, M.M. (1978). Social validity: The case for subjective measurement, *or* how applied behavioral analysis is finding its heart. *Journal of Applied Behavior Analysis, 11,* 203–214.

Bibliography

Roberts, M.C. (Ed.). (1995). *Handbook of pediatric psychology* (2nd ed.). New York: Guilford.

Roberts, M.C., Goocher, G.P., Routh, D.K., & Willis, D.J. (Eds.). (1993). *Readings in pediatric psychology.* New York: Plenum.

Routh, D.K. (Ed.). (1988). *Handbook of pediatric psychology.* New York: Guilford.

17

Cognitive Behavior Therapy for Eating Disorders

DONALD A. WILLIAMSON, LESLIE G. WOMBLE, AND NANCY L. ZUCKER

Introduction

Definition

The criteria for a diagnosis of anorexia nervosa are summarized in Table 1. It is generally believed that fear of weight gain and body image disturbances are central features of anorexia nervosa that motivate extreme weight control methods such as fasting or purging (Williamson, 1990). The *Diagnostic and Statistical Manual for Mental Disorders,* 4th ed. (*DSM-IV;* American Psychiatric Association, 1994) designates two subtypes of anorexia nervosa. The restricting subtype describes anorexic patients who lose weight by restrictive eating and do not binge eat or purge. The binge eating/purging subtype describes anorexic patients who binge eat and/or purge. The *DSM-IV* criteria for a diagnosis of bulimia nervosa are summarized in Table 2. A central feature of bulimia nervosa is binge eating in which the individual uncontrollably eats a large amount of food in a short period of time. Compensatory behaviors such as self-induced vomiting, laxative and/or diuretic abuse, compulsive exercising, or fasting are presumed to be motivated by fear of weight gain and body image disturbances (Williamson, 1990). Two subtypes of bulimia ner-

vosa are designated in *DSM-IV.* The purging subtype describes persons who binge eat, but use self-induced vomiting, laxative abuse, or diuretic abuse to prevent weight gain. The nonpurging subtype describes persons who binge eat, but use other forms of compensatory behavior such as dieting or excessive exercise to prevent weight gain. It is our experience that these patients are usually 10 to 15 pounds overweight. In addition to anorexia nervosa and bulimia nervosa, *DSM-IV* designates a subclinical eating disorder category, eating disorder not otherwise specified (American Psychiatric Association, 1994). Examples of this diagnosis include subthreshold anorexics who are not emaciated and obese binge eaters who binge eat but do not use vomiting or exercise to prevent weight gain (Williamson, Gleaves, & Savin, 1992).

Prevalence

The prevalence of anorexia nervosa and bulimia nervosa in the general population is estimated to be approximately 1% for the former and 1% to 3% for the latter. These prevalence ratings do not take into account the disordered eating that encompasses the subclinical forms of eating disorders (Wilson & Eldredge, 1992). This consideration is important, given that 40% to 50% of patients referred for treatment in our program are diagnosed with eating disorder not otherwise specified (Williamson, Sebastian, & Varnado, 1995).

DONALD A. WILLIAMSON, LESLIE G. WOMBLE, AND **NANCY L. ZUCKER** • Department of Psychology, Louisiana State University, Baton Rouge, Louisiana 70803-3103.

Handbook of Child Behavior Therapy, edited by Watson and Gresham. Plenum Press, New York, 1998.

TABLE 1. Summary of *DSM-IV* Diagnostic Criteria for Anorexia Nervosa

A. Refusal to maintain minimal normal body weight

B. Intense fear of gaining weight or becoming fat

C. Body image distortion

D. Amenorrhea, for at least three consecutive menstrual cycles.
   Restricting type: The person does not regularly engage in binge eating behavior.
   Binge eating/Purging type: The person regularly engages in binge eating or purging behavior.

TABLE 2. Summary of *DSM-IV* Diagnostic Criteria for Bulimia Nervosa

A. Recurrent binge eating, characterized by both of the following:
   (1) Eating an amount of food that is larger than what most people would eat.
   (2) A sense of lack of control over eating during the binge episode.

B. Inappropriate compensatory behavior to prevent weight gain, such as vomiting, misuse of laxatives or diuretics, fasting, or excessive exercise.

C. Binge eating and compensatory behavior both occur at least twice a week for three months.

D. Body image distortion.

E. Disturbance does not occur during episodes of Anorexia Nervosa.
   Purging type: The person engages in vomiting or the misuse of laxatives or diuretics.
   Nonpurging type: The person uses other compensatory behaviors, such as fasting or excessive exercise.

Specific Features

Greater than 90% of individuals meeting full criteria for anorexia nervosa and bulimia nervosa are female (American Psychiatric Association, 1994). Unlike the male to female ratio that changes as age increases, research shows that the social class distribution remains stable across ages (Lask & Bryant-Waugh, 1992). Eating disorders are most prevalent among Caucasian girls from middle to upper socioeconomic status families. Anorexia nervosa and bulimia nervosa seem to occur primarily in industrialized cultures in which food is readily available, and the social pressure to be thin is greater (American Psychiatric Association, 1994).

Comorbidity

Other forms of psychopathology have been found to commonly coexist with eating disorders. In particular, depression is comorbid with eating disorders (Hinz & Williamson, 1987). Researchers have identified depression as a potential risk factor leading to the development of eating disorders. For example, in a study of girls in grades 9 through 12, depression was found to be a significant predictor of eating disturbance (Gross & Rosen, 1988). Research has also found anorexia nervosa and bulimia nervosa to be associated with a secondary diagnosis of obsessive–compulsive disorder (Bulik, Beidel, Duchmann, Weltzin, & Kaye, 1991; Kasvikis, Tsakiris, Marks, Basoglu, & Noshirvani, 1986). Anxiety disorders such as panic disorder, simple phobia, and social phobia are also sometimes comorbid with bulimia nervosa (Williamson, Barker, & Norris, 1993). Eating disorders are also frequently associated with the presence of personality disorders. Research studies have found that anorexia nervosa is associated with cluster C personality disorders (avoidant, dependent, compulsive, and passive–aggressive personality disorders). Bulimia nervosa is most commonly associated with cluster B personality disorders, that is, borderline, histrionic, narcissistic, and antisocial personality disorders (Johnson & Wonderlich, 1992).

Differential Diagnosis

Although eating disorders co-occur with a number of other psychiatric disorders, some of the primary symptoms of eating disorders may be present because of problems distinctly different from disordered eating. When assessing for the presence of an eating disorder, it is important to recognize the characteristics that differentiate other psychiatric disorders from eating disorders. For example, weight loss is a common symptom of major depression. In such cases, the individual is not concerned with fear of weight gain as would be the case for anorexia nervosa. Similarly, overeating may occur in major depression and dysthymic disorder as it does in bulimia nervosa. The depressed individual does not generally report a distorted body image nor does the depressed individual typically engage in compensatory behaviors to prevent weight gain. Therefore, the absence of fears related to weight gain and body image disturbances generally favor a diagnosis of depression. Symptoms of anxiety disorders may also resemble eating disordered behavior. For example, an individual may present with a fear of eating in public, which is a characteristic of anorexia nervosa. This avoidant behavior may be more indicative of social phobia than of anorexia if the individual fears being embarrassed in public, e.g., by choking on food. Anorexic patients often obsess about food and may engage in ritualistic behavior, such as counting bites, while eating or preparing food. This behavior would be designated as obsessive–compulsive if the individual exhibits other obsessions that are unrelated to food and does not engage in other behaviors indicative of anorexia nervosa (American Psychiatric Association, 1994).

Prognosis if Treated/Untreated

Very little is known about the prognosis of eating disorders if untreated. Clinical researchers have implied that if eating disorders are not treated, the condition of the disorder worsens. However, little research to date has tested this hypothesis. In a cross-sectional retrospective study, Witcher and Williamson (1992) found that the increased severity of bulimia nervosa at referral for treatment was associated with younger age of onset and longer duration of an eating disorder. Also, Williamson and colleagues (1987) found that higher frequency of purging was related to worsened symptoms of depression, anxiety, interpersonal sensitivity, and impulsivity. Treatment studies for bulimia nervosa have often measured changes in general psychiatric symptoms, for example, depression or anxiety.

These studies have generally reported that improvement of eating disorder symptoms is associated with improved general psychological functioning (Williamson, Netemeyer, et al., 1995). Williamson, Prather, and colleagues (1989) reported that greater psychiatric disturbance at admission to treatment was associated with a poor prognosis. These pieces of circumstantial evidence suggest that there may be some validity to the notion that eating disorders worsen over time and become more resistant to treatment.

Problem Identification

Individuals with eating disorders exhibit behaviors such as binge eating, purging, dieting, exercise, and body dissatisfaction that serve as markers of their disturbed eating patterns. Further, several risk factors that lead to the development of eating disorders have been identified. These risk factors include depression (Gross & Rosen, 1988), teasing about body weight and appearance (Richards, Thompson, & Coovert, 1990), and societal emphasis on thinness (Polivy & Herman, 1995). Each individual exhibiting symptoms of an eating disorder is unique. Therefore, it is important to take an idiographic approach to assessment. Research has identified body dysphoria (or dissatisfaction) as one of the strongest and most consistent risk factors associated with eating disordered symptoms (Attie & Brooks-Gunn, 1989; Stice, Schupak-Neuberg, Shaw, & Stein, 1994). A combination of any of the behaviors can be identified to illustrate the presence of an eating disorder. The process by which this integration occurs is described in more detail in the problem analysis section.

Comprehensive multitrait multimethod assessment instruments and techniques that identify the presence of risk factors leading to the development of eating disorders and the presence of eating disordered behaviors, are most helpful in making an appropriate diagnosis that will ultimately lead to the formation of an effective treatment plan. Among other things, the assessment should include a diagnostic interview, self-report inventories, self-monitoring of eating and purging behavior, behavioral observations, and body composition assessment. Table 3 presents assessment inventories for eating disorder symptoms and the behavioral characteristics that they measure.

TABLE 3. Summary of Assessment Procedures for Eating Disorders

Instrument/reference	Binge eating	Purging	Dieting	Body dissatisfaction	Fear of fat/social pressure	Self-esteem	Depression	Personality
EAT (Garner & Garfinkel, 1979) & ChEAT (Maloney et al., 1989)		X	X					
BULIT-R (Thelen et al., 1991)	X	X						
EDI-2 (Garner, 1991)	X	X		X				X
BSQ (Cooper et al., 1987)				X				
Golfarb Fear of Fat Scale (Golfarb et al., 1985)					X			
Piers-Harris Self Concept Scale (Piers & Harris, 1969)						X		
POTS (Thompson & Cattarin, 1992)					X			
BDI (Beck et al., 1961) CDI (Kovacs & Beck, 1977)							X	
SPPA (Harter, 1988) or SPPC (Harter, 1985)						X		
EDE (Cooper & Fairburn, 1987)	X	X	X	X				
IDED-IV (Williamson et al., 1996)	X	X	X	X				
SCID-II (Spitzer et al., 1987)							X	X
MMPI (Hathaway & McKinley, 1951) MMPI-2 (Harhaway et al., 1989)							X	X

Note: Abbreviations stand for the following—EAT (Eating Attitudes Test); ChEAT (Children's Eating Attitude Test); BULIT-R (Bulimia Test Revised); EDI-2 (Eating Disorders Inventory–2); BSQ (Body Shape Questionnaire); POTS (Perception of Teasing Scale); BDI (Beck Depression Inventory); CDI (Children's Depression Invenory); SPPA (Self Perception Profile for Adolescents); SPPC (Self Perception Profile for Children); EDE (Eating Disorders Examination); IDED-IV (Interview for the Diagnosis of Eating Disorders–IV); SCID-II (Structured Clinical Interview for *DSM-III-R* Personality Disorders); MMPI (Minnesota Multiphasic Personality Inventory)

Due to the fact that individuals with eating disorders often deny that they have a problem, self-report inventories may not be valid. Semistructured interviews that identify the presence of the behaviors necessary for the diagnosis of eating disorders can be very helpful in problem identification. For example, the Eating Disorder Examination (EDE; Z. Cooper & Fairburn, 1987) is a semistructured interview that assesses for the symptoms of anorexia nervosa and bulimia nervosa. The EDE consists of four subscales: Restraint, Eating Concern, Shape Concern, and Weight Concern. Internal consistency of subscales was found to be adequate to high with coefficient alpha ranging from .67 to .90 (Z. Cooper, Cooper, & Fairburn, 1989). Evidence for concurrent and discriminant validity has been established for symptom severity (Fairburn & Cooper, 1993). To date, however, the validity of the EDE as a diagnostic tool corresponding to the *DSM-IV* has not been reported.

The Interview for the Diagnosis of Eating Disorders–IV (IDED–IV; Williamson, Anderson, & Gleaves, 1996) is a semistructured interview designed to identify pathological eating behaviors and to diagnose anorexia nervosa, bulimia nervosa, and eating disorders not otherwise specified using *DSM-IV* criteria. During the interview process, a detailed history regarding weight fluctuations, major life events, and specific foods eaten is obtained. High levels of internal consistency and interrater reliability for diagnosis has been found using the IDED–IV. Convergent and discriminant validity of the IDED–IV have also been established. Other techniques that can be used in conjunction with the self-report inventories and clinical interviews are described below.

Pathological Eating

Pathological eating behaviors such as binge eating, purging, and/or excessive dieting must be evaluated in order to establish a sound treatment plan. In order to assess these behaviors, it is often helpful to instruct the individual to self-monitor eating habits. Self-monitoring procedures typically involve documenting the kind and amount of food eaten, whether the individual subjectively interprets the consumption as a binge, the events and mood that preceded eating, any purgative behavior, and subsequent mood following the use of compensatory mechanisms (Williamson, 1990). Data from self-monitoring forms can be used to evaluate baseline levels of behavior and can be used to evaluate treatment outcome. Further, examination of the relationships among environmental events, feelings, and maladaptive eating behaviors can lead to a well-conceptualized case formulation for each individual patient (Williamson, 1990; Williamson, Barker, et al., 1993; Williamson, Davis, & Duchmann, 1992). Like self-report measures, the self-monitoring of an individual who denies an eating problem may be inaccurate and filled with omissions of data entry. Anorexic patients may maximize what they have eaten. Bulimics may underreport the actual frequency of binges and purges since acknowledgment of such pathological eating behavior may be quite embarrassing. The use of behavioral observations and collateral reports from friends and family members may be very helpful in obtaining a reliable assessment of pathological eating. For example, a binge eater may often consume food at a faster pace than others and in amounts that exceed what one would think of as normal. Family members may observe this eating pattern directly. However, bulimic patients often engage in binge eating only when they are alone. In such cases, family members and friends may notice large quantities of missing food. If the individual does not purge following a binge, rapid weight gain usually occurs. If, however, the individual purges, the presence of bulimia may be harder to detect, because most purging bulimics are at normal weight level. Behavioral observations include: frequent visits to a bathroom following meals; teeth marks above the knuckles (which is caused by abrasions from sticking a finger down the throat); and swollen salivary glands. Individuals may also engage in other compensatory behaviors to prevent weight gain, for example, excessive exercise. In school, the individual may participate on athletic teams as a socially acceptable way to work off calories and thus avoid detection (Bryant-Waugh & Lask, 1995).

Extreme dieting can be observed by refusal to eat and weight loss below a normal weight level. Individuals may choose to eat alone or secretly try to get rid of food that is given to them. Further, those who engage in starvation may exhibit secondary effects such as poor concentration, irritability, mood swings, and impulsivity (Garner, 1995). One of the best ways to assess food avoidance is to watch the individual eat a "test meal." Observations indicative of an eating disorder are the following: eating at an excessively slow pace or alternatively at an excessively fast pace, pushing food around without eating, refusal to eat high fat "forbidden foods," cutting food up into small bites, chewing excessively on food, and making excuses to get out of eating meals.

In addition to self-report inventories, behavioral observations, and the clinical interviews, a physical examination may reveal the presence of pathological eating. Starvation, excessive vomiting, and abuse of laxatives affect a number of organ systems. For example, dehydration may be apparent, hormone levels may be low, electrolyte imbalances may be found, or resting metabolic rate may be reduced (Bennett, Williamson, & Powers, 1989; Devlin et al., 1990; Platte et al., 1994). The physical exam should also include evaluation of body composition in order to estimate total body fat. Measurement of body composition is very helpful in the identification of an eating disorder, particularly anorexia, because low body fat can serve as an objective measure of emaciation. Several techniques such as dual x-ray absorbitometry, underwater weighing, bioelectric impedance, and skinfold assessment can be used to assess body composition. However, because of cost, most of these techniques, with the exception of skinfold assessment, are impractical for most clinicians who are not associated with a research facility (Williamson, Barker et al., 1993). Norms for age and sex are available for skinfold measures (Durnin & Womersley, 1974). Body Mass Index (BMI) is another valid, economical way to assess body fatness. An individual's height in meters and weight in kilograms is used to calculate BMI by using the formula $BMI = weight(kg)/height(m)^2$. The BMI has been validated as an index of adiposity (Garrow, 1983).

Body Dysphoria

Body dysphoria has been defined as extreme dissatisfaction with body size/shape in persons who are normal weight or underweight (Williamson, Barker, Bertman, & Gleaves, 1995). Body dysphoria is both a symptom of eating disorders and a risk factor associated with the development of eating disorders (Attie & Brooks-Gunn, 1992; Bunnell, Cooper, Hertz, & Shinker, 1992; Gross & Rosen, 1988; Williamson, Netemeyer, et al., 1995). Along with self-report inventories, behavioral observations of friends or family members contribute to the assessment of body dysphoria. For example, the individual may often wear baggy clothes, may engage in frequent checking in front of the mirror, or may repeatedly state that or ask if she is fat. Reports of these habits by family members are supportive of the presence of body dysphoria and overconcern with body size/shape.

In the clinic, one can administer the Body Image Assessment Procedure (BIA), which uses nine silhouettes of female body sizes ranging from thin to obese. The individual is asked to select the silhouette that best represents what she looks like (current body size) and then is asked to select the silhouette that best represents what she would like to look like (ideal body size). The discrepancy between current body size (CBS) and ideal body size (IBS) has been shown to be a valid measure of body size dissatisfaction (Gleaves, Williamson, Eberenz, Sebastian, & Barker, 1995; Williamson, Gleaves, Watkins, & Schlundt, 1993). The Body Image Assessment Procedure for Children (BIA–C) is a modification of the BIA procedure developed by Williamson, Davis, Bennett, Goreczny, and Gleaves (1989). This procedure involves four sets of body image cards that correspond to male and female children and preadolescents. Satisfactory reliability coefficients were found for the BIA–C and concurrent validity has been established (Vernon-Guidry & Williamson, 1996).

Affective and Personality Problems

Some individuals with pathological eating behaviors may have additional psychiatric problems which must be evaluated and treated in a comprehensive individualized treatment plan (Williamson, 1990). For example, the individual could be depressed, deficient in social support, or have low self-esteem. Behavioral observations can be used in conjunction with the self-report measures described in Table 3 to evaluate these problem areas. For example, if the individual is depressed, she may experience a decreased interest in activities that she enjoys, concentration problems, restlessness or fidgetiness, frequent fatigue, or a lack of energy. In addition, the individual may tend to isolate herself from others and this may ultimately lead to a lack of social support. Those who are overweight frequently may be teased by their peers due to their excess weight and this may contribute to the person's depression, social isolation, and low self-esteem. Personality disorders can be evaluated using the Structured Clinical Interview for *DSM-III-R* Personality Disorders (SCID-II; Spitzer, Williams, & Gibbon, 1987). Also, personality measures such as the Minnesota Multiphasic Personality Inventory (MMPI; Hathaway & McKinley, 1967) have been used extensively with eating disorders. Research has shown that the most typical MMPI scale elevations for bulimic, anorexic, and binge eating disorder patients are on scales 2 (Depression) and 4 (Psychopathic Deviance). These patients possess poor impulse control and tend to feel anxious and guilty about their impulsive behaviors. Most research examining personality variables uses the original MMPI (Hathaway & McKinley, 1967). The MMPI–2, which is the revised version of the MMPI, is currently available and in widespread use (Hathaway, McKinley, & Butcher, 1989).

Problem Analysis

In formulating a treatment program, it is essential to perform a thorough analysis of the assessment data. Such analysis should lead to a case formulation that explains both the development of the eating problem and the internal and external factors that are maintaining current eating disorder behaviors, so that a treatment plan can be developed. It is important to emphasize that both assessment and problem analysis are ongoing processes that are often revised as treatment progresses.

Careful analysis of the assessment information should lead to a framework for understanding a patient's current behavior and maladaptive thinking patterns. Sharing this conceptualization with the client can help in the information-gathering process. It facilitates the patient's understanding regarding the development of eating disorder symptoms and helps the client to identify important information to add to the current formulation. This problem analysis helps the clinician clarify behavioral excesses, deficits, and historical and environmental factors that have contributed to eating disorder formation. The behavioral and cognitive domains identified in this formulation then become the target areas for treatment.

In their review of the literature examining the risk factors implicated in the etiology of bulimia, Striegel-Moore, Silberstein, and Rodin (1986) concluded that three questions need to be addressed in approaching this problem: (1) Why women? (2) Which women in particular? and (3) Why now? Information gathered during the assessment process should address these questions on a smaller scale, in terms of the individual adolescent being assessed. Several attempts to address these questions have been made through structural modeling studies (Williamson, Netemeyer, Jackman, Anderson, Funsch, & Rabalais, 1995), factor analytic studies (Tobin, Johnson, Steinberg, Staats, & Dennis, 1991; Gleaves, Williamson, & Barker, 1993; Varnado, Williamson, & Netemeyer, 1995) and longitudinal studies (Attie & Brooks-Gunn, 1989; Thompson,

Coovert, Richards, Johnson, & Cattarin, 1995). What has emerged is a complex interaction of factors implicated in the development and maintenance of eating disorders. In analyzing the assessment data, these factors need to be considered along with their role in the maintenance and development of pathology. Several etiological factors are briefly discussed, and an examination of maintaining factors in eating disorder pathology follows.

Analysis of Environmental Influences

Social pressure for thinness has been implicated as an important risk factor in the development of eating pathology. Several studies have indicated that these cultural dictates are strongly endorsed by adolescent girls and young women (Striegel-Moore et al., 1986; Thelen & Cormier, 1995; Thompson et al., 1995). The prevalence of eating disorders among females has been used as one source of evidence in support of sociocultural influences affecting the development of anorexia and bulimia nervosa. Problem analysis must address why the individual in question is so strongly affected by social pressures for thinness. When evaluating the influence of sociocultural factors for each individual with an eating disorder, there are several important considerations. One question is, "Does the adolescent in question live in an environment that strongly emphasizes thinness as the ideal physique?" Living in a competitive atmosphere that rewards beauty or fitness, such as a private school, boarding school, or athletic team increases the importance of a slim physique (Striegel-Moore et al., 1986). Socioeconomic status (Striegel-Moore et al., 1986), familial pressure to maintain a thin body size (Pike & Rodin, 1991; Thelen & Cormier, 1995), a history of teasing about body size (Thompson et al., 1995), and a family or personal history of obesity and subsequent degradation are all environmental elements for the clinician to consider when formulating the development of eating pathology.

Questions that should be asked are, "Do your parents diet? Have you ever been told by your parents or coaches that you need to lose weight? Have you ever been teased about your appearance?" Affirmative answers may indicate that treatment must address not only the concerns about physical appearance expressed by the client but also the attitudes of people in the client's environment (parents, friends, coaches). These people must be educated about the impact of their attitiudes on the client's behavior.

For example, for an anorexic client who has a thin mother who is always skipping meals, the mother will need to be informed about the importance of modeling healthy behavior (e.g., eating on a regular schedule). Attitudes of school coaches toward weight and body shape need to be examined to determine their contribution to the current disorder. The weekly public weighing of athletes, the assignment of a "goal weight" to adolescent student athletes that is not based on body composition, and sport participation based on weight status are practices that need to be examined and modified for treatment to be successful.

Individual Factors

The second question of Striegel-Moore and colleagues (1986)—which women in particular?—necessitates an examination of intrapersonal factors that contribute to eating disorder development. In a factor analysis of characteristics of 245 bulimia nervosa patients, Tobin and colleagues (1991) reported that bulimia nervosa was best described as a multidimensional construct. One primary factor found by Tobin and colleagues (1991) was named "depression, intrapersonal deficits, and interpersonal deficits" (p. 16). Items that loaded on this factor included measures of ineffectiveness, personality disturbance, social adjustment, maturity fears, self-injury, depression, and interpersonal distrust. In a confirmatory factor analysis of this study, Gleaves and colleagues (1993) validated this affective and personality disorder factor.

Such findings have important implications for both the intra- and interpersonal factors to investigate during the problem analysis phase. The following are several examples of questions to be answered by the assessment data for the purpose of treatment planning. In the domain of interpersonal relationships, the following questions should be asked: Does the client exhibit appropriate social skills? and Does the client appear to be comfortable in social situations?

Other affective and personality disturbances also need to be assessed. For example, decrements in domains such as social adjustment and the presence of a high degree of interpersonal distrust provide specific areas for treatment intervention. Some additional personality factors may also contribute to the development of eating disorders. These factors include a competitive need to excel in all aspects, including physical appearance, the presence of low self-confidence, dependency on others for approval,(Striegel-Moore, Silberstein, & Rodin, 1993), and perfectionism (Williamson, 1990). Some questions that tap these dimensions include the following: Does the client's self-concept appear to be determined by the reactions of others? Is the client overly concerned about making a good impression on others? If so, self-management strategies, such as ways to positively reinforce oneself, may need to be a treatment focus. Is the client overly perfectionistic? Do these feelings of perfection extend into views on physical appearance? If so, cognitive restructuring of dysfunctional beliefs regarding achievement may need to be one aspect of treatment.

Though all these factors may contribute to the development of an eating disorder, a core feature found across several studies is body dysphoria (Gleaves et al., 1993, 1995; Killen et al., 1994; Levine & Smolak, 1992; Thompson et al., 1995). Gleaves and colleagues (1995) reported that the construct of body image is multidimensional. This construct was found to have four factors: fear of fatness, body dissatisfaction, body size overestimation, and preference for thinness. Assessment data should be examined to determine the presence or absence of these factors and their influence on behavior. For example, fear of fatness and a preference for thinness may motivate behaviors that will reduce the fear of weight gain, for example, dieting, exercise, or purging. Body size overestimation can cause the individual to misperceive actual body size, for example, feeling fat even when at a normal weight level. This misperception may motivate behaviors to lose weight. Consequently, a cycle is established in which the individual, afraid of gaining weight, engages in restrictive dieting practices. Dieting may in turn lead to feelings of hunger which motivates binge eating (Polivy & Herman, 1995). From this sequence, a cycle of dieting and binge eating can evolve. In order to educate the patient about this cycle, the clinician can explain:

> "By dieting, you are not giving your body all the nutrients it needs to grow and to function.

Because you are depriving your body, when you eat you may have difficulty controlling the amount of food that you consume, so you eat more than you had originally planned. Because you are so afraid of gaining weight, you immediately start your strict dieting again and thus risk the same pattern happening over again."

Analysis of Biological Factors

Biological factors can also contribute to the development of an eating disorder. Factors to examine include the onset of puberty (Thompson et al., 1995), the presence of obesity in the family, and a personal history of obesity (Striegel-Moore et al.,1986; Thompson et al., 1995).

Striegel-Moore and colleagues (1986) reported that the onset of puberty can be very anxiety-provoking for an adolescent female. Social pressure for thinness dictates a prepubescent physique as the cultural ideal. This physique is devoid of both body fat and female sexual characteristics. Weight gain at puberty for females is primarily in the form of an increase in fat stores. Body changes tend to make the feminine body more curvaceous and thus further removed from current cultural ideals. These sudden body changes may make an adolescent female feel unable to control her weight and body shape. The increased need for nutrients during growth periods and the corresponding hunger that ensues could also be very anxiety-provoking under these circumstances. Bulimic symptoms are reported to be rare among prepubertal girls. Therefore, it is probable that binge eating may develop in response to weight gain and body dissatisfaction associated with the onset of puberty. Assessment should examine whether the earliest symptoms of an eating disorder, for example, dieting or overconcern with body size or shape, developed soon after the onset of puberty.

Factors of Onset

Levine and Smolak (1992) proposed that the cumulative effect of several stressful life events during the course of a year may precipitate disordered eating behavior. Such events may include weight gain, beginning to date, and threats to achievement or status, for example, moving to high school or college. Adolescents particularly vulnerable to such stressors have an identity that is built upon high achievement in a variety of realms including social relationships, school, attractiveness, and fitness (Levine & Smolak, 1992). Assessment should attempt to identify these precipitating factors. Once identified these same factors may be targets for prevention. For example, if the onset of an eating disorder followed a breakup of a serious relationship, then skills to cope with interpersonal distress may be one treatment target.

Maintaining Factors

Thus far, problem analysis has considered etiological factors and instigating factors in the development of eating disorder symptoms. Factors maintaining eating disorder symptoms are most important for treatment planning. Identification of the reinforcement contingencies maintaining disturbed patterns of eating, purging, or dieting provide important information regarding the most important targets for treatment.

Body image disturbances and fear of fatness have been implicated as important factors in both the etiology and maintenance of eating disturbances (Williamson, 1990). Body image is viewed as reactive to environments and emotions as opposed to being viewed as a stable phenomenon (McKenzie et al., 1993). Body image concerns will be activated more strongly in some situations and emotional states. Because of the fluctuating nature of body image concerns, it is important for the clinician to assess these concerns across a variety of situations and emotional states. These situations will eventually become targets of exposure techniques as treatment progresses.

As previously mentioned, body image concerns can lead to restrictive eating or purging as a way to reduce the anxiety caused by a fear of fatness. Restrictive eating, in turn, is also a strong risk factor for the development of binge eating (Polivy & Herman, 1995). An individual who breaks dietary restraint will often overeat or binge, and this causes anxiety due to fear of weight gain. Thus, dieting may function as a setting event which serves as a direct antecedent to overeating or binge eating. Assessment data should be examined to determine the situations in which dieting is more or less likely to occur. For example, restrictive eating may occur at some meals but not during others. Breakfast may be skipped due to a lack of parental supervision in the morning; lunch may be prepared at home and then disposed of at school also due to a lack of monitoring. A "normal" dinner may then be consumed at night with the family to give the impression of normal eating.

In addition, feelings of fatness are more pervasive in some situations than others. For example, the client may "feel fat" while wearing a bathing suit, while at a co-ed gathering, or just before an important social event such as a school dance. Such information can be used to show the client that feelings of "fatness" are not biologically based but are actually a function of the way in which the client interprets body size in the context of environmental situations. For example, a client who is feeling fat may interpret the failure of a friend to say "hello" as due to their "unattractive body weight" and not because the friend simply failed to see the client while walking past him or her in the hall at school.

Positive feedback from family and friends can serve as both an etiological and maintaining factor in eating disorder development. Initial positive attention for weight loss may reinforce a desire to lose additional weight. Over time, these external sources of reinforcement may wane. However, over time fear of fatness may develop into a form of overvalued ideation that is independent of social reinforcers. This overvalued ideation may cause the person to disregard the negative feedback that may ensue with continued weight loss.

The Case Formulation: Putting the Information Together

Table 4 presents an outline that can be used to develop a case formulation for a person diagnosed with an eating disorder. By using this five-step approach, the evaluator can present the patient with a conceptualization of problems and lead directly to the treatment plan.

Plan Implementation

Behavioral Therapy

The following sections describe components of behavioral treatment programs for anorexia and bulimia nervosa. These treatment programs have been tested in outpatient and hospital settings. There have been very few attempts to treat persons with eating disorders in the school setting.

Meal Planning

Teaching the patient to plan nutritionally balanced meals is essential to promoting healthy eating

---

TABLE 4. Steps in Preparing the Client for Treatment

I. What made this individual at risk for developing an eating disorder?
   A. Evaluate biological, sociocultural, and intrapersonal factors that contribute to vulnerability for eating disorder formation.
   B. The answer to this question will not be utilized in the initial treatment planning. After eating disorder symptoms have been managed, this information will be used to target areas of skill deficits.
   C. Presenting this information is useful to a client. An understanding of the cause and effect relationship between risk factors and the development of pathology can provide an individual with a framework for understanding the development of her pathology and thus provide a client with a sense of control.

II. What are the factors currently maintaining the disorder?
   A. Look at patterns of eating. How is restrictive eating maintaining dysfunctional patterns? Is restrictive eating promoting binge eating or is it negatively reinforced by reducing anxiety caused by a fear of fatness?
   B. Address with the client how these patterns of eating are maintaining the disordered eating behaviors.
   C. Examine distorted cognitions related to food and weight.
   D. Explain to the client how these thoughts maintain disordered eating behaviors and affect the way in which incoming information is processed. Explain how one goal of treatment is to learn to examine how realistic these cognitions are and to replace them with an accurate assessment of the situation.

III. Explain the relationship between the cognitive distortions, behavioral excesses, and behavioral deficits of the client and your choice of a treatment regimen.

IV. Ask the client to repeat back their understanding of the case formulation.

V. Ask the client if he/she has any questions.

habits (Wilson & Fairburn, 1993). During the initial period of treatment, a dietitian should prepare meal plans to ensure that caloric intake is sufficient for weight gain (for anorexia nervosa patients) and to emphasize the importance of eating three nutritional meals (Beumont, O'Connor, Touyz, & Williams, 1987). Over the course of therapy, the patient may gradually assume responsibility for planning meals after learning how to incorporate a wide variety of foods into the diet.

Eating Behavior Modification

Stimulus control methods (Agras, 1987) are used to control binge eating and purging in bulimia nervosa. Stimulus control procedures are designed to condition eating behavior to specific environment cues. Table 5 summarizes specific techniques used for this purpose. The procedure calls for eating three meals per day at the same time and place. This procedure has the effect of reducing binge eating by decreasing the occurrence of energy depletion and hunger caused by skipping meals and dieting, and by strengthening a normal pattern of eating throughout the day. In addition, environmental stimuli that elicit binge eating can be gradually extinguished through this method.

Other methods that promote eating behavior chanage include (a) teaching the patient to eat at a slower rate, (b) elimination of easy access to binge foods, and (c) planning eating before the opportunity to eat. Food selections and shopping habits, for example, buying groceries when hungry, may also be modified (Fairburn & Wilson, 1993).

Behavioral contracts between the therapist and patient are used to promote adherence to meal plans and specify behavioral goals. Form 17.1 illustrates a behavioral contract for a patient diagnosed with bulimia nervosa.

Gaining weight is the first priority when treating anorexia nervosa. Operant reinforcement contingencies have been found to be an effective way to increase the caloric intake of inpatient anorexic patients (Agras, 1987). Negative consequences such as loss of privileges or tube feeding result if the patient does not achieve goals related to eating. Immediate feedback concerning eating, along with positive and negative reinforcement for behavior change, is required in the modification of anorexic eating habits (Agras, 1987).

Exposure with Response Prevention

Exposure with response prevention (ERP) is used to reduce the anxiety that motivates extreme weight control methods such as purging, fasting, and extreme exercise (Rosen & Leitenberg, 1982; Williamson, 1990). The first step of ERP is the creation of a hierarchy of foods that cause fear and anxiety (Williamson, 1990). These "forbidden" foods are usually high in carbohydrates and/or fat and the foods consumed during binge eating and are then usually purged. The patient is exposed to the foods in a hierarchical manner beginning with foods that evoke the least anxiety. The patient is prevented from purging and encouraged to relax and verbalize thoughts and feelings associated with eating feared foods. The inappropriate methods for

TABLE 5. Stimulus Control Procedures

I. To establish situational control over eating
   A. Try to eat at the same times and places at each meal
   B. Eat three meals per day

II. To slow down eating
   A. Put utensil down between bites
   B. Assess hunger and satiety throughout the meal

III. To reduce the frequency of binge eating
   A. Do not keep binge foods in the house
   B. Do not purchase binge foods
   C. Eat binge foods only when in the company of others

IV. To increase the frequency of meals
   A. Follow the prescribed meal plan
   B. Take foods with you if you are afraid to eat foods in restaurants
   C. Plan ahead so that you will not have to make decisions on the "spur of the moment"

FORM 17.1. Behavioral Contract for Bulimia Nervosa

___Jane Doe___   __5-18-96__
    Name   Date

__Donald A. Williamson, Ph.D.__
    Therapist

I agree to follow the behavioral prescription described below for the next seven days:

1. Monitor my eating and exercise every day

2. Attend group therapy sessions on Tues. and Thurs.

3. Purge only once

4. Binge only once

5. Eat at least two meals every day

6. Refrain from weighing myself outside the clinic

If I am compliant with this behavioral prescription: I will avoid admission to a higher level of care

and will be allowed to exercise for five hours next week.

_____
    Signature   Date

---

coping with body image distortion and physiological feelings of fullness, for example, purging, are also modified during ERP. Exposure to eating usually lasts about thirty minutes and purging or other extreme weight control habits are prevented for the next two hours. This format continues over the course of treatment sessions, and gradually the patient is encouraged to continue exposure to feared foods without the therapist's presence, as homework assignments. Form 17.2 illustrates a hierarchy of forbidden foods to be consumed over a five-week partial (day) hospital program. In a hospital setting each meal and snack provide the opportunity for use of exposure with response prevention. The patient's eating is supervised by staff members and the patient must be observed for two hours after eating in order to prevent purging. In outpatient therapy, we have found group therapy to provide an effective method for using exposure with response prevention. We have group members eat a meal prior to group therapy and then they participate in a group lasting 1.5 hrs, which functions to prevent purging.

Cognitive Therapy

Modification of irrational beliefs and attitudes regarding body size/shape and eating is a crucial component in the treatment of eating disorders. Faulty cognitions pertaining to body shape and weight and nutrition are modified through cognitive restructuring. We use this approach with adolescents and adults.

Fairburn (1981) was the first to apply cognitive–behavioral treatment to bulimia nervosa. There are three stages of treatment: (1) introduction and education, (2) cognitive restructuring, and (3) relapse prevention (Fairburn & Cooper, 1989). The first stage includes presenting the cognitive model, educating the patient about the etiology and maintenance of bulimia nervosa, and discussion of treatment goals. Other components of the first stage

FORM 17.2. Hierarchy of Forbidden Foods

NAME____Jane Doe_____

DATE OF INITIATION OF PROGRAM__4-11-96_

PROJECTED COMPLETION DATE___5-24-96___

		Foods	Week of program to be eaten
Least Forbidden		1.Cereal	one
		2.Turkey	two
		3.Cabbage	one
		4.Okra	one
		5.Baked Potato	two
Modestly Forbidden		6.Hot Dog	two
		7.Beans	two
		8.Corn	three
		9.Spaghetti	three
		10.Mexican Food (tacos)	four
Moderately Forbidden		11.Peanuts/Peanut Butter	four
		12.Chips	three
		13.Fried Chicken	four
		14.Beef	four
		15.Fried Fish	five
Very Forbidden		16.French Fries	five
		17.Fried Shrimp	four
		18.Cheese Cake	five
		19.Pie	four
		20.Chocolate Pudding	four

include nutritional counseling, training in the completion of food diaries, and introduction to basic behavioral techniques such as stimulus control procedures and ERP.

Modeled after A.T. Beck's (1976) cognitive therapy for depression, the second stage focuses on cognitive change. The therapist explains to the patient the relationship between feelings, thoughts and behaviors, emphasizing the emotions produced by eating and by small changes in body size. The patient is taught to monitor and record irrational thoughts and beliefs concerning food, weight gain, and body size/shape. Rational responses are presented by the therapist as substitutions for the patient's misinterpretation of bodily cues related to fatness. The patient is encouraged to consider a rational alternative to interpretations that she has overeaten and will gain weight. Engaging in behaviors that disconfirm dysfunctional beliefs can lead to modification of cognitive distortions as well (Wilson & Fairburn, 1993). For example, consumption of forbidden foods and discovery that weight gain does not occur, can lead to a rejection of beliefs underlying extreme fear of weight gain. Through this process, the patient learns to recognize distorted thoughts and to dispute them with rational statements.

Relapse prevention strategies are the focus of the third stage. A combination of cognitive and behavioral techniques are employed to ensure that treatment gains are maintained. Minor lapses of pathological eating are viewed as acceptable as long as there is a general trend toward recovery of health and normal eating. The patient is encouraged to learn from minor lapses by identifying antecedent "risk factors" that resulted in an episode of binge eating, purging, or extreme dieting.

Cognitive approaches for anorexia nervosa have been modeled after treatment procedures developed for bulimia nervosa (Wilson & Fairburn, 1993). We have found that the treatment of anorexia nervosa requires a multidisciplinary treatment program with several levels of care, for example, inpatient, partial day hospital, and outpatient services (Williamson, Duchmann, Barker, & Bruno, in press).

Development of a Treatment Plan

Inpatient vs. Outpatient Therapy

Treatment of anorexia nervosa typically begins in a hospital setting because of serious medical complications caused by malnutrition. The decision for hospitalization hinges on factors such as low body weight, the extent of unhealthy eating behaviors, the presence and severity of secondary psychopathology, and the failure of less intensive treatment. Before the patient is hospitalized, it is beneficial for the patient and family to be aware of conditions that will determine discharge. Developing a treatment contract can ensure that these goals are clear and specific.

Partial (day) hospitalization usually follows an inpatient stay to minimize risks of relapse and to promote generalization of behavior change to the natural environment. In this setting, the patient is in the restricted environment of the hospital for the majority of the day, and then is allowed to go home at night. All meals are consumed in a structured setting and extreme methods for weight control, such as purging, are prevented. This structure promotes gradual transfer of behavior change to the nonhospital environment.

Outpatient therapy routinely follows partial day hospitalization, with the goal of maintenance of treatment gains. Treatment on an outpatient basis is usually intensive and requires more self-control and responsibility by the patient relative to that required in hospital settings. Bulimic patients can often be successfully treated as outpatients, but if purging occurs several times per day, inpatient or partial hospital treatment may be required (Williamson, Davis, et al., 1992).

Length of Treatment

Cognitive–behavior therapy for eating disorders can vary considerably in length. Controlled studies have reported outpatient treatment programs for bulimia nervosa lasting 2 to 5 months (e.g., Kirkley, Schneider, Agras, & Bachman, 1985; Thackwray, Smith, Bodfish, & Meyers, 1993; Williamson, Prather, et al., 1989). Other studies investigating inpatient cognitive–behavioral treatment of anorexia nervosa have reported treatment lengths of 2 to 5 months (Channon, de Silva, Helmsley, & Perkins, 1989; Kennedy & Garfinkel, 1989). We have found that transfer from inpatient status to a partial hospital program can significantly reduce the length of hospitalization and reduce the total costs of treatment. In an outpatient clinic setting, treatment will often exceed 5 to 6 months and can last as long as 1 to 2 years depending on the severity of the eating disorder and the presence of other psychiatric problems, for example, personality disorder or depression.

Level of Care

The level of care that is initially selected is directly related to the severity of the eating disorder. For example, intensive treatment such as inpatient hospitalization is required for patients with anorexia nervosa who are severely underweight or for individuals suffering from serious medical problems resulting from malnutrition or frequent purging. Table 6 represents an integrated system of care

TABLE 6. Integrated System of Care

	Inpatient	Day Hospital	Outpatient
Level of care	Intensive, restricted, 24 hrs/day	Less restrictive, 10 to 12 hrs of five days/week	Unrestricted therapy conducted twice weekly
Admissions criteria	1. Low body weight 2. Severe medical complications 3. Daily purging 4. Severe personality disorders 5. Failure of less intense treatment 6. Severe depression and anxiety	1. Moderarely low body weight status 2. Uncontrolled binge eating 3. Daily purging 4. Moderate to severe interpersonal problems 5. Significant depression and anxiety	1. Binge eating and purging occur less than once/day 2. Restrictive eating on most days 3. Mild depression and anxiety 4. Body image disturbances 5. Significant fear of fatness
Estimated length of treatment	2–4 weeks	2–6 weeks	4–6 months

that illustrates the various levels of care, criteria for admission to a particular treatment program, and estimated length of treatment. Typically, a patient begins treatment at one level of care and moves up or down to another level of care over the course of treatment, depending upon their response to the therapeutic program.

Effectiveness of Treatment

Research on CBT for bulimia nervosa has expanded over the past 10 years. We were able to identify more than 30 published papers that evaluated the effectiveness of cognitive behavior therapy for bulimia nervosa. Of these studies, 18 could be described as randomized controlled group outcome studies. This type of controlled experiment is the strongest experimental design for answering questions about the effectiveness of a treatment method.

Research on the treatment of anorexia nervosa has generally consisted of reporting the treatment results of relatively large numbers of anorexic patients over a number of years. This type of clinical report is best regarded as an uncontrolled single group experiment (e.g., Williamson, Prather, et al., 1989). The failure to evaluate CBT for anorexia nervosa in controlled experiments is primarily due to the medical dangers associated with a failure to aggressively treat anorexia nervosa. For example, these patients are often emaciated, dehydrated, and in danger of dying. Such dangers preclude the use of no treatment or minimal treatment control

groups when testing CBT for anorexia nervosa. Typical of these single-group treatment experiments for anorexia nervosa is the report of Kennedy and Garfinkel (1989). They reported that about half of their treated subjects had maintained a normal body weight and had regular menses. Another 30% of their sample had improved but remained underweight.

In the following sections we review the research findings pertaining to CBT for bulimia nervosa. All but one of these studies (Williamson, Prather, et al., 1989) were conducted in an outpatient setting. The length of treatment for these studies ranged from 6 sessions (over 6 weeks) to 19 sessions (over 18 weeks). The mean number of therapy sessions was 15 and the average duration of active outpatient therapy was 12 weeks. Most studies reported using individual therapy, though a few reported using a group therapy format (e.g., Kettlewell, Mizes, & Wasylyshyn, 1992; Mitchell et al. 1990; Williamson, Prather, et al., 1989).

Comparison of CBT and No Treatment

Many controlled evaluations have compared CBT to a no-treatment or waiting-list control group (Agras, Schneider, Arnow, Raeburn, & Telch, 1989; Freeman, Barry, Dunkeld-Turnbull, & Henderson, 1988; Lee & Rush, 1986; Leitenberg, Rosen, Gross, Nudelman, & Vera, 1988; Wolf & Crowther, 1992). These studies have consistently found CBT to be more effective than no treatment. It is common for these studies to report reductions in binge eating and purging of about 70% to 90%, relative to baseline (Williamson, Sebastian, et al., 1995).

Comparison of CBT and Placebo/Minimal Treatment

This research question has been addressed in a number of controlled investigations of CBT. These studies have generally contrasted CBT with a relatively inactive form of psychotherapy (e.g., Agras et al., 1989; Lacey, 1983; Thackwray et al., 1993). All of these studies have found CBT to be more effective in comparison to a minimal treatment condition. Also, Mitchell and colleagues (1990) compared CBT to a medication placebo and found CBT to be more effective.

Comparison of CBT and Other Psychotherapies

Three early studies (Fairburn, Kirk, O'Connor, & Cooper, 1986; Freeman et al., 1988; Kirkley et al., 1985) compared CBT to another form of psychotherapy or psychoeducational intervention. The results of these investigations suggested only a slight advantage for CBT over other forms of psychotherapy. In a more controlled evaluation of this question, Fairburn and colleagues (1991) compared CBT with interpersonal therapy (IPT), which did *not* focus upon eating habits or body size/shape concerns. At the end of 19 weeks of therapy, CBT was found to be more effective than IPT. At 12-month follow-up, however, the two types of treatment did not differ (Fairburn, Jones, Peveler, Hope, & O'Connor, 1993). The results of these studies suggest that psychotherapeutic approaches that focus on the interpersonal problems of bulimic patients may be as effective as CBT.

Comparison of CBT and Behavior Therapy

As noted earlier, CBT is composed of behavioral and cognitive components. Behavioral components generally include procedures to directly modify nutrition and eating habits as well as exposure with response prevention (ERP). Cognitive components generally include self-monitoring of cognitions and modification of attitude about dieting and body size/shape. A number of studies have

investigated the contributions of the behavioral and cognitive components to treatment outcome. The results of these studies have yielded somewhat mixed findings. Two studies (Wolf & Crowther, 1992; Yates & Sambrillo, 1984) found no differences between CBT and behavior therapy without the cognitive components. No follow-up data were presented in these studies. Fairburn and colleagues (1991) found CBT to be more effective than behavior therapy at the end of 19 weeks of treatment and at 12-month follow-up (Fairburn et al., 1993). Similarly, Thackwray and colleagues (1993) found CBT to be more effective at 6-month follow-up.

Another series of studies investigated the effects of adding ERP to CBT. Two of these studies found a small advantage for inclusion of ERP with CBT (Leitenberg et al., 1988; Wilson, Rossiter, Kleifield, & Lindholm, 1986). However, Agras et al. (1989) found that an intense form of ERP (flooding) had a detrimental effect upon the effectiveness of CBT.

Taken together, these studies suggest that the complete CBT program is more effective than the basic behavior therapy program, especially at long-term follow-up. Also, it does not appear that ERP substantially adds to the efficacy of CBT.

Comparison of CBT and Pharmacotherapy

Two studies have evaluated the effectiveness of CBT in comparison to pharmacotherapy. Mitchell and colleagues (1990) compared four treatment conditions: (a) imipramine, (b) medication placebo, (c) imipramine plus CBT, and (d) CBT plus placebo medication. The results of this study showed no advantage for adding imipramine to CBT for reducing binge eating and purging. Imipramine was effective for reducing anxiety and depression, however. CBT was more effective than imipramine without CBT and this advantage was maintained at six-month follow-up (Pyle et al., 1990). Agras and colleagues (1992) compared CBT alone and in combination with desipramine with desipramine alone. There was a significant advantage for CBT and the combination of desipramine and CBT (24 weeks of therapy) over pharmacotherapy alone. The primary effects of desipramine (above those achieved by CBT alone) were a reduction of hunger and preoccupation with food.

The results of these studies suggest that CBT is more effective than pharmacotherapy alone. Combining CBT and pharmacotherapy may yield the broadest treatment effects, that is, reduction of bulimic behavior as well as of depression, anxiety, and hunger.

Plan Evaluation

Target Behaviors

Factor analytic studies of the symptoms of eating disorders have found four symptom clusters: (1) restrictive eating, (2) bulimic behaviors (binge eating and purging), (3) body image disturbances, and (4) affective and personality disturbances (Gleaves & Eberenz, 1993; Gleaves et al., 1993; Tobin et al., 1991; Varnado et al., 1995). These findings suggest that the targets for treatment should measure these symptom clusters, at a minimum.

Research Findings Related to Treatment Outcome

In a review of the literature pertaining to evaluation of treatment outcome for eating disorders, Williamson and colleagues (1996) concluded that very few studies have sampled all four symptom clusters identified by factor analytic studies. Furthermore, at the time of the review, there was no single, easily administered measure which evaluated all four symptom clusters. The most comprehensive method for evaluating treatment outcome was a semistructured interview format called the Eating Disorder Examination (EDE; Fairburn & Cooper, 1993). This interview yields therapist ratings for four subscales: (1) dietary restraint, (2) concerns about eating, (3) concerns about body shape, and (4) concerns about body weight. The EDE is somewhat time-consuming and has not been widely adopted outside a few research programs. In response to the research need for a simpler method for evaluating treatment outcome, Anderson, Williamson, Gleaves, and Duchmann (1995) developed a self-report inventory named the Multifactorial Assessment for Eating Disorder Symptoms (MAEDS). The MAEDS has 56 items, answered by the patient using a Likert-type rating scale. Factor analysis was used to derive six subscales: (1) depression, (2) binge eating, (3) purgative behavior, (4) fear of fatness, and (5) restrictive eating, and (6) avoidance of forbidden foods. Subsequent research with the MAEDS has found that it is reliable, valid, and sensitive to behavior changes during treatment. It is our hope that the MAEDS will provide an easy but comprehensive method for measuring treatment outcome for eating disorders. If this occurs, then it will be much easier to evaluate the efficacy of treatment and level of effectiveness can be compared across individuals, treatment approaches, and research studies.

In addition to evaluating changes in symptom clusters, it is important to evaluate generalization of behavior change in settings outside the clinic or hospital. This evaluation can be based upon reports of the patient and family. Also direct observation of eating behavior, for example, at school, can be very helpful in determining the generalization of behavior change.

To ensure integrity of treatment, we have found that the use of treatment manuals is most helpful. Treatment manuals can be used to structure the process of behavior therapy. They also provide a source of information to alter erroneous beliefs about body weight, dieting, and the hazards of extreme weight control methods.

Summary and Directions for Future Research

Research on CBT for bulimia nervosa is quite well developed. Treatment research on CBT for anorexia nervosa has been limited by the medical hazards associated with nonaggressive treatment of anorexia nervosa. We believe that much of the research on bulimia nervosa can be generalized to anorexia nervosa and to cases of eating disorder not otherwise specified.

This research literature shows that CBT is a very effective form of treatment for bulimia nervosa. Treatment can usually be conducted in an outpatient clinic in a time-limited (usually 12 to 16 weeks) format. Treatment outcome research has found CBT to be more effective than (a) no treatment, (b) minimal treatment, (c) medication placebo, (d) imipramine, (e) desipramine, and (f) behavior therapy without cognitive components. Other psychotherapies, especially interpersonal therapy, may be as effective as CBT, but may require more time (Fairburn et al., 1993).

Future research should investigate the long-term effectiveness of CBT and should attempt to identify subject characteristics and treatment methods that are associated with a positive response to treatment. Persons diagnosed with an eating disorder are often resistant to treatment and/or deny that they have an eating disorder (Williamson, 1990). These patients are often difficult to treat and are very prone toward relapse. Identification of this subset of patients and development of effective treatment strategies for them will be a major challenge for the next generation of clinical researchers.

References

Agras, W.S. (1987). *Eating disorders: Management of obesity, bulimia, and anorexia nervosa.* New York: Pergamon.

Agras, W.S., Schneider, J.A., Arnow, B., Raeburn, S.D., & Telch, C.F. (1989). Cognitive–behavioral and response–prevention treatments for bulimia nervosa. *Journal of Consulting and Clinical Psychology, 57,* 215–221.

Agras, W.S., Rossiter, E.M., Arnow, B., Schneider, J.A., Telch, C.F., Raeburn, S.D., Bruce, B., Perl, M., & Koran, L.M. (1992). Pharmacologic and cognitive–behavioral treatment for bulimia nervosa: A controlled comparison. *American Journal of Psychiatry, 149,* 82–87.

American Psychiatric Association. (1994). *Diagnostic and statistical manual of mental disorders* (4th ed.). Washington, DC: Author.

Anderson, D.A., Williamson, D.A., Gleaves, D.H., & Duchmann, E.G. (1995). Developing a treatment outcome measure to determine treatment effectiveness: An alternative to traditional evaluation of cost-effectiveness. *Advances in Health Care Research, 14,* 74–79.

Attie, I., & Brooks-Gunn, J. (1989). Development of eating problems in adolescent girls: A longitudinal study. *Developmental Psychology, 25,* 70–79.

Attie, I., & Brooks-Gunn, J. (1992). Developmental issues in the study of eating problems and disorders. In J.H. Crowther, D.L. Tennebaum, S.E. Hobfoll, and M.A.P. Stephens (Eds.), *The etiology of bulimia nervosa: The individual and familial context* (pp. 35–58). Washington, DC: Hemisphere.

Beck, A., Ward, C., Mendelson, M., Mock, J., & Erbaugh, J. (1961). An inventory for measuring depression. *Archives of General Psychiatry, 4,* 561–571.

Beck, A.T., (1976). *Cognitive therapy and the emotional disorders.* Madison, CT: International Universities Press.

Bennett, S.M., Williamson, D.A., & Powers, S.K. (1989). Bulimia nervosa and resting metabolic rate. *International Journal of Eating Disorders, 8,* 417–424.

Beumont, P.J.V., O'Connor, M., Touyz, S.W., & Williams, H. (1987). Nutritional counseling in the treatment of anorexia and bulimia nervosa. In P.J.V. Beumont, G.D. Burrows, & R.C. Casper (Eds.), *Handbook of eating disorders Part 1: Anorexia and bulimia nervosa* (pp. 349–359). Amsterdam: Elsevier.

Bryant-Waugh, R., & Lask, B. (1995). Childhood-onset eating disorders. In K.D. Brownell & C.G. Fairburn (Eds.), *Eating disorders and obesity: A comprehensive handbook* (pp. 183–188). New York: Guilford.

Bulik, C.M., Beidel, D.C., Duchmann, E., Weltzin, T.E., & Kaye, W.H. (1991). An analysis of social anxiety in anorexic, bulimic, social phobia, and control women. *Journal of Psychopathology and Behavior Assessment, 13,* 199–201.

Bunnell, D.W., Cooper, P.J., Hertz, S., & Shenker, I.R. (1992). Body shape concerns among adolescents. *International Journal of Eating Disorders, 13,* 385–389.

Channon, S., de Silva, P., Helmsley, D., & Perkins, R. (1989). A controlled trial of cognitive–behavioural and behavioural treatment of anorexia nervosa. *Behaviour Research and Therapy, 27,* 529–536.

Cooper, P.J., Taylor, M.J., Cooper, Z., & Fairburn, C.G. (1987). The development and validation of the Body Shape Questionnaire. *International Journal of Eating Disorders, 6,* 485–494.

Cooper, Z., & Fairburn, C.G. (1987). The Eating Disorder Examination: A semi-structured interview of the assessment of the specific psychopathology of eating disorders. *International Journal of Eating Disorders, 6,* 1–8.

Cooper, Z., Cooper, P.J., & Fairburn, C.G. (1989). The validity of the Eating Disorder Examination and its subscales. *British Journal of Psychiatry, 154,* 807–812.

Devlin, M.J., Walsh, T., Kral, J.G., Heymsfield, S.B., Pi-Sunyer, F.X., & Dantzic, S. (1990). Metabolic abnormalities in bulimia nervosa. *Archives in General Psychiatry, 47,* 144–148.

Durnin, J.V.G.A., & Womersley, J. (1974). Body fat assessed from total body density and its estimation from skinfold thickness: Measurement on 481 men and women aged from 16 to 72 years. *British Journal of Psychiatry, 32,* 32–77.

Fairburn, C.G. (1981). A cognitive behavioural approach to the management of bulimia. *Psychological Medicine, 11,* 707–711.

Fairburn, C.G., & Cooper, P.J. (1989). Eating disorders. In K. Hawton, P.M. Salkovskis, J. Kirk, & D.M. Clark (Eds.), *Cognitive behaviour therapy for psychiatric problems* (pp. 277–314). New York: Oxford University Press.

Fairburn, C.G., & Cooper, Z. (1993). The Eating Disorder Examination (12th edition). In C.G. Fairburn & G.T. Wilson (Eds.), *Binge eating: Nature, assessment, and treatment* (pp. 3–14). New York: Guilford.

Fairburn, C.G., & Wilson, G.T. (1993). *Binge eating: Nature, assessment, and treatment.* New York: Guilford.

Fairburn, C.G., Kirk, J., O'Connor, M., & Cooper, P.J. (1986). A comparison of two psychological treatments for bulimia nervosa. *Behaviour Research and Therapy, 24,* 629–643.

Fairburn, C.G., Jones, R., Peveler, R.C., Carr, S.J., Solomon, R.A., O'Connor, M.E., Burton, J., & Hope, R.A. (1991). Three psychological treatments for bulimia nervosa: A comparative trial. *Archives of General Psychiatry, 48,* 463–469.

Fairburn, C.G., Jones, R., Peveler, R.C., Hope, R.A., & O'Connor, M. (1993). Psychotherapy and bulimia nervosa: Longer-term effects of interpersonal psychotherapy, behavior therapy, and cognitive behavior therapy. *Archives of General Psychiatry, 50,* 419–428.

Freeman, C.P.L., Barry, F., Dunkeld-Turnbull, J., & Henderson, A. (1988). Controlled trial of psychotherapy for bulimia nervosa. *British Medical Journal, 296,* 521–525.

Garner, D.M. (1991). *Eating Disorder Inventory–2 manual.* Odessa, FL: Psychological Assessment Resources.

Garner, D.M. (1995). Measurement of eating disorder psychopathology. In K.D. Brownell & C.G. Fairburn (Eds.), *Eating disorders and obesity: A comprehensive handbook.* New York: Guilford.

Garner, D.M., & Garfinkel, P.E. (1979). The Eating Attitudes Test: An index of the symptoms of anorexia nervosa. *Psychological Medicine, 9,* 273–279.

Garrow, J.S. (1983). Indices of adiposity. *Review of Clinical Nutrition, 53,* 697–708.

Gleaves, D.H., & Eberenz, K. (1993). Psychopathology of anorexia nervosa: A factor analytic investigation. *Journal of Psychopathology and Behavioral Assessment, 15,* 141–152.

Gleaves, D.H., Williamson, D.A., & Barker, S.E. (1993). Confirmatory factor analysis of a multidimensional model of bulimia nervosa. *Journal of Abnormal Psychology, 102,* 173–176.

Gleaves, D.H., Williamson, D.A., Eberenz, K.P., Sebastian, S.B., & Barker, S.E. (1995). Clarifying body-image disturbance: Analysis of a multidimensional model using structural equation modeling. *Journal of Personality Assessment, 64,* 478–493.

Goldfarb, L.A., Dykens, E.M., & Gerrard, M. (1985). The Goldfarb Fear of Fat Scale. *Journal of Personality Assessment, 49,* 329–332.

Gross, J., & Rosen, J.C. (1988). Bulimia in adolescents: Prevalence and psychosocial correlates. *International Journal of Eating Disorders, 14,* 59–63.

Harter, S. (1985). Competence as a dimension of self-evaluation. Toward a comprehensive model of self-worth. In R. Leahy (Ed.), *The development of the self.* New York: Academic.

Harter, S. (1988). *Manual for the Self-Perception Profile for Adolescents.* Denver, CO: University of Denver Press.

Hathaway, S., & McKinley, J. (1967). *MMPI manual, Revised edition.* New York: Psychological Corporation.

Hathaway, S., McKinley, J.C., & Butcher, J.N. (1989). *MMPI–2 manual.* New York: Psychological Corporation.

Hinz, L.D., & Williamson, D.A. (1987). Bulimia and depression: A review of the affective variant hypothesis. *Psychological Bulletin, 102,* 150–158.

Johnson, C., & Wonderlich, S. (1992). Personality characteristics as a risk factor in the development of eating disorders. In J. Crowther, D. Tennebaum, S. Hobfoll, & M. Stephens (Eds.), *The etiology of bulimia nervosa: The individual and familial context* (pp. 179–196). Washington, DC: Hemisphere.

Kasvikis, Y.G., Tsakiris, F., Marks, I.M., Basoglu, M., & Noshirvani, H.F. (1986). Past history of anorexia nervosa in women with obsessive–compulsive disorder. *International Journal of Eating Disorders, 5,* 106–109.

Kennedy, S.H., & Garfinkel, P.E. (1989). Patients admitted to a hospital with anorexia nervosa and bulimia nervosa: Psychopathology, weight gain, and attitudes toward treatment. *International Journal of Eating Disorders, 8,* 181–190.

Kettlewell, P.W., Mizes, J.S., & Wasylyshyn, N.A. (1992). A cognitive–behavioral group treatment of bulimia. *Behavior Therapy, 23,* 657–670.

Killen, J.D., Taylor, C.B., Hayward, C., Wilson, D.M., Haydel, K.F., Hammer, L.D., Simmonds, B., Robinson, T.N., Litt, I., Varady, A., & Kraemer, H. (1994). Pursuit of thinness and onset of eating disorder symptoms in a community sample of adolescent girls: A three year prospective analysis. *International Journal of Eating Disorders, 16,* 227–238.

Kirkley, B.G., Schneider, J.A., Agras, W.S., & Bachman, J.A. (1985). Comparison of two group treatments for bulimia. *Journal of Consulting and Clinical Psychology, 53,* 43–48.

Lacey, H. (1983). Bulimia nervosa, binge eating, and psychogenic vomiting: A controlled treatment study and long term outcome. *British Medical Journal, 286,* 1609–1613.

Lask, B., & Bryant-Waugh, R. (1992). Early-onset anorexia nervosa and related eating disorders. *Journal of Child Psychology and Psychiatry, 33,* 281–300.

Lee, N.F., & Rush, A.J. (1986). Cognitive–behavioral group therapy for bulimia. *International Journal of Eating Disorders, 5,* 599–615.

Leitenberg, H., Rosen, J.C., Gross, J., Nudelman, S., & Vera, L.S. (1988). Exposure plus response prevention treatment for bulimia nervosa. *Journal of Consulting and Clinical Psychology, 56,* 535–541.

Levine, M.P., & Smolak, L. (1992). Toward a model of the developmental psychopathology of eating disorders: The example of early adolescence. In J.H. Crowther, D.L. Tennenbaum, S.E. Hobfoll, & M.P. Stephens (Eds.), *The etiology of bulimia nervosa: The individual and family context* (pp. 59–80). Washington, DC: Hemisphere.

Maloney, M.J., McGuire, J., Daniels, S.R., & Specker, B. (1989). Dieting behavior and eating attitudes in children. *Pediatrics, 84,* 482–487.

McKenzie, S.I., Williamson, D.A., & Cubio, B.A. (1993). Stable and reactive body image disturbances in bulimia nervosa. *Behavior Therapy, 24,* 195–207.

Mitchell, J.E., Pyle, R.L., Eckert, E.D., Hatsukami, D., Pomeroy, C., & Zimmerman, R. (1990). A comparison study of antidepressants and structured intensive group psychotherapy in the treatment of bulimia nervosa. *Archives of General Psychiatry, 47,* 149–157.

Piers, E.V., & Harris, D.B. (1969). *The Piers-Harris Children's Self Concept Scale.* Los Angeles: Western Psychological Services.

Pike, K.M., & Rodin, J. (1991). Mothers, daughters, and disordered eating. *Journal of Abnormal Psychology, 100,* 198–204.

Platte, P., Pirke, K.M., Trimborn, P., Pietsch, K., Krieg, J.C., & Fichter, M.M. (1994). Resting metabolic rate and total energy expenditure in acute and weight recovered patients with anorexia nervosa and in healthy young women. *International Journal of Eating Disorders, 16,* 45–52.

Polivy, J., & Herman, C.P. (1995). Dieting and its relation to eating disorders. In K.B. Brownell & C.G. Fairburn (Eds.), *Eating disorders and obesity: A comprehensive handbook.* New York: Guilford.

Pyle, R.L., Mitchell, J.E., Eckert, E.D., Hatsukami, D., Pomeroy, C., & Zimmerman, R. (1990). Maintenance treatment and 6-month outcome for bulimic patients who respond to initial treatment. *American Journal of Psychiatry, 147,* 871–875.

Richards, K.J., Thompson, J.K., & Coovert, M. (1990, March). *Development of body image and eating disturbance in 10–15 year-old females.* Paper presented at the annual meeting of the Southeastern Psychological Association, Atlanta, GA.

Rosen, J.C., & Leitenberg, H. (1982). Bulimia nervosa: Treatment with exposure and response prevention. *Behavior Therapy, 13,* 117–124.

Spitzer, R.L., Williams, J.B.W., & Gibbon, M. (1987). *The structured clinical interview for the DSM-III-R (SCID-II).* New York: New York State Psychiatric Institute, Biometrics Research.

Stice, E.M., Schupak-Neuberg, E., Shaw, H., & Stein, R. (1994). Relation of media exposure to eating disorder symptomology: An examination of mediating mechanisms. *Journal of Abnormal Psychology, 103,* 836–840.

Striegel-Moore, R.H., Silberstein, L.R., & Rodin, J. (1986). Toward an understanding of risk factors for bulimia. *American Psychologist, 41,* 246–263.

Striegel-Moore, R.H., Silberstein, L.R., & Rodin, J. (1993). The social self in bulimia nervosa: Public self-consciousness, social anxiety, and perceived fraudulence. *Journal of Abnormal Psychology, 102,* 297–303.

Thackwray, D.E., Smith, M.C., Bodfish, J.W., & Meyers, A.W. (1993). A comparison of behavioral and cognitive–behavioral interventions for bulimia nervosa. *Journal of Consulting and Clinical Psychology, 61,* 639–645.

Thelen, M.H., & Cormier, J.F. (1995). Desire to be thinner and weight control among children and their parents. *Behavior Therapy, 26,* 85–99.

Thelen, M.H., Farmer, J., Wonderlich, S., & Smith, M. (1991). A revision of the Bulimia Test: The BULIT-R. *Psychological Assessment, 3,* 119–124.

Thompson, J.K., & Cattarin J. (1992). The Perception of Teasing Scale: A revision and extension of the Physical Appearance Related Teasing Scale (PARTS). *The Behavior Therapist, 15,* 230.

Thompson, J.K., Coovert, M.D., Richards, K.J., Johnson, S., & Cattarin, J. (1995). Development of body image, eating disturbance, and general psychological functioning in female adolescents: Covariance structure modeling and longitudinal investigations. *International Journal of Eating Disorders, 18,* 221–236.

Tobin, D.L., Johnson, C., Steinberg, S., Staats, M., & Dennis, A.B. (1991). Multifactorial assessment of bulimia nervosa. *Journal of Abnormal Psychology, 100,* 14–21.

Varnado, P.J., Williamson, D.A., & Netemeyer, R. (1995). Confirmatory factor analysis of eating disorder symptoms in college women. *Journal of Psychopathology and Behavioral Assessment, 17,* 69–79.

Veron-Guidry, S., & Williamson, D.A. (1996). Development of a body image assessment procedure for children and pre-adolescents. *International Journal of Eating Disorders, 20,* 287–293.

Williamson, D.A. (1990). *Assessment of eating disorders: Obesity, anorexia, and bulimia nervosa.* New York: Pergamon.

Williamson, D.A., Prather, R.C., Upton, L., Davis, C.J., Ruggiero, L., & VanBuren, D. (1987). Severity of bulimia: Relationship with depression and other psychopathology. *International Journal of Eating Disorders, 6,* 39–47.

Williamson, D.A., Davis, C.J., Bennett, S.M., Goreczny, A.J., & Gleaves, D.H. (1989). Development of a simple procedure for assessing body image disturbances. *Behavioral Assessment, 11,* 433–446.

Williamson, D.A., Prather, R.C., Bennett, S.M., Davis, C.J., Watkins, P.C., & Grenier, C.E. (1989). An uncontrolled evaluation of inpatient and outpatient cognitive–behavior therapy for bulimia nervosa. *Behavior Modification, 13,* 340–360.

Williamson, D.A., Davis, C.J., & Duchmann, E.G. (1992). Anorexia and bulimia nervosa. In V.B. Van Hasselt & D.J. Kolko (Eds.), *Inpatient behavior therapy for children and adolescents* (pp. 341–364). New York: Plenum.

Williamson, D.A., Gleaves, D.H., & Savin, S.M. (1992). Empirical classification of eating disorder NOS: Support for *DSM-IV. Journal of Psychopathology and Behavioral Assessment, 14,* 201–216.

Williamson, D.A., Barker, S.E., & Norris, L.E. (1993). Etiology and management of eating disorders. In P.B. Sutker & H.E. Adams (Eds.), *Comprehensive handbook of psychopathology* (pp. 505–529). New York: Plenum Press.

Williamson, D.A., Gleaves, D.H., Watkins, P.C., & Schlundt, D.G. (1993). Validation of self-ideal body size discrepancy as a measure of body size dissatisfaction. *Journal of Psychopathology and Behavioral Assessment, 15,* 57–68.

Williamson, D.A., Barker, S.E., Bertman, L.J., & Gleaves, D. (1995). Body image, dysphoria, and dietary restraint: Factor structure in nonclinical subjects. *Behaviour Research and Therapy, 33,* 85–93.

Williamson, D.A., Netemeyer, R.G., Jackman, L.P., Anderson, D.A., Funsch, C.L., & Rabalais, J.Y. (1995). Structural equation modeling of risk factors for the development of eating disorder symptoms in female athletes. *International Journal of Eating Disorders, 17,* 387–393.

Williamson, D.A., Sebastian, S.B., & Varnado, P.J. (1995). Anorexia and Bulimia Nervosa. In A.J. Goreczny (Ed.), *Handbook of Health and Rehabilitation Psychology* (pp. 175–196). New York: Plenum.

Williamson, D.A., Anderson, D.A., & Gleaves, D.H. (1996). Anorexia nervosa and bulimia nervosa: Structured interview methodologies and psychological assessment. In J.K. Thompson (Ed.), *Body image, eating disorders, and obesity: An integrative guide for assessment and treatment* (pp. 205–223). Washington, DC: American Psychological Association.

Williamson, D.A., Duchmann, E.G., Barker, S.E., & Bruno, R.M. (in press). Treatment manual for anorexia nervosa. In V.B. Van Hasselt & M. Hersen (Eds.), *Handbook of psychological treatment protocols for children and adolescents.* Hillsdale, NJ: Erlbaum.

Wilson, G.T., & Eldredge, K.L. (1992). Pathology and development of eating disorders: Implications for athletes. In K.B. Brownell, J. Rodin, & J.H. Wilmore (Eds.), *Eating, body weight, and performance in athletes: Disorders of modern society* (pp. 115–127). Philadelphia: Lea & Febiger.

Wilson, G.T., & Fairburn, C.G. (1993). Cognitive treatments for eating disorders. *Journal of Consulting and Clinical Psychology, 61,* 261–269.

Wilson, G.T., Rossiter, E., Kleifield, E.I., & Lindholm, L. (1986). Cognitive–behavioral treatment of bulimia nervosa:

A controlled evaluation. *Behaviour Research and Therapy, 24,* 277–288.

Witcher, D.B., & Williamson, D.A. (1992). Duration of bulimia nervosa and symptom progression: A retrospective analysis of treatment-seeking bulimics. *Journal of Substance Abuse, 4,* 255–261.

Wolf, E.M., & Crowther, J.H. (1992). An evaluation of behavioral and cognitive–behavioral group interventions for the treatment of bulimia nervosa in women. *International Journal of Eating Disorders, 11,* 3–15.

Yates, A.J., & Sambrillo, F. (1984). Bulimia nervosa: A descriptive and therapeutic study. *Behavior Research and Therapy, 22,* 503–517.

18

Behavioral Treatment of Feeding Disorders in Children

THOMAS R. LINSCHEID

Introduction

Behavioral feeding problems in children are defined as those disorders which lead to the lack of ingestion of a nutritionally or developmentally appropriate diet in children who are not prevented from eating for medical reasons. Onset of the problems usually occurs between 6 months and 5 years of age, with many problems traced to the 6- to 24-month time period. Feeding problems can occur in the normally developing child, but are often found in children with known medical conditions or in the developmentally disabled population. Feeding problems in children can be some of the most troublesome to parents as their ability to feed their child and to have him or her grow normally is used as an index of their effectiveness as parents. Due to the absence of a standard classification system for childhood feeding disorders, incidence and prevalence rates very widely. The prevalence of feeding disorders has been estimated as high as 25% to 35% in younger children (Palmer & Horn, 1978). Dahl (1987) suggests that 1% to 2% of infants and children have eating problems severe enough to result in impaired growth. Surveying a nonclinical sample of 413 parents of infants and toddlers in regard to behavioral problems, O'Brien (1996) found that mealtime difficulties was rated 8th on a list of 20 daily hassles encountered in parenting, and Refus-

ing to Eat Food, an item on the Eyberg Child Behavior Inventory, was endorsed by nearly 33% of parents responding to the survey. In the same sample, when asked about their needs, 35% indicated a need for further information about nutrition and feeding, and 60% needed additional information about behavior problems. These data, from a nonclinical sample, suggest that feeding problems are common and that parents are in need of information about nutrition and feeding practices and about behavioral problems in general.

There are several reasons feeding problems may go undetected. Parents who perceive their child to have limited intake of vegetables may not bring this issue to the attention of a pediatrician or other professional if the child's growth is adequate. In addition, for parents whose child has a medical condition or developmental disability, feeding problems may be seen as less important than other more immediate concerns (Linscheid, 1992).

The etiology of feeding problems encompasses a number of areas (Ginsberg, 1988). Children whose medical conditions preclude normal feeding practices during infancy or their toddler years may not develop chewing, swallowing, and taste preferences generally acquired during normal development. Family factors and practices also play a role in the development of feeding problems. For example, growth failure problems have been reported in infants whose parents were overly concerned about fat intake and therefore restricted their infants' access to high-fat foods (Pugliese, Weyman-Daum, Moses, & Lifshitz, 1987). Impairment of oral–

THOMAS R. LINSCHEID • Division of Psychology/Pediatrics, Children's Hospital/The Ohio State University, Columbus, Ohio 43205.

Handbook of Child Behavior Therapy, edited by Watson and Gresham. Plenum Press, New York, 1998.

motor and swallowing mechanisms certainly is etiologically prominent in the development of feeding problems as well. However, although medical, developmental, motor, or cultural factors may be involved in the original etiology of a feeding problem, ineffective behavioral interactions between child and parent or caregiver become the target for intervention. In this sense, behavior plays a role in every feeding problem.

In order to understand the origins of feeding problems independent of medical and developmental issues, it is important to understand the natural development of feeding and eating in children. There appears to be a critical time for the introduction of solid food (Illingsworth & Lister, 1964) during which infants are more receptive to solid texture and seem to be neurologically "ready" to develop chewing and swallowing skills. Illingsworth and Lister suggested that failure to introduce solid food during this time can lead to behavioral resistance to the introduction of solid food at later times.

An infant's or toddler's natural growth rate affects appetite and willingness to accept food as well. During the first year of life, infants show a consistent appetite and triple their birth weight. Between 12 and 15 months of age this rapid rate of growth slows and the infant who has gained perhaps 12 to 16 pounds during the first year of life will gain only 4 to 6 pounds during the second to fifth years of life (Smith, 1977). For parents whose infant has shown a consistent appetite, relatively consistent food intake, and stable food preferences during the first year of life, the natural slowing of growth rate results in a child with little appetite at some meals, significant appetite at others, and variable food preferences. Complicating this issue further is the onset of the "terrible twos" near the end of the second year of life (Kuczynski, Kochanski, Radke-Yarrow, & Girius-Brown, 1987). This is a period during which tantrums, demands for attention, and inflexibility all increase. The parents who, during the first year of life, judge success in feeding by the amount of food eaten, experience frustration as their child's natural appetite and taste preferences vary dramatically from meal to meal.

These changes in the child's behavior lead to changes in the parent's behavior. Parents may offer better-tasting food or more between-meal snacks in order to get their child to eat. The child's food refusal at mealtimes is then reinforced by access to preferred foods or social interaction in the form of coaxing, begging, pleading, or threatening by a parent who continues to think that he or she must get the child to eat. Not surprisingly, strictly behaviorally based feeding problems are often found in children whose parents report difficulty in behavior management in other areas. Clearly, as indicated earlier, behaviorally based feeding problems often coexist and are closely related and interact with medical conditions, developmental conditions, and neuromotor difficulties.

Spontaneous remission rates are low with feeding problems unless contingencies change naturally. Refusal to accept a wider variety of foods or textures rarely resolves itself, as children actually develop phobic-like responses to new foods (Palmer, Thompson, & Linscheid, 1975). Failure to address a behavioral feeding problem can lead to other more serious problems. These include nutritional deficits and social problems. It is not uncommon for a child who has a very limited diet (e.g., eating only Chicken McNuggets and ice cream) to be afraid to go to events such as birthday parties where they may be offered food that they are afraid to eat. This problem is further compounded if other children begin to tease or ridicule the child.

Depending on the nature of the feeding problem, there is generally a low recurrence rate once the problem is successfully treated. When a child has learned to accept a given food or texture, the natural reinforcers for eating, i.e., hunger reduction and taste, serve to reinforce continued acceptance of the new foods and textures in the absence of the reinforcers that were used to increase acceptance during the feeding treatment. In feeding treatment programs, it is common for food which was originally a nonpreferred food to become a preferred food once the child has eaten it for some time.

Problem Identification

Referral for feeding problems in children most often comes from family physicians or pediatricians or directly from the parents. Physician referrals are prompted when the child is gaining too rapidly, gaining too slowly, showing medical indications of poor nutrition (low hemoglobin level secondary to inadequate intake of foods containing folic acid), or failing to acquire oral feeding following a period of being fed artificially. When parents seek help it is usually for concerns about variety or texture of foods accepted or for mealtime behavior problems.

If the child has a known medical problem, a working knowledge of the normal course of the disorder and its treatment is necessary. For example, gastroesophagial reflex (GER) is not an uncommon problem in children. In this condition gastric contents move upward out of the stomach into the esophagus. Presence of gastric acids in the esophagus can produce discomfort (heartburn?) and over time can result in esophagitis, leading to mild pain and discomfort during and after eating. It is common for children with GER to reduce their intake and become selective of foods most likely based on the attempt to reduce this discomfort. It can easily be seen that behavioral efforts to increase food intake while a child is experiencing these aversive consequences of eating will have little chance of success. Children with juvenile rheumatoid arthritis must take aspirin-like medications on a regular basis to alleviate pain (Kewman, Warschausky, & Engel, 1995). These medications can cause severe stomach upsets unless taken with food. During the toddler and preschool years, when children's appetites are variable, they may not always be interested in eating at times when medication is due. Parents may resort to providing highly palatable foods such as candy, ice cream, and so on, at these times in order to get their child to eat. The child then learns that refusal to eat healthy foods on parents' demand will be reinforced by access to more desirable foods.

A nutritional assessment is often necessary to determine whether a child's eating pattern represents a health problem. To assess nutritional adequacy of a child's diet, nutritionists and dietitians frequently use a three- or seven-day food record in which parents record types and quantities of food consumed by the child over the time periods specified. The record is then analyzed as to the adequacy of overall caloric intake and nutrient balance. The dietary assessment can serve to confirm that a nutritional problem exists and to provide nutritional goals for treatment, or to reassure parents that the child is receiving a balanced diet over time.

The use of standardized behavioral assessment instruments has not proven very helpful in the specification of a feeding problem. Various checklist format measures such as the Child Behavior Checklist (Achenbach & Edelbrock, 1987) or the Child Behavior Inventory (Eyberg & Ross, 1978) can provide information about the child's overall behavior but do not provide specific information that is useful in assessing a feeding problem. It can be important, however, to know whether the feeding problem is an isolated problem or one of many problems the child may be having. If the child is having multiple behavior problems, a more general parent training approach may be taken rather than treatment directed only at the feeding problem. Archer, Rosenbaum, and Streiner (1991) developed the Children's Eating Behavior Inventory. This is the only instrument designed specifically to assess feeding problems in children. It can be useful for comparing the parents' perception of their child's eating and feeding behaviors with perceptions of other parents, but it does not yield specific information about possible causes or maintaining variables for the child in question.

The most important techniques in behavioral assessment of feeding problems are the direct observation of the child during mealtimes, and interviews with parents. During an interview, a three- or seven-day food record used by dietitians can be very informative and can prompt questions helpful in behavioral assessment. For example, questions about who fed, location of feeding, and so on, can be asked about particularly good or bad feeding days or meals. This information may provide clues as to stimulus control issues or possible reinforcers or punishers operating in the feeding situation. Observations of the feeding behavior can be taken in the clinic, home, school, or by reviewing videotapes (Budd & Fabry, 1984). This last technique has proved particularly useful as the child is allowed to remain in the natural setting as opposed to eating in the clinic or having strangers in the home during mealtime. Stark and colleagues (1993) used this technique to assess behavioral problems in the home for children with cystic fibrosis. Werle, Murphy, and Budd (1993) also have found the use of videotape most helpful in assessing feeding problems and then counseling parents to be therapists with their children in the home setting.

During the assessment phase, observation of mealtime behavior yields hypotheses about possible reinforcers and punishers operating in the feeder–child interaction and allows the therapist to define problem behaviors. For home-based treatment in which parents serve as therapists, parents are asked to record various types of information which can be used to further assess and to monitor progress of the feeding treatment. Parents may keep a record of a variety of foods eaten in the course of the week, weigh food before and after meals to assess the quantity of intake, and count behavior such as spitting food out, gagging, or food refusal. Parents should not be asked to record data which requires complex recording techniques (e.g., interval recording). The reliability and validity of data recorded by untrained observers attempting to utilize complex systems is questionable at best. If the feeding problem is inadequate intake, weight and calories consumed, that is, products of changed behavior, may be more important than actual observed behaviors such as bites accepted.

Problem Analysis

Behavioral feeding problems can have multiple functions or causes. In order to determine the function of a behavior in the feeding situation it is important to know the type of feeding problem and the historical and current contingencies and situations which may have led to or may be maintaining the specific problem. Importantly, both operant and respondent conditioning are involved in feeding problems and often are interactive with a medical or developmental condition or stage.

The feeding situation is readily conceptualized in terms of the traditional three-component operant model: antecedent, behavior, and consequence. A high chair, the sight and smell of food, a specific feeding location, are all antecedents, which precede (and may come to signal) specific feeding behaviors. Feeding behaviors include appropriate responses such as food acceptance, chewing and swallowing, and appropriate use of utensil, and inappropriate behaviors such as food refusal, crying, gagging, attempts to leave the situation, or inappropriate manners. Clearly, these are all behaviors that the child may emit and that can vary in rate. Consequences of these behaviors can be categorized as reinforcers or punishers dependent on their effect on the rate of the behaviors in question. For example, food acceptance may be reinforced by accompanying social praise, by reduced feelings of hunger, or by the taste of the food. Likewise, food refusal may be negatively reinforced if the presentation of a

nonpreferred food is withdrawn contingent upon refusal behavior or the feeding situation itself is terminated upon food refusal. Refusal to accept a nonpreferred food could also be punished by withdrawal of social attention and preferred foods.

In a structured feeding setting the therapist (parent?) has control of a number of reinforcers and punishers which can be manipulated to change feeding behavior. The therapist can also control the setting event of hunger through appetite manipulation, which serves to increase the reinforcing value of food. With these factors clearly under the control of the therapist or parent, selected behaviors can be targeted for increase (acceptance of nonpreferred foods) or decrease (pushing spoon away) through contingency manipulation (Linscheid & Rasnake, 1985).

The role of respondent conditioning must also be considered when analyzing feeding problems (Siegel, 1982). As indicated earlier, children who miss the normal period for introduction of solid foods have more difficulty accepting these foods. They appear to have more difficulty in learning to chew the food and to move solid food into position to be swallowed. This leads to anxiety or distress if gagging or choking occurs, and distress can quickly become conditioned to the presence of food in the mouth or even to the presence of food near the mouth. Conditioned anxiety to food presentation also occurs when children's feeding problems have led parents to try to force food into the child's mouth or where there are extremely intense and distressing interactions around food. Through this process, food itself acquires the power to elicit fear, anxiety, and distress in some children. In the classic two-factor model, the process sets the stage for negative reinforcement of food refusal because anxiety is reduced when food is withdrawn contingent on the child's distressed behaviors (crying, gagging, etc.)

In order to analyze feeding problems using learning principles, it is necessary to be aware of the many different types of feeding problems. Babbitt and colleagues (1994) describe two major types of feeding problems that can occur separately or may overlap. These are (1) motivational problems caused and maintained by faulty contingencies and lack of appropriate stimulus control and (2) skill deficit problems in which physiological abilities to feed and swallow may exist but may be underdeveloped from underuse or lack of experience. Examples of problems in the motivational category are refusal to eat an adequate variety of food despite attaining normal weight (limited variety), refusal to eat certain textures despite demonstrated ability to chew and swallow foods of that texture, and mealtime tantrums or disruptive behaviors. Skill deficit problems are often encountered in children who have medical conditions that have prevented or delayed the development of chewing or swallowing. Failure to progress to solid foods from pureed textures, delays in swallowing, failure to resume oral feeds following a period of tube feedings, and immature use of utensils are examples of skill deficit problems.

Feeding problems can also be categorized by specific and discrete behaviors or capabilities. Linscheid (1992) suggests a classification system that includes major problems and possible causes. Problems include mealtime tantrums, bizarre food habits, multiple food dislikes, prolonged subsistence on pureed food, delays in chewing and swallowing, delays in self-feeding, pica, excessive overeating, pronounced underintake of food, and rumination. Possible causes for these problems are behavior mismanagement, neuromotor dysfunction, mechanical obstruction, and medical or genetic abnormalities. To emphasize the multifaceted nature of feeding problems, all ten of the major problems delineated have more than one possible cause.

Functional analysis of feeding problems can best be accomplished by interview, observation and history. Although it is important to ask feeder or caregivers about food or texture preferences, the interview approach may not yield a valid assessment of a child's willingness to accept a specific food or texture. Clinical experience has shown that some children willingly accept foods or textures that parents or caregivers report the child will not eat. This may occur because the stimulus properties of the clinic, hospital, or feeding therapist may not signal the same behaviors as those signaled by the parent of caregiver who identified the problem. In addition, parents often stop offering foods that the child rejects and therefore their reports of likes and dislikes are not current. A more objective and current method of assessing the stimulus control properties of various foods or food textures is to present a variety of foods and food textures with prompts to eat each food. The behavioral reaction (e.g., acceptance, rejection, expulsion, negative behaviors) to each type of food or texture can be recorded (cf.

Babbitt et al., 1994; Munk & Repp, 1994). This method provides evidence of current food and texture preferences. Empirically based procedures to determine reinforcers are also frequently part of the functional assessment process (Babbitt et al., 1994). By interview, the foods that the child is currently accepting can be determined and can be assumed to function as reinforcers in the treatment situation. It is important to know what foods and in what texture are currently being accepted by the child. For the child who is currently not eating by mouth, reinforcers will initially be social in nature and specific types of praise, access to toys, and so on, must be determined prior to initiating treatment.

It is also possible to form hypotheses about operative contingencies by observation or by interview. This involves observing or asking about the response of feeders to certain child behaviors. For example, parents who report that they respond to food refusal by coaxing, lecturing, or reasoning with the child may be inadvertently positively reinforcing food refusal by contingent attention. Positive reinforcement of food refusal may also occur when a parent provides access to a preferred food when a nonpreferred food is rejected.

Plan Implementation

Following problem identification and problem assessment, information should be available to plan an effective treatment. In developing a plan, treatment techniques and strategies are matched to the specific problem(s) and goals are established. In addition, procedures for appetite manipulation should be clearly delineated and understood by all involved.

A major decision to be made in the treatment plan is where the treatment is to be conducted. Linscheid, Budd, and Rasnake (1995) discuss the factors that should be considered in this decision. They suggest that inpatient treatment be considered if the child's weight or nutritional status places the child in medical jeopardy or if appetite manipulation methods necessary to induce hunger could increase the risk of dehydration or dangerous but temporary weight loss. In such cases close medical monitoring may be necessary. Inpatient treatment may also be warranted if attempts at outpatient therapy have proven unsuccessful. Failure of outpatient therapy usually occurs because of limitations on appetite manipulation and inconsistencies in treatment implementation (i.e., lack of treatment integrity). In most outpatient treatments, not all treatment meals are conducted with the therapist present and parents are not always able to provide the needed consistency because of fluctuations in normal daily routines, needs of their other children, or interruptions for phone calls, and so on. In addition, if the parent–child interaction has become so dysfunctional as to preclude effective home-based treatment, inpatient treatment should be considered.

Inpatient treatment may also be considered in cases where the treatment technique itself may require medical monitoring. These techniques, to be described later, include forced feeding procedures or swallowing induction procedures. Aspiration of food into the lungs during these procedures is of some concern.

The advantages of inpatient treatment are the close medical monitoring available and consistency in the application of the treatment, as each meal is conducted or monitored by the therapist. For children whose feeding problems is related to an existing medical condition, inpatient treatment may be the only alternative. The disadvantages, of course, are higher costs, disruption to the family's routine, and threats to generalization to the home setting.

Prerequisites for outpatient treatment suggested by Linscheid and colleagues (1995) are (1) the child's medical status is stable, (2) parents or caregivers are available to participate in outpatient treatment sessions, and (3) the treatment is supported and accepted by all caregivers who will be feeding the child. Outpatient treatment of feeding problems in children often involves the school, especially when these problems occur in children with developmental disabilities (Luiselli, 1989; Sisson & Van Hasselt, 1989). Treatment in more than one setting (e.g., school, group home, natural home) obviously requires coordination and consistency for maximal progress.

Behavioral Procedures

Behavioral procedures used in the treatment of feeding problems are based on operant and respondent conditioning principles and are selected based on results of problem identification and functional analysis procedures. Common procedures will be described in the following sections.

Positive Reinforcement

This procedure, perhaps the most basic component of any feeding treatment program, involves supplying a previously determined reinforcing stimulus event contingent upon a predefined target behavior. Social interaction (praise, clapping, tickling etc.) and access to a preferred food or toy are the most commonly described reinforcers (Babbitt et al., 1994; Linscheid, 1992; Linscheid et al., 1995; Palmer, et al., 1975; Werle et al., 1993). These are delivered immediately upon the occurrence of the behavior and are initially provided on a continuous reinforcement schedule, that is, one reinforcer for each occurrence of the behavior. Later, the ratio is changed so that the reinforcer may be delivered for every second, third, or tenth occurrence of the behavior or on a random basis. In treatment of feeding problems, it is common for a food that was initially determined to be a nonpreferred food to become a reinforcer after repeated acceptances of that food by the child. Therefore, the ratio of reinforcement should not only be "thinned" during treatment but the specific reinforcers should be monitored to determine reinforcing property shifts. For example, It may be necessary to reinforce bites of green beans (initially nonpreferred) with ice cream (preferred) but once the child willingly accepts green beans they may be used to reinforce acceptance of another nonpreferred food (cf. Linscheid, Tarnowski, Rasnake, & Brams, 1987).

Depending on the age and developmental level of the child, token reinforcers have been used effectively. For example, Linscheid and and colleagues (1987) presented one piece of a Mr. Potato Head toy contingent upon each successful meal. When the child had accumulated all of the body parts, he was taken to the hospital's gift shop and allowed to purchase a small toy. Stark and colleagues (1993) used stars, which could be exchanged for a trophy each week, to reward compliance with caloric requirements in children with cystic fibrosis.

Negative Reinforcement

Allowing the child to escape an ongoing aversive situation has been used to increase food acceptance (cf. Ahearn, Kerwin, Eicher, Shantz, & Swearingin, 1996). The feeding situation itself can be an aversive situation for many children with feeding problems. Babbitt et al. (1994) report a treatment in which escape from the feeding situation to a play setting was initially contingent upon the swallowing of one bite of food or liquid. The number of bites of food necessary to terminate the meal was gradually increased until the patient was eating an adequate amount. Blackmon and Nelson (1985) report a procedure for use with children who are dependent on gastrosotomy tube feedings but who have a prior history of normal feeding. They simply force food into the child's mouth and then manually prevent expulsion of the food. It can be assumed that the child who was not eating found the forcing of food into the mouth aversive. Swallowing of the food terminates the aversive restraint situation and thus provides negative reinforcement for the behavior of swallowing. A procedure developed by Riordan, Iwata, Finney, Wohl, & Stanley (1984) involves presenting the food to the child with a prompt to eat ("Johnny, take a bite"). If the food is not accepted within a preset time interval (e.g., 2 seconds) it is inserted into the child's mouth with whatever force is necessary. Assuming that the forced insertion of food is aversive, the child has the opportunity to avoid the aversive consequence by accepting the bite before the time interval expires. Hoch, Babbitt, Coe, Krell, and Hackbert (1994) describe a modification of this procedure they call contingency contacting. Food is presented to the child with the prompt to eat. If the food is not accepted the utensil with the food is kept in contact with the child's lip until it is accepted. Assuming that the child finds the presence of the utensil aversive, escape is possible by opening the mouth and accepting the food. Acceptance is positively reinforced as well with social praise and, if enough food is consumed, hunger reduction.

For medical and social acceptability reasons, negative reinforcement procedures that require forced feeding may not be possible with outpatient or home-based treatments. Forced feeding could lead to aspiration of food (rare) and is not as well accepted by parents (Hoch et al., 1994).

Punishment

The most common punishment technique used in feeding treatment is time-out from positive reinforcement (Linscheid, Oliver, Blyler, & Palmer, 1978; Linscheid, 1992; Linscheid et al., 1995; Singer, 1990). Time-out is a contingent reduction in reinforcement density and is used to decrease the frequency of inappropriate mealtime or feeding behaviors. For example, a child who is seated in a high chair for feeding is turned around to face a blank wall for a predetermined time period (e.g., 30 seconds) based on the occurrence of an undesirable behavior such as pushing the feeder's hand away or tantrumming. While turned away (i.e., in time-out) the child receives no social interaction and does not have access to preferred foods. Assuming that social interaction and identified preferred foods are reinforcers (time-in?) this contingency reduces the probability of inappropriate behaviors. The procedures can also be conducted by having the feeder simply turn away from the child and removing the food for the preset time period. Time-out can be used for brief periods during the meal itself, as just described, but can also be used to punish failure to consume the amount requested during a meal or feeding opportunity. Singer (1990) used a 15-minute time-out when a child with cystic fibrosis refused to consume a preset amount of milk shake required every hour. Linscheid and colleagues (1987) required a six-year-old child to stay in his hospital room without the TV on and without visitors for two hours after each meal in which he did not eat the required amount of food.

Stimulus Control Procedures

Stimulus control develops after a history of differential reinforcement or punishment for specified behaviors. A child may exhibit inappropriate mealtime or feeding behaviors in response to a specific feeder or type of food. In some straightforward cases of this type, the specific food, food groups, or feeder eliciting the behavior can be changed initially so that acceptance of other foods or acceptance of food from another feeder can be reinforced. For example, Werle and colleagues (1993) taught parents to use the verbal prompt "take a bite" for foods the child willingly accepted, and then the prompt was used to increase acceptance of nonpreferred foods.

Shaping and fading are techniques based on stimulus control and are frequently used in feeding treatments (Linscheid et al., 1995). Shaping involves the gradual increase in criteria for reinforcement moving toward the desired behavior. A child who has never consumed food orally may be reinforced for simply allowing a therapist's finger to touch his lips lightly, then a touch with a spoon, then placement of spoon lightly between his lips and so on until reinforcement is given only for accepting the spoon in the mouth with food and swallowing (cf. Luiselli & Luiselli, 1995). This technique has often been used to introduce new texture by initially reinforcing the acceptance of very small amounts of the new texture or taste and then requiring increasing quantities for reinforcement (Johnson & Babbitt, 1993; Linscheid et al., 1987).

Fading, or the gradual removal of physical or verbal prompts, is most often used in teaching independent utensil use or other self-feeding skills. Initially, the feeder may manually guide the child's hand with spoon into the food and then into the child's mouth. The manual guidance is removed gradually, starting with the point at which the spoon enters the mouth and then progressively earlier in the sequence until the child is independently feeding (Linscheid, 1992). Fading can also be used to increase acceptance of textured food (Luiselli & Gleason, 1987). Johnson and Babbitt (1993) taught a child to accept textured foods on a spoon by gradually increasing the textured foods in the infant's baby bottle. The mode of presentation was faded from baby bottle to push bottle to spoon. Reinforcement was provided for acceptance and inappropriate behaviors were placed on extinction.

Swallow induction, while itself not a stimulus control technique, has been used to establish stimulus control of swallowing (Hoch, Babbitt, Coe, Ducan, & Trusty, 1995; Lamm & Greer, 1988). Food is placed in the mouth and then a finger or stimulator is used to elicit a gag response by gently touching the back of the tongue. The gag response is naturally followed by swallowing. Pairing the verbal prompt to swallow with this action can establish stimulus control of swallowing in children who may accept food but not swallow. Eliciting the swallow response provides the opportunity for reinforcement as well.

Appetite Manipulation

Interestingly, appetite manipulation during feeding treatments has received little attention in the literature, and seldom are methods used to increase appetite described in research reports. It is assumed that increasing the motivation to eat by inducing hunger should produce more rapid results. The simplest form of appetite manipulation is to prevent the child from having any access to food or liquids other than water between treatment meals. Children who have been fed artificially via gastrostomy tube or by total parenteral nutrition (TPN) generally receive 100% of their calorie needs via artificial methods. Nutrition provided via tube feedings is usually provided slowly over much of the day. This feeding schedule precludes the children experiencing hunger or sensing hunger and then having the hunger reduced by eating, the natural reinforcement for food consumption. It is necessary to induce hunger in these children if behavioral feeding is to be successful. Appetite manipulation can easily be accomplished by reducing the number of calories delivered via tube feedings. Nonnutritive fluids can be given through the tube so as to keep the child hydrated during treatment and the number of calories given through the tube can be manipulated to produce hunger while avoiding rapid or dangerous weight loss. Because of the need to manipulate tube feeding amounts and to monitor weight loss and hydration status, children who have been fed via artificial means are usually treated in medical inpatient settings (Linscheid et al., 1995).

Simply restricting access to food and nutritive liquids between meals can be used in both inpatient and outpatient treatments. For outpatient treatment, it is important to plan for the possibility that the child may refuse to eat for several days. When this occurs the child may become distressed and parents may begin to question the treatment plan because they are afraid their child will become ill or suffer some longer-term problems. If parents give up and allow the child access to a preferred food, the child's refusal to eat other foods will be reinforced and the problem may actually become worse. It is very important to have a plan for appetite manipulation that is realistic for the setting and type of treatment approach selected (Linscheid et al., 1995).

The Plan

To arrive at an actual treatment plan the preceding assessment information, functional analysis results, and techniques are necessary. The main components of the plan are the goals and the techniques to be used. Goals must be measurable and realistic and relate to the specific feeding problems identified. For a child with underintake of food the goal may state the number of calories to be consumed. For the child whose problem is texture based, the goal may be to produce acceptance of solid foods with a specified consistency, and for the child who eats only two or three foods the goal may be to increase the acceptance of foods to at least thirty foods diverse in taste and texture and representing a balanced diet. Goals specifically related to behavior are included as well (e.g., reduce distressed vocalizations to less than 20% of intervals). The plan should also indicate how decisions regarding changes are made. For example, when teaching texture acceptance, the plan may state that a move to the next level of texture occurs after the child accepts five foods of the current texture on 100% of prompts to eat (cf. Linscheid et al., 1987).

The best and most appropriately planned treatment is only as good as its implementation. The main threats to program integrity are the complexity of the program, the number and type of people involved, the setting in which the program is to be carried out, the child's medical condition, and the willingness of parents or caregivers to be involved and follow through.

Feeding programs should be kept simple, with clearcut goals and objectively defined and detailed procedures. When working with parents or teachers who are not familiar with behavioral assessment, data recording strategies must be "doable" and reflect what the parents or teachers are trying to accomplish. In most home-based programs it is not possible to have a separate data recorder, so the type of data selected to monitor progress must be collectable by the feeder either during the meal itself or after the meal is completed (e.g., weighing the food, number of bites). Asking the parent or teacher to perform more complex activities than the examples given will insure either poor quality data or poor compliance with treatment procedures. When treatments are conducted in a setting where behaviorally trained personnel are available it is still important to keep data collection systems simple, as the complexity of a program is often the result of trying to get too fancy with the type and amount of data collected. While the data are important, in the real world, preoccupation with data can oftentimes spoil an otherwise successful treatment.

The integrity of treatment application is also a function of the setting complexity. Settings where there are other children and much going on (e.g., school cafeteria) are likely to distract the feeder and compromise consistency and the feeder's ability to provide reinforcement immediately. Integrity is also threatened when individuals are involved who are not behavioral in orientation or who do not understand the behavioral principles on which the procedures are based. As an example, physical and occupational therapists often have very different interpretations of a child's resistance to eat, relying more on motor or sensory problems than on behavior per se. Although these disciplines are invaluable for children with known oral–motor problems, varied interpretations of behaviors such as chewing and swallowing or "tactile defensiveness" often lead to disagreements about approaches unless these issues are addressed prior to treatment initiation.

The inclusion of parents or caregivers in the original plan of treatment and in the implementation of the program is crucial for generalization. In-home or outpatient treatment in which the parents are the main therapists and many treatment meals are conducted in the home is probably the best model for insuring generalization. When inpatient treatment is required, parents should still be very much involved by initially observing and then conducting the treatment themselves with "coaching" by the behavior therapist. Allowing the parents to feed with the therapist out of the room is important. The therapist can observe via closed circuit TV or through an observation mirror and can correct the parent immediately if deviations from the prescribed treatment protocol occur. Staging family meals at the hospital with other family members present and eating can be very important, as can conducting treatment meals in settings other than the original treatment setting once the child has progressed sufficiently (hospital cafeteria, ward day room).

Plan Evaluation

Plan evaluation is generally quite straightforward for behavioral feeding problems. Treatment results can be compared to actual behavior baselines, to pretreatment caloric intake and variety of foods accepted, or to the child's actual weight prior to treatment, depending on the most clinically relevant information. The original plan should include fail-safe stipulations that specify a review of treatment procedures if certain subgoals are not achieved at predetermined times. Failure to meet subgoals are not achieved at predetermined times. Failure to meet subgoals should require a review of the appropriateness of the techniques selected for use, the effectiveness of reinforcers and punishers, the techniques for appetite manipulation, and the child's medical condition. Also to be examined is the integrity with which the program has been conducted.

Failure of a program that has been implemented correctly in all aspects should prompt several questions. For example, does the child have an undiagnosed medical condition which may be limiting appetite or causing discomfort upon feeding? This author was involved in treating two children who showed little interest in food despite intense behavioral efforts to increase intake. In both cases the attending physician was informed of the failure of the behavioral intervention and pursued a more intensive medical workup. Both of these children were subsequently diagnosed with brain tumors located in the hypothalamus. It was hypothesized that the tumors were so small as to cause no visible neurological abnormalities and they were not detected until advanced technology was utilized. In effect, failure of the behavioral program functioned as a symptom to prompt additional medical workup for these children who had not shown traditional symptoms of neurological involvement. A close working relationship with competent medical personnel is important in these situations. For children who are artificially fed, treatment failure may led to a decision to discontinue behavioral treatment temporarily so as to allow additional growth and maturation of oral–motor function if these factors are judged to be related to treatment failure. Occasionally, treatment fails because a parent or caregiver does not consider the treatment important enough to implement consistently or correctly. In these cases, medical neglect charges or the involvement of social service agencies can sometimes be considered if the child's medical condition is jeopardized. This is especially true when the treatment has been shown to be effective under controlled conditions.

Summary and Directions for Future Research

Behavioral feeding treatments for feeding problems in children have proved very effective. Treatment success depends on a thorough knowledge of the child's medical condition, the specifics of the feeding problems, the ability to manipulate appetite, potential reinforcers and punishers, and a willingness of parents or caregivers to participate in the treatment process. Assessment procedures and functional analysis procedures yield information useful in goal setting and treatment planning. Treatment can be conducted in the child's home setting, school, clinic, or in an inpatient medical setting. Success of the treatment program often depends on fitting the setting in which the treatment is to be conducted to the needs of the child and the requirements of the treatment plan.

Perhaps the most pressing issue for future research on behavioral treatment of feeding disorders and, for that matter, behavioral treatment in general, relates to making behavioral treatment more efficient. Babbitt and colleagues (1994) report that patients treated in the behavioral feeding program at the Kennedy Krieger Institute at Johns Hopkins University are treated for 30 to 60 days as inpatients. At Children's Hospital in Columbus, Ohio, the average length of stay for inpatient treatment of a feeding disorder is 8.7 days. The difference may be in the severity of cases treated or it may be due to different practice patterns. With managed care companies setting priorities to reduce inpatient admissions and the length of inpatient stays, it will become crucially important to demonstrate that these treatments either cannot be conducted on an outpatient basis with any comparable degree of success or that treatment success leads to long-term cost reductions justifying inpatient treatment. If inpatient treatment can be justified by these arguments, efficiency must be addressed.

The state of the art has advanced to the point that behavioral interventions for feeding problems can be said to be effective in a large number of cases; however, it remains to be shown that they are being conducted in the most efficient manner. Demonstrations of the necessity to conduct long baselines or detailed functional analyses currently do not exist in the area of feeding disorders. We do not know that collecting detailed data on each treatment case, thus incurring additional expense, adds anything to the effectiveness of treatment. We must question our most basic assumptions about the essential components of behavioral interventions in the era of managed care, capitation and health care reform.

To become more efficient we must also develop home-based treatment strategies. Can behavioral feeding treatments be effectively and efficiently conducted in the patient's home? If so, what types of cases are best treated in the home, what supports are needed for parents or caregivers, what type of medical monitoring is necessary, and who will do this? These are the questions that need to be addressed as health care delivery models change. Ideally these questions will be answered by systematic research designed to demonstrate comparative effectiveness and efficiency.

References

Achenbach, T.M., & Edelbrock, C. (1987). *Manual for the Child Behavior Checklist and Revised Child Behavior Profile.* Burlington: University of Vermont, Department of Psychiatry.

Ahearn, W.H., Kerwin, M.E., Eicher, P.S., Shantz, J., & Swearingin, W. (1996). An alternating treatments comparison of two intense interventions for food refusal. *Journal of Applied Behavior Analysis, 29,* 321–332.

Archer, L.A., Rosenbaum, P.L., & Streiner, D.L. (1991). The Children's Eating Behavior Inventory: Reliability and validity results. *Journal of Pediatric Psychology, 16,* 629–642.

Babbitt, R.L., Hoch, T.A., Coe, D.A., Cataldo, M.F., Kelly, K.J., Stackhouse, C., & Perman, J.A. (1994). Behavioral assessment and treatment of pediatric feeding disorders. *Journal of Behavioral and Developmental Pediatrics, 15,* 278–291.

Blackmon, J.A., & Nelson, C. (1985). Reinstituting oral feedings in children fed by gastrostomy tube. *Clinical Pediatrics, 24,* 234–238.

Budd, K.S., & Fabry, P.L. (1984). Behavioral assessment in applied parent training: Use of a structured observation system. In R.F. Dangel & R.A. Polster (Eds.), *Parent training: Foundations of research and practice* (pp. 417–442). New York: Guilford.

Dahl, M. (1987). Early feeding problems in an affluent society: III. Natural course health, behavior, development. *Acta Paediatrica Scandinavia, 76,* 872–880.

Eyberg, S., & Ross, A.W. (1978). Assessment of child behavior problems: The validation of a new inventory. *Journal of Clinical Child Psychology, 7,* 113–116.

Ginsberg, A.J. (1988). Feeding disorders in the developmentally disabled population. In D.C. Russo & J.K. Kedesty (Eds.), *Behavioral medicine with the developmentally disabled* (pp. 21–41). New York: Plenum.

Hoch, T.A., Babbitt, R.L., Coe, D.A., Krell, D.M., & Hackbert, L. (1994). Contingency contacting: Combining positive reinforcement and escape extinction procedures to treat persistent food refusal. *Behavior Modification, 18,* 106–128.

Hoch, T.A., Babbitt, R.L., Coe, D.A., Ducan, A., & Trusty, E.M. (1995). A swallow induction procedure to establish eating. *Journal of Behavior Therapy and Experimental Psychiatry, 26,* 41–50.

Illingworth, R.S., & Lister, J. (1964). The critical or sensitive period, with special reference to certain feeding problems in infants and children. *Journal of Pediatrics, 65,* 834–851.

Johnson, C.R., & Babbitt, R.L. (1993). Antecedent manipulation in the treatment of primary solid food refusal. *Behavior Modification, 17,* 510–521.

Kewman, D.G., Warschausky, S.A., & Engel, L. (1995). Juvenile rheumatoid arthritis and neuromuscular conditions: Scoliosis, spinal cord injury, and Muscular dystrophy. In M.C. Roberts (Ed.), *Handbook of pediatric psychology* (2nd ed., pp. 384–402). New York: Guilford.

Kuczynski, L., Kochanski, G., Radke-Yarrow, M., & Girius-Brown, O. (1987). A developmental interpretation of young children's noncompliance. *Developmental Psychology, 23,* 799–806.

Lamm, N., & Greer, R.D. (1988). Induction and maintenance of swallowing responses in infants with dysphagia. *Journal of Applied Behavior Analysis, 21,* 143–156.

Linscheid, T.R. (1992). Eating problems in children. In C.E. Walker & M.C. Roberts (Eds.), *Handbook of clinical child psychology* (2nd ed., pp. 451–473). New York: Wiley.

Linscheid, T.R., & Rasnake, L.K. (1985). Behavioral approaches to the treatment of failure to thrive. In D. Drotar (Ed.), *New directions in failure to thrive: Implications for research and practice* (pp. 279–294). New York: Plenum.

Linscheid, T.R., Oliver, J., Blyler, E., & Palmer, S. (1978). Brief hospitalization in the behavioral treatment of feeding problems in the developmentally disabled. *Journal of Pediatric Psychology, 3,* 72–76.

Linscheid, T.R., Tarnowski, K.J., Rasnake, L.K., & Brams, J.S. (1987). Behavioral treatment of food refusal in a child with short-gut syndrome. *Journal of Pediatric Psychology, 12,* 451–460.

Linscheid, T.R., Budd, K.S., & Rasnake, L.K. (1995). Pediatric feeding disorders. In M.C. Roberts (Ed.), *Handbook of pediatric psychology* (2nd ed., pp. 501–515). New York: Guilford.

Luiselli, J.K. (1989). Behavior analysis and treatment of pediatric feeding disorders in developmental disabilities. In M. Hersen, R.K. Eisler, & P.M. Miller (Eds.), *Progress in behavior modification* (Vol. 24, pp. 91–131). Newbury Park, CA: Sage.

Luiselli, J.K., & Gleason, D.J. (1987). Combining sensory reinforcement and texture fading procedures to overcome chronic food refusal. *Journal of Behavior Therapy and Experimental Psychology, 18,* 149–155.

Luiselli, J.K., & Luiselli, T.E. (1995). A behavioral analysis approach toward chronic food refusal in children with gastrostomy-tube dependence. *Topics in Early Childhood Special Education, 1,* 1–18.

Munk, D.D., & Repp, A.C. (1994). Behavioral assessment of feeding problems of individuals with severe disabilities. *Journal of Applied Behavior Analysis, 27,* 241–250.

O'Brien, M. (1996). Child-rearing difficulties reported by parents of infants and toddlers. *Journal of Pediatric Psychology, 21,* 433–446.

Palmer, S., & Horn, S. (1978). Feeding problems in children. In S. Palmer & S. Ekvall (Eds.), *Pediatric nutrition in developmental disorders* (pp. 107–129). Springfield, IL: Thomas.

Palmer, S., Thompson R.J., & Linscheid, T.R. (1975). Applied behavior analysis in the treatment of childhood feeding problems. *Developmental Medicine and Child Neurology, 17,* 333–339.

Pugliese, M.T., Weyman-Daum, M., Moses, N., & Lifshitz, F. (1987). Parental health beliefs as a cause of nonorganic failure to thrive. *Pediatrics, 80,* 175–182.

Riordan, M.M., Iwata, B.A., Finney, J.W., Wohl, M.K.,& Stanley, A.E. (1984). Behavioral assessment and treatment of food refusal by handicapped children. *Journal of Applied Behavior Analysis, 17,* 327–341.

Siegel, L.J. (1982). Classical and operant procedures in the treatment of a case of food aversion in a young child. *Journal of Clinical Child Psychology, 11,* 167–172.

Singer, L. (1990). When a sick child won't—or can't—eat. *Contemporary Pediatrics, 7,* 60–76.

Sisson, L.A., & Van Hasselt, V.B. (1989). Feeding disorders. In J.K. Luiselli (Ed.), *Behavioral medicine and developmental disabilities* (pp. 45–73). New York: Springer-Verlag.

Smith, D.W. (1977). *Growth and its disorders.* Philadelphia: Saunders.

Stark, L.J., Knapp, L.G., Bowen, A.M., Powers, S.W., Jelalian, E., Evans, S., Passero, M.A., Mulvihill, M.M., & Hovell, M. (1993). Increasing calorie consumption in children with cystic fibrosis: Replication with 2-year follow-up. *Journal of Applied Behavior Analysis, 26,* 435–450.

Werle, M.A., Murphy, T.B., & Budd, K.S. (1993). Treating chronic food refusal in young children: Home-based parent training. *Journal of Applied Behavior Analysis, 26,* 421–433.

ment and treatment of pediatric feeding disorders. *Journal of Behavioral and Developmental Pediatrics, 15,* 278–291.

Budd, K.S., & Fabry, P.L. (1984). Behavioral assessment in applied parent training: Use of a structured observation system. In R.F. Dangel & R.A. Polster (Eds.), *Parent training: Foundations of research and practice* (pp. 417–442). New York: Guilford.

Linscheid, T.R., Budd, K.S., Rasnake, L.K. (1995). Pediatric feeding disorders. In M.C. Roberts (Ed.), *Handbook of pediatric psychology* (2nd ed., pp. 501–515). New York: Guilford.

Luiselli, J.K. (1989). Behavior analysis and treatment of pediatric feeding disorders in developmental disabilities. In M. Hersen, R.K. Eisler, & P.M. Miller (Eds.), *Progress in behavior modification* (Vol. 24, pp. 91–131). Newbury Park, CA: Sage.

Riordan, M.M., Iwata, B.A., Finney, J.W., Wohl, M.K., & Stanley, A.E. (1984). Behavioral assessment and treatment of food refusal by handicapped children. *Journal of Applied Behavior Analysis, 17,* 327–341.

Stark, L.J., Knapp, L.G., Bowen, A.M., Powers, S.W., Jelalian, E., Evans, S., Passero, M.A., Mulvihill, M.M., & Hovell, M. (1993). Increasing calorie consumption in children with cystic fibrosis: Replication with 2-year follow-up. *Journal of Applied Behavior Analysis, 26,* 435–450.

Werle, M.A., Murphy, T.B., & Budd, K.S. (1993). Treating chronic food refusal in young children: Home-based parent training. *Journal of Applied Behavior Analysis, 26,* 421–433.

Bibliography

Babbitt, R.L., Hoch, T.A., Coe, D.A., Cataldo, M.F., Kelly, K.J., Stackhouse, C., & Perman, J.A. (1994). Behavioral assess-

V

Cross-Setting Problems

The problems addressed in this section are those that occur across settings and are not usually considered school, home, or medical problems in the traditional and more restrictive sense. That is, although they may occur more frequently in one setting than in another, treatment is usually conducted in several environments. For example, although anxiety (Chapter 19 by Laurent and Potter) may occur in response to a specific stimulus or class of stimuli, treatment is often conducted in multiple settings, particularly for individuals who respond anxiously to a wide variety of stimuli. Depression and self-injurious behaviors (Chapters 20 by Watson and Robinson and 21 by Mace, Vollmer, Progar, and Boyajian) are two prime examples of problems that are manifested, and treated, across environments. It is common for a child to exhibit depressed or self-injurious behavior in several settings and in the presence of many varied, yet more specific, discriminative stimuli.

Tics and habits (Chapter 22 by Watson and Sterling) represent an interesting challenge for behavior analysts. Because highly effective treatments exist for these behaviors (e.g., habit reversal), some may question the necessity of conducting functional analyses to derive treatment. Watson and Sterling do not challenge the empirical basis of habit reversal, rather they present examples of how functional analysis methodology may help in prescribing more streamlined treatments in cases of habits and tics.

Although antisocial behavior of individuals certainly occurs across settings, Sprague, Sugai, and Walker (Chapter 23) note the difficulty in describing and implementing an interdisciplinary model for addressing this most pressing problem. They focus on utilizing the school environment as a context for building change, because of the consistency and predictability of the school routine and the empirical basis for strategies that can be applied in the school setting. An area related to the development of antisocial behavior is social competence (Chapter 24 by Gresham). Children who experience social difficulties often grow up to show more serious problems such as delinquency, depression, and suicide, to name just a few. Thus, building social competency in young children is an important job for the behavior analyst.

19

Anxiety-Related Difficulties

JEFF LAURENT AND KIRSTEN I. POTTER

Introduction

Our understanding of childhood anxiety has evolved significantly over the last 10 to 15 years. A defining event in this evolution was the advent of the third edition of the *Diagnostic and Statistical Manual of Mental Disorders* (*DSM-III;* American Psychiatric Association, 1980). Until the release of the *DSM-III,* much of our knowledge about childhood anxiety dealt with fears and phobias. The *DSM-III,* and its successors, the *DSM-III-R* (American Psychiatric Association, 1987) and the *DSM-IV* (American Psychiatric Association, 1994), have facilitated research in childhood anxiety by providing a common classification system. Changes have occurred between *DSM-III-R* and *DSM-IV* that suggest that the symptoms associated with anxiety are consistent across children, adolescents, and adults, although the specific manifestations of these symptoms may reflect developmental differences. These changes include removing Avoidant Disorder from the section of the *DSM* dealing with disorders first evidenced in infancy, childhood, and adolescence, and considering Avoidant Disorder as a form of Social Phobia; it is no longer an available diagnosis. The other change was allowing Overanxious Disorder, another category previously presented with disorders first evidenced in infancy, childhood, and adolescence, to be subsumed under Generalized Anxiety Disorder. The symptoms of *DSM-IV* anxiety disorders that have been examined with children (i.e., Generalized Anxiety Disorder/Overanxious Disorder, Separation Anxiety Disorder, Obsessive–Compulsive Disorder, Panic Disorder, Phobias) are presented in Table 1. It is important to note that to receive a *DSM-IV* diagnosis of an anxiety disorder, symptoms must be present for a specified period of time (e.g., 4 weeks, 6 months), and to such a significant extent that the anxiety interferes with the child's functioning. Children who demonstrate symptoms of anxiety, but not to the extent that would warrant a *DSM-IV* diagnosis, may still experience distress.

Although *DSM-IV* provides guidelines for diagnosing anxiety disorders, the use of this system is not without controversy. As early as *DSM-III,* Achenbach (1980) was questioning the utility of a diagnostic system that was developed on an intuitive rather than an empirical basis. Laurent, Landau, and Stark (1993) examined the most efficient inclusion and exclusion criteria for the differential diagnosis of depression and anxiety in children using conditional probabilities. Base rates, sensitivity, specificity, positive predictive power, and negative predictive power rates were derived from child interview data based on *DSM-III-R* diagnostic criteria. Symptoms describing worries served as the most efficient inclusion criteria for anxiety disorders, especially worries about future events and competence in academics. Recently, others have written about the important role worry plays in childhood anxiety (Vasey, 1993; Vasey, Crnic, & Carter, 1994). Laurent and colleagues (1993) found that the other *DSM-III-R* symptoms associated with anxiety did not differentiate children with anxiety from children with depression. As a result, it may be more accurate to

JEFF LAURENT AND KIRSTEN I. POTTER • Department of Psychology, Illinois State University, Normal, Illinois 61790-4620.

TABLE 1. Symptoms Associated with *DSM-IV* Anxiety Disorders

	GAD	SAD	OCD	PD	PH
Worry					
about work	√				
about school performance	√				
about relationships with others	√				
about someone close to them being harmed or dying		√			
about being separated from someone they are close to or a significant person		√			
Recurrent and persistent thoughts, impulses, images, or behaviors			√		
Actual or perceived physical symptoms					
restlessness	√				
being easily fatigued	√				
difficulty concentrating	√				
irritability	√				
muscle tension	√				
sleep disturbance—insomnia, too much sleep, or restless sleep	√				
pounding heart or accelerated heart rate				√	
sweating for no obvious reason				√	
trembling or shaking				√	
shortness of breath or feelings of smothering				√	
feeling of choking				√	
chest pain or discomfort				√	
nausea or abdominal distress		√		√	
feeling dizzy, lightheaded, or faint				√	
numbness or tingling sensations				√	
chills or hot flashes				√	
Fears and/or Phobias					
fear of losing control				√	
fear of dying				√	
fear when separated or in anticipation of separation		√			
fear of being home alone without adults present		√			
fear of being in a social situation where there are unfamiliar people					√[1]
fear related to an object or situation (e.g., heights, animals, flying, blood)					√[2]
Other Symptoms					
refusal to go to school or to participate in outside activities because of separation		√			
nightmares about being separated from others		√			
refusal to sleep away from home or insistence on sleeping near someone they are close to		√			
feelings of unreality or being detached from themselves				√	

Note: GAD = Generalized Anxiety Disorder/Overanxious Disorder; SAD = Separation Anxiety Disorder; OCD = Obsessive–Compulsive Disorder; PD = Panic Disorder; PH[1] = Social Phobia, PH[2] = Specific Phobia.

view *DSM* symptoms associated with anxiety, other than worry, as indicative of general distress or the broader construct of internalizing disorder.

Epidemiological studies and prevalence figures are closely tied to definitional issues. Most epidemi-ological studies of children's anxiety before the advent of *DSM-III* focused on fears and phobias. Typical prevalence rates reported ranged from 8% (Agras, Sylvester, & Oliveau, 1969) to 43% (Lapouse & Monk, 1959). These early studies relied on reports from mothers (Agras et al., 1969; Lapouse & Monk, 1959) or teachers (Werry & Quay, 1971); children themselves were not interviewed. More recent studies using *DSM-III* or *DSM-III-R* criteria and child interviews have found varying prevalence rates, ranging from 3% (Anderson, Williams, McGee, & Silva, 1987; Bowen, Offord, & Boyle, 1990) to 38% (Last, Hersen, Kazdin, Finkelstein, & Strauss, 1987), depending on the anxiety disorder of interest and the population surveyed. Moreau and Weissman (1993) and Costello and Angold (1995) provide summaries of recent prevalence studies in community and school samples. Acknowledging limitations in available measures, samples, and informants used to examine the prevalence of anxiety disorders, Costello and Angold (1995) report relatively consistent patterns that have emerged across these samples. First, anxiety disorders are not uncommon; estimates in non-clinical samples range from 6% to 18%. Additionally, children report symptoms associated with anxiety disorders much more frequently than parents do about their children. The prevalence of anxiety disorders seems to increase slightly with age, with the exception of Separation Anxiety, which decreases with age. Finally, anxiety disorders appear more common among girls than among boys in non-clinical samples.

The impact of anxiety on children's functioning has been demonstrated in a frequently cited series of studies conducted by Strauss and colleagues (Strauss, Frame, & Forehand, 1987; Strauss, Lahey, Frick, Frame, & Hynd, 1988). Anxious children experienced a broad range of psychosocial difficulties compared to their nonanxious peers. Specifically, anxious children exhibited impaired peer relations, higher levels of depression, poorer self-concepts, attention problems, and teacher-reported deficits in academic performance (Strauss et al., 1987). Strauss and colleagues (1988) also reported that children with clinically significant anxiety disorders were less liked by their peers than nonreferred youngsters. In fact, children with anxiety disorders were as disliked by their peers as were children with conduct disorders. These children also tended to be socially neglected by their classmates. These potentially adverse consequences make early identification of anxiety and anxiety disorders important, so that appropriate interventions may occur.

Because it is a relatively common phenomenon, the major theoretical orientations within psychology have attempted to explain the occurrence of anxiety. However, no school of thought has completely or satisfactorily explained the underpinnings of anxiety. As a result, there has been room for new theories and interpretations regarding the genesis and nature of anxiety. Each of the major theoretical orientations within psychology continues in one form or another and has not been replaced, because it is difficult to accumulate evidence that totally disproves any particular theory. However, different schools and their theories have been more or less popular at different times.

According to Delprato and McGlynn (1984), the use of the term *anxiety* falls into one of two categories in the behavior therapy literature; a label for an inferential construct used to explain symptomatic behaviors, or a simple categorical concept denoting the occurrence of designated behaviors in specific situations. Delprato and McGlynn (1984) believe that the task of the modern behaviorist is to account for "situationally cued verbal and/or physiologic and/or motoric behaviors that by convention are said to either 'reflect' anxiety or to 'manifest' it" (p. 3).

Historically, behavior/learning theories posited that fear or anxiety resulted from the pairing of an unconditioned stimulus with a conditioned stimulus in such a manner that fear became a conditioned response (Shaffer, 1986). J.B. Watson and Rayner (1920) provided the classic behavioral paradigm for the acquisition of anxiety when they conditioned the emotional response of fear in Little Albert. Fear, the unconditioned response to a loud noise, also became the conditioned response when the unconditioned stimulus (i.e., the loud noise) was paired with a conditioned stimulus (a white rat).

The application of this conditioning paradigm has undergone revision over time. For example, Mowrer (1939) used this paradigm in developing a two-factor fear-mediation theory of anxiety. In his theory, anxiety developed as a learned or conditioned response to a conditioned stimulus that was paired or associated with a painful or aversive unconditioned stimulus. Anxiety was anticipatory in nature, occurring in reaction to danger signals that motivated a person to prepare for the impending traumatic events (i.e., unconditioned stimulus). Anxiety also became reinforcing in that this preparation diminished the traumatic effects, reduced tension, and brought about a state of relief. In the two-factor fear-mediation model, anxiety has both motivating and reinforcing aspects (Mowrer, 1939). Mowrer's work was later challenged by those who believed in the "approach–withdrawal" or avoidance theories to explain anxiety (see Delprato & McGlynn, 1984, for a summary of this position).

Cognitive-expectancy theories of anxiety represent recent adaptations of the conditioning paradigm. For example, Reiss's (1980) expectancy model of fear proposed that what was learned in the conditioning paradigm was an expectation regarding the occurrence, magnitude, or duration of an unconditioned stimulus. In this model the conditioned stimulus provided information regarding the unconditioned stimulus. Reiss's model demonstrated how the relationship between the unconditioned stimulus and the conditioned stimulus had evolved from one of temporal contiguity learning to stimulus-expectancy learning (see Hilgard & Marquis, 1940, for the historical precursor to Reiss's model).

In their dissatisfaction with behaviorism, cognitive psychologists reexamined and eventually accepted the notion that internal processes, coupled with external determinants, influenced human behavior (Lachman & Lachman, 1986). From the perspective of cognitive psychology, it is people's interpretation of events, not the events themselves, that are responsible for negative emotions. Perhaps the most influential cognitive theory of emotional disorders is that presented by Beck (1976). According to Beck (1976; Beck & Emery, 1985), the anxious person's thinking is dominated by themes of danger or threat to his or her domain (i.e., self, family, property, status, or other valued intangibles). The reaction of a person with an anxiety disorder differs from that of a person exposed to a realistic threat because the former perceives danger in a situation where it is truly nonexistent, distorts the magnitude of the danger, is preoccupied with the idea of danger, and consistently misinterprets innocuous stimuli as indicative of danger (Beck, 1976; Beck & Emery, 1985). In addition, anxious individuals do not believe they have the ability to perform or cope adequately with the situation they perceive as dangerous or threatening. It is important to remember that in Beck's theory the cognitive component plays a significant role in determining behavioral and affective responses (Beck, 1976; Beck & Emery, 1985). In an anxiety disorder, the affective response, anxiety (i.e., worry), and its behavioral components

(e.g., social withdrawal, attention problems) are the product of excesses or deficits within the cognitive apparatus (Beck, 1976).

A hybrid of behavior/learning and cognitive theories is the cognitive–behavioral model of childhood psychopathology (Kendall, 1985). Within this model, both the learning process and the influence of behavioral contingencies and models in the child's environment, and internal, cognitive processes are considered important in understanding childhood anxieties. In other words, from the cognitive–behavioral perspective, thoughts, feelings, and behaviors are linked. Kendall and Gosch (1994) state, "cognitive activities such as expectations, attributions, self-statements, problem-solving skills, and schemata are needed to produce, understand, and treat psychopathological behavior such as anxiety disorders" (pp. 415–416).

Problem Identification

Self-Report Measures

Many self-report measures exist to assess anxiety among children. Perhaps the two most popular measures are the Revised Children's Manifest Anxiety Scale (RCMAS; Reynolds & Richmond, 1978, 1985) and the State–Trait Anxiety Inventory for Children (STAIC; Spielberger, 1973). Other, more specific measures of anxiety also exist, including the Fear Survey Schedule for Children–Revised (FSSC–R; Ollendick, 1983), and the Social Anxiety Scale for Children–Revised (LaGreca & Stone, 1993), to name a few. These measures have been reviewed extensively in other chapters and articles dealing with the assessment of childhood anxiety (e.g., Finch & McIntosh, 1990; James, Reynolds, & Dunbar, 1994; Strauss, 1991), so they will not be reviewed here. However, it is important to note that, although measures of anxiety typically report good convergent validity, they do not exhibit very good discriminant validity. In fact, there is growing recognition that paper-and-pencil self-report measures of anxiety overlap considerably with those instruments that are used to assess depression (Brady & Kendall, 1992; Wolfe, Finch, Saylor, Blount, Pallmeyer, & Carek, 1987).

A paper-and-pencil self-report measure that has been useful in differentiating anxiety and depression in adults is the Positive and Negative Affect Schedule (PANAS; D. Watson, Clark, & Tellegen, 1988). According to Watson and his colleagues (D. Watson & Clark, 1984; D. Watson et al., 1988), positive affect (PA) reflects the extent to which a person feels enthusiastic, active, and alert; high PA is a state of high energy, full concentration, and pleasurable engagement, whereas low PA is characterized by sadness and lethargy. Negative affect (NA) is a general dimension of subjective distress and unpleasantness that is reflected in a variety of aversive mood states, including anger, disgust, guilt, and nervousness; low NA reflects a state of calmness and serenity. An elevated level of NA is common to both depression and anxiety; popular self-report measures of anxiety and depression tend to assess NA. What distinguishes these disorders is PA; depressed individuals exhibit low positive affectivity when compared to anxious individuals.

Recently, Laurent, Potter, and Catanzaro (1994) have been working to develop a measure of positive-negative affect for children consistent with the work of D. Watson and colleagues (1988), the Positive and Negative Affect Scale for Children (PANAS–C). From the research version of the PANAS–C, which consists of 30 items, these authors have derived a 20-item scale similar to the adult PANAS. The Positive Affect (PA) scale consists of 10 items: excited, happy, strong, energetic, cheerful, active, proud, joyful, delighted, and lively. The Negative Affect (NA) scale contains 10 items: sad, upset, nervous, guilty, scared, miserable, afraid, lonely, mad, and gloomy. On the PANAS–C youngsters are instructed to indicate how often they have felt interested, sad, and so forth on a 5-point Likert scale (1 = very slightly or not at all to 5 = extremely).

In an initial study (Laurent, Potter, & Catanzaro, 1994), the PANAS–C was administered to 100 children in Grades 4 through 8. Principal components analyses of the two 10-item scales resulted in strong one-factor solutions for each scale. Alpha and item-total correlations for the PA and NA scales also were promising (PA alpha = .91, item-total correlations range from .49 to .78; NA alpha = .88, item-total correlations range from .36 to .80). In addition, correlations obtained between the PA scale, NA scale, the Children's Depression Inventory (CDI; Kovacs, 1980/1981), and trait portion of the STAIC (Spielberger, 1973) were consistent with those reported for a normal population of adults (D. Watson

et al., 1988). The PANAS–C appears to be a promising self-report measure that will help identify and differentiate children who are experiencing anxiety from those who are suffering from depression.

In addition to the PANAS–C, other self-report instruments that may be useful in assessing anxiety in children include the Thought Checklist for Children (TCC; Laurent & Stark, 1993), the Negative Affect Self-Statement Questionniare (NASSQ; Ronan, Kendall, & Rowe, 1994), and measures of anxiety sensitivity (Laurent & Stark, 1993; Silverman, Fleisig, Rabian, & Peterson, 1991). The TCC (Laurent & Stark, 1993), patterned after the Cognition Checklist (CCL; Beck, Brown, Eidelson, Steer, & Riskind, 1987) used with adults, is a self-report instrument designed to assess depressive and anxious cognitions of children and adolescents. The TCC contains two 18-item scales, one measuring depressive cognitions, the other anxious cognitions. A youngster rates how often each thought typically occurs on a 4-point scale ranging from 0 (never) to 3 (all the time) in the context of one of four scenarios (attending a party, with a friend, experiencing pain or physical discomfort, taking a test) and on a fifth section in which they rate the frequency of thoughts regardless of the situation. Each situation contains items that are intended to sample anxious or depressed cognitions. Unlike the CCL, which presents situations in the form of a sentence stem (e.g., "When I have to attend a social occasion I think:"), the TCC presents situations in the context of a scenario. The alpha coefficients for the Depression and Anxiety scales of the TCC are .91 and .88, respectively. Corrected item-total correlations for the TCC-Depression Scale (TCCD) range from .33 to .73 (M = .57). For the TCC-Anxiety Scale (TCCA), the corrected item-total correlations range from .33 to .66 (M = .50). The TCC is a brief theory-based self-report measure that is designed to differeniate youngsters who are experiencing anxiety from those experiencing depression, based on their cognitions.

The NASSQ (Ronan et al., 1994) was developed to assess self-statements associated with negative affect in children and adolescents. Youngsters report how often the thoughts listed on the NASSQ "pop into [their] head" over the past week using a 5-point Likert scale. The NASSQ contains an 11-item anxiety-specific scale for 7–10-year-olds, and a 21-item anxiety-specific scale for 11–15-year-olds, along with depression-specific scales, and a negative affect scale for the 11–15-year-old group. The Spearman-Brown reliablity coefficient for the 7–10-year-old version anxiety-specific scale was .87, while the alpha was .89. For the 11–15-year-old version anxiety-specific scale, the Spearman-Brown reliability coefficient was .94, and coefficient alpha was .96. Test–retest reliability over a 2-week interval was .96 and .78 for the 7–10-year-old version and the 11–15-year-old version, respectively. Although a relatively new measure, the NASSQ, like the TCC, potentially addresses some shortcomings of traditional self-report measures of anxiety.

The ASIC (Laurent & Stark, 1993) is a 13-item measure designed to identify youngsters with high anxiety sensitivity. In the most basic terms, anxiety sensitivity is the degree to which an individual is afraid of becoming anxious. Anxiety sensitivity also concerns beliefs about the consequences of anxiety. The occurrence or maintenance of anxiety disorders has been associated with high anxiety sensitivity in adults (Peterson & Reiss, 1987; Reiss, 1980, 1987). On the ASIC, children select the one phrase that best represents the extent to which they agree with the item. Each item is scored on a 0 to 3 point scale; not true (0), sometimes true (1), mostly true (2), true (3). Examples of items from the ASIC include, "When I am nervous, I worry that I might be crazy," and "I must stay in control of my emotions." The alpha coefficient for the ASIC was .90 with corrected item-total correlations ranging from .39 to .71 (M = .61). Silverman and colleagues (1991) present a similar measure of anxiety sensitivity, the Childhood Anxiety Sensitivity Index (CASI).

Generally, self-report measures of symptoms of anxiety (e.g., RCMAS, STAIC) are best used in a multiple gate procedure for screening purposes because of their poor discriminant validity. The other measures described in this section (e.g., PANAS–C, ASIC) are promising alternatives that are theory-based and designed to be sensitive to the discriminant validity issue. If the intent of the assessment is to screen individuals as a preventive activity (i.e., for possible treatment) or for research purposes (i.e., to identify anxious and nonanxious groups), then self-report measures may be sufficient. However, if the reason for the assessment is to provide a clinical diagnosis, self-report measures should not be used.

Clinical Interviews

There are a number of diagnostic interviews that either contain a section on anxiety disorders or are devoted entirely to assessing anxiety. Among the more popular global interviews that include a section assessing anxiety are the Child Assessment Schedule (CAS; Hodges, Kline, Stern, Cytryn, & McKnew, 1982), and the Schedule for Affective Disorders and Schizophrenia in School-Age Children (K–SADS; Puig-Antich & Ryan, 1986). Examples of interviews specific to anxiety include the Anxiety Disorder Interview Schedule for *DSM-IV:* Parent and Child Version (ADIS–P & C; Silverman & Albano, 1995) and the Children's Anxiety Evaluation Form (CAEF; Hoehn-Saric, Maisami, & Wiegand, 1987).

The diagnostic interview with which we are most familiar is the K–SADS (Puig-Antich & Ryan, 1986). The K–SADS is a clinical interview appropriate for use with children 6 to 16 years of age. The measure contains both unstructured and structured interview items. The structured portion of the interview includes questions on approximately 200 specific symptoms or behaviors relevant to most Axis I *DSM-III* diagnoses (Orvaschel, 1985). Although the *DSM* has undergone modifications since the development of the K–SADS, many of the diagnostic criteria for the anxiety disorders have remained the same. Therefore, we continue to use the K–SADS with only slight modification to items. Most items on the structured interview are rated on a 6- or 7-point range of severity, with specific criteria indicated for scoring levels. Sample questions are provided for all items to be rated. However, the interviewer is encouraged to ask whatever questions are necessary to arrive at an accurate rating for each specific item (Orvaschel, 1985). In general, studies have demonstrated moderate to very good agreement between raters on the K–SADS items (e.g., Ambrosini, Metz, Prabucki, & Lee, 1989; Laurent, Hadler, & Stark, 1994).

There are several advantages to diagnostic interviews. First, they allow the interviewer to gather more detailed information from the child about particular feelings and/or behaviors associated with anxiety than do self-report measures. For example, we once interviewed a youngster with the K–SADS who indicated that she had a fear of cows. If taken at face value, she would possibly have been diagnosed with a simple phobia. However, given that she attended a school district that was becoming suburbanized, we questioned her further about this fear. It turned out that she had never seen a real cow, but thought that she would be afraid of a cow if she ever saw one up close. Although she may in fact be frightened in the presence of a cow, without ever seeing one, it was difficult to say that she had a cow phobia and should be viewed as a youngster with a simple phobia. On the other hand, there were several youngsters who vividly told of their fear of dogs and the physical manifestations that occurred when they encountered neighborhood dogs. Diagnostic interviews provide an opportunity to discover valuable information that is not available with paper-and-pencil self-report instruments.

Another advantage of diagnostic interviews is that they allow the person using them to derive or rule out a diagnosis, typically based on the criteria from some version of the *DSM*. Determining whether a youngster displays symptoms significant enough to warrant a clinical diagnosis has treatment implications, and may determine the course of intervention for that child. Being able to determine whether a child has symptoms severe enough to receive a diagnosis of an anxiety disorder also has implications for research. Research that relies solely on the use of symptom-oriented self-report measures of anxiety (e.g., RCMAS), and then draws conclusions about children with anxiety disorders, is suspect. Not all youngsters who obtain high scores on self-report measures of anxiety are suffering from an anxiety disorder (Laurent, Hadler, & Stark, 1994). The only legitimate means of determining whether a youngster suffers from an anxiety disorder is the use of a diagnostic interview.

As is the case with self-report measures, several existing chapters provide detailed information regarding clinical interviews that can be used with children (e.g., Hodges & Cools, 1990; Silverman, 1994). Interested readers are directed to these resources.

Rating Scales and Symptom Checklists

There are a number of rating scales and symptom checklists available for teachers and parents that include anxiety subscales. Among the more popular measures are the earlier versions of the Child Behavior Checklist and Teacher Report Form

(CBCL and TRF; Achenbach & Edelbrock, 1983, 1986)—the revision (Achenbach, 1991a, b) includes an anxiety/depression subscale; there is no separate subscale for anxiety. Other popular instruments that include anxiety subscales are the Personality Inventory for Children (PIC; Wirt, Lachar, Klinedinst, & Seat, 1984), the Revised Behavior Problems Checklist (RBPC; Quay & Peterson, 1987), and the Depression and Anxiety in Youth Scale (DAYS; Newcomer, Barenbaum, & Bryant, 1994). Again, there are a number of resources available to readers interested in further discussion of rating scales and symptom checklists (e.g., Daugherty & Shapiro, 1994).

When considering rating scales and symptom checklists, it is important to keep in mind research examining informant variance. When dealing with externalizing behaviors such as hyperactivity, oppositional behaviors, and inattention, the literature suggests that children are not very accurate reporters of their own behaviors (e.g., Christensen, Margolin, & Sullaway, 1992; Loeber, Green, & Lahey, 1990). However, the opposite appears to be true with regard to symptoms associated with internalizing behaviors. In these situations, children are viewed as accurate reporters of their behaviors and feelings (R.G. Klein, 1991; LaGreca, 1990; Loeber et al., 1990). In fact, many theories dealing with internalizing disorders, especially those concerned with anxiety and depression, acknowledge the key role of cognitions in these disorders (Beck, 1971; Ellis, 1962; Reiss, 1980). It is unlikely that a parent or teacher is aware of a child's cognitions, whereas the nature of internalizing disorders makes the individual dwell on cognitions or self-statements. Loeber et al. (1990) found that children were perceived as more useful informants than teachers when it came to internalizing problems, although parents were useful informants. It is important to remember that it is not uncommon to find low correspondence among informants when dealing with internalizing disorders (see Achenbach, McConaughy, & Howell, 1987, for a review). Because of this low level of agreement, rating scales are best viewed as providing supporting evidence. It is likely that the more debilitating the symptoms of anxiety that a child is experiencing, the more likely parent and/or teacher reports will be accurate. However, if the symptoms reported by the child are not consistent with the observations or ratings provided by parents and/or teachers, the child's report should not be dismissed. In such a case, further evaluation is warranted to understand the discrepancies.

Observation and Physiological Assessment

In addition to self-report, interviews, and rating scales, other potentially useful approaches to assessment exist. These include observation techniques and physiological assessment. Observation techniques are widely used to assess children's behavior in naturalistic settings (e.g., home, school). When target behaviors are suitably identified, a wide variety of possible observational systems exist (e.g., Alessi, 1980). However, one of the difficulties in using observation techniques with anxiety disorders is the fact that often one of the most important symptoms, worry, is difficult to observe. Certainly there are instances where verbal cues are available to indicate that a child is worried. For instance, the child might talk with his or her parents, peers, or teachers regarding concerns about performance. Other children, however, might not share these concerns or worries with others. In the case of suspected phobias or specific fears, behavioral avoidance tasks might be used. Generally, behavioral avoidance tasks require the individual to enter a room that contains the feared stimulus. The individual's approach behavior is scored objectively (e.g., steps taken to feared stimulus, reponse latency). Interested readers are referred to Dadds, Rapee, and Barrett (1994), and Kendall and Ronan (1990) for discussions of behavior observation techniques.

Although somewhat controversial, physiological assessment is another technique available to assess anxiety. The controversy surrounding these techniques (e.g., heart rate, arousal, galvanic skin response) generally concerns their accuracy. In defense of physiological assessment techniques, it is noted that they are often misused and misinterpreted. King (1994), Tomarken (1995), and Beidel (1991) provide discussions of issues surrounding physiological assessment for interested readers.

Assessment Process

The purpose of assessment should be considered in choosing appropriate techniques for assessment. If the purpose is to confirm a suspected diagnosis in a clinical setting, a diagnostic inter-

view may be most appropriate. If the purpose is to share impressions with a concerned teacher, perhaps an observational technique would be helpful. If the purpose is early identification, a screening procedure may be appropriate.

With regard to screening, Laurent, Hadler, and Stark (1994) examined the usefulness of a multiple-stage procedure in the identification of youth experiencing elevated levels of anxiety. Children in grades four through seven completed a three-stage screening procedure. During the first and second stages, children completed a paper-and-pencil self-report measure of trait anxiety; the third stage involved a clinical interview with the child.

In the first stage screening, 17.55% of the sample met the cutoff criterion on the RCMAS (i.e., one standard deviation above the mean, or a T-score ≥ 60). At the second stage screening, 69.35% continued to score at or above the cutoff criterion; this was roughly 11% of the original 758 students initially screened. During the third stage screening, 40.96% of those identified as anxious at the second stage screening were identified as anxious via the clinical interview; 4.48% of the original sample.

Generally, Laurent, Hadler, and Stark (1994) viewed the multiple-stage screening procedure as a useful technique in the identification of children experiencing anxiety. They noted that additional reports from other informants could be gathered after the second stage of screening and used as corroborating evidence. They reason that it is likely that children passing through two screening stages are experiencing some emotional discomfort that may be observable to others in their environment. Data obtained from multiple sources may provide a broader understanding of a child's anxiety (e.g., does the anxiety cross situations; is it observable to others in the child's environment?), and would be helpful in planning the most appropriate intervention (e.g., involvement of parents and/or teachers in treatment).

Problem Analysis

The person who is anxious selectively attends to stimuli that indicate possible danger and ignores stimuli that indicate that there is no danger. The individual also has difficulty concentrating because he or she is hypervigilant, scanning the environment for the danger that is perceived as being just around the corner. In addition, anxious individuals make arbitrary inferences and overgeneralize. The anxious individual dwells on thoughts of catastrophes, often exaggerating the possible outcomes. Because danger is perceived as imminent, the anxious person is continuously on guard; this results in a constant state of emotional distress.

From the cognitive perspective, anxiety is related to the threat of loss or danger. This could be the perceived threat of losing someone close to the individual, social status, confidence in oneself, or the perceived threat of losing anything that the individual values. The actions or behaviors that an individual exhibits are the reaction to this perceived threat. Perhaps the most common reaction is to avoid the situation or stimulus that is perceived as threatening and that elicits the anxiety. From a behavioral perspective, avoiding the situation or stimulus can be viewed as negatively reinforcing. If the perception of threat is diminished or removed by avoiding the situation, it is likely that this avoidance behavior will continue. In other situations, the anxious behaviors are negatively reinforced. For instance, a youngster who is experiencing anxiety, complains of a stomachache, and is then pampered by a parent may seek this attention from an adult in other anxiety-provoking situations. More typically, a child's reaction to anxiety is likely to act as both a positive and negative reinforcer. For instance, if a child is given a challenging assignment (i.e., one that is perceived to be difficult or beyond the child's ability), he or she may experience the threat of failure. As a result, the child may begin to cry or display some other physiological symptom of anxiety. This may gain the attention of the teacher, who tries to comfort the child by patting the back, using a soothing voice, or, in an extreme case, reducing or eliminating the assignment. In the short term, this anxiety-related behavior results in avoiding the assignment, thus acting as a negative reinforcer and reducing the immediate threat of failure. At the same time, the soothing voice and the pat on the back from the teacher could act as positive reinforcers for the anxious behavior. To help a youngster who is suffering from anxiety, one must deal with the distorted perceptions or cognitions that result in particular situations being viewed as threatening, and the resulting avoidant behavior.

Plan Implementation

Once assessment has been completed, interventions can be designed to help the child or adolescent. Common interventions used to treat anxiety disorders in children and adolescents include behavior therapy, cognitive–behavior therapy, pharmacotherapy, and family therapy. The focus in this chapter will be on behavior and cognitive–behavior therapy.

Systematic Desensitization

Developed by Wolpe (1958), systematic desensitization has become a widely used intervention for treating anxiety in children (Ollendick & Cerny, 1981). Systematic desensitization is designed to be a graduated deconditioning technique consisting of three steps. The first step, relaxation training, was developed by Jacobson (1938) to achieve deep muscle relaxation and used by Wolpe (1958) to inhibit the anxiety response while conducting systematic desensitization. The second step in the process is to construct a hierarchy of anxiety-producing stimuli, starting with the least anxiety-producing and ending with the most anxiety-producing. The final step in systematic desensitization is the pairing of each anxiety-inducing stimulus on the hierarchy with relaxation. This gradual exposure to anxiety-producing situations while engaging in an incompatible activity, such as muscle relaxation, may occur in vivo or through the use of images. For example, the child is asked to think of the least anxiety-provoking stimulus while simultaneously relaxing. As the anxiety-inducing stimulus becomes no longer disturbing to the child, higher-level stimuli are presented until the child can visualize the strongest anxiety-inducing stimulus with no disturbance.

Wolpe (1958) stresses that individuals who are not able to achieve a relaxed state will have difficulty with this technique. Ollendick and Francis (1988) report that younger children who experience anxiety may have difficulty pairing relaxation and imagery, due to problems attaining the desired muscular response to relaxation and difficulty in producing a clear image of anxiety-provoking stimuli.

Due to the difficulty that children have in learning relaxation techniques, Koeppen (1974) and Ollendick (1978) have developed relaxation scripts specific to children. Francis and Beidel (1995) note that the difference between relaxation scripts for children and relaxation scripts for adults is that children's scripts are often shorter and do not require the isolation of as many distinct muscle groups. Koeppen (1974) has developed a specific relaxation script that is appealing to children and may help to induce deep muscle relaxation. For example, in teaching the child to recognize the difference between relaxed and tense muscles, the child may be asked to imagine using the jaw to bite down on a jawbreaker and then asked to relax the muscles. Practice in tensing and relaxing separate muscle groups allows the child to recognize tension and to use this as a cue to use the relaxation exercises that they have learned. In addition, Ollendick and Cerny (1981) provide a relaxation script to be used with older children and recommend that children receive two relaxation training sessions per week, introducing no more than three muscle groups per session. Children may practice the relaxation techniques they have learned at home and keep a record of the number of times and with what muscle groups they have practiced.

A recent, controversial variation of systematic desensitization is the eye movement desensitization and reprocessing (EMDR) technique introduced by Shapiro (1989a, b, 1991). Originally used to deal with the negative affect associated with traumatic memories, EMDR is an imaginal exposure and cognitive reprocessing technique. EMDR requires the individual to imagine the traumatic event and focus on associated affect, cognitions, and body sensations, while performing rapid lateral eye movements by following the repetitive motion of the therapist's hand/finger. After the eye movement set (usually 20 seconds), the individual briefly reports on any changes in the image or concurrent experiences (i.e., affect, cognitions, body sensations). The individual then engages in the next eye movement set, during which he or she is to focus on any new or spontaneous material that has been generated. This cycle—imaginal exposure in conjunction with eye movement followed by the individual's feedback—is repeated until the individual no longer generates new or spontaneous material, is comfortable, and reports that the original traumatic memory fails to elicit discomfort. At this point, a positive cognition is paired with the original scene by having the inividual imagine the original scene, rehearse the positive statement covertly, and simultaneously engage in eye movement.

Support for EMDR is mixed. Goldstein and Feske (1994) report success using this technique with seven adults suffering from Panic Disorder. Muris and Merckelbach (1995) found mixed support for EMDR in their study of two spider phobic adults. While the individuals' self-reported discomfort lessened, behavioral measures did not change significantly from pre- to posttest. Finally, Acierno, Hersen, Van Hasselt, Tremont, and Meuser (1994) were critical of the technique, finding most studies supporting EMDR poorly designed, whereas sounder studies did not support the procedure. At this point, EMDR has not been widely used with children or evaluated in the child anxiety literature.

Flooding/Implosion

Flooding and implosion techniques are based on classic extinction theory. Whereas systematic desensitization uses a gradual exposure method to extinguish the anxiety-inducing response, flooding and implosion therapy exposes the child immediately to the most anxiety-producing stimulus on their hierarchy of fears in order to extinguish the anxiety response. The rationale behind the therapy is that through continued exposure to anxiety-producing cues, without negative reinforcement, the fearful response should decrease and finally be extinguished. In order to measure the decrease in anxious symptoms, children may be asked to give anxiety ratings while being exposed to the anxiety-inducing stimulus until the self-reported level of anxiety has decreased. Differences in flooding therapy and implosion therapy are minimal; flooding therapy focuses on the situational or environmental cues in imagery, while implosion therapy focuses on the cues that elicit the conditioned response (internal representations of the feared stimuli). Flooding and implosion interventions may use visualization techniques as well as in vivo exposure to treat anxiety disorders in children. For example, a child who has a fear of dogs may visualize being in the presence of a dog or the child may actually expose herself or himself to dogs in order to overcome the anxiety.

Francis and Beidel (1995) warn that flooding and implosion therapy can produce a great deal of distress in children, especially younger children, so it is important that the child receives an explanation and understands the rationale behind the treatment. In addition, positive results with flooding and implosion therapy are most likely to occur when the child is presented with the fear-producing stimulus that was conditioned to produce an anxious response (Ollendick & Cerny, 1981). Determining the conditioned stimulus may be difficult when relying on the self-report of the child. Therefore, the clinician may wish to interview the parents or teacher in order to gain more information.

Flooding procedures have been primarily used in the treatment of Obsessive–Compulsive Disorder (OCD). McCarthy and Foa (1988) demonstrated the effectiveness of flooding in the treatment of a 13-year-old male suffering from OCD. The obsessive thoughts were related to failure in school, causing harm to family members, and ridicule by his coach and friends. The child's compulsive behaviors were related to the action that he was performing at the time of the thought. For instance, if he was combing his hair when he thought about causing injury to his family, he would repeat the motion of combing his hair 20 more times. The treatments used included imaginal flooding, in vivo flooding, and response prevention over the course of 15 sessions. In addition, during the last week of treatment, the child's therapy was conducted for eight hours over the course of two days and took place in his home. Imaginal flooding consisted of gradual exposure to anxiety-producing images, and included images of the consequences anticipated if the rituals were not performed. In vivo flooding consisted of gradual exposure to the anxiety-producing stimulus without participation in ritualistic behavior following the feared stimulus. Response prevention consisted of instructing the child that no ritualistic behaviors were to be performed during the course of the intervention. To ensure success, the patient was monitored by his mother, and the school was contacted to inform personnel of the treatment the child was receiving. In addition, the child was rewarded for compliance during the therapy session and at home. Imaginal and in vivo exposures were assigned as homework each day and consisted of listening to taped imaginal scenes and facing anxiety-provoking stimuli presented during treatment sessions. The results of the treatment indicated that the rituals were decreased and treatment gains were maintained one year after therapy. McCarthy and Foa (1988) believe that it is necessary to involve the primary caregiver as well as school personnel to promote a successful treatment outcome.

Modeling

Modeling, in general, refers to the learning that occurs through observation of another person's behavior (Bandura, 1977). The use of modeling to help a child overcome anxious feelings may occur through filmed, live, or participant observation of behavior. Filmed modeling requires that the child observe a videotape demonstrating nonfearful behavior and appropriate responses to stimuli that produce anxiety in the child. Live observation requires that the child observe a live model who is demonstrating nonfearful and appropriate behavior to anxiety-inducing stimuli. Participant modeling uses the live model to demonstrate and engage the child in appropriate behaviors when faced with an anxiety-inducing stimulus. In addition, once the child has learned the appropriate behaviors, she or he is encouraged to perform the responses alone. In this approach, not only does the child observe the behaviors of the model, but the child is also given the opportunity to practice nonfearful responses. Finally, reinforcement and feedback are given for appropriate behaviors in the anxiety-producing situation (Ollendick & Francis, 1988).

Johnson and McGlynn (1988) demonstrated the use of modeling in the treatment of a six-year-old female suffering from a simple phobia of balloons. The child was referred by her mother who was concerned after noticing that her daughter avoided situations in which she would come in contact with balloons. This fear affected her ability to participate in activities when balloons were present, and had caused nightmares. Treatment of the child's phobia occurred through filmed and guided participant modeling. During the filmed modeling, the child watched a young female interact with balloons, gradually, after initial fearful responses. Graduated participant modeling consisted of using the child model in the videotape to help the patient overcome her fear of balloons. The model gradually interacted with the balloons in the room and asked the patient to imitate each of her behaviors. Subsequent sessions used the therapist as the model interacting with balloons. Treatment was terminated by the mother before completion of the intervention. However, the mother reported that the fear of balloons had decreased so that the child could come in contact with balloons without an anxious response. Follow-up two years after termination revealed no further difficulties associated with her simple phobia of balloons.

Cognitive–Behavioral Intervention

Cognitive–behavioral theory maintains that individuals respond to their environment indirectly; their responses are mediated by their cognitions (Kendall & Gosch, 1994). A situation leads to different responses depending on the content of the child's thoughts and the manner of cognitive processing. Cognitive–behavioral therapy uses techniques that seek to change cognitive activities through correction of maladaptive cognitions, and this results in changes in behavior. Therefore, cognitive–behavioral treatment combines the techniques of behavior therapy with the emphasis on thought processes found in cognitive therapy.

Evidence in the literature examining anxiety disorders in children suggests that the key symptom that identifies anxious children is a cognitive symptom, worrying (Laurent et al., 1993). Based on this finding, it is logical that therapy for children suffering from anxiety problems would focus on not only behavior, but also cognitions related to anxiety. Thus, cognitive–behavioral interventions for children may focus on the development of cognitive strategies, including self-instruction training, correction of maladaptive self-talk, and problem solving (Hart & Morgan, 1993).

Kendall, Kane, Howard, and Siqueland (1989) developed a cognitive–behavioral treatment program for use with anxious children. Kendall and colleagues (1992) describe the treatment program in detail in their book on cognitive–behavioral interventions, and Kendall (1994) demonstrated the effectiveness of the intervention program with a sample of children, ages 9 to 13, who were diagnosed with an anxiety disorder.

The components of the intervention developed by Kendall and colleagues (1989) are aimed at identifying anxious feelings and somatic reactions due to anxiety, at identifying negative or unrealistic expectations and attributions in anxiety-inducing situations, at developing a coping plan to deal with an anxiety-inducing situation, and at appraising performance in anxious situations and administering self-reinforcement for appropriate performance. The intervention program uses a combination of behavioral and cognitive techniques over the course of 16 sessions. The

first 8 sessions are aimed at developing the necessary skills for children to overcome the anxiety, and the last 8 sessions are used to practice the skills they have learned in anxiety-provoking situations. Kendall (1990) has developed a workbook, the *Coping Cat Workbook,* that may be used in conjunction with the cognitive–behavioral treatment program. In addition, during the intervention the child is assigned "Show That I Can" (STIC) tasks that are completed outside the therapy sessions as a means to reinforce the skills learned during the intervention program (Kendall et al., 1992). These tasks are reviewed at the beginning of each therapy session and provide the therapist with a tool to review past learning and assimilate new learning throughout the 16-week intervention.

The initial eight sessions of the intervention program are directed at skill areas designed to decrease anxious reactions (Kendall et al., 1992). The first skill area involves teaching the child to be aware of feelings and physical symptoms that are due to anxiety. The second skill area requires that the child be familiar with and evaluate what they are thinking when they are in an anxiety-provoking situation. The third skill area focuses on the development of problem-solving skills such as making coping plans and modification of anxious thoughts. The final skill area focuses on the child's evaluating and rewarding himself or herself for nonanxious behavior in an anxiety-producing situation. The following is a brief description of the Kendall and colleagues (1989, 1992) program.

Session 1

The first session is designed as a period during which the clinician builds rapport with the child and gathers information from the child about anxious feelings experienced. This information may include what stimuli or experiences evoke anxious responses in the child and the response to the anxiety. Kendall and colleagues (1992) stress the importance of developing a therapeutic relationship or sense of rapport with children suffering from anxiety. The idea of therapy may evoke considerable anxiety in an already anxious child, making it difficult to proceed with treatment. The STIC assignment for Session 1 includes asking the child to keep a diary of times during the week when he or she feels good. This includes activities at the time and ways of recognizing the good feeling.

Session 2

The goal of the second session is to help the child identify different types of feelings through behavioral cues such as facial expressions or body posture. This may be accomplished by using pictures out of a magazine or books and asking the child to determine what the person is feeling based on cues in the picture. Next, the child is asked to identify emotions that members of their family or friends may be experiencing based on behavioral cues.

Session 3

During the third session, the child is asked to identify different feelings and the physical reactions associated with these feelings. The therapist helps the child identify anxious feelings by discussing anxiety-producing situations. In addition to discussing the situation, the therapist will describe the physical symptoms related to the situation, so that the child understands the connection between the anxiety and the physical symptoms. The STIC tasks for Sessions 2 and 3 require the child to identify pleasant and anxious experiences and write them down in a diary. The child is asked to focus on the physical reactions to experiences and to record them as well.

Session 4

Once the child has learned to identify the physical symptoms related to the anxiety, the therapist can teach the child relaxation exercises using the physical reactions as cues. The exercises developed by Koeppen (1974) and Ollendick (1978), mentioned earlier in this chapter, provide relaxation scripts which can be used by the therapist to teach deep muscle relaxation. The STIC task for the child after Session 4 is to practice the relaxation exercises at home, and to keep a record in a diary of the beneficial aspects of the relaxation and any difficulties experienced with the exercises.

Session 5

The fifth session focuses on teaching children to recognize what they say to themselves when they are feeling anxious (i.e., identifying anxious cognitions). Kendall and colleagues (1992) call this self-

talk, and state that "self-talk includes the child's expectations and attributions about herself, others, and situations" (p. 84). According to Kendall and colleagues (1992), the expectations and attributions that the anxious child is experiencing "focus around catastrophic appraisals of future events, negative self-evaluation, perfectionistic standards for performance, heightened self-focused attention or concern about what others are thinking about her, concerns about failure or not coping adequately, and sometimes accompanying feelings of worthlessness" (p. 84). Once the child recognizes the self-talk they use in anxiety-provoking situations, he or she can begin to monitor and reduce the negative statements. The STIC task used with Session 5 includes asking the child to identify two anxiety-provoking situations during the week, and to record thoughts or self-talk.

Session 6

During the sixth session, the children are taught problem-solving skills and how to apply them in anxiety-provoking situations. The therapist may begin by choosing a situation or problem that does not produce anxiety, and ask the child to develop different strategies for dealing with the problem. Once the child has become comfortable with generating alternative solutions, the therapist may introduce more anxiety-provoking scenarios and let the child develop different ways to solve the problem. At this point in therapy, the therapist begins to develop an anxiety hierarchy to be used in Sessions 9 to 16. The STIC task for Session 6 requires the child to write down two anxiety-provoking experiences, and to identify the situation in which they occurred, the feelings that the child had during the experience, and the thoughts or self-talk used. This provides the child with a review of the tasks completed in the earlier sessions.

Session 7

The seventh session consists of the therapist helping children evaluate themselves and reward success or partial success. Kendall and colleagues (1992) suggest that anxious children can be perfectionistic and perceive success as "all or nothing." Therefore, it is important to teach an anxious child that success can include partial successes. The key here is for the child to see that how people evaluate their performance has a direct impact on how they feel (Kendall et al., 1992). To help the child identify rewards, the therapist and child can collaborate and make a list of rewards that may be used to self-reinforce when successful.

Session 8

The eighth session is a review of the concepts and skills learned during the first seven sessions. The anxious child reviews the four steps taught by the therapist including recognizing physical symptoms, recognizing self-talk, using problem-solving strategies, and using self-evaluation and self-reward. Kendall and colleagues (1992) suggest using an acronym such as FEAR to remind the child of the steps used in reducing anxiety. The letters in the acronym stand for the following:

> F—Feeling frightened? (recognizing physical symptoms of anxiety)
> E—Expecting bad things to happen? (recognizing self-talk and what you are worried about happening)
> A—Actions and attitudes that will help. (different behaviors and coping statements the child can use in the anxiety-provoking situation based on problem solving)
> R—Results and rewards. (self-evaluation and self-reward) (Kendall et al., 1992, p. 93)

Sessions 9–16

At this point in therapy, the therapist uses the anxiety hierarchy developed after Session 6 to present low levels of anxiety to the child and allow practice of the skills developed during the first part of the intervention. For each anxiety-provoking stimulus that is presented, the therapist and child examine the situation and rate it from 1 to 10 based on the level of anxiety, use coping approaches to deal with the anxiety, and evaluate and reward performance in the situation. As the child develops ability to deal with anxious situations, the therapist presents situations that provoke an increased level of anxiety. The presentation of the anxiety-provoking stimulus occurs first through images and then through in vivo exposure. The last session is used to discuss the therapy, to review the skills that were

developed, and to consider real-life situations that may occur outside therapy. The STIC tasks for the second half of the intervention require that the child practice FEAR skills outside the therapy sessions and record successful use of the skills, as well as any difficulties experienced. Toward the end of the intervention, the child develops a project to inform other children about anxiety and how to cope in anxious situations. Subjects who participated in Kendall's (1994) study developed projects such as commercials, poems, rap songs, radio spots, and TV commercials. A taped copy of this project was given to the child at the end of the intervention to take home and show to family and friends.

Kane and Kendall (1989) used the cognitive–behavioral treatment program outlined here to provide therapy for four children diagnosed with Overanxious Disorder. Treatment efficacy was demonstrated through parent reports, clinician ratings, and child self-reports. Follow-up data indicated that gains made during treatment were maintained for two of the children based on parent and child reports. The remaining two children continued to indicate improvement, although parent reports indicated some difficulties. In addition to the study conducted by Kane and Kendall (1989), Kendall (1994) conducted a study using the cognitive–behavioral treatment program to provide therapy for 47 children suffering from anxiety disorders. Results from the study indicated that the treatment program produced considerable change in the reported difficulties due to anxiety. Furthermore, treatment gains due to the cognitive–behavioral intervention were maintained at one-year follow-up.

March and Mulle (March & Mulle, 1995; March, Mulle, & Herbel, 1994) have developed a manual-based approach to treat Obsessive–Compulsive Disorder (OCD) in children and adolescents. Their treatment involves a series of steps over 16 weekly sessions. The first step involves an informational session on the first visit. During this session, OCD is placed within a medical model (i.e., a neurobehavioral disorder), which allows the therapist, child, and family to align against an illness, thus avoiding blaming the child and/or parent(s) for the disorder. A treatment rationale, framed in social learning theory, is also presented, as are definitions of relevant behavioral terminology. The next step, which typically occurs over Weeks 2 and 3, involves making or identifying the OCD as the problem. This is highlighted by having the child choose a "nasty nickname" for their OCD. A stimulus hierarchy is also generated during this step, and the child selects graded exposure targets. Next, during Weeks 4 to 16, the child is provided anxiety management training along with exposure and response prevention (E/PR) experiences. Anxiety management training focuses on relaxation techniques, diaphragmatic breathing, cognitive restructuring, and constructive self-talk. The intent of this training is to provide the child with a "tool kit" for dealing with the E/PR experiences. Each session during Weeks 4 to 16 includes review of the preceding week; a statement of goals; new information and selection of E/PR targets; within-session imaginal and/or in vivo E/PR; "nuts and bolts" practice; defining E/PR homework for the coming week; and, monitoring progress (March & Mulle, 1995). After the Week 16 session, there is a "graduation ceremony," which is followed by a booster session at a later date.

March and Mulle (1995) provide evidence that this manualized approach to providing cognitive–behavioral therapy has been successful in treating an 8-year-old female suffering from OCD. Within 11 weeks of treatment, there was complete resolution of OCD symptoms. These treatment gains were maintained at 6-month follow-up. Similarly, March and colleagues (1994) used this manualized approach to cognitive–behavioral psychotherapy with 15 children and adolescents with OCD. Analyses revealed a significant benefit for treatment immediately posttreatment and at follow-up. Nine participants experienced at least a 50% reduction in symptoms at posttreatment; six were asymptomatic. No participants relapsed at follow-up intervals.

Kendall and Southam-Gerow (1995) have suggested that there are advantages to using manual-based treatment programs such as those just described. These advantages include the methodological control the therapist has over the intervention, the ease of focusing training, and the verification of treatment integrity.

Generalization

Manual-based treatment programs are particularly sensitive to the generalization of skills learned in the sessions. Two approaches used to maximize generalization are parental involvement in treatment and the use of homework. Parental involvement can be an important component of the cognitive–behavioral therapy program for anxious children. In addition to providing parents with a greater understanding of the therapy, their participation allows the therapist to gather information about the child's functioning outside the sessions. In Kendall and colleagues' (1992) program, parents are more formally involved after their child has been seen for three sessions. During the last 15 minutes of Session 4, the therapist allows the parent to participate in a relaxation exercise with their child. This training provides parents with an opportunity to learn and practice techniques that may be used in helping their children with relaxation activities at home. To help generalize the skills learned in treatment to the home environment, it is suggested that parents read the relaxation script to the child while the child relaxes. The parent and child may also make a relaxation tape that recites the relaxation script and then practice relaxation together while listening to the tape. Or, the child could practice relaxation exercises alone using this tape, with the parent nearby to help if necessary. Parents should be encouraged to keep a diary with the child, recording when relaxation exercises are completed and who participated in the activity (parent, child, therapist). Near the end of the program (Sessions 15 and 16), the therapist discusses strategies with parents to help their child continue to generalize the learned skills outside of therapy.

Similarly, in March and Mulle's (1995) manualized treatment program parents are included at different stages of the intervention. During Week 1, parents participate in a session that focuses on eduction and treatment planning. Parents are also involved during Weeks 6 and 12, which are devoted to incorporating targets for parental response prevention or extinction.

Another important component of cognitive–behavioral treatment programs is the weekly homework assignments. These homework assignments help children practice the skills that they learn during the intervention program. Homework assignments provide the therapist with a tool with which to monitor progress throughout the 16-week intervention. If parents are aware of the assignments and understand them, they may be able to help their children complete the STIC task outside the session. In fact, after Session 8 in Kendall and colleagues' (1992) program, the child's homework assignment is to explain the FEAR steps to the parents. In addition to helping the child better understand and generalize these skills, making parents aware of these steps allows them to encourage their use in anxiety-provoking situations. By helping their child practice these steps, parents are facilitating the generalization of these coping skills. Kendall and colleagues (1992) note that many parents welcome the opportunity to help their child master the FEAR steps because they offer an alternative to unsuccessful strategies that may have been used in the past. In the treatment program described by March and Mulle (1995), weekly homework assignments are described on written information sheets for parents. Parents also receive written "tips" on how to manage their own behaviors with respect to their child's anxiety; these tips are keyed to the child's treatment goals.

Helping children recognize the signs of anxiety during the treatment sessions, practicing what is learned in the sessions outside the treatment setting through homework assignments, and involving parents in the treatment of their child's anxiety disorder all increase the likelihood of generalization beyond the treatment sessions.

Pharmacotherapy

In addition to the approaches described previously, drugs are often used in the treatment of anxiety. D.F. Klein, Rabkin, and Gorman (1985) reviewed eight studies comparing the effect of anxiolytics (i.e., antianxiety agents) versus antidepressants in the treatment of anxiety. The patients in these studies were adults and the participants formed a diagnostically heterogeneous group. D.F. Klein et al. (1985) concluded that no obvious superiority of either anxiolytics or antidepressants emerged in these studies. Nevertheless, they stated that since antidepressants were sometimes more and never less effective, they probably were the more active drug. However, they believed it was not possible, on the basis of their review, to recommend differentially prescribing one type of drug over the other for the treatment of anxiety. Gittelman and Koplewicz (1986) found a similar equivocal situation when reviewing the research concerning pharmacological treatment of childhood anxiety. Research both supports and contradicts the use of

anxiolytics in treating childhood anxiety, whereas antidepressants are effective in reducing depressive and anxious symptomatology. Readers interested in the pharmacological treatment of childhood anxiety are referred to Allen, Leonard, and Swedo (1995), Kutcher, Reiter, and Gardner (1995), and Bernstein (1994).

Plan Evaluation

Once an intervention has been selected and implemented, the clinician must demonstrate the effectiveness of the treatment. As treatment is occurring, the integrity of the treatment plan must be evaluated. In the March and Mulle (1995) study, one of the investigators provided treatment, while the other reviewed the weekly goals of the treatment plan and evaluated whether these goals were being addressed. In terms of the interventions described in the previous section, the same measures used to diagnose the individual with an anxiety disorder typically are used in posttreatment comparisons to evaluate effectiveness. Self-report measures, parent and teacher reports, and structured interviews all may be used to measure treatment efficacy.

Self-report measures can be administered to children to assess the child's level of improvement during treatment and after the intervention has been completed. In his study examining the effectiveness of his cognitive–behavioral treatment program, Kendall (1994) used the RCMAS as well as Trait and State scales of the STAIC to measure anxiety at pretreatment and posttreatment. Other self-report measures used in this study included the FSSC–R, the Coping Questionnaire for Children (CQ–C), the CDI, and the NASSQ. Results from these self-report measures indicated a decrease in anxiety symptoms posttreatment.

Parent and teacher reports may also be used in the evaluation of treatment efficacy. In conjunction with child reports, parent reports may provide a more complete picture of treatment gains, and/or parent satisfaction with the treatment. Similar to child self-reports, parent reports may be used to compare child behavior before and after the intervention. Kendall (1994) used the internalizing score from the CBCL, and the trait anxiety scales from the State–Trait Anxiety Inventory for Children–Parent form (STAIC–P). Teacher reports of anxiety will be specific to the classroom, academics, and the school evironment, and will provide the clinician with a viewpoint in addition to that of the parents. In order to obtain information from the teacher, Kendall (1994) utilized the internalizing score from Teacher Rating Form.

It is to be expected that, even after treatment, the child will not be able to deal effectively with every anxiety-producing stimulus. Ollendick and Cerny (1981) acknowledge that maintenance and generalization of interventions do not occur spontaneously. The clinician needs to be aware of this and to prepare the child for "life after treatment." The focus of treatment, to help the child overcome anxieties, will not generalize to all situations in which they face anxiety outside the therapy session. The goal of the cognitive–behavioral treatment program described earlier (Kendall et al., 1992) is to teach the child how to cope when confronted with anxiety-provoking situations. Kendall and colleagues (1992) suggest that early in the intervention process children should be taught, and reminded, that once therapy ends the problem is not automatically cured; there is effort involved after therapy to maintain the skills that have been learned. Throughout treatment, children should be taught to evaluate, monitor, and regulate their own behavior outside the therapy situation (Ollendick & Cerny, 1981). The treatment protocol developed by Kendall et al. (1989) instituted the FEAR plan to prepare children to assess and monitor their behavior after treatment. The FEAR plan is designed to help children consider alternatives and choose appropriate solutions in anxiety-producing situations. Practicing the four steps in the FEAR plan during therapy sessions, as well as in everyday situations, helps maintain and generalize skills (Kendall et al., 1992).

It is inevitable that the child will experience failure and make mistakes during and after treatment. The clinician can use these setbacks as opportunities to teach the child that learning occurs through mistakes and failures, as well as through success. Kendall and colleagues (1992) encourage the examination of errors in the therapy process to help children identify different ways to solve problems, and to allow the child to practice learned coping strategies.

It may be necessary for the clinician to meet with the child after treatment has been terminated to provide continued support. The final therapy session does not mean that further contact with the child will not be necessary. Children should know that the therapist is available if they need further help in dealing with anxiety difficulties (Kendall et al., 1992). Posttreatment contact may sometimes be referred to as a booster session. Booster sessions allow the therapist to evaluate the progress made by the child since the termination of therapy sessions. Specific to the cognitive–behavioral treatment program provided by Kendall and colleagues (1992), booster sessions may be used to review the steps in the FEAR plan. Kendall and colleagues (1992) identify two situations in which booster sessions are recommended. The first is when the child has encountered a difficult situation in which they need outside help to problem solve. The child may be led through the problem-solving steps by the therapist to gain a better understanding of the situation. In addition, modeling, role-plays, and further experience with problem solving should be part of the booster session (Kendall et al., 1992). The second situation in which a booster session takes place is when the therapist takes a proactive stance and provides support before the anxiety-producing event takes place. In this instance, the therapist helps the child problem solve and generate solutions for an anticipated problem.

The more similar the therapy experiences are to anticipated posttreatment experiences, the more likely maintenance and generalization will occur (Ollendick & Cerny, 1981). Practice during the therapy session is necessary for the development of skills. In addition to practice, use of stimuli in the therapy session that are likely to be encountered in everyday situations will help the child generalize skills across settings (Ollendick & Cerny, 1981).

Concluding Remarks

The past decade has seen significant progress made in our understanding of the nature of anxiety disorders among children. In addition to a clearer symptom picture, there is the recognition that children are susceptible to many of the anxiety problems experienced by adults. With a clearer understanding of the symptoms associated with anxiety, there have been several studies examining the prevalence of various anxiety disorders among children. We also know more about the detrimental effects of anxiety on children's functioning.

Despite these important gains in the description of anxiety disorders, there is much to be done in the area of treatment. Although treatment of children with anxiety disorders or anxiety-related problems occurs daily in clinics, schools, and other settings, relatively few treatment studies exist in the literature. There are several possible explanations for this state of affairs. First, practitioners may not have the time or inclination to systematically collect data regarding the effectiveness of their interventions. It is hoped that this is not the case, since evaluation of treatment efficacy would dictate some form of accountability in regard to intervention implementation. If evaluation is not intrinsically motivated, soon managed health care may dictate such accountability.

Another possible explanation for the scarcity of treatment studies in the literature may be an "eclectic" approach to intervention. Certainly, the child's improvement is the focus of any treatment activity. Rather than adhere to any one approach, clinicians may borrow from several approaches that they feel will benefit the child. Cognitive–behavioral therapy demonstrates the value of combining treatment philosophies. Although this is a defensible approach to treatment, again, we would hope that some form of evaluation would be included as part of any treatment program. Subjective feelings on the part of the clinician that the child is "getting better" may not satisfy parents, teachers, insurance companies, or the child. Regardless of the philosophical or theoretical orientation of the clinician, some means of empirically testing the hypothesis that the child will improve as a result of treatment should be included in the treatment plan.

It is likely that some treatment studies are not included in the literature because they are difficult to do. The majority of existing studies that do appear in the child anxiety literature are single subject designs. In addition to making sense, especially when dealing with specific phobias, single subject studies are easier to design and implement methodologically. Well-controlled group studies demand resources that may not be available to many clinicians. A matched control group and a waiting list group, in addition to the treatment group, are typically needed to demonstrate the efficacy of group interventions. The number of participants necessary to conduct such research may be prohibitive in many situations. Perhaps screening activities, such as those outlined by Laurent, Hadler and colleagues (1994), provided in school settings, would allow identification of children who suffer from elevated levels of anxiety. These children, although perhaps not experiencing levels of anxiety significant enough to receive a *DSM-IV* diagnosis, likely would benefit from treatment. A school screening program might provide large enough numbers of students suffering from anxiety to conduct group treatment studies. The manualized treatment approaches provided by Kendall and colleagues (1992) and March and Mulle (1995; March et al., 1994) are potentially useful resources in providing therapy in such settings. In addition, manualized treatment approaches may promote research with children suffering from anxiety, because they provide a structured framework for intervention.

It is likely that interest in childhood anxiety will continue to grow. In addition to studies examining characteristics of children suffering from various anxiety disorders, it is hoped that those working with these children will share their successes with others working with these youngsters.

References

Achenbach, T.M. (1980). DSM-III in light of empirical research on the classification of child psychopathology. *Journal of the American Academy of Child Psychiatry, 19,* 395–412.

Achenbach, T.M. (1991a). *Manual for the CBCL/4-18 and 1991 profile.* Burlington, VT: University Associates in Psychiatry.

Achenbach, T.M. (1991b). *Manual for the TRF and 1991 profile.* Burlington, VT: University Associates in Psychiatry.

Achenbach, T.M., & Edelbrock, C. (1983). *Manual for the Child Behavior Checklist.* Burlington, VT: University of Vermont Department of Psychiatry.

Achenbach, T.M., & Edelbrock, C. (1986). *Manual for the Teacher's Report Form.* Burlington, VT: University of Vermont Department of Psychiatry.

Achenbach, T.M., McConaughy, S.H., & Howell, C.T. (1987). Child/adolescent behavioral and emotional problems: Implications of cross-informant correlations for situational specificity. *Psychological Bulletin, 101,* 213–232.

Acierno, R., Hersen, M., Van Hasselt, V.B., Tremont, G., & Meuser, K.T. (1994). Review of the validation and dessemination of eye-movement desensitization and reprocessing: A scientific and empirical dilemma. *Clinical Psychology Review, 14,* 287–299.

Agras, S., Sylvester, D., & Oliveau, D. (1969). The epidemiology of common fears and phobias. *Comprehensive Psychiatry, 10,* 151–156.

Alessi, G.J. (1980). Behavioral observation for the school psychologist: Reponsive-discrepancy model. *School Psychology Review, 9,* 31–45.

Allen, A.J., Leonard, H., & Swedo, S.E. (1995). Current knowledge of medications for the treatment of childhood anxiety disorders. *Journal of the American Academy of Child and Adolescent Psychiatry, 34,* 976–986.

Ambrosini, P.J., Metz, C., Prabucki, K., & Lee, J. (1989). Videotape reliability of the third revised edition of the KSADS. *Journal of the American Academy of Child and Adolescent Psychiatry, 28,* 723–728.

American Psychiatric Association. (1980). *Diagnostic and statistical manual of mental disorders* (3rd ed.). Washington, DC: Author.

American Psychiatric Association. (1987). *Diagnostic and statistical manual of mental disorders* (3rd ed., rev.). Washington, DC: Author.

American Psychiatric Association. (1994). *Diagnostic and statistical manual of mental disorders* (4th ed.). Washington, DC: Author.

Anderson, J.C., Williams, S., McGee, R., & Silva, P.A. (1987). DSM-III disorders in preadolescent children. *Archives of General Psychiatry, 44,* 69–76.

Bandura, A. (1977). *Social learning theory.* Englewood Cliffs, NJ: Prentice Hall.

Beck, A.T. (1971). Cognition, affect, and psychopathology. *Archives of General Psychiatry, 24,* 495–500.

Beck, A.T. (1976). *Cognitive therapy and the emotional disorders.* New York: International Universities Press.

Beck, A.T., & Emery, G. (1985). *Anxiety disorders and phobias: A cognitive perspective.* New York: Basic Books.

Beck, A.T., Brown, G., Eidelson, J.I., Steer, R.A., & Riskind, J.H. (1987). Differentiating anxiety and depression: A test of the cognitive content-specificity hypothesis. *Journal of Abnormal Psychology, 96,* 179–183.

Beidel, D.C. (1991). Determining the reliability of psychophysiological assessment in childhood anxiety. *Journal of Anxiety Disorders, 5,* 139–150.

Bernstein, G.A. (1994). Psychopharmacological interventions. In T.H. Ollendick, N.J. King, & W. Yule (Eds.), *International handbook of phobic and anxiety disorders in children and adolescents* (pp. 439–451). New York: Plenum.

Bowen, R.C., Offord, D.R., & Boyle, M.H. (1990). The prevalence of overanxious disorder and separation anxiety disorder: Results from the Ontario Child Health Study. *Journal of the American Academy of Child and Adolescent Psychiatry, 29,* 753–758.

Brady, E.U., & Kendall, P.C. (1992). Comorbidity of anxiety and depression in children and adolescents. *Psychological Bulletin, 111,* 244–255.

Christensen, A., Margolin, G., & Sullaway, M. (1992). Interparental agreement on child behavior problems. *Psychological Assessment, 4,* 419–425.

Costello, E.J., & Angold, A. (1995). Epidemiology. In J.S. March (Ed.), *Anxiety disorders in children and adolescents* (pp. 109–124). New York: Guilford.

Dadds, M.R., Rapee, R.M., & Barrett, P.M. (1994). Behavioral observation. In T.H. Ollendick, N.J. King, & W. Yule (Eds.), *International handbook of phobic and anxiety disorders in children and adolescents* (pp. 349–364). New York: Plenum.

Daugherty, T.K., & Shapiro, S.K. (1994). Behavior checklists and rating forms. In T.H. Ollendick, N.J. King, & W. Yule (Eds.), *International handbook of phobic and anxiety disorders in children and adolescents* (pp. 331–347). New York: Plenum.

Delprato, D.J., & McGlynn, F.D. (1984). Behavioral theories of anxiety disorders. In S.M. Turner (Ed.), *Behavioral theories and treatment of anxiety* (pp. 1–49). New York: Plenum.

Ellis, A. (1962). *Reason and emotion in psychotherapy.* New York: Stuart.

Finch, A.J., Jr., & McIntosh, J.A. (1990). Assessment of anxieties and fears in children. In A.M. LaGreca (Ed.), *Through the eyes of the child: Obtaining self-reports from children and adolescents* (pp. 234–258). Boston: Allyn & Bacon.

Francis, G., & Beidel, D. (1995). Cognitive–behavioral psychotherapy. In J.S. March (Ed.), *Anxiety disorders in children and adolescents* (pp. 321–340). New York: Guilford.

Gittelman, R., & Koplewicz, H.S. (1986). Pharmacotherapy of childhood anxiety disorders. In R. Gittelman (Ed.), *Anxiety disorders of childhood* (pp. 188–203). New York: Guilford.

Goldstein, A.J., & Feske, U. (1994). Eye movement desensitization and reprocessing for panic disorder: A case series. *Journal of Anxiety Disorders, 8,* 351–362.

Hart, K.J., & Morgan, J.R. (1993). Cognitive–behavioral procedures with children: Historical context and current status. In A.J. Finch, Jr., W.M. Nelson III, & E.S. Ott (Eds.), *Cognitive–behavioral procedures with children and adolescents: A practical guide.* Needham Heights, MA: Allyn & Bacon.

Hilgard, E.R., & Marquis, D.G. (1940). *Conditioning and learning.* New York: Appleton-Century.

Hodges, K., & Cools, J.N. (1990). Structured diagnostic interviews. In A.M. LaGreca (Ed.), *Through the eyes of the child: Obtaining self-reports from children and adolescents* (pp. 109–149). Boston: Allyn & Bacon.

Hodges, K., Kline, J., Stern, L., Cytryn, L., & McKnew, D. (1982). The development of a child assessment interview for research and clinical use. *Journal of Abnormal Child Psychology, 10,* 173–189.

Hoehn-Saric, E., Maisami, M., & Wiegand, D. (1987). Measurement of anxiety in children and adolescents using semistructured interviews. *Journal of the American Academy of Child and Adolescent Psychiatry, 26,* 541–545.

Jacobson, E. (1938). *Progressive relaxation.* Chicago: University of Chicago Press.

James, E.M., Reynolds, C.R., & Dunbar, J. (1994). Self-report instruments. In T.H. Ollendick, N.J. King, & W. Yule (Eds.), *International handbook of phobic and anxiety disorders in children and adolescents* (pp. 317–329). New York: Plenum.

Johnson, J.H., & McGlynn, F.D. (1988). Simple phobia. In M. Hersen & C.G. Last (Eds.), *Child behavior therapy casebook* (pp. 43–53). New York: Plenum.

Kane, M.T., & Kendall, P.C. (1989). Anxiety disorders in children: A multiple-baseline evaluation of a cognitive–behavioral treatment. *Behavior Therapy, 20,* 499–508.

Kendall, P.C. (1985). Toward a cognitive–behavioral model of child psychopathology and a critique of related interventions. *Journal of Abnormal Child Psychology, 13,* 357–372.

Kendall, P.C. (1990). *Coping cat workbook.* Temple University, Department of Psychology, Philadelphia, PA 19122.

Kendall, P.C. (1994). Treating anxiety disorders in children: Results of a randomized clinical trial. *Journal of Consulting and Clinical Psychology, 62,* 100–110.

Kendall, P.C., & Gosch, E.A. (1994). Cognitive–behavioral interventions. In T.H. Ollendick, N.J. King, & W. Yule (Eds.), *International handbook of phobic and anxiety disorders in children and adolescents* (pp. 415–438). New York: Plenum.

Kendall, P.C., & Ronan, K.R. (1990). Assessment of children's anxieties, fears, and phobias: Cognitive–behavioral models and methods. In C.R. Reynolds & R.W. Kamphaus (Eds.), *Handbook of psychological and educational assessment: Personality, behavior, and context* (pp. 223–244). New York: Guilford.

Kendall, P.C., & Southam-Gerow, M.A. (1995). Issues in the transportability of treatment: The case of anxiety disorders in youths. *Journal of Consulting and Clincial Psychology, 63,* 702–708.

Kendall, P.C., Kane, M.T., Howard, B., & Siqueland, L. (1989). *Cognitive–behavioral therapy for anxious children: Treatment manual.* Temple University, Department of Psychology, Philadelphia, PA 19122.

Kendall, P.C., Chansky, T.E., Kane, M.T., Kim, R.S., Kortlander, E., Ronan, K.R., Sessa, F.M., & Siqueland, L. (1992). *Anxiety disorders in youth: Cognitive-behavioral interventions.* Needham Heights, MA: Allyn & Bacon.

King, N.J. (1994). Physiological assessment. In T.H. Ollendick, N.J. King, & W. Yule (Eds.), *International handbook of phobic and anxiety disorders in children and adolescents* (pp. 365–379). New York: Plenum.

Klein, D.F., Rabkin, J.G., & Gorman, J.M. (1985). Etiological and pathophysiological inferences from the pharmacological treatment of anxiety. In A.H. Tuma & J. Maser (Eds.), *Anxiety and the anxiety disorders* (pp. 501–532). Hillsdale, NJ: Erlbaum.

Klein, R.G. (1991). Parent–child agreement in clinical assessment of anxiety and other psychopathology: A review. *Journal of Anxiety Disorders, 5,* 187–198.

Koeppen, A.S. (1974). Relaxation training for children. *Elementary School Guidance and Counseling, 9,* 14–21.

Kovacs, M. (1980/1981). Rating scales to assess depression in school-aged children. *Acta Paedopsychiatrica, 46,* 305–315.

Kutcher, S., Reiter, S., & Gardner, D. (1995). Pharmacotherapy: Approaches and applications. In J.S. March (Ed.), *Anxiety disorders in children and adolescents* (pp. 341–385). New York: Guilford.

Lachman, R., & Lachman, J.L. (1986). Information processing psychology: Origins and extensions. In R.E. Ingram (Ed.), *Information processing approaches to clinical psychology* (pp. 23–49). San Diego, CA: Academic.

LaGreca, A.M. (1990). Issues and perspectives on the child assessment process. In A.M. LaGreca (Ed.), *Through the eyes of the child: Obtaining self-reports from children and adolescents* (pp. 3–17). Needham Heights, MA: Allyn & Bacon.

LaGreca, A.M., & Stone, W.L. (1993). Social Anxiety Scale for Children–Revised: Factor structure and concurrent validity. *Journal of Clinical Child Psychology, 22,* 17–27.

Lapouse, R., & Monk, M.A. (1959). Fears and worries in a representative sample of children. *American Journal of Orthopsychiatry, 29,* 803–818.

Last, C.G., Hersen, M., Kazdin, A.E., Finkelstein, R., & Strauss, C.C. (1987). Comparison of DSM-III separation anxiety and overanxious disorders: Demographic characteristics and patterns of comorbidity. *Journal of the American Academy of Child and Adolescent Psychiatry, 26,* 527–531.

Laurent, J., & Stark, K.D. (1993). Testing the cognitive content-specificity hypothesis with anxious and depressed youngsters. *Journal of Abnormal Psychology, 102,* 226–237.

Laurent, J., Landau, S., & Stark, K.D. (1993). Conditional probabilities in the diagnosis of depressive and anxiety disorders in children. *School Psychology Review, 22,* 98–114.

Laurent, J., Hadler, J.R., & Stark, K.D. (1994). A multiple-stage screening procedure for the identification of childhood anxiety disorders. *School Psychology Quarterly, 9,* 239–255.

Laurent, J., Potter, K., & Catanzaro, S.J. (1994, March). *Assessing positive and negative affect in children: The development of the PANAS–C.* Paper presented at the 26th annual convention of the National Association of School Psychologists, Seattle, WA.

Loeber, R., Green, S.M., & Lahey, B.B. (1990). Mental health professionals' perception of the utility of children, mothers, and teachers as informants on childhood pathology. *Journal of Clinical Child Psychology, 19,* 136–143.

March, J.S., & Mulle, K. (1995). Manualized cognitive–behavioral psychotherapy for obsessive–compulsive disorder in childhood: A preliminary single case study. *Journal of Anxiety Disorders, 9,* 175–184.

March, J.S., Mulle, K., & Herbel, B. (1994). Behavioral psychotherapy for children and adolescents with obsessive–compulsive disorder: An open trial of a new protocol driven treatment package. *Journal of the American Academy of Child and Adolescent Psychiatry, 33,* 333–341.

McCarthy, P.R., & Foa, E.B. (1988). Obsessive–compulsive disorder. In M. Hersen & C.G. Last (Eds.), *Child behavior therapy casebook* (pp. 55–69). New York: Plenum.

Moreau, D.L., & Weissman, M.M. (1993). Anxiety symptoms in nonpsychiatrically referred children and adolescents. In C.G. Last (Ed.), *Anxiety across the lifespan: A developmental perspective* (pp. 37–62). New York: Springer.

Mowrer, O.H. (1939). A stimulus–response analysis of anxiety and its role as a reinforcing agent. *Psychological Review, 46,* 553–565.

Muris, P., & Merckelbach, H. (1995). Treating spider phobia with eye-movement desensitization and reprocessing: Two case reports. *Journal of Anxiety Disorders, 9,* 439–449.

Newcomer, P.L., Barenbaum, E.M., & Bryant, B.R. (1994). *Depression and Anxiety in Youth Scale.* Austin, TX: PRO-ED.

Ollendick, T.H. (1978). *Relaxation techniques with hyperactive, aggressive children.* Unpublished manuscript, Indiana State University.

Ollendick, T.H. (1983). Reliability and validity of the Revised Fear Survey Schedule for Children (FSSC–R). *Behaviour Research and Therapy, 21,* 685–692.

Ollendick, T.H., & Cerny, J.A. (1981). *Clinical behavior therapy with children.* New York: Plenum.

Ollendick, T.H., & Francis, G. (1988). Behavioral assessment and treatment of childhood phobias. *Behavior Modification, 12,* 165–204.

Orvaschel, H. (1985). Psychiatric interviews suitable for research with children and adolescents. *Psychopharmacology Bulletin, 21,* 737–745.

Peterson, R.A., & Reiss, S. (1987). *Anxiety sensitivity index manual.* Palos Heights, IL: International Diagnostic Systems.

Puig-Antich, J., & Ryan, N. (1986). *Schedule for Affective Disorders and Schizophrenia for School-Age Children* (4th working draft). Pittsburgh, PA: Western Psychiatric Institute and Clinic.

Quay, H.C., & Peterson, D.R. (1987). *Manual for the Revised Behavior Problem Checklist.* Coral Gables, FL: Author.

Reiss, S. (1980). Pavlovian conditioning and human fear: An expectancy model. *Behavior Therapy, 11,* 380–396.

Reiss, S. (1987). Theoretical perspectives on the fear of anxiety. *Clinical Psychology Review, 7,* 585–596.

Reynolds, C.R., & Richmond, B.O. (1978). What I think and feel: A revised measure of children's manifest anxiety. *Journal of Abnormal Child Psychology, 6,* 271–280.

Reynolds, C.R., & Richmond, B.O. (1985). *Revised Children's Manifest Anxiety Scale (RCMAS) manual.* Los Angeles: Western Psychological Services.

Ronan, K.R., Kendall, P.C., & Rowe, M. (1994). Negative affectivity in children: Development and validation of a self-statement questionnaire. *Cognitive Therapy and Research, 18,* 509–528.

Shaffer, D. (1986). Learning theories of anxiety. In R. Gittelman (Ed.), *Anxiety disorders of childhood* (pp. 157–167). New York: Guilford.

Shapiro, F. (1989a). Efficacy of the eye movement desensitization procedure in the treatment of traumatic memories. *Journal of Traumatic Stress, 2,* 199–223.

Shapiro, F. (1989b). Eye movement desensitization: A new treatment for posttraumatic stress disorder. *Journal of Behavior Therapy and Experimental Psychiatry, 20,* 211–217.

Shapiro, F. (1991). The eye movement desensitization and reprocessing procedure: From EMD to EMDR—A new treatment for anxiety and related traumata. *Behavior Therapist, 14,* 133–136.

Silverman, W.K. (1994). Structured diagnostic interviews. In T.H. Ollendick, N.J. King, & W. Yule (Eds.), *International handbook of phobic and anxiety disorders in children and adolescents* (pp. 293–315). New York: Plenum.

Silverman, W.K., & Albano, A.M. (1995). *Anxiety Disorders Interview Schedule for DSM-IV: Parents & Child Version* (ADIS-P & C). San Antonio: Psychological Corporation.

Silverman, W.K., Fleisig, W., Rabian, B., & Peterson, R. (1991). The Childhood Anxiety Sensitivity Index. *Journal of Clinical Child Psychology, 20,* 162–168.

Spielberger, C.D. (1973). *Preliminary manual for the State–Trait Anxiety Inventory for Children ("How I Feel Questionnaire").* Palo Alto, CA: Consulting Psychologists Press.

Strauss, C.C. (1991). Assessment of anxiety in children. In R.J. Prinz (Ed.), *Advances in behavioral assessment of children and families* (Vol. 5, pp. 83–111). London: Jessica Kingsley.

Strauss, C.C., Frame, C.L., & Forehand, R. (1987). Psychosocial impairment associated with anxiety in children. *Journal of Clinical Child Psychology, 16,* 235–239.

Strauss, C.C., Lahey, B.B., Frick, P., Frame, C.L., & Hynd, G.W. (1988). Peer social status of children with anxiety disorders.

Journal of Consulting and Clinical Psychology, 56, 137–141.

Tomarken, A.J. (1995). A psychometric perspective on psychophysiological measures. *Psychological Assessment, 7,* 387–395.

Vasey, M.W. (1993). Development and cognition in childhood anxiety: The example of worry. In T.H. Ollendick & R. Prinz (Eds.), *Advances in clinical child psychology* (Vol. 15, pp. 1–39). New York: Plenum.

Vasey, M.W., Crnic, K.A., & Carter, W.G. (1994). Worry in childhood: A developmental perspective. *Cognitive Therapy and Research, 18,* 529–549.

Watson, D., & Clark, L.A. (1984). Negative affectivity: The disposition to experience aversive emotional states. *Psychological Bulletin, 96,* 465–490.

Watson, D., Clark, L.A., & Tellegen, A. (1988). Development and validation of brief measures of positive and negative affect: The PANAS scales. *Journal of Personality and Social Psychology, 54,* 1063–1070.

Watson, J.B., & Rayner, R. (1920). Conditioned emotional reactions. *Journal of Experimental Psychology, 3,* 1–14.

Werry, J.S., & Quay, H.C. (1971). The prevalence of behavior symptoms in younger elementary school children. *American Journal of Orthopsychiatry, 41,* 136–143.

Wirt, R.D., Lachar, D., Klinedinst, J.K., & Seat, P.D. (1984). *Multidimensional description of child personality: A manual for the Personality Inventory for Children.* Los Angeles: Western Psychological Services.

Wolfe, V.V., Finch, A.J., Jr., Saylor, C.F., Blount, R.L., Pallmeyer, T.P., & Carek, D.J. (1987). Negative affectivity in children: A multitrait-multimethod investigation. *Journal of Consulting and Clinical Psychology, 55,* 245–250.

Wolpe, J. (1958). *Psychotherapy by reciprocal inhibition.* Stanford, CA: Stanford University Press.

Bibliography

Gittelman, R. (Ed.). (1986). *Anxiety disorders of childhood.* New York: Guilford. This is one of the first contemporary books devoted to childhood anxiety disorders, and forms the foundation of much of the work that has occurred over the past 10 years. Many of the authors of this volume are still influential in the field of childhood anxiety disorders.

Kendall, P.C., Chansky, T.E., Kane, M.T., Kim, R.S., Kortlander, E., Ronan, K.R., Sessa, F.M., & Siqueland, L. (1992). *Anxiety disorders in youth: Cognitive–behavioral interventions.* Boston: Allyn & Bacon. A well-articulated guide to cognitive–behavioral interventions with children who suffer from anxiety. This book provides chapters on the cognitive–behavioral perspective on treatment, assessment, and diagnostic issues, an integrated approach to treatment, and case illustrations. Chapters dealing with treatment results, maintenance, and working with families are also provided.

March, J. (Ed.). (1995). *Anxiety disorders in children and adolescents.* New York: Guilford.

Ollendick, T.H., King, N.J., & Yule, W. (Eds.). (1994). *International handbook of phobic and anxiety disorders in children and adolescents.* New York: Plenum. Successors to Gittelman's (1986) work, these texts provide the most recent perspective on anxiety disorders in youth.

Reynolds, W.M. (Ed.) (1992). *Internalizing disorders in children and adolescents*. New York: Wiley. A book dealing with internalizing disorders (i.e., anxiety and depression) among youth more generally. Several chapters are devoted to anxiety disorders. The juxtaposition of anxiety and depressive disorders nicely captures the comorbidity issues that exist in the literature today.

A Behavior Analytic Approach for Treating Depression

T. STEUART WATSON AND SHERI L. ROBINSON

Introduction

The interest in mood disorders among children has ballooned in the past 15 years as evidenced by the increase in published articles addressing the issue. Amid the surge of interest has been controversy, however. Specifically, proponents of psychoanalytic theory have questioned the existence of mood disorders in children due to their lack of a developed superego (Digdon & Gotlib, 1985), while others have contended that if mood disorders do exist in children, then they are "masked" in the form of other problem behaviors, such as aggression or anxiety (Cytryn & McKnew, 1974; Hammen & Compas, 1994). The current popular view of childhood mood disorders contends that the essential features of depression are similar among children, adolescents, and adults with allowances for developmental differences (Kazdin, 1990).

Mood disturbances encompass a variety of symptoms and disorders including major depressive disorder, dysthymia, bipolar disorder, and cyclothymia. Because there is no diagnosis by treatment interaction, this chapter focuses on depressive *behaviors* exhibited by children, regardless of the diagnosis. That said, however, understanding diagnosis is critical for behavior therapists who may be called on to defend their diagnosis before a managed care review panel or to secure necessary ancillary services for their client.

Diagnosis

Diagnosis of childhood depression and related disorders are most frequently rendered using criteria outlined in the *Diagnostic and Statistical Manual of Mental Disorders* (*DSM-IV;* American Psychiatric Association, 1994) under the major category of Mood Disorders. Other criteria such as the Weinberg criteria (Weinberg, Rutman, Sullivan, Penick, & Dietz, 1973) for childhood depression and the Research Diagnostic Criteria (RDC; Spitzer, Endicott, & Robins, 1978) are also used for research and clinical purposes. In general, the term childhood depression in this chapter will be used to describe *depressive behaviors* as well as the clinical diagnoses of Major Depressive Disorder (MDD) and Dysthymic Disorder (DD) identified in the *DSM-IV.* According to *DSM-IV,* five out of nine identified symptoms must be present, one of which must be depressed mood or loss of interest or pleasure, for at least two weeks in order to receive a diagnosis of MDD (see Table 1). Dysthymic disorder is characterized by an overall depressed mood that is chronic but with less severe symptoms than found with MDD. Similar symptoms are included in the Weinberg criteria and RDC criteria (see Tables 2 and 3); however, the Weinberg criteria are less stringent and less exclusionary than *DSM* criteria.

Unfortunately, for those hoping to make exact diagnoses, differential diagnosis using *DSM* criteria

T. STEUART WATSON AND SHERI L. ROBINSON • School Psychology Program, Mississippi State University, Mississippi State, Mississippi 39762.

Handbook of Child Behavior Therapy, edited by Watson and Gresham. Plenum Press, New York, 1998.

TABLE 1. Summary of *DSM-IV* Symptoms for Major Depressive Episode

At least five of the following symptoms present for the same 2-week period. One of the symptoms must be either (a) depressed mood or (b) loss of interest or pleasure.

1. Depressed or irritable mood most of the day, nearly every day.
2. Markedly diminished interest or pleasure in all or most activities.
3. Significant weight loss or gain or failure to make expected weight gains, or decrease or increase in appetite most days.
4. Insomnia or hypersomnia most days.
5. Psychomotor agitation or retardation most days which is observable by others.
6. Fatigue or loss of energy most days.
7. Feelings of worthlessness or excessive or inappropriate guilt most days.
8. Diminished ability to think or concentrate or indecisiveness most days.
9. Recurrent thoughts of death, suicidal ideation with or without a plan, or a suicide attempt.

Note: From *Diagnostic and Statistical Manual of Mental Disorders* (4th ed.) (p. 327). American Psychiatric Association, 1994, Washington, DC: Author. Copyright 1994 by American Psychiatric Association. Adapted by permission.

TABLE 2. Summary of Weinberg Criteria for Childhood Depression

Both dysphoric mood and self-deprecatory ideation must be present.

1. Dysphoric mood
2. Self-deprecatory ideation

Two or more of the following symptoms must be present.
3. Aggressive behavior (agitation)
4. Sleep disturbance
5. Change in school performance
6. Diminished socialization
7. Change in attitude toward school (negative attitude)
8. Somatic complaints
9. Loss of usual energy
10. Unusual change in appetite and/or weight

Note: From *Assessment and Treatment of Depression in Children and Adolescents* (2nd ed.) (pp. 24–25), by Harvey F. Clarizio, 1994, Brandon, VT: Clinical Psychology Publishing Co. Copyright 1994 by John Wiley & Sons.

TABLE 3. Summary of Research Diagnostic Criteria Symptoms for Major Depressive Disorder

Five or more of the following symptoms for definite and four for probable must be present.

1. Poor appetite or weight loss or increased appetite and weight gain.
2. Sleep difficulty or sleeping too much.
3. Loss of energy, fatigability, or tiredness.
4. Psychomotor agitation or retardation.
5. Loss of interest or pleasure in usual activities.
6. Feeling of self-reproach or excessive or inappropriate guilt.
7. Complaints or evidence of diminished ability to think or concentrate, such as slowed thinking or indecisiveness.
8. Recurrent thoughts of death or suicide, or any suicidal behavior.

Note: From "Research Diagnostic Criteria," by Robert Spitzer, Jean Endicott, and Eli Robins, 1978, *Archives of General Psychiatry, 35*, p. 776. Copyright 1978 by American Medical Association.

alone is complicated by symptom overlap with other disorders such as separation anxiety disorder, adjustment disorder, and bereavement. Fortunately for the behavior analyst, differential diagnoses among disorders is secondary and relatively unimportant, as effective treatment is not predicated by a diagnosis. From a behavioral perspective, depression is a term used to refer to *a set of specific behaviors and events that tend to occur together as opposed to a disease involving consistent internal/physiological/biochemical events with certain behavioral manifestations.* This is not to say that certain biochemical events (e.g., changes in serotonin availability/uptake) do not occur concurrently with depressive behavior. However, these biochemical changes are difficult or impossible to measure on a momentary basis and their role as causes of depressive behavior is not established. With the behavioral definition in mind, behavior analysts search for behaviors described in the *DSM* as well as additional behaviors and events (e.g., negative social interactions, lack of response contingent reinforcement) that may be related to the depressive behavior and that are important for treatment planning.

Prevalence

Determining the extent to which children experience depressive symptoms is largely confounded by (a) the variety of inventories, sources (e.g., parent, child), and criteria used for determining the presence of depression, (b) the lack of agreement on definition, and (c) populations studied (Kazdin, 1990). However, the majority of researchers addressing prevalence rates have identified subsamples of children experiencing relatively extreme degrees of depressive symptoms (i.e., 2 standard deviations above the mean on standardized measures), resulting in more homogenous populations. For example, Lefkowitz and Tesiny (1985) sampled 3,000 normal children, grades 3 through 5, using a peer-based measure, and found that 5.2% evidenced severe depression. In another study, 2% of children ages 7–12 years from the general population were identified as depressed, using *DSM* criteria, compared to clinical populations having prevalence rates ranging from 2% to 60%, with an average between 10% and 20% (Puig-Antich & Gittelman, 1982).

Differences in prevalence rates related to sex and age have also been identified. Although there is minimal support for sex differences for children ages 6–12 years, differences have been found among adolescents, with females diagnosed twice as often as males. With regard to age, in one study, 13% of children ages 9–12 years referred for treatment were diagnosed with depression compared to 1% of children ages 1–6 years (Kashani, Ray, &

Carlson, 1984). More recent studies conducted with adolescents and children indicate higher rates of depression at the time of the study and higher lifetime prevalence for adolescents (Garrison, Addy, Jackson, McKeown, & Waller, 1992; Lewinsohn, Hops, Roberts, Seeley, & Andrews, 1993). In addition, depression among preschoolers is considered rare, with prevalence increasing from grade school to adolescence (Clarizio, 1994).

Comorbidity

A wide range of disorders have been found to coexist with depression in children, including conduct disorder (Harrington, Fudge, Rutter, Pickles, & Hill, 1991; Puig-Antich, 1982), eating disorders (Hendren, 1983; Rastam, 1992; Smith & Steiner, 1992), Attention-Deficit/Hyperactive Disorder (ADHD; Biederman & Steingard, 1989; Biederman, Newcorn, & Sprich, 1991; Carlson & Cantwell, 1980; Milberger, Biederman, Faroane, Murphy, & Tsuang, 1995), substance abuse (Angold & Costello, 1993; Buckstein, Glancy, & Kaminer, 1992; Deykin, Levy, & Wells, 1987; Fleming & Offord, 1990), and anxiety disorders (Brady & Kendall, 1992; Kovacs, 1990; Kovacs et al., 1984). Reviews of existing literature have resulted in estimation of comorbidity rates of depression with other disorders. For example, Fleming and Offord (1990) found depressive disorders to coexist with behavioral disorders such as conduct disorder (17%–79%), oppositional defiant disorder (0%–50%), ADHD (0%–57%), and substance abuse (23%–25%). Rohde, Lewinsohn, and Seeley (1991) collapsed occurrences of conduct disorder and oppositional defiant disorder and found a comorbidity rate of 8% in depressed children compared to 1.6% of the nondepressed sample. Comorbidity rates of depressive and anxious symptoms are particularly high. Kovacs (1990) found that 30%–75% of depressed children and adolescents could also be diagnosed with anxiety disorders and that as many as 70% displayed anxiety symptoms. Brady and Kendall (1992) reported comorbidity rates of depression and anxiety among children ranging from 15.9% to 61.9%. It has even been suggested that anxiety and depression are not distinguishable in children and adolescents and attempts to do so do not result in different treatment protocols or outcomes (Finch, Lipovsky, & Casat, 1989).

It is often difficult to differentiate children presenting with depressive symptoms from other childhood problems such as learning disabilities, ADHD, and anxiety (Clarizio, 1994). Behaviors common among children identified as learning disabled and depressed include difficulty concentrating, poor academic performance, and poor social skills. Typically, anhedonia in children with learning disabilities is limited to school-related activities, whereas depressed children are more likely to report lack of enjoyment in most previously enjoyed activities across settings. Learning disabled children show a marked discrepancy between ability and achievement and the academic disability tends to be specific; no such relationship has been found in children diagnosed with depression. Finally, learning disabilities are usually identified before second grade. It is relatively rare for a child to be diagnosed with depression before the second grade. Similarly, ADHD is usually identified during the preschool or early elementary years (see Chapter 6).

Anxiety and depressive symptoms are perhaps the most difficult to differentiate. This is partially due to shared symptom criteria and poor discrimination on standardized measures; however, some differences have been noted. Anxious children are more likely to verbalize concerns about potential threats and future events whereas depressed children are more likely to make verbalizations regarding loss or failure. Although children with both diagnoses may display negative affect, depressed children are more likely to report anhedonia. Finally, children displaying anxious behaviors engage in an increase in activity in the form of escape or avoidance compared to depressed children who have an overall decrease in activity. In most cases of depressive symptoms in nondepressed populations, the symptoms tend to be mild, but chronic compared to the episodic nature of symptoms in depressed children. Because of the high degree of comorbidity and symptom overlap among children diagnosed with depression, one may prefer to view depression as a set of maladaptive behaviors that may or may not be functionally equivalent to, or members of the same response class with, other problem behaviors.

Etiology

Behavioral theories of childhood depression are derived from preexisting adult models that are concerned primarily with the analysis of overt behavior and verbalizations (Digdon & Gotlib, 1985). Reinforcement, learning, skill deficits, and environmental events preceding and following depressive behaviors provide the basis for behavioral etiology and treatment. Although several behavioral explanations of depression exist, the lack of or reduction in reinforcement plays a primary, though sometimes different, role in most of the explanations.

Loss or Reduction of Reinforcement

Lewinsohn (1974, 1975) proposed that depression is the result of a loss or reduction of reinforcement from the environment, which he referred to as response-contingent positive reinforcement (RCPR). RCPR refers to reinforcement that is the result of a child's actions and not merely the number of available reinforcers. In addition, RCPR is a function of *both* reinforcing activities and a child's interpersonal skills (i.e., the ability to evoke reinforcement and minimize punishment from the environment). Children who lack interpersonal skills not only receive less reinforcement, but the skill deficit may prevent the child from finding appropriate methods of handling problem situations and accessing alternative sources of reinforcement (Kennedy, Spence, & Hensley, 1989).

The change in rate of reinforcers may be slow and/or discrete. For example, a child may initially receive praise for a newly acquired academic skill, such as reading, but as time goes by, the parents no longer comment on the skill (reduction and removal of reinforcement). Conversely, the change in rate of reinforcement may also be due to the removal of a highly visible and pivotal reinforcer, as happens with parental attention due to divorce. Whether the change is discrete or overt, if the reinforcement is not reinstated, depressive symptoms may emerge. In addition, although in some situations such as divorce when short-term depressive behavior would be considered normal, the behaviors may be maintained by social attention or exacerbated by limiting opportunities to receive reinforcement from the environment over time (e.g., social withdrawal). Little research specifically addressing the theory has been conducted with children, but support for the model has been found in studies with depressed adults (e.g., Strack & Coyne, 1983; Youngren & Lewinsohn, 1980).

Social Skills Deficits

Another view of depression closely related to Lewinsohn's (1974) theory focuses entirely on the child's inability to evoke reinforcement from the environment due to a skill deficit. This differs from Lewinsohn's theory in that the problem lies not solely in the environmental situation (which is often out of the child's control), but in the child's lack of skill; however, social skills deficits may be an antecedent to a low rate of RCPR. The skill deficit may also prevent the child from avoiding or escaping negative interactions with others. Research specifically addressing the relationship between social skills and depression supports the premise that social skill deficits are related to childhood depression although causality cannot be assumed. For example, Wierzbicki and McCabe (1988) found that self- and parental reports of social skills were significantly related to the child's current level of depression and predictive of future depressive behaviors. In addition, a negative correlation has been found between peer popularity and depression (Jacobsen, Lahey, & Strauss, 1983; Lefkowitz & Tesiny, 1985). Kennedy and colleagues (1989) compared the social skills of depressed children (ages 8–12 years) to nondepressed children and identified specific interpersonal deficits among the depressed group. Results revealed that the depressed group reported lower levels of assertiveness and greater submissiveness (i.e., inability to escape negative interactions), poorer social skills, and were less popular than the nondepressed group. Finally, Altmann and Gotlib (1988) found that depressed children spent more time alone and less time interacting with peers. When they did interact with peers, depressed children engaged in more negative behaviors (e.g., aggression) than did their nondepressed peers. Thus, research supports the notion that social skills deficits (e.g., less assertive) or excesses (e.g., more aggressive) play a role in childhood depression because these deficits result in both peer rejection and withdrawal.

Self-Control Model

Rehm (1977) proposed a model of depression based on Kanfer's (1971) more general self-control theory. According to Rehm, depression is the result of three maladaptive self-regulatory processes: self-monitoring, self-evaluation, and self-reinforcement.

Self-monitoring is observing one's own behavior as well as antecedents and consequences surrounding the behavior. Rehm proposed that depressed children lack the ability to identify situations that result in reinforcement and those that result in punishment, and tend to selectively attend to poor outcomes and underestimate positive outcomes.

Self-evaluation refers to evaluating one's own behavior against a self-imposed standard of performance. According to Rehm's (1977) model, a child may lack the ability to appropriately evaluate his or her own behavior due to overly stringent expectations; this inability results in little self-reinforcement. For example, a child receives a 95% on a spelling test, but because his self-set goal is 100%, he may consider the still excellent grade a failure. By inappropriately evaluating his behavior, the child has denied himself reinforcement through the use of positive self-statements. However, it may also be the case that a child is extremely accurate in self-evaluation and becomes depressed due to failed expectations. For example, a child may evaluate her performance at soccer and determine that she is the worst player on the team. It is possible that she really is the worst player on the team. Treatment would then focus on possibly improving soccer skills or identifying other existing skills rather than changing the expectation.

A final feature of self-control theory is self-reinforcement. Self-reinforcement serves as a supplement to naturally occurring reinforcement and as immediate reinforcement when external reinforcers are not available. Rehm (1977) suggested that depression is related to too little self-reinforcement and too much self-punishment. This is evident in the example provided earlier regarding the expectation of perfect test performance. Not only did the child not self-reinforce (which would have been appropriate considering the grade), but he self-punished for not achieving his goal. This is not to suggest that when planning treatment with a depressed child one should simply lower expectations and goals, but instead one should help the child determine the appropriateness of goals and identify opportunities for reinforcement. We would be remiss not to mention that some behaviorists contend that the "self" cannot be reinforced, as in the term self-reinforcement. We conceptualize the term to mean self-administered reinforcers, which removes the negative connotations associated with the word "self".

Familial Interactions

There is evidence to suggest that parental behavior is related to childhood depression in a number of ways. First, parents who are depressed are more likely than nondepressed parents to have children with maladaptive behaviors including depressed symptoms (Brody & Forehand, 1986; Dodge, 1990; Downey & Coyne, 1990). Weissman, Fendrich, Warner, and Wickramaratne (1992) found that more than 50% of children of depressed parents were diagnosed with depression before the age of 20. Depressed mothers displayed more negative affect and less positive affect than nondepressed mothers when interacting with their children (Cole & Rehm, 1986; Garrison, Jackson, Marstellar, McKeown, & Addy, 1990; Goodman & Brumley, 1990). Second, depressed children regard their families more negatively than do normal peers and their families spend less time in recreational activities (Puig-Antich et al., 1993). Finally, researchers have found that poor family interactions were the strongest predictor of depression in children and adolescents (Cole & Rehm, 1986; Garrison et al., 1990; Goodman & Brumley, 1990). Specifically, mothers of depressed children have been found to provide fewer reinforcers for accomplishments, have higher standards for reinforcement, and were much more punitive than were controls.

Establishing causality poses the greatest difficulty in interpreting research findings of family interaction models. One could argue that there is little difference between the family interaction model and other models because it is difficult to determine whether the child's behavior evokes negative parental responses or if parental behaviors precede depressive behavior in children. The relationship between family interactions and childhood depression could be the result of (a) parental psychopathology (e.g., parental modeling of depressed behaviors), (b) poor parenting skills (e.g., detached, punitive, low rates of reinforcement), or (c) parental response to characteristics and behavior of the child (e.g., positive reinforcement of negative affect or removal/reduction of reinforcement due to unpleasant affect).

Learned Helplessness Model

Seligman's (1975) original model was developed through research with animals and adults leading to the conclusion that depressive symptoms were the result of learning that one's actions did not influence one's environment (i.e., learned helplessness). This model was later revised to focus on attributions, the way in which a depressed individual explains the causes of positive and negative events (Abramson, Seligman, & Teasdale, 1978). Although traditionally viewed as cognitive in nature, attributions can be explained behaviorally as intraverbal or rule governed behavior (i.e., what people say about their own behavior). There are three factors contributing to the revised helplessness model: (a) did the individual's behavior result in an outcome (internal), (b) will the cause of the outcome always exist (stable), and (c) did the cause affect all areas of a specific outcome (global). According to the model, people displaying depressive symptoms attribute negative events to internal, stable, and global factors, whereas positive events are attributed to external, transient, and specific factors. For example, if a depressed child flunks a test, she may make verbal statements that she flunked the test because she is stupid. Intelligence is internal, stable, and affects all academic areas. A nondepressed child who flunks a test may say he failed because the test was unfair. Someone else created the test (external), the next one could be better (transient), and it was just one test (specific). Although we are not particularly concerned with the attributions per se, we might target the negative verbalizations for change.

Developmental Differences and Considerations

Developmental issues must be taken into account when identifying depressive symptoms in children. Although the *DSM-IV* allows for some developmental differences in depression criteria for children and adults (e.g., irritability in children), it is important to have a clear understanding of child development. Certain behaviors in childhood may be unpleasant, but developmentally appropriate. For example, a preschool child who cries frequently is probably not suffering from depression, yet the same frequency and duration of the behavior may be considered a symptom of depression in an adolescent. The cognitive ability of a child must also be taken into account when attempting to diagnose a child with depression. Reports of guilt or hopelessness are less likely to be found among young children, who tend to be oriented in the present and to be concrete thinkers (Weiss et al., 1992). Young children may also lack the experience and verbal ability to report abstract, internalizing symptoms.

Differences in reported symptoms have been found between children and adolescents. For example, using a standardized diagnostic interview, Ryan and colleagues (1987) found that children displayed more overt depressed expressions and somatic complaints than did adolescents. Conversely, adolescents expressed greater hypersomnia, hopelessness, weight change, and suicide attempts. Kovacs and Gatsonis (1989) also found hypersomnia to be a distinguishing feature between adolescents and children, with adolescents seven times more likely to report hypersomnia than were children. Weiss and colleagues (1992) found a number of similarities as well as differences among 515 children and 515 adolescents diagnosed with depression. Children (ages 8–12) reported higher levels of anxiety than did adolescents (ages 13–16) and lower levels of irritability. Overall, symptoms of depression for children and adolescents are more alike than not, but important differences do exist that can be useful in determining behaviors that are developmentally appropriate and inappropriate.

Problem Identification

When children are referred for problems related to depression, the first job of the clinician is to determine suicide risk, especially in older children and adolescents. If the child is exhibiting suicidal ideation (e.g., preoccupation with death, plan for committing suicide), presuicidal behaviors (e.g., giving away possessions, overwhelming sense of hopelessness, sudden change in behavior or academic functioning) or has made a previous attempt to commit suicide, the clinician must take any necessary and appropriate steps to make certain that the child is safe until the risk of suicide is diminished.

If there is no suicide risk or after the risk has diminished, the clinician must then identify the specific behaviors of concern. To aid in this task, a number of tools are available to assist in both diagnosing and estimating frequency, severity, and duration of symptoms. In this section, we describe the most effective methods for identifying behaviors associated with problems of depression. The three

primary methods are interviews, rating scales, and behavioral observations. In some instances, permanent product data may be of assistance in identifying target behaviors and evaluating outcome.

Typically, we begin the problem identification process by first interviewing the parents and then interviewing the client (child). Then, we may use rating scales as an adjunct or supplement to our interview data. Occasionally, we use rating scales as a means of guiding our interviews with parents and children. We also include direct observations by parents, teachers, and/or clinicians wherever appropriate.

Parent Interview

We interview parents and, where appropriate, teachers, because (a) they are crucial sources of information in identifying depressive symptoms in children, (b) they are typically responsible for initial referrals based upon overt behavioral symptomology, (c) they are usually easily accessible and can describe the child's behavior across a variety of settings and situations, and (d) children rely on adult intervention because they most likely do not know symptoms of depression and may be unaware that they should tell someone about their symptoms (Kazdin, 1990). We begin parent interviews by first obtaining general information regarding social, developmental, medical, and academic histories.

Next, we ask specific questions regarding the immediate behaviors of concern, such as when the behavior was first noticed, in what situations the behavior occurs, and how often the behavior occurs. We are also careful to ask about corollary behaviors, such as changes in activity level, appetite, sleep patterns, overt expressions of sadness, and negative self-statements (what the layperson might refer to as low self-esteem), that parents may not realize are functionally related. At this point, we also begin asking analysis-type questions regarding the possible function of the behavior(s) and evocative stimuli so that during problem analysis we can test the hypothesized functions derived from the problem identification stage.

Child Interview

It is important to obtain self-report information because many symptoms are not easily observable and are subjective to the child. When gathering information from children, one must take into account a child's capability of accurately reporting the presence of symptoms. Children are better reporters of covert and intraverbal behavior, whereas parents and teachers tend to be more accurate reporters of overt behavior and are better able to estimate duration, frequency, and intensity of symptoms (Edelbrock, Costello, Dulcan, Conover, & Kalas, 1986; Shain, Naylor, & Alessi, 1990). Because children may have difficulty comprehending questions regarding the frequency, severity, and duration of affective responses (e.g., sadness, hopelessness, somatic complaints, negative self-statements), the clinician must ask questions that are concrete and situation specific (e.g., "When your parents reprimand you, what do you say to yourself?" or "How much of the time between breakfast and lunch does your stomach hurt?"). For many helpful guidelines on interviewing children, see Witt, Cavell, Heffer, Carey, and Martens (1988).

There are also many standardized interviews commonly used by both researchers and clinicians and these typically have parallel forms for child and parent (see for review, Kazdin, 1990). Format of the interviews varies from highly structured (i.e., less experience needed to administer) to semistructured (i.e., requires highly skilled professional). The Schedule for Affective Disorders and Schizophrenia for School-Age Children (K–SADS; Puig-Antich & Chambers, 1978), a modification of the Schedule for Affective Disorders and Schizophrenia (Endicott & Spitzer, 1978), is intended for use with children and adolescents ages 6 to 17 years. It is among the most widely used standardized interview for childhood depression. There are two versions of the K–SADS: an epidemiological version (K–SADS–E) and the Present Episode version (K–SADS–P). The K–SADS–E is intended to identify current symptoms and their onset. The K–SADS–P is used to identify symptoms at their worst in addition to severity of symptoms within the past week. It is composed of an unstructured section designed to gather information regarding chronicity of the problem and a semistructured section used to identify symptoms. The K–SADS has been found to be a reliable instrument for identifying symptoms of depression and conduct disorder (Kolvin et al., 1991). It is recommended that the parent be interviewed first in order to gain infor-

mation to guide and direct the interview with the child.

The Interview Schedule for Children (ISC; Kovacs, 1978) is a semistructured interview and, like the K–SADS, was originally developed for use in a research project with depressed children. Because the ISC is one of the few instruments developed specifically for research with depressed children, it has a high concentration of depressive symptoms and symptom duration items. The ISC is used to identify symptoms of depression in children ages 8 to 17 years, but is not intended for making differential diagnoses. As recommended for most of the interviews described, the parent should be interviewed first, followed by the child. The interview begins in an unstructured format and then focuses on symptoms that are rated on a 0 to 8 scale. Each item is rated by the interviewer three times (parent, child, both). The ISC and the K–SADS may be the interviews of choice for young children due to the flexibility in presentation and wording.

The Child Assessment Schedule (CAS; Hodges, McKnew, Cytryn, Stern, & Kline, 1982) is a semistructured interview reflecting *DSM* criteria and is intended to be administered by clinicians. There are three editions of the CAS, each designed for different age groups (i.e., ages 5–7, 7–12, adolescents). The interview consists of four sections with 11 topic areas (e.g., family, school, activities, and somatic complaints). The CAS has been found to be especially useful in identifying depressive symptoms in younger children (Verhulst, Bieman, Ende, Berden, & Sanders-Woudstra, 1990).

The Diagnostic Interview for Children–Revised (DICA–R; Herjanic & Reich, 1982) consists of two interviews, one for children ages 6 to 12 years and another for adolescents. The two versions are virtually the same except for age-appropriate wording and examples. The revised version was adapted to include *DSM* criteria and is highly structured. Symptoms are coded dichotomously as "yes" or "no." The parallel parental form includes questions regarding medical and developmental history

Like the DICA–R, the Diagnostic Interview Schedule for Children–Revised (DISC–R; Costello, Edelbrock, Dulcan, Kalas, & Klaric, 1984) is a highly structured interview and may be administered by a trained layperson. The DISC was originally developed for epidemiological research. The interview begins with general questions and then becomes more specific to match *DSM* criteria. The response format is "yes," "no," and "sometimes." It is not recommended for use with children under 10 years of age, as it tends to overdiagnose this population.

Rating Scales

When using rating scales to supplement or guide interviews, it is imperative to remember that most instruments either focus on criteria necessary to meet a formal diagnosis according to *DSM* criteria or measure frequency, intensity, and duration of depressive symptoms (severity measure). Both are potentially useful for problem identification. Most scales and interviews have items reflecting thoughts and feelings which need not be disregarded by the behavior analyst. These items should be regarded as covert behaviors from which more information can be obtained (springboard). For example, if a child says "I am sad," instead of assuming that this statement in and of itself indicates a symptom of depression, look for the function of such verbal behaviors (e.g., positive reinforcement from others).

Some of the more common rating scales used to assess depression and depressive symptomology in children are the Children's Depression Inventory (CDI; Kovacs & Beck, 1977), the Child's Depression Rating Scale–Revised (CDRS–R; Pozanski et al., 1984), the Children's Depression Scale (Lang & Tisher, 1978), Child Depression Scale (Tisher & Lang, 1983), and the Children's Affective Rating Scale (McKnew, Cytryn, Efron, Gershon, & Bunney, 1979). The CDI, derived from the Beck Depression Inventory (Beck, Ward, Mendelson, Mock, & Erbaugh, 1961), is one of the most frequently used self-report measures. The CDI is a symptom-oriented scale with 27 items reflecting intraverbal behavior and overt behavioral indicators. Each item describes three levels of increasing severity and the child is to indicate which statement most closely reflects symptoms over the previous two weeks. This instrument is not particularly useful for identifying specific target behaviors.

The CDRS–R is a depression severity scale derived from the Hamilton Depression Rating Scale for adults (Hamilton, 1967). It is composed of 17 items, 14 of which are rated by the clinician based on parent and child responses and 3 that are scored based on clinician observation of nonverbal behavior. The CSRS–R is easy to use and often is used in conjunction with interviews. It, too, does not assist the clinician in identifying behaviors to change during intervention.

In some situations, we also use the child's peers as a source of information. Peer ratings are useful because children spend large portions of the day in a variety of social situations with other children. Information derived from peer reports can be used for comparison with self-report of social interactions as well as indicating problems to be followed up in interviews and direct observation. For example, knowing that a child is unpopular provides preliminary information that, through further analysis, may identify inappropriate behavioral excesses or deficits in social interactions contributing to depressive behaviors.

The Peer Nomination Inventory for Depression (PNID; Lefkowitz & Tesiny, 1980) is a standardized measure of peer-reported depression. It is a 19-item sociometric scale consisting of 13 depression items, 4 happiness items, and 2 popularity items. Children are asked to identify the peer(s) representing certain characteristics (e.g., Who often looks sad?). A child's score is determined by the proportion of nominations received for the three areas (i.e., depression, happiness, popularity). Although the PNID has relatively low correspondence with teacher and self-reports, which is consistent with the meta-analytic work of Achenbach, McConaughy, and Howell (1987), it has been found to correlate moderately well with teacher ratings of social behavior and with other peer ratings of popularity (Kazdin, 1990). This suggests that peer ratings are useful in identifying peer-specific social problems (e.g., social interaction, peer rejection).

Direct Observations

Whenever possible, we conduct behavioral observations in the natural setting to estimate the strength of the problem behavior, to determine whether there are other behaviors contributing to the problem, and to gather preliminary functional assessment information. Our observation also allows us to determine whether the parent's and child's reports of the problem are accurate. In addition to observations in natural settings, we conduct clinic-based observations, particularly in cases where we suspect that the parent–child interaction is an antecedent for depressive behavior. We frequently have the parents and/or teachers observe and record specific behaviors to assess symptoms across settings and people and to identify other potential target behaviors.

Permanent Products

Although it may be difficult to determine whether poor academic performance leads to depressive behavior or whether depression leads to academic deficits, schoolwork may serve as permanent product data. In either case, if there is a functional relationship between depressive behavior and academic performance, improvements in one should result in improvements in the other. In addition, school performance may also serve as a socially valid outcome measure of improvements in depressive behavior. Some children experience either weight gain or loss as a function of changes in appetite. Measuring weight is one of the most direct methods for assessing positive changes in appetite.

One criticism of obtaining data from different sources is the low level of agreement between sources, with correlations ranging from .20 to .39 compared to correlations of .50 to .60 for same-source reporting on different measures (Achenbach et al., 1987; Crowley & Worchel, 1993). Although not all differences can be accounted for, the low correspondence has been attributed to the use of different measures (item type and format) by different reporting sources. In fact, Crowley, Worchel, and Ash (1992) found that three of the most widely used measures of depression (i.e., CDI, PNID, & CBCL–Teacher) measure different constructs. Among the disagreements, parents tend to report fewer symptoms than do children (Fleming, Boyle, & Offord, 1993). For example, Barrett and colleagues (1991) compared child and parent ratings on the Kiddie–SADS and found that agreement regarding the presence or absence of symptoms ranged from 40% to 60%. As would be expected, *observable symptoms* resulted in greater agreement. Children reported 39 out of 52 symptoms more often than did parents and 17 of the symptoms were reported 2 to 3 times more often by children. Only four symptoms were reported more often by parents: hypersomnia, increased appetite, anhedonia, and exaggerated illness behaviors.

Although low levels of agreement may be considered a problem by some, it need not be for the behavior analyst. Rating scales and interviews should be viewed as a guide to help determine if the behaviors reported constitute a problem and to identify behaviors to further analyze in the problem analysis phase. It is also likely that behaviors occurring in one setting do not occur in other settings (e.g., sleep) and that different behaviors are expected (therefore considered important) in different settings. Despite low correlations between sources, all sources have been shown to be valid across specific correlates (e.g., popularity), and may also provide unique insight into the functions of depressive behavior (Kazdin, 1990). Information from parents and teachers should be compared to identify behaviors considered most important by both, to look for behaviors that generalize across settings, and to specify those that occur in one setting but not another. All this information is useful for problem analysis and treatment planning. Information from parents, teachers, and children should be used by the clinician to guide direct observations and future interviews.

Problem Analysis

After specific behaviors have been identified and preliminary hypotheses generated in the problem identification stage, the clinician must conduct a more thorough assessment to determine the function of the depressive behavior. Considering the seriousness of depressive behavior, particularly for adolescents, we deem a descriptive functional *assessment* an appropriate and ethically correct means of ascertaining function. That is, in order to conduct a functional *analysis*, depressive behavior must be intentionally reinforced to determine the function of the behavior, which may result in a worsening of the depressive behavior, obviously an undesirable consequence. Therefore, we use direct observations, self-recording, and interviews to assess function. Despite the importance of assessing function in designing treatment for depression, most studies use rating scales or *DSM* criteria to diagnose depression and then select a treatment package based on what has worked for similar problems, mostly with adults, in the past. Hence, there is scant available data linking the function of depressive behavior to treatment.

When engaging in problem analysis, it is important to first determine whether the problem behavior of a child deviates substantially from the behavior of peers. Although certain behaviors, such as frequent crying or complaining, may be upsetting or indicative of depressed symptoms, it may be normal relative to other children of that age. Second, the clinician must determine what behaviors are expected or needed in particular settings. Finally, it must be determined whether the target problem behavior is a skill deficit or a performance deficit. In other words, does the child need to be taught a skill or taught to use a skill that is already in his or her repertoire.

In a typical problem analysis of depressive behaviors, the goal is to determine whether social attention, tangible reinforcers, and/or avoidance or escape from aversives are maintaining the behavior. Analyzing depressive behaviors sometimes, however, necessitates a slight deviation in the analysis procedures. For example, the clinician must also determine which of the contingencies is noticeably absent from the child's environment either as a result of behaviors which fail to evoke reinforcers or from a lack or reduction in reinforcers available in the environment.

Social Attention

Social attention is a likely maintaining variable of much depressive symptomology, especially somatic complaints, negative verbalizations, and negative affective expression. Parents and teachers may inadvertently reinforce such behaviors by attending to them. For example, a child may make a statement such as "I'm so stupid" to a parent while working on homework. A typical response to such a statement would be, "No, don't say that. I think you are very smart." From our experience at the clinic, parents tend to be very vulnerable to self-deprecating statements made by their children and seldom let such statements pass without comment. Also, children often develop somatic complaints, typically stomachaches and headaches, which tend to draw attention without drawing negative reactions. This is not to say that reactions must be positive in order to reinforce a behavior. For example, children displaying dysphoric mood characterized by crying, negative or flat affect, and complaining may draw negative social attention from adults and peers; the negative attention also maintains the depressive behavior. In order to determine whether or not behav-

iors are reinforced by social attention, parents and teachers must record instances of the target behavior and responses to the behavior by others (see the A-B-C tracking form in Chapter 22, as one example).

The lack or absence of social attention or opportunities to obtain social attention may also contribute to the development of depressive behaviors. For example, a child whose family has just moved may become depressed because he has few or no friends at the new school or neighborhood. Thus, the move itself did not cause depressive behavior, rather, it was the abrupt removal or reduction of social attention. Some children may lack many necessary social skills, thus preventing them from obtaining social reinforcers that are readily available in the environment. Still, in other cases, the child may have the requisite social skills but does not demonstrate them or their responses fail to evoke social reinforcement from adults and peers in their environment.

In conducting a descriptive assessment of depressive behaviors, the clinician must take care to analyze both social attention possibilities: (a) social attention as a reinforcer for depressive behavior and (b) the lack of social attention as an antecedent for depressive behavior. This information is best obtained by interviewing the parents and child, by observing the child's interactions with his or her parents, peers, and teacher(s), and asking parents and teachers to record data.

Escape or Avoidance

It may be that, in certain instances, children display behaviors associated with depression, such as hypersomnia, decreased motor activity, school refusal, and social withdrawal in order to escape or avoid aversive situations. It is often difficult to determine whether a child is refusing school because they are allowed to do things that are fun when home from school (social or tangible reinforcement), because they are avoiding unpleasant stimuli associated with the school setting (negative reinforcement by avoidance), or for both reasons simultaneously (i.e., multiple-function behavior). Assessing this function is sometimes problematic because (a) parents and teachers do not recognize that a behavior that results in the absence or cessation of an aversive contingency may increase in strength (negative reinforcement), (b) the behaviors may occur with such low frequency and long duration that they do not readily lend themselves to repeated observation, and (c) parents and teachers are often unaware of the aversive contingencies that are available for certain behaviors, making careful interviewing a must. The clinician must ask questions that directly seek to determine whether a particular function is maintaining a behavior (e.g., "When your child stays home from school, what does she do during the day?" "When your child complains of a stomachache and does not go to school, does his stomachache disappear shortly after school begins?" and "Does your child make negative statements about school or have other specific complaints about his teacher, peers, a particular subject, etc.?"). Answers to these questions do not guarantee accurate identification of function, but they do allow the clinician to make inferences about the predominant function of a behavior.

Tangible Reinforcement

In some cases, parents or peers may unintentionally reinforce depressive behaviors with tangible reinforcers. In an effort to "cheer up" their child who has been moping around the house, parents may provide known reinforcers or preferred stimuli for their child. For example, if a parent typically says something like, "Let's go get some ice cream" to their child who verbalizes that they are sad or lonely, negative verbalizations may increase. The response of negative verbalizations may then generalize in topography (response generalization) and to new stimuli (stimulus generalization).

To assess the function(s) of depressive behavior, several types of information must be collected. Typically we begin problem analysis by interviewing parents to determine their usual responses to their child's depressive behavior. We are careful to ask questions that help to identify situations or other stimuli that occasion depressive behavior. It is, however, often extremely difficult to pinpoint antecedents that reliably precede depressive behavior, especially when those behaviors occur within several response domains (e.g., negative verbalizations, somatic complaints, decreased motor activity, increased or decreased appetite). Therefore, we concentrate more heavily on identifying the consequences that maintain depressive behavior. After interviewing parents, we typically interview the child

for several reasons: (a) they are the only ones who can provide information regarding covert events, (b) to corroborate the parent's information regarding typical responses, (c) to obtain the child's perspective about environmental events that may be influencing their behavior, and (d) to obtain information regarding the role of peers in the maintenance of the behavior.

Upon collecting interview data, we then instruct the parents and child to record their behavior for a period of at least one week, taking special care to note antecedents and consequences (one appropriate form is the A-B-C tracking form found in Chapter 22). Recording behavior in the natural setting allows us to compare interview and self-observation data and to discuss and explore discrepancies and similarities between the two sources. Examining data from these sources permits us to draw strong inferences about the function(s) of the depressive behavior. Once function is determined, we are then able to design a treatment plan based on the results of our analysis.

Plan Implementation

After analyzing the specific problem behavior(s), we begin treatment by discussing with the parents and, if appropriate, the child, the relationship between the analysis information and treatment procedures. We are careful not to blame the parents when describing the functional relationship between their behavior and their child's depressive behavior. We also make sure that the rationale for treatment is understood by all parties involved in treatment prior to actually implementing an intervention.

There are two broad approaches to planning treatment for depressive behavior: the shotgun approach and the functional approach. The shotgun approach, also referred to as a "treatment package" (see, for example, Asarnow & Carlson, 1988; Lewinsohn, Clarke, Hops, & Andrews, 1990), combines several different treatment strategies at once and is usually tied to a particular theory of depression. Each theoretical model tends to emphasize a different core symptom (e.g., self-control theory emphasizes overly stringent expectations and little self-reinforcement). The difference between package and functional approaches is that packages assume certain behaviors are problematic and that all of the behaviors have a similar function. A functional-based treatment approach, on the other hand, relies on data collected during the analysis to guide intervention and focuses on behaviors identified as problematic only during problem identification. Some of the treatment components will be the same, but they are selectively used in a functional approach, whereas they are always used in a package approach. There are several advantages of a functional-based treatment approach: (a) it is systematic and thus likely to be more cost- and time-efficient, (b) it is likely that some skills are prerequisites to other skills, (c) treatment of one symptom may result in improvements in other symptoms, and (d) improvements in one symptom may prove to be incompatible with other problem behaviors (e.g., teaching a child to smile is incompatible with frowning).

In a review of the pharmacological and cognitive–behavioral treatment literature on childhood depression, Dujovne, Barnard, and Rapoff (1995) reported that there is support for the use of cognitive and behavioral approaches, but they also noted the scarcity of research and the methodological limitations of the research that does exist. Because treatment outcome studies of children with depression are scant in general, and virtually nonexistent using a functional approach, the following section will focus on the methods of treatment employed in the treatment packages as they would be applied to specific behaviors identified during problem identification and selected based on the problem analysis. Although we briefly describe some of the more prominent treatment packages, we will focus primarily on linking analysis data to specific intervention techniques. Full descriptions of package approaches are easily found in most other behavior therapy texts and journal articles. At this point, it is imperative for us to reiterate that *we are not treating depression.* Depression is a hypothetical construct and, as such, cannot be targeted for intervention. Instead, we are treating depressive behaviors, which are appropriate targets for intervention. In addition, it is not feasible to describe treatment for every possible depressive behavior evidenced by children. Rather, one may focus on a keystone behavior that, when changed, will have positive effects on other behaviors in the same response class (Barnett, Bauer, Ehrhardt, Lentz, & Stollar, 1996).

Social Attention

Research supports a consistent relationship between depressive behaviors and social competence (e.g., Altman & Gotlib, 1988; Patterson & Stoolmiller, 1991; Wierzbicki & McCabe, 1988). Children identified as depressed have been found to be more impulsive, lack assertiveness, and receive low teacher and peer acceptance ratings. In addition, Rudolph, Hammen, and Burge (1994) found that depressive symptoms in children were related to problems with social problem solving, conflict resolution, and peer rejection. If poor peer relations is identified as a contributing factor resulting in or maintaining depressive behavior, social skills training may be the treatment of choice (see Chapter 24, this volume, for a description).

If social attention is found to be a maintaining variable for depressive behavior, the treatment goal is to differentially reinforce nondepressive behavior while extinguishing depressive behavior. For example, an eight-year-old female was referred to our clinic for excessive sadness (operationally defined as verbalizing negative self-statements) and extended crying episodes. The analysis revealed that the crying occurred primarily in the presence of the mother (discriminative stimulus) and resulted in comforting (e.g., hugging, positive statements) from the mother. Therefore, to reduce the depressive behavior, we instructed the mother to hug and say positive things to her child when she was exhibiting nondepressive behavior and to ignore the crying and negative statements. After several weeks of intervention, the mother reported that the child no longer seemed sad and that her "depression has lifted."

Peer attention may maintain depressive behavior, as was found in the case of an adolescent female who reported not having friends and being depressed. When questioned about what precluded her from having friends, she reported that she frequently made negative comments about herself around her peers; this at first resulted in positive comments but eventually alienated her friends from her. Thus, treatment focused on prompting positive comments and this increased the likelihood that her peers would attend to her appropriate behavior. We designed an intervention in which examples of positive statements were written on individual 3 × 5 index cards. The client was instructed to look at the cards during transitions between classes and then use the positive statements during the next class period to evoke positive interactions with her peers. The strategy was immediately successful and the cards were unnecessary after a couple of weeks. The client reported no depression after three weeks of intervention.

Escape/Avoidance

When the analysis indicates that a child's depressive behavior results in escape or avoidance of aversive stimuli, the treatment goal is to prevent escape and teach more appropriate skills that are situationally adaptive. In some cases, the child may lack appropriate skills to terminate unpleasant events, and this results in escape or avoidance behavior. For example, a child referred to our clinic suddenly refused to attend school and engage in school-related activities that were once enjoyed. During problem analysis, which consisted of interviews with the teacher, parents, and child, it was discovered that a peer was threatening the child during recess and lunch. The child's response to the threat was to cry and run away from the situation. In this example, the depressive symptoms (school refusal and anhedonia) were maintained by avoidance of a highly aversive event (being bullied). Thus, treatment focused on teaching appropriate responses to threats; these responses resulted in discontinuation of the threats and a willingness to return to school. In cases where school refusal is the primary, or one of the primary, symptoms, an intervention directly targeted at returning the child to school may be indicated (see Chapter 8, this volume, for a full description).

In other instances, the child may withdraw or evidence other depressive behaviors simply to avoid engaging in performance situations or activities such as schoolwork. In these situations, treatment is not necessarily focused on teaching a skill, but on preventing escape from the aversive situation. Escape is made contingent upon demonstrating nondepressive behavior. For example, a child who successfully avoids schoolwork by making somatic complaints and negative verbalizations about their academic ability may be allowed to escape schoolwork only after they have completed increasingly larger percentages of work (shaping) without making somatic complaints or negative verbalizations.

Tangible Reinforcers

Although it would be unusual for tangible reinforcers by themselves to maintain depressive behavior, they may play a role in conjunction with social attention and escape/avoidance. For example, peers, parents, or other adults may be inclined to deliver preferred tangible stimuli contingent upon the demonstration of depressive behavior. In such cases, it is important for the clinician to arrange a reinforcement schedule whereby tangible stimuli are delivered for behaviors incompatible with depressive behavior.

Treatment Packages

Stark, Reynolds, and Kaslow (1987) compared a self-control treatment (S-C) to behavioral problem-solving therapy (BPS), and a wait-list control group using 28 school-age children identified as depressed. The S-C therapy was derived from treatment implemented with adults by Rehm and colleagues (1981). The S-C group was taught (a) to self-monitor pleasant activities, positive self-statements, and self-reinforcement of log sheet completion, (b) to make adaptive attributions, and (c) to set realistic standards through didactic presentations, role-playing, and behavioral homework assignments. The BPS treatment was partially based on work by Lewinsohn and associates (e.g., Lewinsohn, Sullivan, & Grosscup, 1980), which consisted of a combination of self-monitoring, pleasant activity scheduling, and problem-solving training. The children were taught to self-monitor the type and frequency of their activities. Problem-solving skills were modeled by the therapists and applied by the children in developing strategies for increasing pleasant activities and decreasing unpleasant activities. Results of the comparison indicated that improvements in both treatment groups were clinically and statistically significant and superior to control, but there were no significant differences between the two treatments. The BPS treatment did receive better parental reports than the S-C treatment, however.

Butler, Meizitis, Frieman, and Cole (1980) compared the efficacy of a cognitive restructuring intervention to a problem solving/social skills training approach, control group, and attention placebo group. Children in the cognitive restructuring group were taught to recognize irrational thoughts, to improve listening skills, and to recognize the relationship between thoughts and feelings. The other treatment group engaged in behavioral role-playing emphasizing social skills and problem solving. The problem solving/social skills was found to be superior to the cognitive restructuring group, attention placebo group, and control group.

Lewinsohn and colleagues (1990) compared the efficacy of a multicomponent cognitive–behavioral intervention with adolescents alone, adolescents and their parents, to a wait-list control. The intervention was a modification of the Coping with Depression Course (CDC) originally used with adults. The course was designed to address common depressive behaviors including anxiety, negative verbalizations, poor social skills, and a low rate of engagement in pleasant activities, through the use of relaxation training, social skills training, and problem-solving techniques. Both treatment groups improved significantly more than the wait-list control and maintained improvements at two-year follow-up.

In another study, 68 middle-school children were randomly assigned to one of four conditions: CDC (without relaxation training), relaxation training, self-modeling interventions, or control (Kahn, Kehle, Jenson, & Clark, 1990). The self-modeling intervention targeted behaviors such as appropriate eye contact, posture, positive affect, and positive verbalizations. Participants in the self-modeling group were videotaped during baseline and then instructed to exhibit behaviors that were incompatible with the target behaviors. A videotape was taken and edited in order to produce a final tape of the participants behaving in a nondepressed manner. Treatment consisted of simply watching the three-minute tape of themselves. Findings were consistent with that of other treatment package comparisons in that there were significant differences for treatment groups compared to the control group, but no substantial differences between treatments.

Plan Evaluation

Evaluating the effectiveness of an intervention is a natural extension of the problem identification phase. Behaviors that are targeted for intervention are observed and their frequency (or duration) recorded to serve as baseline data. These same behaviors are then assessed and charted throughout the treatment process to determine whether the intervention is effective. In determining effectiveness, we also attend to other measures, such as parent and teacher reports of general functioning, child and peer reports of affect and mood, and possibly permanent product data. We are especially concerned that changes in the child's behavior have ecological validity. For example, if one of our goals was to increase smiling, we assess to determine whether an increase in smiling resulted in more positive interactions with peers, teachers, and parents. If it did, then the increased smiling probably had ecological validity; if it did not, then smiling probably did not have ecological validity in that it is not a functional behavior in the child's environment.

Occasionally, treatment will not result in either immediate improvements in a behavior or in enough improvement in a behavior. In such cases, the first question that must be asked is, "Was the correct target behavior(s) identified?" It may be that there are more salient behaviors that need to be targeted or that there are other behaviors that are antecedents to the target behavior or behaviors that must be addressed. If the clinician is reasonably certain that the correct behavior or behaviors have been targeted, the next obvious question is, "Was the function of the behavior correctly identified?" This question is particularly important when basing treatment on the function of the behavior and is less important when using a treatment package approach. If, for example, a child's decreased motor activity was determined to be maintained by social attention during the analysis phase, the treatment might involve differential reinforcement, extinction, contingency contracting, and prompting. If the actual function of the decreased motor activity is escape/avoidance, then the treatment is likely to be ineffective or less than maximally effective. Therefore, the clinician must determine whether the function of the behavior was correctly identified.

In some cases, where the behavior has been correctly identified and analyzed, the treatment may not be of sufficient strength. That is, (a) the reinforcers available for nondepressive behavior may not be as strong as reinforcers available for depressive behavior (quality), (b) the effort required to obtain reinforcement for nondepressive behavior may be greater than the effort required to obtain reinforcement for depressive behavior (response effort), or (c) there is a thicker schedule of reinforcement for depressive than for nondepressive behaviors (rate of reinforcement). Each of these, quality and rate of reinforcement and amount of response effort required, must be examined when attempting to determine why treatment was not effective.

Directions for Future Research

This section is in some ways the easiest and the most difficult to write. It is easy because there is clearly a lack of empirical evidence linking functional assessment of depressive behavior to intervention. On the other hand, because of the limited research base, it is difficult to identify one or even several areas where further work is most urgently needed. It should be relatively clear, from the research cited in this chapter, that most of the empirical work in childhood depression has focused on diagnosing depression, identifying etiological variables, and validating the effectiveness of treatment package approaches. The lack of research on a function-based treatment approach represents what is perhaps the largest and most important gap in the behavioral literature on childhood depression. The need for this type of research may be evidenced by the consistent findings of no differences between various active treatment approaches (Lewinsohn et al., 1990). That is, behavior therapy and variations of cognitive–behavioral therapy have been found to be equally effective for reducing depression in children and adolescents. The literature does not specify, however, why particular treatment strategies were used nor which component within a particular treatment package was functionally related to amelioration of the depressive behavior. These omissions in the treatment literature on depression, from a behavior analyst's view, are quite glaring and must be addressed before meaningful conclusions can be reached about the components of effective therapy.

If behavior analysis is to gain widespread acceptance in the professional and lay communities, then behavior analysts and the organizations that represent behavior analysis (e.g., Association for Behavior Analysis) must commit to, promote, and advocate research that focuses on behaviors that are generally thought of as internalizing behaviors. The

behavior analysis literature is replete with studies on the functional assessment and treatment of overt (i.e., externalizing) behaviors such as self-injury, stereotypy, and feeding, to name just a few. Analysis and treatment of overt behaviors is important and should continue. However, there is a conspicuous absence in the behavior analysis literature on the analysis and treatment of behaviors related to depression, anxiety, somatic complaints, as examples. As a wise behavior analyst once opined, "Behavior is behavior is behavior." Behavior analysts should embrace this credo and go into the great unforeseen darkness known only as "behaviors within the skin."

References

Abramson, L.Y., Seligman, M.E.P., & Teasdale, J. (1978). Learned helplessness in humans: Critique and reformulation. *Journal of Abnormal Psychology, 87,* 49–74.

Achenbach, T.M., McConaughy, S.H., Howell, C.T. (1987). Child/adolescent behavioral and emotional problems: Implications of cross-informant correlations for situational specificity. *Psychological Bulletin, 101,* 213–232.

Altmann, E.O., & Gotlib, I.H. (1988). The social behavior of depressed children: An observational study. *Journal of Abnormal Child Psychology, 16,* 29–44.

American Psychiatric Association. (1994). *Diagnostic and statistical manual of mental disorders* (4th ed.). Washington, DC: Author.

Angold, A., & Costello, E. (1993). Depressive comorbidity in children and adolescents: Empirical, theoretical, and methodological issues. *American Journal of Psychiatry, 150,* 1779–1791.

Asarnow, J.R., & Carlson, G.A. (1988). Childhood depression: Five-year outcome following combined cognitive–behavior therapy and pharmacotherapy. *American Journal of Psychotherapy, 42,* 456–464.

Barnett, D.W., Bauer, A.M., Ehrhardt, K.E., Lentz, F.E., & Stollar, S.A. (1996). Keystone targets for change: Planning for widespread positive consequences. *School Psychology Quarterly, 11,* 95–117.

Barrett, M.L., Berney, T.P., Bhate, S., Famuyiwa, O.O., Fundudis, T., Kolvin, I., & Tyrer, S. (1991). Diagnosing childhood depression: Who should be interviewed—parent or child? *British Journal of Psychiatry, 159*(Suppl. 11), 22–27.

Beck, A.T., Ward, C., Mendelson, M., Mock, J., & Erbaugh, J. (1961). An inventory for measuring depression. *Archives of General Psychiatry, 4,* 561–571.

Biederman, J., & Steingard, R. (1989). Attention-deficit hyperactivity disorder in adolescents. *Psychiatric Annals, 19,* 587–596.

Biederman, J., Newcorn, J., & Sprich, S. (1991). Comorbidity of attention deficit hyperactivity disorder with conduct, depressive, anxiety, and other disorders. *American Journal of Psychiatry, 148,* 564–577.

Brady, E.U., & Kendall, P.C. (1992). Comorbidity of anxiety and depression in children and adolescents. *Psychological Bulletin, 111*, 244–255.

Brody, G.H., & Forehand, R. (1986). Maternal perceptions of child maladjustment as a function of the combined influence of child behavior and maternal depression. *Journal of Consulting and Clinical Psychology, 54*, 237–240.

Buckstein, O.G., Glancy, L.J., & Kaminer, Y. (1992). Pattern of affective comorbidity in a clinical population of dually diagnosed adolescent substance abusers. *Journal of the American Academy of Child and Adolescent Psychiatry, 31*, 1041–1045.

Butler, L., Miezitis, S., Frieman, R., & Cole, E. (1980). The effects of two school-based intervention programs on depressive symptoms in preadolescents. *American Education Research Journal, 17*, 111–119.

Carlson, C.A., & Cantwell, D.P. (1980). A survey of depressive symptoms and disorder in a child psychiatric population. *Journal of Child Psychology and Psychiatry, 21*, 19–25.

Clarizio, H.F. (1994). *Assessment and treatment of depression and children and adolescents* (2nd ed.). Brandon, VT: Clinical Psychology Publishing.

Cole, D.A., & Rehm, L.P. (1986). Family interaction patterns and childhood depression. *Journal of Abnormal Child Psychology, 14*, 297–314.

Costello, A.J., Edelbrock, L.S., Dulcan, M.K., Kalas, R., & Klaric, S.H. (1984). *Report on the NIHM Diagnostic Interview Schedule for Children (DISC)*. Washington, DC: National Institute of Mental Health.

Crowley, S.L., & Worchel, F.F. (1993). Assessment of childhood depression: Sampling multiple data sources with one instrument. *Journal of Psychoeducational Assessment, 11*, 242–249.

Crowley, S.L., Worchel, F.F., & Ash, M.J. (1992). Self-report, peer-report, and teacher-report measures of childhood depression: An analysis by item. *Journal of Personality Assessment, 59*, 189–203.

Cytryn, L., & McKnew, D. (1974). Factors influencing the changing clinical expression of the depressive process in children. *American Journal of Psychiatry, 131*, 879–881.

Deykin, E.Y., Levy, J.C., & Wells, V. (1987). Adolescent depression, alcohol and drug abuse. *American Journal of Public Health, 77*, 178–182.

Digdon, N., & Gotlib, I.H. (1985). Developmental considerations in the study of childhood depression. *Annual Progress in Child Psychiatry and Child Development, 5*, 162–199.

Dodge, L. (1990). Developmental psychopathology in children of depressed mothers. *Developmental Psychology, 26*, 3–6.

Downey, G., & Coyne, J. (1990). Children of depressed parents: An integrative review. *Psychological Bulletin, 108*, 50–76.

Dujovne, V.F., Barnard, M.U., & Rapoff, M.A. (1995). Pharmacological and cognitive–behavioral approaches in the treatment of childhood depression: A review and critique. *Clinical Psychology Review, 15*, 589–611.

Edelbrock, C.S., Costello, A.J., Dulcan, M.K., Conover, N.C., & Kalas, R. (1986). Parent–child agreement on child psychiatric symptoms assessed via structured interview. *Journal of Child Psychology and Psychiatry, 27*, 181–190.

Endicott, J., & Spitzer, R.L. (1978). A diagnostic interview: The schedule for affective disorders and schizophrenia. *Archive of General Psychiatry, 35*, 837–844.

Finch, A.J., Lipovsky, J.A., & Casat, C.D. (1989). Anxiety and depression in children and adolescents: Negative affectivity or separate constructs? In P.C. Kendall & D. Watson (Eds.), *Anxiety and depression: Distinctive and overlapping features*. New York: Academic.

Fleming, J.E., & Offord, D.R. (1990). Epidemiology of childhood depression disorders: A critical review. *Journal of the American Academy of Child and Adolescent Psychiatry, 29*, 571–580.

Fleming, J.E., Boyle, M.H., & Offord, D.R. (1993). The outcome of adolescent depression in the Ontario child health study follow-up. *Journal of the American Academy of Child and Adolescent Psychiatry, 32*, 28–33.

Garrison, C.Z., Jackson, K.L., Marstellar, F., McKeown, R.E., & Addy, C. (1990). A longitudinal study of depressive symptomatology in young adolescents. *Journal of the American Academy of Child and Adolescent Psychiatry, 29*, 581–585.

Garrison, C.Z., Addy, C.L., Jackson, K.L., McKeown, R., & Waller, J.L. (1992). Major depressive disorder and dysthymia in young adolescents. *American Journal of Epidemiology, 135*, 792–802.

Goodman, S., & Brumley, H. (1990). Schizophrenic and depressed mothers: Relational deficits in parenting. *Developmental Psychology, 26*, 31–39.

Hamilton, M.A. (1967). Development of a rating scale for primary depressive illness. *British Journal of Social and Clinical Psychology, 6*, 278–296.

Hammen, C., & Compas, B.E. (1994). Unmasking unmasked depression in children and adolescents: The problem of comorbidity. *Clinical Psychology Review, 14*, 585–603.

Harrington, R., Fudge, H., Rutter, M., Pickles, A., & Hill, J. (1991). Adult outcomes of childhood and adolescent depression. II. Links with antisocial disorder. *Journal of the American Academy of Child and Adolescent Psychiatry, 30*, 434–439.

Hendren, R.L. (1983). Depression in anorexia nervosa. *Journal of the American Academy of Child Psychiatry, 122*, 59–65.

Herjanic, B., & Reich, W. (1982). Development of a structured psychiatric interview for children: Agreement between child and parent on individual symptoms. *Journal of Abnormal Child Psychology, 10*, 307–324.

Hodges, K., McKnew, D., Cytryn, L., Stern, L., & Kline, J. (1982). The Child Assessment Schedule (CAS) diagnostic interview: A report on reliability and validity. *Journal of the American Academy of Child Psychiatry, 21*, 468–473.

Jacobsen, R.H., Lahey, B.B., & Strauss, C.C. (1983). Correlates of depressed mood in normal children. *Journal of Abnormal Child Psychology, 11*, 29–40.

Kahn, J.S., Kehle, T.J., Jenson, W.R., & Clark, E. (1990). Comparison of cognitive–behavioral, relaxation, and self-modeling interventions for depression among middle-school students. *School Psychology Review, 19*, 196–211.

Kanfer, F.H. (1971). The maintenance of behavior by self-generated stimuli and reinforcement. In A. Jacobs & L. Sachs (Eds.), *The psychology of private events: Perspectives on covert response systems* (pp. 39–59). New York: Academic.

Kashani, J.H., Ray, J.S., & Carlson, G.A. (1984). Depression and depression-like states in preschool-age children in a child development unit. *American Journal of Psychiatry, 141*, 1397–1402.

Kazdin, A.E. (1990). Childhood depression. *Journal of Child Psychology and Psychiatry, 31,* 121–160.

Kennedy, E., Spence, S.H., & Hensley, R. (1989). An examination of the relationship between childhood depression and social competence amongst primary school children. *Journal of Child Psychology and Psychiatry, 30,* 561–573.

Kolvin, I., Barrett, M.L., Bhate, S.R., Berney, T.P., Famuyiwa, O.O., Fundusis, T., & Tyrer, S. (1991). The Newcastle Child Depression Project: Diagnosis and classification of depression. *British Journal of Psychiatry, 159*(Suppl. 11), 9–21.

Kovacs, M. (1978). *Interview Schedule for Children (ISC).* Pittsburgh, PA: University of Pittsburgh School of Medicine.

Kovacs, M. (1990). Comorbid anxiety disorders in childhood-onset depressions. In J.D. Maser & C.R. Cloninger (Eds.), *Comorbidity of mood and anxiety disorders* (pp. 272–281). Washington, DC: American Psychiatric Press.

Kovacs, M., & Beck, A.T. (1977). An empirical-clinical approach toward a definition of childhood depression. In J.G. Schulterbrandt & A. Raskin (Eds.), *Depression in childhood: Diagnosis, treatment, and conceptual models* (pp. 1–25). New York: Raven.

Kovacs, M., & Gatsonis, C. (1989). Stability and change in childhood-onset depressive disorders: Longitudinal course as a diagnostic validator. In L.N. Robins & J.E. Barrett (Eds.), *The validity of psychiatric diagnosis* (pp. 57–73). New York: Raven.

Kovacs, M., Feinberg, T.L., Crouse-Novak, M.A., Paulauskas, S., Pollack, M., & Finkelstein, R. (1984). Depressive disorders in childhood: II. A longitudinal study of the risk for a subsequent major depression. *Archives of General Psychiatry, 41,* 643–649.

Lang, M., & Tisher, M. (1978). *Children's Depression Scale.* Victoria, Australia: Australian Council for Educational Research.

Lefkowitz, M.M., & Tesiny, E.P. (1980). Assessment of childhood depression. *Journal of Consulting and Clinical Psychology, 48,* 43–50.

Lefkowitz, M.M., & Tesiny, E.P. (1985). Depression in children: Prevalence and correlates. *Journal of Consulting and Clinical Psychology, 53,* 647–656.

Lewinsohn, P.M. (1974). A behavioral approach to depression. In R.J. Freidman & M.M. Katz (Eds.), *The psychology of depression: Contemporary theory and research,* (pp. 157–186). New York: Wiley.

Lewinsohn, P.M. (1975). The behavioral study and treatment of depression. In M. Hersen, R.M. Eisler, & P.M. Miller (Eds.), *Progress in behavior modification* (Vol. 1, pp. 19–55). New York: Academic.

Lewinsohn, P.M., Sullivan, J.M., & Grosscup, S.J. (1980). Changing reinforcing events: An approach to the treatment of depression. *Psychotherapy: Theory, Research, and Practice, 17,* 322–334.

Lewinsohn, P.M., Clarke, G.N., Hops, H., & Andrews, J. (1990). Cognitive–behavioral treatment for depressed adolescents. *Behavior Therapy, 21,* 385–401.

Lewinsohn, P.M., Hops, H., Roberts, R.E., Seeley, J.R., & Andrews, J.A. (1993). Adolescent psychopathology. I. Prevalence and incidence of depression and other DSM-III-R disorders in high school students. *Journal of Abnormal Psychology, 102,* 133–144.

McKnew, D.H., Jr., Cytryn, L., Efron, A.M., Gershon, E.S., & Bunney, W.E., Jr. (1979). Offspring of patients with affective disorders. *British Journal of Psychiatry, 134,* 148–152.

Milberger, S., Biederman, J., Faroane, S., Murphy, J., & Tsuang, M. (1995). Attention deficit hyperactivity disorder: Issues of overlapping symptoms. *American Journal of Psychiatry, 152,* 1793–1799.

Patterson, G.R., & Stoolmiller, M. (1991). Replications of a dual failure model for boys' depressed mood. *Journal of Consulting and Clinical Psychology, 59,* 491–498.

Pozanski, E.O., Grossman, J.A., Buchsbaum, Y., Banegas, M., Freeman, L., & Gibbons, R. (1984). Preliminary studies of the reliability and validity of the Children's Depression Rating Scale. *Journal of the American Academy of Child Psychiatry, 23,* 191–197.

Puig-Antich, J. (1982). Major depression and conduct disorder in prepuberty. *Journal of the American Academy of Child Psychiatry, 21,* 118–128.

Puig-Antich, J., & Chambers, W. (1978). *The Schedule for Affective Disorders and Schizophrenia for School-age Children (Kiddie–SADS).* New York: New York State Psychiatric Institute.

Puig-Antich, J., & Gittelman, R. (1982). Depression in childhood and adolescence. In E.S. Paykel (Ed.), *Handbook of affective disorders* (pp. 379–392). New York: Guilford.

Puig-Antich, J., Kaufman, J., Ryan, N.D., Williamson, D., Dahl, R.E., Lukens, E., Todak, G., Ambrosini, P., Rabinovich, H., & Nelson, B. (1993). The psychosocial functioning and family environment of depressed adolescents. *Journal of the American Academy of Child and Adolescent Psychiatry, 32,* 244–253.

Rastam, M. (1992). Anorexia nervosa in 51 Swedish adolescents: Premorbid problems of comorbidity. *Journal of the American Academy of Child and Adolescent Psychiatry, 31,* 819–829.

Rehm, L.P. (1977). A self-control model of depression. *Behavior Therapy, 8,* 787–804.

Rehm, L.P., Kornblith, S.J., O'Hara, M.W., Lamparski, D.M., Romano, J.M., & Volkin, J.I. (1981). An evaluation of major components in a self-control therapy program for depression. *Behavior Modification, 5,* 459–489.

Rohde, P., Lewinsohn, P.M., & Seeley, J.R. (1991). Comorbidity of unipolar depression: II. Comorbidity with other disorders in adolescents and adults. *Journal of Abnormal Psychology, 54,* 653–660.

Rudolph, K.D., Hammen, C., & Burge, D. (1994). Interpersonal functioning and depressive symptoms in childhood: Addressing the issues of specificity and comorbidity. *Journal of Abnormal Child Psychology, 22,* 355–371.

Ryan, N.D., Puig-Antich, J., Ambrosini, P., Rabinovich, H., Robinson, D., Nelson, B., Iyengar, S., & Twomey, J. (1987). The clinical picture of major depression in children and adolescents. *Archives of General Psychiatry, 44,* 854–861.

Seligman, M.E. (1975). *Helplessness: On depression, development, and death.* San Francisco: Freeman.

Shain, B.N., Naylor, M., & Alessi, N. (1990). Comparison of self-rated and clinician-rated measures of depression in adolescents. *American Journal of Psychiatry, 147,* 793–795.

Smith, C., & Steiner, H., (1992). Psychopathology in anorexia nervosa and depression. *Journal of the American Academy of Child and Adolescent Psychiatry, 31,* 841–843.

Spitzer, R.L., Endicott, J., & Robins, E. (1978). Research Diagnostic Criteria: Rationale and reliability. *Archives of General Psychiatry, 35,* 773–782.

Stark, K.D., Reynolds, W.M., & Kaslow, N.J. (1987). A comparison of the relative efficacy of self-control therapy and a behavioral problem-solving therapy for depression in children. *Journal of Abnormal Child Psychology, 15,* 91–113.

Strack, M.A., & Coyne, J.C. (1983). Social confirmation of dysphoria: Shared and private reactions to depression. *Journal of Personality and Social Psychology, 44,* 806–814.

Tisher, M., & Lang, M. (1983). The Children's Depression Scale: Review and further developments. In D.P. Cantwell & G.A. Carson (Eds.), *Affective disorders in childhood and adolescence: An update* (pp. 375–415). New York: Spectrum.

Verhulst, F.C., Bieman, H.V., Ende, H.V.D., Berden, G.F.M.G., & Sanders-Woudstra, J. (1990). Problem behavior in international adoptees. III. Diagnosis of child psychiatric disorders. *Journal of the American Academy of Child and Adolescent Psychiatry, 29,* 420–428.

Weinberg, W., Rutman, J., Sullivan, L., Penick, E., & Dietz, S. (1973). Depression in children referred to an educational diagnostic center: Diagnosis and treatment. *Journal of Pediatrics, 83,* 1066.

Weiss, B., Weisz, J.R., Politano, M., Carey, M., Nelson, W.M., & Finch, A.J. (1992). Relations among self-reported depressive symptoms in clinic-referred children versus adolescents. *Journal of Abnormal Psychology, 101,* 391–397.

Weissman, M., Fendrich, M., Warner, V., & Wickramaratne, P. (1992). Incidence of psychiatric disorder in off-spring at high and low risk for depression. *Journal of the American Academy of Child and Adolescent Psychiatry, 31,* 640–648.

Wierzbicki, M., & McCabe, M. (1988). Social skills and subsequent depressive symptomatology in children. *Journal of Clinical Child Psychiatry, 17,* 203–208.

Witt, J.C., Cavell, T.A., Heffer, R.W., Carey, M.P., & Martens, B.K. (1988). Child self-report: Interviewing techniques and rating scales. In E.S. Shapiro & T.R. Kratochwill (Eds.), *Behavioral assessment in schools: Conceptual foundations and practical applications* (pp. 384–454). New York: Guilford.

Youngren, M.A., & Lewinsohn, P.M. (1980). The functional relationship between depression and problematic interpersonal behaviour. *Journal of Abnormal Psychology, 89,* 333–341.

Bibliography

Abramson, L.Y., Seligman, M.E.P., & Teasdale, J. (1978). Learned helplessness in humans: Critique and reformulation. *Journal of Abnormal Psychology, 87,* 49–74.

Clarizio, H.F. (1994). *Assessment and treatment of depression and children and adolescents* (2nd ed.). Brandon, VT: Clinical Psychology Publishing.

Kazdin, A.E. (1990). Childhood depression. *Journal of Child Psychology and Psychiatry, 31,* 121–160.

Lewinsohn, P.M. (1974). A behavioral approach to depression. In R.J. Freidman & M.M. Katz (Eds.), *The psychology of depression: Contemporary theory and research,* (pp. 157–186). New York: Wiley.

Lewinsohn, P.M. (1975). The behavioral study and treatment of depression. In M. Hersen, R.M. Eisler, & P.M. Miller (Eds.), *Progress in behavior modification* (Vol. 1, pp. 19–55). New York: Academic.

Rehm, L.P. (1977). A self-control model of depression. *Behavior Therapy, 8,* 787–804.

21

Assessment and Treatment of Self-Injury

F. CHARLES MACE, TIMOTHY R. VOLLMER, PATRICK R. PROGAR, AND AMY B. MACE

Introduction

Self-injurious behavior (SIB) is among the most serious behavior disorders affecting children. The disorder consists of a highly heterogeneous set of repetitive behaviors that can produce tissue and sensory damage in a single act, or more often, have cumulative effects that can be debilitating or life threatening in severe cases. These self-injurious responses include, but are not limited to, head banging, face slapping, skin picking and scratching, body punching, ingestion of inedible objects, hair pulling, and eye, ear, and nose poking and gouging. Although SIB is occasionally observed in individuals with normal intellectual development, the disorder is most commonly associated with mental retardation. Prevalence studies indicate that up to 25,000 United States citizens suffer from serious forms of the disorder (National Institutes of Health, 1989), constituting 2.6% of the school age (Griffin et al., 1987) and 10% to 17% of the institutionalized population of persons with mental retardation (Baumeister & Rollings, 1976; Schroeder, Schroeder, Smith, & Dalldorf, 1978). The social and medical consequences of SIB, which can be enormous, include institutionalization, hospitalization, aversive treatment, and chemical or mechanical restraint (Favell et al., 1982).

Much of the research on SIB has focused on its environmental determinants and behavioral treatment (Iwata, Dorsey, Slifer, Bauman, & Richman, 1982/1994; Mace, Lalli, & Shea, 1992). In a seminal review of experimental behavioral research, E.G. Carr (1977) found support for three bases for the disorder: (1) SIB is an operant behavior maintained by social positive reinforcement (e.g., disapproval, sympathy); (2) SIB is an operant behavior maintained by the termination or avoidance of aversive events (e.g., task demands); and (3) SIB is maintained by the production of sensory stimulation. In the two decades since Carr's review, numerous studies have confirmed that SIB can be maintained by environmental contingencies. Most contemporary approaches to behavioral treatment use this information to discontinue reinforcement of SIB while arranging similar reinforcement for adaptive replacement behaviors (e.g., E. Carr & Durand, 1985).

The disproportionate prevalence of SIB in individuals with severe to profound mental retardation and its association with specific developmental syndromes has also spawned considerable research on neurobiological factors in self-injury (Harris, 1992). For example, SIB occurs in children with Pervasive Developmental Disorder (PDD) and autism at higher rates than in children without these disorders

---

F. CHARLES MACE, TIMOTHY R. VOLLMER, AND PATRICK R. PROGAR • The University of Pennsylvania and Children's Seashore House, Philadelphia, Pennsylvania 19104. AMY B. MACE • School Psychology Program, Lehigh University, Bethlehem, Pennsylvania 18015-3094.

Handbook of Child Behavior Therapy, edited by Watson and Gresham. Plenum Press, New York, 1998.

but with similar IQs. The disorder is highly correlated with the syndromes Lesch-Nyhan, Cornelia de Lange, Riley-Day, Rett, and Fragile-X. All but Riley-Day Syndrome are associated with specific topographies of self-injury suggesting the involvement of syndrome-specific types of neurobiologic disorders. Several neurobiologic models of SIB have been developed and tested in mice, rats, and rabbits, with varying degrees of success (Breese, et al. 1995; Harris, 1992; Tessel, Schroeder, Stodgell, & Loupe, 1995). These models have, in turn, provided a basis for psychopharmalogic treatment of SIB aimed at remediation of the underlying neurobiological disturbance (Aman, 1993; Farber, 1987; Mace & Mauk, 1995).

At present, the majority of researchers and clinicians agree that SIB can be maintained by environmental or biologic factors, or some combination of the two. In this chapter, we present a functional analysis and treatment model of SIB that accommodates both behavioral and biologic factors. Although our emphasis here will be on behavioral assessment and treatment methods, interested readers will find detailed summaries of neurobiological models and psychopharmacologic treatment of SIB in Harris (1992), Aman (1993), and Mace and Mauk (1995).

Problem Identification and Analysis

Problem identification is the first step in assessment and treatment of any behavioral disorder. Unlike other behavioral disturbances, SIB is often conspicuous and of great concern to parents, teachers, and other care providers. The disorder thus is readily identifiable and less likely to go underreported. The chief concerns related to problem identification and SIB are (1) specification of the environmental conditions surrounding occurrences of SIB; (2) estimation of the frequency, intensity, and duration of SIB episodes; and (3) differentiation of clinical from subclinical forms of the disorder. Concerns (1) and (2) can be addressed via indirect and direct forms of behavioral assessment, whereas identification of SIB of clinical severity is accomplished by medical examination or administration of the Self-Injury Trauma (SIT) Scale (Iwata, Pace, Kissel, Nau, & Farber, 1990).

Indirect Methods

Interviews

An efficient means of obtaining information about the presence of behavior problems and the conditions of their occurrence is for the behavior therapist to conduct a problem identification interview with an adult who has had numerous opportunities to observe the target child. Iwata, Wong, Riordan, and Lau (1982) and Kratochwill and Bergan (1990) have developed similar structured behavioral interview formats for this purpose. Both interview formats are generally used in conjunction with a behavior checklist that surveys a wide range of problem behaviors that have been reported in children with and without disabilities. Once surveyed and prioritized, the interviewer focuses on the two or three behavior problems of greatest concern to the care provider. Descriptions of the behavior are solicited to operationally define the problem and permit its accurate measurement. Estimates of the frequency and intensity of the behavior are obtained and preliminary goals for intervention are set. The behavior therapist then obtains detailed accounts of events immediately antecedent and subsequent to occurrences of the target behavior to formulate tentative hypotheses concerning the environmental influences on the problem.

Behavioral interviews of this sort can be very useful at the initial stage of assessment to clarify the nature of the problem, estimate its severity, and understand how it affects the child's home and school environments in general. However, because interviews are an indirect form of assessment, they have significant limitations in their capacity to provide full and accurate accounts of behavior and its maintaining conditions. Research directly comparing information obtained via structured behavioral interview with direct measurement of behavioral and environmental events under natural or analog conditions has yet to be done (Gresham & Davis, 1988). We suspect, however, that the results of research comparing rating-scale findings with direct methods of assessment are applicable to interview data as well.

Rating Scales

Several standardized rating scales have been developed specifically to identify deficits in adaptive behavior, including the presence of behavior problems, in individuals with developmental disabilities. The Vineland Adaptive Behavior Scales (Sparrow, Balla, & Cicchetti, 1985) and the AAMD Adaptive Behavior Scale—School Edition (Lambert, 1981) are among the most widely used standardized scales. Their sections on problem behaviors provide a survey of behavioral difficulties that are commonly seen in this population and permit comparison of a target child's ratings with those of a normed group.

The Motivational Assessment Scale (MAS) (Durand & Crimmins, 1988) is the only rating scale developed specifically to identify the behavioral function of self-injury. The scale consists of 16 items with 4 items each devoted to the assessment of the four known reinforcement functions of SIB: attention, access to materials, escape from demands, and sensory stimulation. Using a Likert-type format, care providers rate each item according to their experience observing an individual's SIB in various situations. Ratings are summed and a behavioral function for SIB is identified for the function with the highest rating. Although the MAS is both convenient and easy to use, independent reliability studies have reported low interrater reliability for the instrument when used in the assessment of self-injury or aggression (Newton & Sturmey, 1991; Sigafoos, Kerr, & Roberts, 1994; Zarcone, Rodgers, Iwata, Rourke, & Dorsey, 1991). These studies call into question the use of the MAS as the sole method for assessing the behavioral function of SIB. We recommend its use be limited to the generation of possible hypotheses to be tested via experimental functional analysis.

Direct Methods

Descriptive Analysis

Almost three decades ago, Bijou and his associates presented a descriptive assessment methodology to identify environmental influences on behavior that could provide useful information for the designing of behavioral interventions (Bijou, Peterson, & Ault, 1968; Bijou, Peterson, Harris, Allen, & Johnson, 1969). The assessment method involved operational definition of target behaviors and antecedent and subsequent environmental events capable of occasioning and reinforcing target behaviors. These events were recorded during continuous 5- or 10-s time intervals over repeated sessions. The resulting data were expressed as percentage of time a child or care provider engaged in various behaviors in different situations. The advent of portable computers and behavioral data collection software (e.g., Repp, Harman, Felce, Van-Acker, & Karsh, 1989) has permitted behavior therapists to record a greater number of behavioral and environmental events in real time with a high degree of accuracy.

We routinely conduct descriptive analyses on parent–child interactions during the first three to five days of a child's inpatient hospitalization at Children's Seashore House. Data are collected via laptop computer on (1) the onset and offset of potential establishing operations (low attention, restricted access to materials or activities, task demands, and low environmental stimulation), (2) the frequency of distinct topographies of SIB and other problem behaviors, and (3) the frequency of potentially reinforcing events occurring subsequent to SIB (attention, return of restricted materials/activities, discontinuation of task demands). The resulting data are analyzed in two ways. First, conditional frequencies of SIB are calculated for each of the potential establishing operations to assess whether the probability of observing SIB is consistently higher following one or more of these events. A second analysis is then performed for possible establishing operations highly correlated with SIB. The proportion of self-injurious responses followed within a short time period by a given event that could reinforce SIB is calculated (e.g., during task demands, the proportion of self-injurious responses followed by a break from demands). This latter analysis permits estimation of the natural schedule of reinforcement that may maintain SIB (Lalli, Browder, Mace, & Brown, 1993; Mace & Lalli, 1991; Sasso et al., 1992).

Although an improvement over indirect measures, descriptive methods of assessment have their own limitations that suggest they are poor substitutes for experimental functional analysis. Because events are free to vary during assessment, multiple environmental events capable of influencing SIB can occur concurrently, thereby obscuring the separate effects of any of the events. For example, a father may be preoccupied with a competing activity (low attention) and then observe his child climbing onto a countertop. When father removes the child from the countertop (restricted access), a self-injurious tantrum ensues followed by a reprimand for climbing and head banging. In this example, it is unclear whether SIB occurs in response to low attention or to restricted access to climbing. Even when a single environmental event covaries naturally with SIB, the relationship is only a *correlational* one. It remains unclear whether SIB and the event are *functionally* related. For instance, a child who engages in high rates of SIB during periods of minimal adult attention may be doing so to produce reactions from his care providers or, alternatively, SIB may produce reinforcing sensory stimulation when other forms of stimulation are not readily available. These limitations were examined in a study by Lerman and Iwata (1993) that compared assessment outcomes for descriptive and experimental analyses conducted on the same individuals. Their study found that descriptive analyses and experimental analyses were in agreement in only 16.7% of the cases.

In view of these limitations, we believe that descriptive analyses should be used in conjunction with experimental analyses to enhance the external validity of functional analysis findings in two key ways. First, repeated observation of adult–child interactions affords the opportunity to identify idiosyncratic and specific forms of establishing operations or reinforcing reactions to SIB that would not necessarily be included in standard analog conditions. For example, we may observe that a parent gives multistep and vague instructions repeatedly during tasks, or that in response to SIB following restriction of a child's access to an object, the parent offers a list of attractive substitutes for the restricted item. Similarly, there may be important functional differences in various forms of attention such as disapproval, sympathy, and redirection (Fisher, Ninness, Piazza, & Owen-DeSchryver, 1996). To the extent that SIB is a function of such idiosyncratic circumstances, including specific intermittent schedules of reinforcement, standard analog conditions may not reliably produce SIB. Thus, narrative information collected during the descriptive analysis can be used to design analog experimental conditions that better represent the individual child's interactional history.

A second use of descriptive analysis (DA) data is to aid in the interpretation of experimental analysis (EA) findings. The discordant results reported by Lerman and Iwata (1993) raise some questions about the validity of either form of assessment; these questions may require qualification of the assessment results. There are three possible outcomes when DA and EA assessments are conducted on a given individual: (1) the DA suggests a function not replicated in the EA; (2) the EA identifies a function not observed in the DA; and (3) both assessments identify a given function. Maximum confidence in the assessment results is warranted in Situation 3. In Situation 1, the failure to replicate a function in the EA implicated by the DA suggests that the relationship observed in the DA was likely spurious or accidental, and that treatment decisions should follow from the EA findings. However, in Situation 2, the possibility exists that the consistent application of a particular contingency in the EA established a functional relation that did not previously exist (see Carr, Newsom, & Binkoff, 1980, Experiment 4). If SIB is never observed to covary naturally with a given environmental condition, EA results showing that same condition is functionally related to SIB should be interpreted cautiously.

Experimental Analysis

Over the past 15 to 20 years, the experimental analysis of self-injury has emerged as an exemplar for behavioral research. The models of analysis developed for SIB have not only answered many basic questions about SIB, but have also influenced our understanding of a range of other behavioral disorders both within developmental disabilities (e.g., aggression) and related to other clinical concerns (e.g., ADHD). An experimental analysis (or functional analysis) of behavior is intended to identify behavior/environment relations. In operant SIB research and clinical practice, experimental analysis is used to evaluate the effects of hypothesized reinforcement contingencies and antecedent variables on SIB rates. The logic of an experimental analysis is straightforward: If reinforcement contingencies for SIB are identified, they can be withheld or modified during treatment and presented contingent on desired alternative behavior.

Methodology

Iwata et al. (1982/1994) published the first study that empirically evaluated a range of potential reinforcement contingencies for SIB. Four analog conditions were arranged to test the operant hypotheses outlined by E.G. Carr (1977). The analog conditions were designed to simulate events that may take place in the extra-experimental environment. A series of 15-min sessions were conducted using a multielement experimental design on a case-by-case basis to test the possibility that SIB was maintained by negative reinforcement (in the form of escape from instructional activity), positive reinforcement (in the form of caregiver attention), and/or sensory reinforcement (such as automatically produced stimulation). A fourth condition was called "play," and served as a control.

The test for *negative reinforcement* was conducted in a "demand" condition, during which the client received instructional demands once every 30 s throughout each 15-min session. Demands were presented using a three-prompt instructional hierarchy (Horner & Keilitz, 1975), and SIB produced a brief break from the instructional demands and instructional activity. If response rates were differentially high in the demand condition, Iwata and colleagues (1982, 1994) concluded SIB was maintained by escape (negative reinforcement). The test for *positive reinforcement* was conducted during a "reprimand" condition, during which a therapist acted as if he or she was engaged in work or reading activities. The client was offered alternative activities such as toys. Contingent upon SIB, a therapist provided statements of disapproval and concern. If response rates were differentially high in the reprimand condition, the authors concluded SIB was maintained by positive reinforcement. The test for *sensory reinforcement* was conducted during an "alone" condition, during which the client was observed alone with no attention or toys. No programmed consequences were delivered contingent on SIB. If response rates were differentially high in the alone condition, the authors concluded SIB was maintained by sensory reinforcement (independent of the social environment). During play (control), the client received attention approximately once every 30 seconds, received no instructions, and had free access to preferred toys and activities. Typically, low rates of SIB were observed in the play condition.

The results of Iwata and colleagues' (1982/ 1994) study were mixed, showing that the function of SIB appeared highly idiosyncratic across individuals. However, the goal of the study was not to show that all SIB occurs for the same reason for all cases; rather, the study may be viewed as a methodological advancement that delineated procedures for identifying reinforcement contingencies on a case-by-case basis. Further, the study supported the hypotheses set forth by E.G. Carr (1977) in his seminal paper: SIB rates fluctuated as a function of environmental events. In 1994, Iwata and colleagues published a summary study providing an overview of the outcomes for 144 experimental analyses using methods either identical or very similar to those methods described above (Iwata, Pace, et al., 1994): 38.1% of the assessments showed a behavioral responsiveness to the negative reinforcement contingency, 26.3% showed a behavioral responsiveness to positive reinforcement, 25.7% were elevated during the alone condition, 5.3% showed multiply controlled behavior, and 4% to 10% of the assessments yielded undifferentiated outcomes.

Perhaps because the Iwata et al. (1982/1994) study was the first empirical evaluation of its kind, the methods were replicated rigorously across individuals without reference to idiosyncratic differences in home, classroom, or residential environments. The focus of the study was to identify particular classes of reinforcement (e.g., positive versus negative) rather than specific forms of reinforcement (e.g., reprimands versus comfort statements). However, now that the utility of the general analytic method has been demonstrated and replicated in dozens of studies and in hundreds of single case analyses, there has been a shift in clinical focus to identify behavioral and environmental features as they occur in the natural environment. For example, Mace and Lalli (1991) demonstrated the utility of incorporating descriptive information into an experimental analysis. "Social attention," for instance, can take numerous forms (e.g., reprimands, comfort statements, physical contact) and descriptive observation may direct the experimenter or clinician to select the form of attention most commonly correlated with a given client's aberrant behavior (see the section on descriptive assessment). Similarly, whereas reprimands were tested as potential reinforcers in Iwata and colleagues' (1982/1994) study, numerous recent studies have demonstrated that positive reinforcement in the form of access to materials (e.g., favorite foods or toys) may be equally likely to maintain aberrant behavior. For example, Vollmer, Marcus, Ringdahl, and Roane (1995) found that aberrant behavior was maintained by tangible positive reinforcement for 7 out of 20 functional analysis participants, although none of these participants showed responsiveness to attention in the form of reprimands or comfort statements. Thus, the general functional analysis methods can be adjusted to incorporate information garnered from interviews and descriptive observations, such as forms of positive or negative reinforcement. Also, assessments can incorporate naturally occurring schedules of reinforcement (e.g., intermittency, delay to reinforcement), naturally occurring antecedent events (e.g., specific instructions used in the participants' environment), and naturally occurring establishing operations (e.g., diverted social attention), among other potentially idiosyncratic variables.

Interpretation of Results

When functional analysis results show elevated rates of SIB in one condition but not in others, the implications for treatment are relatively clear. But, not all functional analyses yield differentiated results. Various factors may account for undifferentiated results; we will address four possibilities. First, the assessment may not include the relevant environmental features responsible for evoking and/or reinforcing aberrant behavior. For example, a child may engage in SIB only when he is hungry because the behavior has historically produced access to food; if the assessment takes place when the child is reasonably satiated, no SIB would be expected. Second, the rates of aberrant behavior in one condition could be a result of the contingencies in effect during another condition (interaction effects). For example, attention-maintained behavior may persist in an alone session that follows an attention session. Third, the behavior may produce its own source of reinforcement, independent of contingencies in effect in the ambient environment. For example, eye poking may produce visual stimulation that does not depend on the presence or absence of a caregiver (Kennedy & Souza, 1995). Fourth, the behavior may be maintained by more than one source of reinforcement and both (or all) sources of reinforcement may yield elevated rates during experimental test conditions.

Over the past several years we have been working (independently and in collaboration) on assess-

ment models that may address some of the factors leading to undifferentiated functional analysis outcomes. An assessment model is depicted in Figure 1.

The first phase of assessment involves obtaining descriptive information through interview and direct observation (Mace & Lalli, 1991). Descriptive information should increase the likelihood that idiosyncratic factors are incorporated into a subsequent experimental analysis. For example, if SIB is maintained by food reinforcement, a descriptive analysis might show that problem behavior occurred following periods without food or when access to food was otherwise restricted, and should show that problem behavior at least intermittently produces access to food. In the absence of information about the naturally occurring context and contingencies in effect, it is unlikely that an experimental analysis would uncover such idiosyncratic establishing operations and reinforcement contingencies. The upper panel of Figure 2 shows hypothetical data from a functional analysis that does not incorporate descriptive information (in this example, food reinforcement). The lower panel of Figure 2 shows hypothetical data from a functional analy-

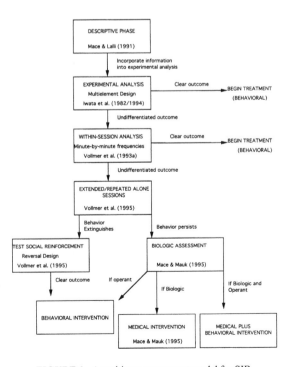

FIGURE 1. A multistep assessment model for SIB.

sis that includes a food reinforcement condition under periods of relative food deprivation. In the hypothetical example, the assessment conducted without the incorporation of descriptive information (i.e., the aberrant behavior/food relation) would have been inconclusive.

In the initial stages of an experimental analysis, we suggest evaluating within-session response patterns to address the possibility of interaction effects (Vollmer, Iwata, Zarcone, Smith, & Mazaleski, 1993a; Vollmer, Marcus, Ringdahl, & Roane, 1995). The upper panel of Figure 3 shows hypothetical data from an experimental analysis using overall session means as the dependent measure. Note that response rates are high in various conditions and the overall outcome of the analysis is undifferentiated. The lower panel of Figure 3 shows hypothetical *within-session* response frequencies on a minute-by-minute basis. In this hypothetical example, high rates of behavior occur in all sessions following the "attention" condition; further, the

behavior decreases following an initial burst of responding. Results such as these may suggest that the target behavior is maintained (reinforced) by attention and the effects of reinforcement influence behavior during ensuing sessions.

If behavior rates are relatively high in two or more experimental conditions, it is possible that behavior is maintained by more than one source of reinforcement. The upper panel of Figure 4 shows hypothetical assessment data in which SIB rates are high in attention and escape conditions. One analytic strategy is to compare the behavior rates to the control condition. The center panel shows elevated rates in the attention condition (from the assessment in the upper panel) compared to the control condition, suggesting a reinforcement effect of attention. The lower panel shows elevated rates in the escape condition (from the assessment in the upper panel) compared to the control condition, suggesting a reinforcement effect of escape. Another strategy to detect multiple control is to sequentially

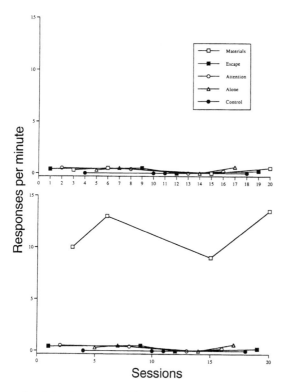

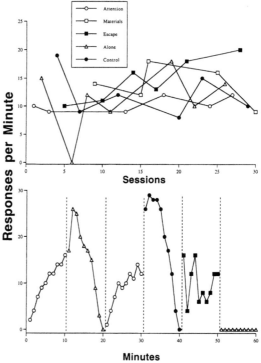

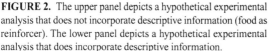

FIGURE 2. The upper panel depicts a hypothetical experimental analysis that does not incorporate descriptive information (food as reinforcer). The lower panel depicts a hypothetical experimental analysis that does incorporate descriptive information.

FIGURE 3. The upper panel depicts a hypothetical undifferentiated experimental analysis. The lower panel depicts a hypothetical analysis of the within-session response patterns, which suggest an attention function for SIB.

impose an attention-based intervention on the attention baseline (e.g., differential positive reinforcement) and an escape-based intervention on the escape baseline (e.g., differential negative reinforcement) (Repp, Felce, & Barton, 1988). The positive reinforcement-based treatment should influence only behavior maintained by attention and the negative reinforcement-based treatment should influence only behavior maintained by escape (R.G. Smith, Iwata, Vollmer, & Zarcone, 1993).

If behavior remains undifferentiated across assessment sessions and within-session patterns do not reveal reinforcement effects, we recommend either of two strategies to test for interaction effects: (a) conduct repeated alone sessions (Vollmer, Marcus, Ringdahl, & Roane, 1995), or (b) conduct one or more long-duration alone sessions (Mace & Mauk, 1995). The logic of repeated or extended alone sessions is that socially reinforced behavior should extinguish if it is no longer reinforced. Extinction may require an extended period of time, so repeated observations (or lengthy observations) may be needed. If behavior does extinguish eventually, social reinforcement contingencies could be tested next (e.g., attention, escape, access to materials, etc.). The upper panel of Figure 5 depicts hypothetical undifferentiated functional analysis results. The center panel depicts a hypothetical assessment during which behavior extinguished after repeated alone sessions. The next step in assessment should be to reinstitute social reinforcement contingencies in a reversal design (Vollmer, Marcus, Ringdahl, & Roane, 1995).

If behavior does not extinguish during extended or repeated alone sessions, it is reasonable to assume that the behavior is not maintained by social reinforcement contingencies. The lower panel of Figure 5 depicts hypothetical data show-

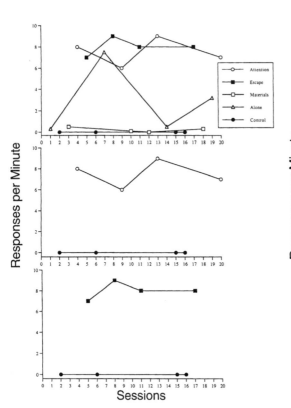

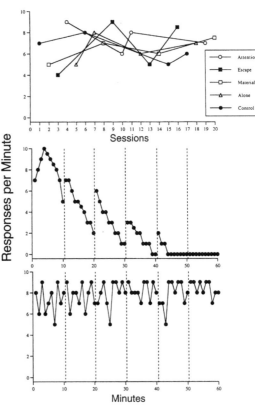

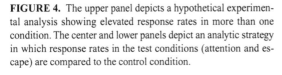

FIGURE 4. The upper panel depicts a hypothetical experimental analysis showing elevated response rates in more than one condition. The center and lower panels depict an analytic strategy in which response rates in the test conditions (attention and escape) are compared to the control condition.

FIGURE 5. The upper panel depicts a hypothetical undifferentiated functional analysis. The center panel depicts hypothetical repeated alone sessions, during which behavior extinguishes. The lower panel depicts hypothetical repeated alone sessions, during which behavior persists.

ing persistent behavior during an extended alone condition (i.e., no extinction effect is seen). The behavioral implications for treatment development are less clear for behavior that is not maintained by social reinforcement, and the model for assessment requires an integrated biologic and behavioral evaluation.

Biobehavioral Model of Self-Injury

A significant portion of SIB functional analyses fail to isolate one or more specific reinforcement contingencies maintaining the behavior (Iwata, Pace, et al., 1994; Vollmer, Marcus, Ringdahl, & Roane, 1995). Absent a clear maintaining condition exogenous to the individual, it is reasonable to formulate plausible hypotheses of endogenous maintaining processes. Two general classes of endogenous processes have been studied. As discussed above, the endogenous process behavior therapists have focused upon is automatic reinforcement, a hypothetical reinforcement process that presumes SIB produces sensory changes capable of reinforcing and maintaining it. Vollmer, Marcus, Ringdahl, & Roane, (1995) and Kennedy and Souza (1995) have presented two approaches to gathering evidence in support of an automatic reinforcement account of an individual's SIB.

A second class of endogenous processes involves a variety of neurobiologic disturbances believed to lead to the occurrence of self-injurious responses (Harris, 1992). Mace and Mauk (1995) have developed a biobehavioral model of assessment and intervention for SIB. The model relies on the use of functional analysis assessment to classify individual cases. SIB is classified as *operant* when SIB rates are consistently higher in one or more test condition(s) and low in the control condition (see bottom panel of Figure 2). If SIB is elevated in all conditions without differentiation among conditions, SIB is classified as *possibly biologic* (see top panel of Figure 3). Finally, a classification of *mixed operant and possibly biologic* is supported when SIB rates are elevated in all conditions, but occur at consistently higher rates in at least one test condition.

Mace and Mauk (1995) described decision rules for assigning clinical subtype classifications for possibly biologic and mixed cases of SIB. These subtypes are based on observable clinical features of self-injury that implicate specific neurotransmit-

ter disturbances that may be involved in particular individuals. The goal of subtyping is to empirically identify individuals who may be responsive to certain medications aimed at remediating or countering the underlying disorder. *Subtype 1: Extreme Self-Inflicted Injury* is assigned when evidence of deep wounds and scarring is apparent. Several researchers have hypothesized that a subset of individuals with SIB may be partially analgesic due to congenital factors or may engage in extreme forms of SIB to produce endogenous β-endorphins (Sandman, 1991). Individuals with this subtype may be responsive to opiate antagonists such as naltrexone. *Subtype 2: Repetitive and Stereotypic SIB* is characterized by the presence of high-rate but low-intensity behaviors that produce tissue damage with repeated occurrences such as skin rubbing and hand mouthing. Repetitive stereotypies have been associated with elevated dopamine and have been responsive to dopamine antagonists such as neuroleptics (Evenden, 1988). *Subtype 3: High-Rate SIB with Agitation if Interrupted* has the appearance of compulsive behavior and may be related to Obsessive–Compulsive Disorder (OCD) in adults with normal intellectual functioning. Several clinical studies have reported success in treating SIB with medications used to treat OCD (e.g., fluoxetine) (King, Bass, & Belhs, 1991). Finally, *Subtype 4: Co-Occurrence of SIB with Agitation,* is characterized by SIB with concomitant agitation including pacing, hyperventilation, screaming, and tachycardia. This elevated arousal suggests that such individuals may be responsive to lithium carbonate and related medications used to treat stress and overarousal (Chandler, Gualtieri, & Fahs, 1988).

The biobehavioral model described by Mace and Mauk (1995) is in its preliminary stage of development and will undergo considerable refinement as results of clinical studies warrant. Our preliminary data indicate that most SIB cases are operant in nature and will be responsive to the kinds of behavioral interventions discussed below.

Plan Implementation

Treatments for SIB are developed based on the information obtained during assessment. When reinforcers maintaining SIB have been identified, the general objectives of treatment are to withhold reinforcers when aberrant behavior occurs (extinction), to present reinforcers contingent on alternative behaviors (differential reinforcement), to alter the reinforcing value of consequent stimuli via manipulation of antecedent stimuli (e.g., modify the establishing operations or modify discriminative stimuli), or to integrate some combination of these three general strategies. The specific form of treatment varies based on the operant function of behavior.

Extinction

Extinction involves discontinuing the contingency between a behavior and its reinforcing consequence resulting in a decrease in the target behavior to zero or near-zero levels if extinction is achieved. In clinical research and practice, extinction is most often accomplished by withholding the stimulus that previously had been reinforcing aberrant behavior. If a behavior is maintained by positive reinforcement (attention or access to materials), extinction would involve ensuring that aberrant behavior does not produce access to those reinforcers (e.g., Lovaas & Simmons, 1969). If a behavior is maintained by negative reinforcement (escape from or avoidance of ambient aversive stimulation), extinction would involve ensuring that aberrant behavior does not produce escape or avoidance (e.g., Iwata, Pace, Kalsher, Cowdery, & Cataldo, 1990).

A variant of extinction is the response-independent schedule, sometimes termed noncontingent reinforcement (NCR). Response-independent schedules involve the presentation of a stimulus on a time-based schedule that is not influenced by the occurrence or nonoccurrence of a target behavior. Time-based schedules can be considered a variant of extinction because the contingency between aberrant behavior and the reinforcing consequence is eliminated (Rescorla & Skucy, 1969). For example, Vollmer, Iwata, Zarcone, Smith, and Mazaleski (1993b) presented attention on an escalating fixed-time (FT) schedule as treatment for attention-maintained SIB; the treatment produced a reduction in SIB relative to baseline and the FT schedule was thinned from continuous attention to FT 5 minutes. When behavior is maintained by escape, noncontingent escape can be presented as treatment using an escalating FT schedule (Vollmer, Marcus, & Ringdahl, 1995). One concern with NCR or FT schedules is the possibility of accidental reinforcement

resulting from reinforcer presentations occurring temporally contiguous to the target behavior. Although contiguous pairings of a response and a reinforcer do occur with FT schedules, contiguous pairings are unlikely to produce reinforcement effects if reinforcers are often presented in the absence of behavior *and* a reinforcer is sometimes delivered when no target response has occurred (Hammond, 1980).

Another variant of extinction, known as "sensory extinction," may be used when problem behavior is thought to be maintained by sensory consequences. For example, Rincover (1978) carpeted a table top to eliminate the sound produced by stereotypic object twirling displayed by a child with autism. Presumably the auditory stimulation had been reinforcing the twirling, a hypothesis supported by extinction-like reductions in aberrant behavior. Sensory extinction procedures have been replicated in several studies (e.g., Dorsey, Iwata, Reid, & Davis, 1982), but it is sometimes unclear whether extinction is the operant process responsible for behavior change. For example, response blocking may reduce self-injury because the blocking is an aversive stimulus (punishment) or because the blocking eliminates sensory stimulus products (extinction). Also, it is sometimes difficult to ascertain which response products are reinforcing the aberrant behavior (e.g., with mouthing, oral or tactile stimulation may serve as reinforcement). More research is clearly needed to evaluate components of sensory extinction procedures.

Differential Reinforcement

Differential reinforcement involves withholding reinforcement contingent on aberrant behavior but delivering reinforcers contingent upon either the omission of the target response or upon the commission of some alternative behavior. Delivery of positive reinforcers contingent on the omission of a target response is known as differential reinforcement of other behavior (DRO). Differential reinforcement of alternative behavior (DRA) consists of delivery of positive reinforcers contingent on the commission of alternative behaviors. The specific response topography that is differentially reinforced usually depends on the individual client's needs (e.g., communication, self-care, daily living skills, academics). Differential negative reinforcement has also been used in the treatment of escape-maintained SIB in both DNRO and DNRA forms (e.g., Roberts, Mace, & Dagget, 1995).

As with extinction, the effects of differential reinforcement depend on matching treatment to the operant function of behavior. If a behavior is maintained by contingent attention, attention should be delivered contingent on some alternative response. If behavior is maintained by escape, escape should be made contingent on some alternative response. If self-injury produces its own source of reinforcement, alternative stimulation can be designed to compete with the automatically produced reinforcers.

A common example of differential reinforcement is functional communication training (FCT) (E. Carr & Durand, 1985). In FCT, the reinforcer maintaining aberrant behavior is delivered contingent upon some alternative, communicative, response (such as a vocalization or sign language). For example, if self-injury is maintained by attention, a participant may be taught a new attention-producing behavior (E. Carr & Durand, 1985). If aberrant behavior is maintained by escape, a participant may be taught a new escape response (Steege et al., 1990). The communicative response may then functionally replace the aberrant behavior, especially if the aberrant behavior no longer produces the reinforcer (i.e., extinction). Several studies have shown that extinction is a critical component of differential reinforcement (Mazaleski, Iwata, Vollmer, Zarcone, & Smith, 1993; Wacker et al., 1990): If problem behavior is still reinforced, it may persist even though reinforcement is available for alternative behavior.

As a general rule, most individuals with SIB can benefit from communication training. At times, however, FCT should be packaged with additional intervention components to achieve clinically significant reductions in SIB. For example, if an individual displays escape-maintained SIB and learns an alternative escape behavior (i.e., communication), he or she may begin to request escape from all instructional activity and hence rarely participate (Marcus & Vollmer, 1995). One possible solution is to make escape contingent on task completion and communication. For example, Lalli, Casey, and Kates (1995) made escape from instructional activities contingent on an escalating ratio of task-related activities chained with a request to "take a break." Results showed that engagement with activities increased and use of alternative escape communication maintained. Similar applications could be used to teach individuals to "wait" prior to receiving attention or materials. That is, it may not always be appropriate to request and receive access to positive reinforcers at all times (e.g., food before a meal, attention when someone is busy); interval schedules could be used to ensure that time elapses prior to reinforcement.

Antecedent Interventions

Antecedent interventions are designed to reduce aberrant behavior by altering environmental events that occur prior to behavior. Most generally, antecedent interventions involve manipulating establishing operations (EOs), manipulating discriminative stimuli (S^Ds), or manipulating factors that make problem behavior less likely and alternative behavior more likely. To experimentally evaluate the effects of antecedent interventions, the reinforcing consequence identified during baseline should be delivered during intervention so that evaluation of antecedent manipulations are not confounded with extinction.

Establishing operations are events that alter the reinforcing value of a stimulus and the momentary probability of responding (Michael, 1982). For example, if SIB is maintained by contingent access to food, food deprivation (such as preceding mealtime) would increase the reinforcer value of food and increase the probability of SIB. Similarly, if SIB is maintained by attention, frequent attention delivered on NCR schedules may compete with SIB by reducing the "motivation" to obtain attention. However, to evaluate NCR effects as establishing operations, attention would still be delivered contingent on SIB during treatment (otherwise the effects may be attributed to extinction). Lalli, Casey, and Kates (1997) recently showed that NCR is effective in some circumstances even when aberrant behavior continues to be reinforced. If reinforcement contingencies remain in effect, the effects of NCR are likely due to a change in establishing operations.

Aversive stimulation establishes escape and avoidance as reinforcement (Michael, 1993). Variables such as illness, allergies, fatigue, demand frequency, and task novelty have been shown to establish instructional activities as aversive events, which can, in turn, temporarily increase the reinforcing value of escape (O'Reilly, 1995; Kennedy & Meyer, 1996; R.G. Smith, Iwata, Goh, & Shore, 1995). For example, O'Reilly (1995) showed that instructions produced more escape behavior on days following nights with less than five hours of sleep. Presumably, sleep altered the aversive properties of instructions. Similarly, R.G. Smith and colleagues (1995) showed that, for some individuals, instructional demands produced low levels of escape behavior unless the demands were presented at a high rate. Thus, frequency of instructions altered the value of escape as reinforcement and, hence, may be viewed as an establishing operation. When the establishing operations have been appropriately identified, they may be modified during treatment (e.g., reducing the rate of instructions).

Some individuals with self-injury also display a general resistance to following instructions. Several investigators have shown that compliance varies inversely with serious behavior problems, including SIB (e.g., Parrish, Cataldo, Kolko, Neef, & Egel, 1986). When a pervasive pattern of noncompliance with instructions is present, a potentially useful antecedent intervention for SIB and noncompliance is the high-p treatment (Mace et al., 1988). Derived from basic research on behavioral momentum (Nevin, 1996), the high-p treatment involves the presentation of a set of instructions that are likely to yield compliance immediately before issuing an instruction that the individual is unlikely to perform. Mace and Belfiore (1990) reported concomitant decreases in SIB following the high-p treatment. Replication studies found that these collateral effects can depend on the conjunctive use of extinction and the high-p treatment (Zarcone, Iwata, Mazaleski, & Smith, 1994).

Finally, there are some cases of escape-maintained self-injury that place the individual at very high risk for permanent physical injury or that co-occur with serious aggression. In such severe cases, clinicians may be unwilling to endure an escape-extinction process or to place themselves at risk for injury due to aggression. A procedure known as instructional fading has proven useful in such cases to gradually introduce demands at a pace that will result in minimal SIB (Pace, Iwata, Cowdery, Andree, & McIntyre, 1993; Zarcone et al., 1993). Through fading, instructional control is gradually transferred from a relatively low-demand situation to situations of increasing demands. In at least one report, the conjunctive use of escape-extinction procedures was necessary to sustain decreases in SIB resulting from instructional fading (Zarcone, Iwata, Smith, Mazaleski, & Lerman, 1994).

Plan Evaluation

Intervention effects are evaluated using single subject experimental designs, including reversal, multielement, and multiple baseline designs. During intervention, some measurable dimension of SIB or stereotypy (usually rate of response) is compared either to baseline levels or to levels in another type of treatment. In SIB research, baseline conditions usually are environmental situations that were shown (via functional analysis) to produce the highest levels of aberrant behavior. It is important to demonstrate that behavioral changes are correlated with the onset of intervention and it is also important to demonstrate that observed behavioral changes can be replicated. Examples of single subject designs are presented in Figures 6 through 8.

The upper panel of Figure 6 is a standard reversal design (ABAB), in which experimental control is demonstrated by observing response rates during baseline and treatment. The effects of treatment are replicated by returning to baseline conditions and

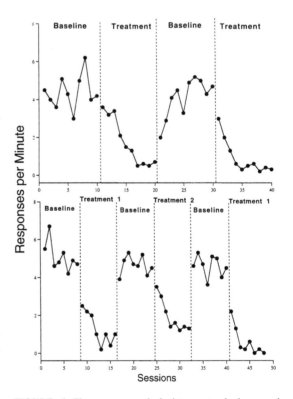

FIGURE 6. The upper panel depicts a standard reversal (ABAB) design, often used to test treatment effects. The lower panel depicts a reversal design (ABACAB) in which the effects of two treatments are tested.

then returning to treatment. The lower panel of Figure 6 shows that reversal designs can become progressively more complex if two or more treatments are compared (ABACAB). The advantage of a reversal design is that it yields a convincing demonstration of treatment effects because those effects are replicated within subjects.

Disadvantages of the reversal design include the undesired effects of returning to baseline conditions, and irreversibility. It is not always desirable to place an individual in the circumstances that previously had supported SIB (baseline). Thus, reversals are often kept to a minimum number of observational sessions in order to ensure the safety of the participant while still obtaining experimental control. Despite the potential risk, reversals are justified from a clinical perspective because it is important to know with certainty that behavioral changes result as a function of treatment. Irreversibility sometimes occurs when behavior changes dramatically and an individual's behavior contacts new sources of reinforcement, making alternative behavior unlikely to extinguish. A good example is reading. Once a child is taught to read, it is unlikely she will "unlearn" to read because reading is naturally reinforced in a wide range of social and nonsocial contexts. Similarly, functional communication is likely to contact reinforcement at least intermittently and may not extinguish once a good behavioral intervention is implemented with integrity.

Figure 7 depicts a standard multiple baseline design, in which experimental control is demonstrated by observing response rates during baseline and treatment conditions when treatment is implemented sequentially (either across people, situations, or behaviors). In the example, treatment is implemented at home, school, and then in day care. Changes in behavior rates are correlated with the implementation of treatment. The advantage of a multiple baseline design is that there is no need to reverse to baseline conditions. However, a strong demonstration of experimental control is sacrificed because there is no within subject replication per se. In other words, even though an intervention may appear to influence behavior across three contexts, the effects of intervention are never withdrawn and replicated in any single context. One possible solution may be to use a brief reversal in one setting.

The upper panel of Figure 8 depicts a standard multielement design, in which treatment response

rates are compared to baseline (no treatment) response rates. The preceding baseline condition is not necessarily required to demonstrate experimental control. Experimental control is demonstrated by the separation in data paths. The lower panel of Figure 8 depicts a multielement designs in which two treatments are compared. It is important to ensure that idiosyncratic features of one treatment are not responsible for differential treatment effects. For example, if one therapist is correlated with Treatment A only and one therapist is correlated with Treatment B only, each therapist should participate in baseline sessions to control for therapist-specific effects. The advantage of multielement designs is that they can produce a rapid demonstration of experimental control. The disadvantage is that interaction effects may result from the rapidly alternating conditions. If interaction effects occur, we recommend considering within-session data analysis such as that depicted in Figure 2.

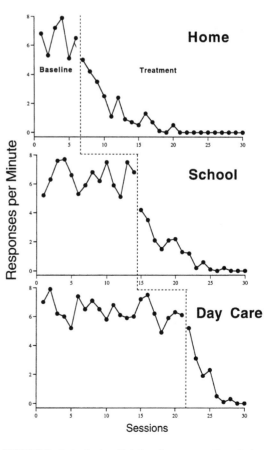

FIGURE 7. A standard multiple baseline across settings design.

426 CHAPTER 21

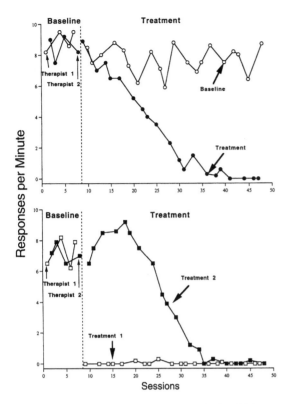

FIGURE 8. The upper panel depicts a standard multielement design, in which response rates during a treatment condition are compared to response rates during a baseline condition.

Maintenance and Generalization of Treatment Effects

General strategies and procedures used to promote generalization and maintenance of treatment effects within behavior analysis are also applicable for SIB. However, due to the severe nature of the behavior and the corresponding effects on care providers, unique risks exist for the maintenance of treatment gains (Shore, Iwata, Lerman, & Shirley, 1994). Maintenance of reduction in SIB generally requires the care provider to maintain extinction procedures, which for some care providers may be difficult to sustain. By contrast, maintenance of a new skill presumably comes into contact with the naturally occurring contingencies in the environment (e.g., teaching a child to raise his hand in class, rather than shout out the answer).

Stokes and Baer (1977) identified nine techniques used in designing or assessing program gen-

eralization. A more recent conceptualization (Kirby & Bickel, 1988) has suggested that "generalization" as used by Stokes and Baer (1977) is really a function of stimulus control and reinforcement processes. Kirby and Bickel (1988) identified six tactics for manipulating stimulus control and reinforcement processes, all of which include one or more of the generalization techniques cited by Stokes and Baer. The six techniques are (1) repeated presentation of naturally occurring stimuli (e.g., use several different therapists in training), (2) repeatedly present supplemental members (e.g., use of written instructions or recording devices), (3) vary extraneous stimuli (e.g., room location, time of day), (4) maximize common features between training and generalization, (5) alter the training schedule by moving from continuous to intermittent reinforcement, and (6) arrange reinforcement in the generalization setting (e.g., train; test for generalization; if generalization doesn't occur, train in that situation; and test for generalization in another setting).

Research on the generalization and maintenance of treatment for SIB may be examined in terms of the preceding taxonomy. Unfortunately, a paucity of data exists on the generalization and long-term maintenance of reductions in SIB. However, the results available have been generally positive. For example, follow-up data have been collected from 17 months (Northup et al., 1994) to 6 years (Williams, Kirkpatrick-Sanchez, & Crocker, 1994) after reaching initial treatment success.

Durand and Carr (1991) is representative of those studies reporting favorable outcomes. Functional communication training and extinction were used to successfully treat severe SIB in three individuals. The intervention reduced rates of SIB to low levels and increased rates of unprompted requests for attention or escape from a task. These gains were maintained for two individuals; however, the third individual developed an articulation problem midway through the follow-up, which led to increased rates of SIB. When the articulation problem was corrected, rates of SIB were again reduced. By not responding to his requests, the alternative response to SIB was functionally subject to extinction.

In terms of the stimulus control and reinforcement taxonomy (Kirby & Bickel, 1988), several techniques were used to promote generalization and maintenance. By teaching an alternative response to

SIB that would have a high probability of being reinforced, Durand and Carr (1991) arranged for high rates of reinforcement in the generalization setting. They implicitly presented naturally occurring members by using different therapists throughout training. Common features of the environment were maximized by conducting the training in the actual classroom.

Williams and colleagues (1994) also attributed the generalization and maintenance of treatment gains using the self-injurious behavior inhibiting system (SIBIS) to the presence of DRA and DRO components in the treatment package. Again, in terms of stimulus control and reinforcement, high rates of naturally occurring reinforcers were delivered for alternative responses, and programming for common features also occurred by using the same therapists in the training and generalization settings.

One study (T. Smith, Parker, Taubman, & Lovaas, 1992) found no improvement in the behavior management skills used by direct-care staff following a one-week workshop. The negative results are somewhat difficult to interpret because individual subject data were not reported. In addition, of three methods used to assess the effectiveness of the workshop, only one involved direct measures of staff behavior. The other two methods consisted of observing role-playing and the results of a paper-and-pencil test.

A change in the function of SIB may be an additional reason for failures of generalization and maintenance of treatment gains. Lerman, Iwata, Smith, Zarcone, and Vollmer (1994) conducted additional functional analyses for four individuals with SIB who relapsed two months to two years after being successfully treated. For three of the individuals, the additional functional analyses showed that their SIB had acquired new or additional functions. The results of these repeated analyses suggest that failures to generalize and maintain treatment effects may be due to more than stimulus control and reinforcement processes.

Summary and Future Directions

Most clinicians and researchers presently recognize that SIB can be maintained by separate or combined effects of biologic and environmental factors. This chapter presented a behavior-analytic assessment and treatment model of SIB that accommodates both behavioral and biologic influences on the disorder.

We described the various direct (e.g., descriptive analysis) and indirect (e.g., interviews, rating scales) assessment methods involved in problem identification. The purpose of this step is to obtain descriptive information in order to (1) specify the environmental conditions surrounding occurrences of SIB; (2) estimate the frequency, intensity, and duration of SIB episodes; and (3) differentiate clinical from subclinical forms of SIB. The direct observation method is often most valuable in helping to formulate hypotheses regarding the possible function(s) of SIB.

Descriptive analyses should be used in conjunction with experimental analyses to enhance the external validity of functional analysis findings by (a) affording the opportunity to identify specific forms of establishing operations and reinforcement that would not necessarily be included in standard analog conditions, and (b) aiding in the interpretation of experimental analysis (EA) findings and offering appropriate qualifications. We identified three possible outcomes when DA and EA assessments are conducted on a given individual: (1) the DA suggests a function not replicated in the EA; (2) the EA identifies a function not observed in the DA; and (3) both assessments identify a given function.

Most functional analyses result in identification of one or more of the following behavioral functions for SIB: positive reinforcement by attention, positive reinforcement by materials, negative reinforcement by escape from performance demands, and/or sensory or automatic reinforcement. For inconclusive results, we discussed various approaches to improve interpretation of functional analysis data. If SIB remains undifferentiated across assessment sessions and within-session patterns do not reveal reinforcement effects, repeated or extended alone sessions may be warranted in order to rule out social contingencies.

Treatments for SIB should be developed based on the information obtained during descriptive and functional assessments. Effective treatment strategies are extinction, noncontingent reinforcement, differential reinforcement, antecedent manipulations, or some combination of these. The specific form of treatment varies based on the operant function of behavior. In the final sections of this chapter, we detailed the advantages and disadvantages of reversal, multielement, and multiple baseline designs, and described procedures for maintenance and generalization of treatment gains.

Our hope is that these assessment and treatment procedures can help therapists develop interventions for SIB that focus on teaching alternative adaptive behaviors that serve a function similar to SIB. Over the past 15 to 20 years, the field of behavior analysis has seen many advances in the assessment and treatment of SIB. As we look to the future, one important area for additional research is the further development of biobehavioral models of SIB. Another key area for investigation is the refinement of assessment procedures for SIB maintained by automatic or sensory reinforcement. A third important area for future research involves distinguishing when behavioral and pharmacological therapies are indicated separately, and when they can best be combined.

ACKNOWLEDGMENTS

Preparation of this chapter was supported in part by a grant awarded to the first author by the National Institute of Mental Health (RO1 MH50358).

References

Aman, M.G. (1993). Efficacy of psychotropic drugs for reducing self-injurious behavior in the developmental disabilities. *Annals of Clinical Psychiatry, 5,* 171–178.

Baumeister, A., & Rollings, J.P. (1976). Self-injurious behavior. *International Review of Research in Mental Retardation, 8,* 1–34.

Bijou, S.W., Peterson, R.F., & Ault, M.H. (1968). A method to integrate descriptive and experimental field studies at the level of data and empirical concepts. *Journal of Applied Behavior Analysis, 1,* 175–191.

Bijou, S.W., Peterson, R.F., Harris, F.R., Allen, K.E., & Johnson, M.S. (1969). Methodology for experimental studies of young children in natural settings. *Psychological Record, 19,* 177–210.

Breese, G.R., Criswell, H.E., Duncan, G.E., Moy, S.S., Johnson, K.B., Wong, D.F., & Mueller, R.A. (1995). Model for reduced brain dopamine in Lesch-Nyhan syndrome and the mentally retarded: Neurobiology of neonatal-6-hydroxy-dopamine-lesioned rats. *Mental Retardation and Developmental Disabilities Research Reviews, 1,* 111–119.

Carr, E., & Durand, V.M. (1985). Reducing behavior problems through functional communication training. *Journal of Applied Behavior Analysis, 18,* 111–126.

Carr, E. G. (1977). The motivation of self-injurious behavior: A review of some hypotheses. *Psychological Bulletin, 84,* 800–816.

Carr, E.G., Newsom, C.D., & Binkoff, J.A. (1980). Escape as a factor in the aggressive behavior of two retarded children. *Journal of Applied Behavior Analysis, 133,* 101–117.

Chandler, M., Gualtieri, C.T., & Fahs, J.J. (1988). Other psychotropic drugs: Stimulants, antidepressants, anxiolytics, and lithium carbonate. In M.G. Aman & N.N. Singh (Eds.), *Psychopharmacology of the developmental disabilities* (pp. 119–145). New York: Springer-Verlag.

Dorsey, M.F., Iwata, B.A., Reid, D.H., & Davis, P.A. (1982). Protective equipment: Continuous and contingent application in the treatment of self-injurious behavior. *Journal of Applied Behavior Analysis, 15,* 217–230.

Durand, V. M., & Carr, E. G. (1991). Functional communication training to reduce challenging behavior: Maintenance and applications in new settings. *Journal of Applied Behavior Analysis, 24,* 251–264.

Durand, V.M., & Crimmins, D.B. (1988). Identifying the variables maintaining self-injurious behavior. *Journal of Autism and Developmental Disorders, 18,* 99–117.

Evenden, J. (1988). Issues in behavioral pharmacology: Implications for developmental disorders. In M.G. Aman & N.N. Singh (Eds.), *Psychopharmacology of the Developmental Disabilities* (pp. 216–238). New York: Springer-Verlag.

Farber, J. (1987). Psychopharmacology of self-injurious behavior in the mentally retarded. *Journal of the American Academy of Child and Adolescent Psychiatry, 26,* 296–302.

Favell, J.E., Azrin, N.H., Baumeister, A.A., Carr, E.G., Dorsey, M.F., Forehand, R., Foxx, R. M., Lovaas, O.I., Rincover, A., Risley, T.R., Romanczyk, R.G., Russo, D.C., Schroeder, S.R., & Solnick, J.V. (1982). The treatment of self-injurious behavior. *Behavior Therapy, 13,* 529–554.

Fisher, W.W., Ninness, H.A.C., Piazza, C.C., & Owen-DeSchryver, J.S. (1996). On the reinforcing effects of the content of verbal attention. *Journal of Applied Behavior Analysis, 29,* 235–238.

Gresham, F.M., & Davis, C.J. (1988). Behavioral interviews with teachers and parents. In E.S. Shapiro & T.R. Kratochowill (Eds.), *Behavioral assessment in schools* (pp. 455–493). New York: Guilford.

Griffin, J.C., Ricketts, R.W., Williams, D.E., Locke, B.J., Altmeyer, B.K., & Stark, M.T. (1987). A community survey of self-injurious behavior among developmentally disabled children and adolescents. *Hospital and Community Psychiatry, 38,* 959–963.

Hammond, L.J. (1980). The effect of contingency upon the appetitive conditioning of free-operant behavior. *Journal of the Experimental Analysis of Behavior, 34,* 297–304.

Harris, J.C. (1992). Neurobiological factors in self-injurious behavior. In J.K. Luiselli, J.L. Matson, & N.N. Singh (Eds.), *Self-injurious behavior: Analysis, assessment, and treatment* (pp. 59–92). New York: Springer-Verlag.

Horner, R.D., & Keilitz, I. (1975). Training mentally retarded adolescents to brush their teeth. *Journal of Applied Behavior Analysis, 8,* 301–309.

Iwata, B.A., Wong, S.E., Riordan, M.M., & Lau, M.M. (1982). Assessment and training of clinical interviewing skills:

Analogue analysis and field replication. *Journal of Applied Behavior Analysis, 15,* 191–203.

Iwata, B.A., Pace, G.M., Kalsher, M.J., Cowdery, G.E., & Cataldo, M.F. (1990). Experimental analysis and extinction of self-injurious escape behavior. *Journal of Applied Behavior Analysis, 23,* 11–27.

Iwata, B.A., Pace, G.M., Kissel, R.C., Nau, P.A., & Farber, J.M. (1990). The self-injury trauma (SIT) scale: A method for quantifying surface tissue damage caused by self-injurious behavior. *Journal of Applied Behavior Analysis, 23,* 99–110.

Iwata, B.A., Dorsey, M.F., Slifer, K.J., Bauman, K.E., & Richman, G.S. (1994). Toward a functional analysis of self-injury. *Journal of Applied Behavior Analysis, 27,* 197–209. (Reprinted from *Analysis and intervention in developmental disabilities,* Vol. 2, pp. 3–20, 1982, Kidlington, UK: Elsevier Science Ltd.

Iwata, B.A., Pace, G.M., Dorsey, M.F., Zarcone, J.R., Vollmer, T.R., Smith, R.G., Rodgers, T.A., Lerman, D.C., Shore, B.A., Mazaleski, J.L., Goh, H.L., Cowdery, G.L., Kalsher, M.J., McCosh, K.C., & Willis, K.D. (1994). The function of self-injurious behavior: An experimental-epidemiological analysis. *Journal of Applied Behavior Analysis, 27,* 215–240.

Kennedy, C.H., & Meyer, K.A. (1996). Sleep deprivation, allergy symptoms, and negatively reinforced problem behavior. *Journal of Applied Behavior Analysis, 29,* 133–135.

Kennedy, C.H., & Souza, G. (1995). Functional analysis and treatment of eye poking. *Journal of Applied Behavior Analysis, 28,* 27–37.

King, B., Bass J., & Belhs, J. (1991). Fluoxetine reduced self-injurious behavior in an adolescent with mental retardation. *Journal of Child and Adolescent Psychopharmacology, 1,* 321–329.

Kirby, K.C., & Bickel, W.K. (1988). Toward an explicit analysis of generalization: A stimulus control interpretation. *Behavior Analyst, 11,* 115–129.

Kratochowill, T.R., & Bergan, J.R. (1990). *Behavioral consultation in applied settings.* New York: Plenum.

Lalli, J.S., Browder, D.M., Mace, F.C., & Brown, K. (1993). Teacher use of descriptive analysis data to implement interventions to decrease students' maladaptive behavior. *Journal of Applied Behavior Analysis, 26,* 227–238.

Lalli, J.S., Casey, S., & Kates, K. (1995). Reducing escape behavior and increasing task completion with functional communication training, extinction, and response chaining. *Journal of Applied Behavior Analysis, 28,* 261–268.

Lalli, J.S., Casey, S., & Kates, K. (1997). Noncontingent reinforcement as treatment for severe problem behavior: Some procedural variations. *Journal of Applied Behavior Analysis, 30,* 127–137.

Lambert, N.M. (1981). *AAMD Adaptive Behavior Scale, School Edition: Diagnostic and technical manual.* Monterey, CA: Publishers Test Service.

Lerman, D.C., & Iwata, B.A. (1993). Descriptive and experimental analyses of variables maintaining self-injurious behavior. *Journal of Applied Behavior Analysis, 26,* 293–319.

Lerman, D.C., Iwata, B.A., Smith, R.G., Zarcone, J.R., & Vollmer, T.R. (1994). Transfer of behavioral function as a contributing factor in treatment relapse. *Journal of Applied Behavior Analysis, 27,* 357–370.

Lovaas, O.I., & Simmons, J.Q. (1969). Manipulation of self-destruction in three retarded children. *Journal of Applied Behavior Analysis, 2,* 143–157.

Mace, F.C., & Belfiore, P. (1990). Behavioral momentum in the treatment of escape-motivated stereotypy. *Journal of Applied Behavior Analysis, 23,* 507–514.

Mace, F.C., & Lalli, J.S. (1991). Linking descriptive and experimental analyses in the treatment of bizarre speech. *Journal of Applied Behavior Analysis, 24,* 553–562.

Mace, F.C., & Mauk, J.E. (1995). Bio-behavioral diagnosis and treatment of self-injury. *Mental Retardation and Developmental Disabilities Research Reviews, 1,* 104–110.

Mace, F.C., Hock, M.L., Lalli, J.S., West, B.J., Belfiore, P., Pinter, E., & Brown, D.K. (1988). Behavioral momentum in the treatment of noncompliance. *Journal of Applied Behavior Analysis, 21,* 123–141.

Mace, F.C., Lalli, J.S., & Shea, M. (1992). Functional analysis and treatment of self-injury. In J.K. Luiselli, J. L. Matson, & N.N. Singh (Eds.), *Self-injurious behavior: Analysis, assessment and treatment* (pp. 122–152). New York: Springer-Verlag.

Marcus, B.A., & Vollmer, T.R. (1995). Effects of differential negative reinforcement on disruption and compliance. *Journal of Applied Behavior Analysis, 28,* 229–230.

Mazaleski, J.L., Iwata, B.A., Vollmer, T.R., Zarcone, J.R., & Smith, R.G. (1993). Analysis of the reinforcement and extinction components in DRO contingencies with self-injury. *Journal of Applied Behavior Analysis, 26,* 143–156.

Michael, J. (1982). Distinguishing between the discriminative and motivational functions of stimuli. *Journal of the Experimental Analysis of Behavior, 37,* 149–155.

Michael, J. (1993). Establishing operations. *Behavior Analyst, 16,* 191–206.

National Institutes of Health. (1989). *NIH consensus development conference on the treatment of destructive behaviors in persons with developmental disabilities.* Bethesda, MD: U.S. Department of Health and Human Services.

Nevin, J.A. (1996). The momentum of compliance. *Journal of Applied Behavior Analysis, 29,* 535–547.

Newton, J.T., & Sturmey, P. (1991). The Motivation Assessment Scale: Interrater reliability and internal consistency in a British sample. *Journal of Mental Deficiency Research, 35,* 472–474.

Northup, J., Wacker, D.P., Berg, W.K., Kelly, L., Sasso, G., & DeRaad, A. (1994). The treatment of severe behavior problems in school settings using a technical assistance model. *Journal of Applied Behavior Analysis, 27,* 33–47.

O'Reilly, M.F. (1995). Functional analysis and treatment of escape-maintained aggression correlated with sleep deprivation. *Journal of Applied Behavior Analysis, 28,* 225–226.

Pace, G.M., Iwata, B.A., Cowdery, G.E., Andree, P.J., & McIntyre, T. (1993). Stimulus (instructional) fading during extinction of self-injurious escape behavior. *Journal of Applied Behavior Analysis, 26,* 205–212.

Parrish, J.M., Cataldo, M.F., Kolko, D.J., Neef, N.A., & Egel, A.L. (1986). Experimental analysis of response covariation among compliant and inappropriate behaviors. *Journal of Applied Behavior Analysis, 19,* 241–254.

Repp, A.C., Felce, D., & Barton, L.E. (1988). Basing the treatment of stereotypic and self-injurious behaviors on hypotheses of their causes. *Journal of Applied Behavior Analysis, 21,* 281–289.

Repp, A.C., Harman, M.L., Felce, D., VanAcker, R., & Karsh, K.L. (1989). Conducting behavioral assessments on computer collected data. *Behavioral Assessment, 2,* 249–268.

Rescorla, R.A., & Skucy, J.C. (1969). Effect of response–independent reinforcers during extinction. *Journal of Comparative and Physiological Psychology, 67,* 381–389.

Rincover, A. (1978). Sensory extinction: A procedure for eliminating self-stimulatory behavior in developmentally disabled children. *Journal of Abnormal Child Psychology, 6,* 299–310.

Roberts, M.L, Mace, F.C., & Dagget, J.A. (1995). Preliminary comparison of two negative reinforcement schedules to reduce self-injury. *Journal of Applied Behavior Analysis, 28,* 579–580.

Sandman, C. (1991). The opiate hypothesis in autism and self-injury. *Journal of Child and Adolescent Psychopharmacology, 1,* 237–248.

Sasso, G.M., Reimers, T.M., Cooper, L.J., Wacker, D., Berg, W., Steege, M., Kelly, L., & Allaire, A. (1992). Use of descriptive and experimental analyses to identify the functional properties of aberrant behavior in school settings. *Journal of Applied Behavior Analysis, 25,* 809–821.

Schroeder, S. R., Schroeder, C.S., Smith, R., & Dalldorf, J. (1978). Prevalence of self-injurious behaviors in a large state facility for the retarded: A three-year follow-up study. *Journal of Autism and Childhood Schizophrenia, 8,* 261–269.

Shore, B.A., Iwata, B.A., Lerman, D.C., & Shirley, M.J. (1994). Assessing and programming generalized behavioral reduction across multiple stimulus parameters. *Journal of Applied Behavior Analysis, 27,* 371–384.

Sigafoos, J., Kerr, M., & Roberts, D. (1994). Interrater reliability of the motivation assessment scale: Failure to replicate with aggressive behavior. *Research in Developmental Disabilities, 15,* 333–342.

Smith, R.G., Iwata, B.A., Goh, H.L., & Shore, B.A. (1995). Analysis of establishing operations for self-injury maintained by escape. *Journal of Applied Behavior Analysis, 28,* 515–535.

Smith, R.G., Iwata, B.A., Vollmer, T.R., & Zarcone, J.R. (1993). Experimental analysis and treatment of multiply controlled self-injury. *Journal of Applied Behavior Analysis, 26,* 183–196.

Smith, T., Parker, T., Taubman, M., & Lovaas, O.I. (1992). Transfer of staff training from workshops to group homes: A failure to generalize across settings. *Research in Developmental Disabilities, 13,* 57–71.

Sparrow, S.S., Balla, D.A., & Cicchetti, D.V. (1985). *Vineland Adaptive Behavior Scales, Classroom Edition.* Circle Pines, MN: American Guidance Service.

Steege, M.W., Wacker, D.P., Cigrand, K.C., Berg, W.K., Novak, C.G., Reimers, T.M., Sasso, G.M., & DeRaad, A. (1990).

Use of negative reinforcement in the treatment of self-injurious behavior. *Journal of Applied Behavior Analysis, 23,* 459–467.

Stokes, T.F., & Baer, D.M. (1977). An implicit technology of generalization. *Journal of Applied Behavior Analysis, 10,* 349–367.

Tessel, R.E., Schroeder, S.R., Stodgell, C.J., & Loupe, P.S. (1995). Rodent models of mental retardation: Self-injury, aberrant behavior, and stress. *Mental Retardation and Developmental Disabilities Research Reviews, 1,* 99–103.

Vollmer, T.R., Iwata, B.A., Zarcone, J.R., Smith, R.G., & Mazaleski, J.L. (1993a). Within-session patterns of self-injury as indicators of behavioral function. *Research in Developmental Disabilities, 14,* 479–492.

Vollmer, T.R., Iwata, B.A., Zarcone, J.R., Smith, R.G., & Mazaleski, J.L. (1993b). The role of attention in the treatment of attention-maintained self-injurious behavior: Noncontingent reinforcement (NCR) and differential reinforcement of other behavior (DRO). *Journal of Applied Behavior Analysis, 26,* 9–21.

Vollmer, T.R., Marcus, B.A., & Ringdahl, J.E. (1995). Noncontingent escape as treatment for self-injurious behavior maintained by negative reinforcement. *Journal of Applied Behavior Analysis, 28,* 15–26.

Vollmer, T.R., Marcus, B.A., Ringdahl, J.E., & Roane, H.S. (1995). Progressing from brief assessments to extended functional analyses in the evaluation of aberrant behavior. *Journal of Applied Behavior Analysis, 28,* 561–576.

Wacker, D.P., Steege, M.W., Northup, J., Sasso, G., Berg, W., Reimers, T., Cooper, L., Cigrand, K., & Donn, L. (1990). A component analysis of functional communication training across three topographies of severe behavior problems. *Journal of Applied Behavior Analysis, 23,* 417–429.

Williams, D.E., Kirkpatrick-Sanchez, S., & Crocker, W.T. (1994). A long-term follow-up of treatment for severe self-injury. *Research in Developmental Disabilities, 15,* 487–501.

Zarcone, J.R., Rodgers, T.A., Iwata, B.A., Rourke, D.A., & Dorsey, M.F. (1991). Reliability analysis of the Motivation Assessment Scale: A failure to replicate. *Research in Developmental Disabilities, 12,* 349–360.

Zarcone, J.R., Iwata, B.A., Vollmer, T.R., Jagtiani, S., Smith, R.G., Mazaleski, J.L. (1993). Extinction of self-injurious escape behavior with and without instructional fading. *Journal of Applied Behavior Analysis, 26,* 353–360.

Zarcone, J.R., Iwata, B.A., Mazaleski, J.L., & Smith, R.G. (1994). Momentum and extinction effects on self-injurious escape behavior and noncompliance. *Journal of Applied Behavior Analysis, 27,* 649–658.

Zarcone, J.R., Iwata, B.A., Smith, R.G., Mazaleski, J.L., & Lerman, D.C. (1994). Reemergence and extinction of self-injurious escape behavior during stimulus (instructional) fading. *Journal of Applied Behavior Analysis, 27,* 307–316.

22

Habits and Tics

T. STEUART WATSON AND HEATHER ELISE STERLING

Introduction

The goal of this chapter is to present a clinician-friendly guide to the identification, functional assessment, treatment, and evaluation of habit and tic behaviors. We combined tics and habits into a single chapter because of the topographical and functional similarities between tics and habits. For example, people who repeatedly shrug their shoulders may do so because they have learned that the specific response of shrugging releases muscle tension (an operant behavior that is maintained by automatic negative reinforcement, also called a habit) or because it is elicited by an internal stimulus as part of an organic disorder (e.g., Tourette's) which results in a feeling of relief or escape from aversive somatic sensation. In both instances, the topography (i.e., shrugging shoulders) and the function (i.e., negative reinforcement by escape) are the same. Regardless of whether the shoulder shrugging is labeled a tic or a habit, the general assessment and treatment procedures will be identical.

Habits

Although there is no agreed upon definition of what constitutes a habit, perhaps the most comprehensive definition is that a habit is a benign, learned, persistent, volitional, topographically repetitive behavior that is maintained by reinforcement (positive, negative, or automatic), and evoked by many discriminative stimuli. Most individuals engage in some form of habit behavior (e.g., hand or foot tapping, eye blinking and squinting, hair twirling) during some part of their life. As most habits are considered benign (i.e., not accompanied by more serious psychopathology), they usually go untreated unless there is considerable cost to the person in terms of physical, social, academic/occupational, and/or psychological discomfort or risk (Hansen, Tishelman, Hawkins, & Doepke, 1990). Because habits may result in negative interactions between parents and child, negative social consequences (e.g., avoidance by peers), physical damage (e.g., malocclusions), and other negative consequences, they are an important concern for parents and the individuals responsible for treatment (e.g., family doctors, pediatricians, and psychologists), as well as for the child who engages in the habit.

At present, the *Diagnostic and Statistical Manual of Mental Disorder,* 4th ed. (*DSM-IV;* American Psychiatric Association, 1994) does not have a separate diagnostic category for behaviors that could be classified as habits, but instead characterizes certain habit behaviors, specifically trichotillomania, as an "Impulse-Control Disorder Not Elsewhere Classified." Other habit behaviors are not included in the *DSM-IV* classification system. Although most behavior analysts are not concerned with *DSM* diagnoses, it is important to be knowledgeable of diagnostic categories and criteria, particularly in this age of managed care where even brief behavioral treatment is carefully scrutinized and most insurance carriers require a diagnosis before reimbursing for treatment.

T. STEUART WATSON AND HEATHER ELISE STERLING
• School Psychology Program, Mississippi State University, Mississippi State, Mississippi 39762.

Handbook of Child Behavior Therapy, edited by Watson and Gresham. Plenum Press, New York, 1998.

Prevalence Rates and Etiology

Because habit disorders cover a wide range of behaviors with different topographies, it is extremely difficult to estimate the overall prevalence in the population. However, approximate prevalence rates for specific habits have been reported. Peterson, Campose, and Azrin (1994) surveyed the literature and summarized the prevalence rates and sex ratios for the major types of habits (see Table 1).

The exact etiology of habits is unclear. Early theories suggested that children who engaged in habits did so as a sign of psychopathology (Freud, 1965; S. Shapiro & Shannon, 1966). More recent research suggests, however, that habits are learned behavior not linked to underlying emotional disturbance or psychopathology (Hunt, Matarazzo, Weiss, & Gentry, 1979). Research has also found that children who engage in habit behaviors are not significantly different in terms of deviant behavior from their peers on measures such as the Child Behavior Checklist (CBCL; Achenbach, 1991) or Eyberg Child Behavior Inventory (Friman, Larzelere, & Finney, 1994). Some authors have suggested that habits are the result of poor impulse control (Leonard, Lenane, Swedo, Rettew, & Rapoport,

1991), reactions to decrease stress (Azrin & Peterson, 1990), or neurologically based (Azrin & Peterson, 1990). It has even been suggested that some habits are nonfunctional (Glaros & Melamed, 1992).

From an operant perspective, it is likely that some behaviors become conditioned reinforcers or are directly reinforced and, as a result, persist for long periods of time and become correlated with many discriminative stimuli. For instance, a three-year-old may suck her thumb (a developmentally normal behavior) before going to sleep, while watching television, and/or during a bath. Sucking her thumb, which hastens the onset of sleep, is consistent with Fantino's delay reduction hypothesis (Fantino, 1969), which states that stimuli that occur temporally closer to positive reinforcers become *conditioned reinforcers.* Sucking her thumb while engaging in another reinforcing activity (e.g., taking a bath, watching TV) may also establish thumb sucking as a conditioned reinforcer. She may also suck her thumb when she becomes upset or frightened, and learns that thumb sucking results in a reduction in physiological discomfort (as with the case of Little Albert, who sucked his thumb while being emotionally conditioned, a situation that resulted in an attenuation of his emotional behavior;

TABLE 1. Prevalence Rates and Sex Ratios of Common Habits Seen in Clinical Settings

Habit	Prevalence rate	Sex ratio
Tics		
Tourette's	0.046%	More common in males
Transient	0.25%	Unknown; assumed to be similar to Tourette's
Bruxism	7%–88% (depending on definition used) Highest rate occurs in 7- to 15-year-olds with mixed dentition	Unknown
Trichotillomania	10% of adults Unknown for children, but assumed to be higher than that of adults	More common in females, except during preschool years when more common in males
Nail biting	Rates increase from preschool age to adolescence where peaks at 45%, then drops steadily to a rate of 4.5% in adults	More common in females
Thumbsucking	30%–40% during preschool years 10%–20% of 6-year-olds or older	Unknown

Note. Some data in the table are from "Behavioral and Pharmacological Treatments for Tics and Habit Disorders," by A.L. Peterson, R.L. Campose, & N.H. Azrin, 1994, *Journal of Developmental and Behavioral Pediatrics, 15,* pp. 430–441.

J.B. Watson & Rayner, 1920). Thus, thumb sucking has been *negatively reinforced* because she escaped unpleasant physiological stimulation contingent on thumb sucking. In other cases, parents may comment on or reprimand a child's thumb sucking and this provides contingent *social attention* for the behavior. T.S. Watson and Allen (1993) proposed that the sucking action produces tactile and kinesthetic stimulation of the oral tissue which may also maintain thumb sucking, a hypothesis that is consistent with *automatic reinforcement*. Because thumb sucking has been reinforced, albeit unintentionally, in various ways over a period of time, it persists and generalizes to new stimuli.

Mechanical theories may help to explain some habits, particularly bruxism. Mechanical theories suggest that individuals brux due to deviations from ideal occlusion. Because of these deviations, bruxers attempt to maintain a more ideal occlusion by grinding or clenching their teeth. There is some evidence to support this theory in that the highest rates of bruxing occur in youth with mixed dentition (Glaros & Melamed, 1992). Psychological theories have suggested a wide variety of reasons for bruxism, ranging from oral fixation to anxiety. Although psychodynamic theories have long been discarded, theories regarding the role of anxiety and stress are still addressed in the literature. It appears, at least in adults, that the anticipation of stress is a better predictor of bruxism than the amount of stress in an individual's life (Glaros & Melamed, 1992). Systemic and neurological theories have also been put forth to explain the maintenance of bruxism, as higher rates of bruxism have been noted in individuals with allergies and hyperthyroidism and in individuals with disabilities, especially those with mental retardation, Down's syndrome, and cerebral palsy. It has also been suggested that children on stimulant medication may be at higher risk for bruxism (Glaros & Melamed, 1992). A slightly different explanation for bruxism has been suggested, but is limited only to nocturnal bruxism. Nocturnal bruxism has been associated with transitions from heavier to lighter sleep stages, leading some researchers to suggest that the function of nocturnal bruxism is to maintain sleep (T.S. Watson, 1993).

Although it is fun to speculate about the specific origins of a particular habit, it is much more important to analyze the specific current antecedents and consequences that evoke and maintain the behavior.

In other words, it is relatively unimportant to know that a child began nail biting after the death of a pet six months ago; it matters more to determine the stimuli that evoke nail biting and the function(s) of the behavior at the present time. In addition, the function(s) of the behavior at its onset may be quite different from the current function(s) of the behavior.

Common Habits Seen in Referrals

Trichotillomania is a disorder that involves the repetitive pulling out of hair from the body. Although the scalp is reported as the most common area from which hair is removed, individuals may pull hair from any part of the body, including the eyelashes, eyebrows, or pubic areas. Adults who engage in hair pulling report high levels of psychological distress associated with this behavior and may go to great lengths to disguise or hide their behavior (Christenson, Mackenzie, & Mitchell, 1991). Alopecia (baldness) is the most often reported side effect of trichotillomania. To receive a *DSM-IV* diagnosis of trichotillomania, the person must (a) have a history of hair pulling with a noticeable loss of hair and (b) report a "need" or urge to pull hair and a sense of relief once the hair has been removed. This second criterion may not be applicable to young children because they are not sufficiently aware of the antecedent physiological stimuli that are reduced by hair pulling. In addition, for a trichotillomia diagnosis the alopecia may not be better accounted for by another mental or medical disorder such as alopecia areata or the ingestion of medication for which a side effect is hair loss.

Although there are no medical concerns directly associated with pulling hair, trichopagia (hair eating) is often a comorbid behavior which may result in significant gastrointestinal difficulties. If excessive hair is swallowed, a trichobezoar (hair ball) may become stationary in the large intestine and block the passage of feces, causing abdominal pain, anemia, vomiting of blood, nausea, and bowel perforation.

Oral habits are not clearly defined in the literature and include a wide range of behaviors such as teeth clenching or grinding (bruxism), chewing, biting, or licking of lips, tongue, or the inside of the mouth (Peterson et al., 1994). Common side effects associated with oral habits are tenderness in mouth and face, chapped and/or raw lips, and infectious unhealed sores on the lips or in the mouth. The most widely researched and treated oral habit is bruxism, which includes teeth grinding (diurnal or nocturnal), clenching, gnashing, or similar behaviors. Bruxism, if left untreated, often leads to irregular and premature wear on the teeth, malocclusion, and facial damage, especially to the temporomandibular joint. In addition to the dental concerns associated with bruxing behaviors, patients who brux also report muscle tenderness in the face and neck.

Two other habits mentioned in this chapter, thumb sucking and nail biting, are common habits seen in children. Persistent thumb sucking, if left untreated, may lead to impaired dental health (e.g., overbites, malocclusions, and narrowing of the dental arches) as well as deformities of the thumb or other fingers (Peterson et al., 1994). Nail biting may lead not only to cosmetic unattractiveness, but also to scarring and infection of the nail bed and/or cuticles, as well as potential dental problems such as the shortening of tooth roots due to excessive pressure.

Covariance with Other Problems

As previously mentioned, habits are usually benign behaviors that are not accompanied by more serious pathology. However, certain habits may occur, or covary, with other habits and this covariance may aid in the treatment process. Covariance is said to exist when the frequency of one behavior changes as a function of changes in another behavior (Balsam & Bondy, 1985). For example, it is not unusual for trichotillomania to be accompanied by thumb sucking. In such cases, it may be easier to observe and treat thumb sucking than it is to treat trichotillomania, which may be a more covert response (T.S. Watson & Allen, 1993). In some instances, a habit is made up of a chain of responses in which one habit behavior serves as a discriminative stimulus for the next habit behavior (e.g., ear lobe rubbing—head scratching—thumb in mouth). Careful observation and interviewing allows the clinician to determine whether there are covarying behaviors for a particular habit or if the habit is a response within a sequence of responses.

Differential Diagnoses

There are only a few organic/physiological conditions from which habit behavior must be distinguished. With trichotillomania and its accompanying hair loss, the primary medical condition that produces hair loss is alopecia areata. Examination by a dermatologist is usually required to rule out these as causes of hair loss. In addition, some medications can cause an alopecia that may mistakenly be interpreted as a sign that the child is hair pulling. Because we are not pharmacologists, we obtain the generic and trade names of all medications that the person is taking so that we may refer to the *Physicians Desk Reference* (*PDR*), for example, to look up possible side effects of medications. If hair loss is a possible side effect of a medication the child is currently taking, we immediately refer to a physician before embarking on treatment. Other habits (e.g., thumb sucking, bruxism, nail biting) do not have any usual medical or organic conditions from which they must be distinguished.

Prognosis

Thumb sucking, a very common behavior of early childhood, spontaneously remits at a rate of about 5%–10% per year. Approximately 45% of 2-year-olds suck their thumbs, whereas only 5% of 11-year-olds suck their thumbs (Lichstein & Kachmarik, 1980). Despite the fact that most children will quit sucking their thumbs without treatment, it is generally unwise to allow thumb sucking to continue after age 5 or 6 due to the heightened possibility of malocclusion caused by the pressure of the thumb on the back of the upper front teeth.

Although Stroud (1983) reported that most cases of trichotillomania spontaneously remit, our experience is that children who pull intensively (defined as pulling with such frequency and severity so as to produce bald spots from the depiled area) rarely spontaneously remit without direct intervention. Various authors have recognized that although only about 1% of referrals to mental health professionals are for trichotillomania, the actual prevalence rate in the general population is substantially higher (Azrin & Nunn, 1978), especially among adults. Thus, it is likely that children who pull their hair do so more discreetly and covertly as they get older and are careful not to create a noticeable bald spot or depiled area.

Nail biting rarely occurs before age 4 but evidences a dramatic increase around age 6; this results in approximately 33%–50% of preadolescents biting their nails. Without intervention, the rate drops to about 24% by age 17–18 and progressively declines after age 40 (Westling, 1988).

The prevalence rate of bruxism in the general population is estimated to be 5%–18% (Redig, Rubright, & Zimmerman, 1966). Cash (1988) found that 35% of those who bruxed as children continue bruxing into adulthood. For the medical reasons mentioned previously, it is wise to seek treatment for bruxism before there is permanent damage to the teeth and oral muscles and tissue.

Tics

Tics are rapid, brief, stereotyped movements or vocalizations that are generally considered to be under involuntary control. Like habits, tics may be elicited or evoked by certain stimuli (e.g., somatic sensations, muscle tension, stress, fatigue) and maintained by reinforcement. Motor tics involve the recurrent contraction of one or more of the body's muscle groups, whereas vocal tics involve recurrent vocal sounds (e.g., throat clearing), words, and/or phrases. Due to the frequency of most tics and the negative attention they almost certainly evoke (e.g., stares, rude comments, teasing), treatment is usually sought more rapidly than it is for habits.

Three classifications of tics that occur along a continuum are listed in the *DSM-IV. Transient tics,* on one end of the continuum, are single or recurrent episodes of motor and/or vocal tics that do not last longer than 12 months at a time (American Psychiatric Association, 1994). *Chronic motor or vocal tics* require the presence of motor or vocal tics, but not both, that have occurred for over one year. Finally, the most severe tic disorder, *Tourette's Disorder,* is characterized by the presence of multiple motor and vocal tics that have existed for over one year.

Prevalence and Etiology

TS affects roughly .05% of the population and is more common in males (A.K. Shapiro and Shapiro, 1982). Transient tics are estimated to affect about .25% of the population, which may be an underestimate given their transient nature. In fact, LaPouse and Monk (1964) and Torup (1972) reported a 12%–16% rate of transient tics among children. According to Peterson and colleagues (1994), the prevalence of chronic motor and vocal tics is un-

known, but is assumed to be somewhere between the rates for Tourette's Disorder and those for transient tics. Pray, Kramer, & Lindskog (1986) reported a rate of 12%–24% in school-age children without differentiating type of tic. Wagaman, Miltenberger, & Williams (1995) reported the frequency of tics in school-age children to be 5%–24%, which seems to be a more conservative, and reasonable, estimate than that provided by Pray and colleagues. All three tic disorders affect three times as many males as females. In addition, it is estimated that chronic vocal tics occur at a much lower rate than do motor tics (Leckman & Cohen, 1988).

As for habits, a number of hypotheses for the emergence and maintenance of tics have been put forth in the literature, but the exact etiology of tics remains unknown. Considerable debate continues over the influence of organic and behavioral factors in the etiology of tic disorders (King & Ollendick, 1984; Pray et al., 1986). Organic explanations of tic disorders are sometimes based on the premise that drugs such as haloperidol (A.K. Shapiro & Shapiro, 1984) are effective in reducing tics; therefore, the disorder must be biological in nature. However, neurological measures such as EEGs and other brain-imaging techniques for neurological abnormalities have failed to provide consistent evidence for possible biological markers of tics (Robertson, Trimble, & Lees, 1988; Robertson, 1989; A.K. Shapiro & Shapiro, 1981, 1982). In addition, genetic studies examining familial history, and twin concordance rates, have been inconclusive in providing evidence for a biological basis for tic disorders (King & Ollendick, 1984; A.K. Shapiro & Shapiro, 1982).

Behavioral explanations of tics, on the other hand, approach the etiology of the disorder from a learning perspective. Essentially, tics are considered to be a normal movement or vocalization, which for a variety of reasons (e.g., social reinforcement, negative reinforcement such as pain reduction) increase in frequency over time and assume an unusual topographical form through shaping and response generalization (Houlihan, Hofschulte, & Patten 1993; Pray et al., 1986). Let's say that a child awoke one morning with a painful, stiff neck after a spill on his bike the previous day. Early in the morning, he stretched his neck from side to side one time and found that stretching resulted in a temporary relief from pain and stiffness. Throughout the day, he intermittently stretched his neck and the stretching response generalized (i.e., the stretching now involves a slight shrugging of shoulders and head thrusting forward). After a couple of days, the "tic" behavior became more efficient because he performed these behaviors in half the amount of time. Because the response has generalized and is executed rapidly, the behavior takes on the appearance of a jerky, uncontrollable, repetitive motion. Initially, the behavior of neck stretching may have been elicited by muscle pain and stiffness. However, the behavior now occurs in the presence of many discriminative stimuli and the behavior that was once maintained primarily by automatic negative reinforcement (i.e., relief from muscle soreness or the avoidance of muscle soreness) does not appear to have a discernible function.

Covariance with Other Problems

As with habits, tics are usually not accompanied by other problems. Although the child with TS, or other tic behaviors, may sometimes appear to have social difficulties, it may be that they have the necessary social skills but limited opportunity to display them because of reduced interactions with peers. It is certainly not uncommon for children with tic disorders to find themselves excluded from interactions with their peers because of their unusual behavior. It is incorrect to assume, however, that tics are *causes* of social problems.

Previous research has suggested that ADHD, obsessive–compulsive disorders, conduct disorders, sleep disorders, headache disorders, and other somatic complaints are associated in some way with tics and TS (Barabas, Matthews, & Ferrari, 1984a, b; Bruun, 1984; Comings & Comings, 1985; Frank, Sieg, & Gaffney, 1991; Messiha & Carlson, 1983; Steingard, Goldberg, Lee, & DeMaso, 1994). Although behavior consistent with a diagnosis of Attention-Deficit/Hyperactive Disorder (ADHD) is often noted in children with tics, it is important to emphasize that research indicates ADHD behaviors are not temporally related to tics themselves (Nolan, Gadow, & Sverd, 1994). That is, the emergence of a tic and ADHD behaviors typically do not occur at the same time and do not cause each other, but rather a correlation exists among tics and ADHD. Thus, the interrelationships between these disorders remain unclear and there is even some question whether they are more likely to occur in children with a tic or TS disorder.

Differential Diagnoses

Tic-like movements often occur in schizophrenia, static and progressive degenerative neurological disorders, general paresis, multiple sclerosis, organically based mental disorders, and as a side effect of some medications, including stimulants such as dextroamphetamine, pemoline, and methylphenidate, which are used to treat ADHD, and prolonged used of neuroleptics. Other disorders from which tic-like movements must be differentiated include Lesch-Nyhan syndrome, amphetamine intoxication, and Sydenham's chorea (Bruun, 1984; Messiha & Carlson, 1983). Stereotypical behavior often resembles tics but occurs predominantly in children with severe developmental disabilities (see Chapter 21). Yates (1970) noted questions to ask regarding the principal features that differentiate tics from organic problems: (a) Can the tic be voluntarily controlled? (b) Is the motor behavior painful? (c) Does the tic occur during sleep? and (d) Are the muscles that are involved in the tic atrophied? Generally, if the tic can be controlled, is not painful, does not occur during sleep, and the muscles are not atrophied, the behavior is indicative of a tic disorder without organic problems.

Prognosis

Transient tics, by their very definition, remit without specific intervention. If another tic occurs, then treatment should be sought to prevent the tic from returning. If a single tic appears and then remits, there is no cause for concern. The primary problem associated with transient tics is that one tic will disappear and another tic will appear shortly thereafter (Werry, 1986). Without treatment of any kind, it is unlikely that the movements associated with chronic motor or vocal tics or TS will cease (Matthews, Leibowitz, & Matthews, 1992).

Problem Identification

When a habit or tic becomes sufficiently frustrating or embarrassing to the child or his parents, treatment is sought. Sometimes, a long period of time elapses between the first appearance of a habit and when parents request help. In one case, a child referred to our clinic had been hair pulling for six years before her parents became sufficiently concerned to seek professional assistance. In other situations, parents are overly concerned about a "potential" habit behavior and seek treatment when none is needed. For example, a girl of seven was referred because she frequently twirled her hair and shook her leg and her mother was concerned that the child was "nervous" or "hyper."

To accurately and operationally identify habit and tic behaviors, we use multiple direct and indirect methods, including interviews, direct observation, and permanent products, where possible.

Interviews

In our first meeting with parent/s and child, which usually lasts about two hours, we conduct a basic family interview to gather social, developmental, medical, and academic histories (if the child is of school age). Any one of the many available, published and nonpublished, standard interviews is acceptable for gathering general background information. During the medical section of the interview, we are careful to ask about any medications the child is currently taking or has taken in the past (including both prescription and nonprescription medications) and if the child has been evaluated by a family physician/pediatrician, dermatologist, or neurologist to rule out possible organic causes for the habit or tic.

During this first interview, we gather in-depth information regarding the history of the problem behavior. Questions such as when the behavior was first noticed, what the behavior looks like (i.e., the topography of the behavior), previous treatment attempts (either by professionals or parents), and other problems of concern (i.e., covarying behaviors), are typically asked. We also begin asking "analysis-type" questions in order to form preliminary hypotheses about the function of the behavior to be tested during problem analysis: (a) When does the behavior occur? (b) Are there times when the habit occurs more frequently? (c) What events typically precede and follow the behavior? (d) What is the parent(s) response to the behavior? and (e) How do siblings or peers respond to the behavior? If the client is an adolescent, we usually question them

about the behavior, particularly in terms of physiological stimuli that may precede and follow the behavior. For example, an adolescent female who pulls her hair may get a tingling feeling in her scalp immediately before pulling, which goes away after the hair is pulled. This type of information is accessible only through the verbal report of the client. It is vital to note that, although such verbal report information is potentially valuable, it must be considered cautiously because the person may be misidentifying such stimuli or may not be aware of more salient stimuli. In certain cases where the habit is performed covertly (e.g., nail biting, hair pulling), we also ask the client to describe the behavior, show it to us, and tell us when they exhibit the behavior.

In one case from our clinic, parents referred their three-year-old child for repeated coughing (sometimes labeled as a vocal tic, habit cough, or psychogenic cough). After obtaining historical information, we questioned at considerable length the child's medical history and were assured that her pediatrician had found no physical reason for the repeated cough. Consistent with other reports of habit cough, this child's cough had begun shortly after a respiratory infection (T.S. Watson & Heindl, 1996). After the behavior had been adequately described by the parent(s), at least in terms of topography, we began asking questions regarding when the cough occurred and discovered that the parents noticed her coughing while eating. Thus, we formed a hypothesis that the ingestion of food was a discriminative stimulus for coughing. The parents were unable to identify any consistent consequence for the cough, so we knew that during problem analysis we would have to manipulate the specific consequences that followed coughing during naturally occurring situations, especially those that involved food.

Finally, we spent a few minutes at the end of the first session educating the parents about normal developmental habits and tics, the "causes" of habit and tic behaviors (from an operant perspective, of course), and emphasize that children who exhibit habits and tics are not necessarily suffering from emotional or nervous problems. If the habit or tic is developmentally appropriate or appears transient in nature, we take a position of judicious restraint. That is, we tell the parents that the behavior is not unreasonable for a child of his or her age and suggest that no intervention be implemented because the behavior will probably spontaneously remit.

It is important to mention that, in school-age children, we conduct an interview similar to that just described with the child's teacher(s), but omitting the background information (i.e., developmental, medical, and social histories). If the behavior also occurs in the school setting, we also work with the teacher to collect baseline data in that setting, whether or not we actually intervene during school hours. Collecting data and conducting a descriptive assessment in the school setting allows us to assess for generalization of treatment results and to determine whether the behavior has the same function across settings and people.

Direct Observation

Prior to conducting a functional assessment/analysis, the parents collect baseline data at home and we collect data in the clinic setting. As one example, a five-year-old overt hair puller was reported by her mother to pull her hair and suck her thumb, especially while watching TV. Therefore, we arranged for the child to watch TV for 20 minutes in the clinic while recording both behaviors using a 10-second partial interval recording system. These clinic observations may serve as both probe and generalization measures.

When asking parents to record data at home, we try to design the most simple, efficient, yet accurate system possible. Therefore, in most situations, we use a simple frequency count within a specified time frame so that we can compute a rate measure. In addition, data recording during a specified time frame does not require parents to spend an entire day observing and recording. An example of one such recording system, used for the five-year-old child who was a thumb sucker and hair puller, is found in Form 22.1.

FORM 22.1. Frequency Recording Form for Habits or Tics

Behavior to be Observed: _____

		TIME	Frequency (please put a tally mark for each occurrence of the behavior)
Monday		6:30 am–7 am	
		2:30 pm–3 pm	
Tuesday		6:30 am–7 am	
		2:30 pm–3 pm	
Wednesday		6:30 am–7 am	
		2:30 pm–3 pm	
Thursday		6:30 am–7 am	
		2:30 pm–3 pm	
Friday		6:30 am–7 am	
		2:30 pm–3 pm	
Saturday		6:30 am–7 am	
		2:30 pm–3 pm	
Sunday		6:30 am–7 am	
		2:30 pm–3pm	

Permanent Products

Another direct means of identifying, and ultimately measuring change in, habit behaviors is collecting permanent product data. With trichotillomania, one can measure the size of the bald spots on the head to determine whether hair is being pulled from that region. In some instances, such as when the child pulls her hair while going to sleep, the parents may be able to collect hairs from the bedsheet after the child has gone to sleep. In cases of nail biting, the clinician can measure the length of the nails on each of the hands to measure nail growth. When assessing and treating the eyelash pulling of a client at our clinic, we measured the length, in millimeters, of her eyelashes. This provided us with a validity measure for the client's self-recording of pulling, and was also a means of measuring treatment success. Tic behaviors typically do not produce observable permanent products and thus are not particularly useful to the clinician when assessing and treating tics.

Rating Scales and Checklists

Although we typically do not use rating scales and checklists in our clinic when treating habits and tics, several rating scales have been constructed for the purpose of determining the rate, frequency, and severity of tics and habits. The currently available scales rely upon clinical judgment based on historical information and evaluative responses provided by the patient and/or parent. The majority of scales and questionnaires that are available to clinicians are used to assess tics.

The Yale Global Tic Severity Scale (YGTSS; Leckman et al., 1989) is a rating scale designed to measure the severity of tics along five dimensions—number, frequency, complexity, intensity, and interference. The Hopkins Scale (Walkup, Rosenberg, Brown, & Singer, 1992) is a scale based on a 10-point linear analog to measure the severity of a client's tic(s). The Hopkins scale is completed by the examiner and parents and assesses the intensity, impairment, interference, and frequency of the tics. The Tourette's Syndrome Severity Scale (TSSS), developed by A.K. Shapiro and Shapiro (1982), is a five-item questionnaire that provides ordinal ratings on the social and personal impairment associated with the tic. Finally, the Clinical Global Impression Scale (CGI) has an adapted form for use with tics (TS–CGI). The TS–CGI is a 7-point ordinal scale that ranks the severity of tics (Leckman et al., 1989).

Walkup and colleagues (1992) found adequate reliability among rating scales for tics and suggest that the scales are equally effective in measuring the overall severity of tics. However, the scales differ in the information provided to the clinician. The TSSS and TS–CGI are the quickest and simplest to administer, but provide information regarding only the overall severity of the tic and are based solely on judgments. In other words, there is no actual behavioral measurement conducted. On the other hand, the Hopkins and YGTSS focus on the tics themselves and the resulting impairment, as well as operationally defining tics, thus making these scales easier to use in a semistructured format. Walkup and colleagues (1992) suggest that the Hopkins and YGTSS scales may better help the clinician evaluate tics than do other scales.

A relatively new instrument that has promise in assessing trichotillomania is the Psychiatric Institute Trichotillomania Scale (PITS; Winchel et al., 1992). This instrument is used in a semistructured interview format and addresses the history and current severity of hair pulling behaviors. The PITS is scored on six items (site, severity, duration, resistance, distress, and interference) by rating each item on an Likert-type scale (0–7).

Leonard and colleagues (1991) have adapted scales used to assess trichotillomania for the purposes of determining the severity of nailbiting (Nail Biting Severity Scale). The scale consists of five items, including the amount of time spent each day biting nails, intensity of urge to bite nails, resistance exerted against biting nails, distress, and degree of interference from biting nails.

Special Considerations

Oftentimes, identifying habit and tic behaviors is rather easy because the behavior is overt (tics) or there is observable damage (alopecia in trichotillomania or absence of nails from the hands) caused by the behavior. However, clinicians often encounter cases where children have learned to discriminate the settings in which they engage in the habit behavior. For example, a child may have learned to avoid negative interactions with his or her parents by engaging in hair pulling only when parents are not present. In addition, some habit behaviors occur only in situations in which it is difficult to monitor the behavior. For example, many children who brux may only do so at night (nocturnal bruxism). The clinician must then create methods by which to identifiy such covert habits. For example, if a young child is suspected of nocturnal bruxism, the parents may use a sound-activated tape recorder placed on a table near the head of the bed to capture the child's bruxing.

As another example, a two-year-old child was referred to our clinic because his parents suspected that his hair loss was due to hair pulling but they had not observed him pulling his hair during the day. Therefore, a reasonable hypothesis was that he was pulling his hair while in his crib going to sleep. In order to directly measure this behavior, we set up a videocamera in the child's bedroom and videotaped him during naptime and at night. The videotapes revealed that he reliably rubbed his teddy bear, pulled his hair, and then sucked his thumb. Without the videotape, we likely would not have captured this sequence of responses and probably would have implemented a less than maximally effective intervention.

Problem Analysis

Regardless of the event(s) that caused the behavior to emerge in the individual's repertoire, one of the most important roles of the behavior therapist is to determine the stimuli that presently evoke and maintain the tic or habit. Information gathered in the problem identification stage leads to hypotheses regarding the function of the behavior that can be tested during problem analysis. Both descriptive assessments and functional analyses will be discussed in this section, as either procedure can yield valuable data that leads directly to intervention.

Antecedent Assessment/Analysis

Lauterbach (1990) suggested that discriminative stimuli exist in the environment that set the stage for, or evoke, habit behaviors. In addition, and just as important, inhibitive stimuli also exist in the environment and stop the behavior from occurring. It is important for the clinician to identify potential discriminative and inhibiting stimuli for treatment to be maximally effective. For example, the child may be more likely to engage in the habit or tic in the presence of the father than in the presence of the mother or siblings because the presence of the father has been correlated with social attention. The most time-efficient methods for identifying evocative stimuli are interviewing and data collection logs based on direct observation (descriptive assessments). Both the parents and child can be questioned regarding the situations, events, and so on, that seem to precede the behavior, or they can keep a log taking care to note specific antecedents.

For example, a young child brought to our clinic for a motor tic was observed by his mother to tic more frequently when she gave him a direct command (e.g., "Willy, go pick up your toy"). This information was gathered by the mother keeping a behavior tracking log regarding what happened before and after the behavior occurred (see Form 22.2).

After obtaining this descriptive information, we then set up an experimental situation in the clinic in which the mother, in random order, issued direct commands, asked questions, made neutral comments, or asked the child to pick up toys. In one 20-minute functional analysis session, the experimental data confirmed the information obtained in the descriptive assessment, that direct commands were functionally related to tic behavior. Thus, at least a portion of our treatment would be based on the combined results from the assessment/analysis of antecedent stimuli.

If children are capable of self-recording, we have them keep a log noting both the external and internal stimuli that precede the habit or tic (see Form 22.3). Some radical behaviorists may be concerned about our having the client note the internal stimuli that precede the behavior. However, because only the child has access to these stimuli and identification of these stimuli may be related to treatment, we have the child record them. If the internal stimuli do not appear functional, we disregard them.

We consider the combination of descriptive and functional information as the optimal and most time-efficient means of assessing the functional effects of antecedent stimuli on habit and tic behavior. A brief experimental functional procedure, like that described above, was made possible by the data obtained during the descriptive assessment. In addi-

FORM 22.2. Behavior Tracking Log for Parents or Teacher

BEHAVIOR TO BE OBSERVED: **COUGHING**

INSTRUCTIONS: RECORD THE BEHAVIOR DURING THE SPECIFIED TIME BY BRIEFLY DESCRIBING THE SET-TING IN WHICH THE BEHAVIOR OCCURRED AND NOTING WHAT HAPPENED IMMEDIATELY BEFORE AND IMMEDIATELY AFTER THE BEHAVIOR OCCURRED. WE HAVE FILLED IN THE TOP BOX AS AN EXAMPLE FOR YOU TO FOLLOW.

Time of Day	Description of setting	What happened before	Briefly describe the behavior	What happened after
About 7:45 at night, we had just finished eating supper and putting away the dishes.	The family was in the family room watching television.	A commercial came on and Bobby's brother (Jake) began talking to dad.	Bobby coughed loudly several times in a row.	Dad told Bobby to stop coughing, that it was getting on his nerves. And Jake laughed at Bobby.

FORM 22.3. Self-Monitoring Recording Form

BEHAVIOR TO BE OBSERVED: **COUGHING**

INSTRUCTIONS: EVERY TIME THE BEHAVIOR OCCURS, TAKE A MINUTE TO FILL OUT THE SPACES ON THIS CHART. BE AS SPECIFIC AS YOU CAN AND REMEMBER TO RECORD EVERY OCCURRENCE OF THE BEHAVIOR.

Setting	What were others doing before the behavior occurred?	What was I doing or feeling before the behavior occurred?	What did others do after the behavior occurred?	What did I do or feel after the behavior occurred?
In the family room, watching TV.	Watching TV.	Watching TV and I felt a little tickle in my throat.	Bobby laughed at me and Dad told me to stop coughing.	Dad fussed at me and told me to stop coughing, Jake laughed at me, and the tickle went away.

tion, the analysis procedure we used is easily replicable in a typical outpatient setting where the clinician is often pressed for time and does not have access to multiple observers, materials, and so on.

Consequent Analysis

Although there are four general classes of maintaining stimuli (i.e., tangible reinforcement, social attention, negative reinforcement, and automatic reinforcement), we have found that social attention, negative reinforcement, and automatic reinforcement are the most common functions for tics and habits. Therefore, we will limit our discussion to these three. It is important to mention that published reports of functional analyses of habits and tics are extremely rare, if they exist.

The most effective and efficient means for determining the function of a habit or tic behavior is to first conduct a descriptive assessment via interviews, direct observation by the clinician, or data recording by the parents or teachers using the behavior tracking log. If the child is of an appropriate age, self-recording may be used. As stated previously, after a function is preliminarily identified through the descriptive assessment, we conduct a brief functional analysis to confirm the results. This practice of using a brief, confirmatory functional analysis may be used when the behavior has one, or more than one, function. If a behavior has more than one potential function, as identified during the descriptive assessment, then the functional analysis will take more time.

Social Attention

Attention from parents, siblings, peers, teachers, and other adults may maintain habit or tic behavior. In our experience, the most common forms of social attention for habits or tics consist of verbal statements intended to stop the behavior (e.g., "Stop shrugging your shoulders," "Don't squint your eyes") or questions intended to display concern (e.g., "Do you need to get a drink of water for your cough?" "Are you all right?"). Siblings can also socially reinforce habits or tics by calling the parent's attention to the behavior (e.g., "Mommy, Billy is pulling his hair again"). The clinician must make sure to ask about the reaction of peers, siblings, and other adults in order to thoroughly assess

the role of social attention in the maintenance of habits and tics.

To experimentally analyze the effects of social attention, a brief assessment may be conducted in which the parent, siblings, peers, teacher, clinician, and so on, provide social attention contingent on demonstration of the tic or habit. We include several different people in the analysis because different results across people and type of comment are common (Fisher, Ninness, Piazza, & Owen-DeSchryver, 1996).

Negative Reinforcement

In some instances, children exhibit habit or tic behavior to escape or reduce aversive stimulation. For example, parents who are reprimanding their child for a misbehavior may stop when the child engages in the habit or tic. Thus, the habit or tic has been negatively reinforced because it resulted in a cessation of an aversive event (reprimanding). This function is somewhat more difficult to identify in a descriptive assessment because parents or teachers may not consider the cessation of an event a consequence. During the interview portion of the descriptive assessment, the clinician must ask direct questions that relate to a negatively reinforcing function.

In one case of a motor and vocal tic in a nine-year-old male that occurred primarily in the school setting, we first conducted a baseline assessment of the frequency of tics that occurred during the school day. We then conducted a descriptive assessment (observation) which indicated that tiquing was followed by the teacher calling the child's name and allowing him to go to his "relaxation chair" and "chill out" for two minutes. On the average, he was tiquing about 20 times per day, which meant that he was missing at least 40 minutes of instruction or learning time each day. Thus, the tic could have been maintained either by social attention (calling the child's name) or by negative reinforcement (escape from academic assignments). We then tested which function or functions were maintaining the tic by recording the frequency of tics when the teacher allowed him to escape by nonverbally signaling him to go to the relaxation chair, or when she called out his name but did not allow him to escape the assignment. Results indicated that social attention had almost no effect on the tiquing whereas negative reinforcement by escape maintained the tic at high levels. After discerning the function, we found designing treatment quite simple because we knew that escape from academic assignments was maintaining the tic.

Automatic Reinforcement

Automatic reinforcement is said to occur when the behavior itself is reinforcing or produces the reinforcement. For example, thumb sucking may be automatically reinforcing because of the kinesthetic stimulation of the soft tissue of the mouth. The most common means of determining whether a behavior is automatically reinforcing is to document the occurrence of the behavior in the absence of other observable contingencies. For example, we assessed the role of automatic reinforcement in the maintenance of thumb sucking by leaving the client alone in a room and observing, through camera monitoring, the rate of thumb sucking. There was no social attention contingent upon the behavior nor access to any tangible reinforcer. Thus, if the thumb sucking persisted during this period of time, it is likely that the function of the behavior was automatic reinforcement. Conceptually, we acknowledge that automatic reinforcement may be either positive or negative. That is, the behavior may produce sensory stimulation of some kind (positive) or it may result in the removal of unpleasant physiological sensations or an aversive condition (negative). The resulting treatment will depend, in part, on whether the automatic reinforcement is positive or negative.

Plan Implementation

Based on the information gathered during the problem analysis stage regarding evocative and maintaining stimuli, treatment plans can be constructed in which the function, not the topography, of the behavior is the focus of change. There are many empirically based behavioral treatments for habits and tics, including punishment (Silber & Haynes, 1991), differential reinforcement (Wagamanaet al., 1995), contingency management (Peterson & Azrin, 1993), relaxation training (Azrin & Peterson, 1990), biofeedback (Cassisi & McGlynn, 1988), self-monitoring (Anthony, 1978), and treatment package approaches such as habit reversal

(Azrin & Nunn, 1973). However, many of these interventions have been applied without particular emphasis on the function of the behavior. That is, the treatments applied to habits and tics typically have not been based on a functional assessment/analysis, but rather on building effective treatments regardless of function.

This section will link assessment/analysis data to interventions. Determining the antecedent stimuli and the function of the habit or tic greatly increases the probability that the intervention will be effective. We will also discuss interventions that have been found to be effective for habits and tics.

Stimulus Control (Antecedent Interventions)

When there is evidence that a specific stimulus or common set of stimuli evoke the habit or tic, the following procedure may be used. First, identify similar stimuli that do not evoke the behavior (for purposes of this section, we will call such stimuli nonevocative stimuli because they do not evoke habits or tics, but acknowledge that these stimuli are evoking other behavior). Then, arrange the environment such that there are numerous opportunities for the nonevocative stimuli to occur, and heavily reinforce all appropriate behaviors other than the habit or tic (differential reinforcement of other, alternative, or incompatible behaviors). Finally, the evocative stimuli may be gradually reintroduced to occur with the nonevocative stimuli as the alternative or other behavior continues to be reinforced.

Using the example cited in the "Antecedent Assessment" section, in which the child exhibited a motor tic when his mother gave him a direct command, our analysis had identified both the evocative and nonevocative stimuli. Therefore, we prompted the mother to restate commands using one of the nonevocative stimuli so that tic behavior was less likely. When an appropriate non-tic behavior occurred (defined in this case as compliance with the request without tiquing), the mother reinforced the behavior with social praise. Points earned for each day no tiquing occurred were charted. The points could be exchanged for items from a reinforcement menu constructed by the mother and child.

After four weeks of no observed tiquing, we began gradually reintroducing the commands and continued reinforcing compliant behaviors. For example, the mother would say "Willy, it sure is a nice day today, go pick up your toys." The neutral comment preceded the command and exerted stronger stimulus control which resulted in no tiquing. We then gradually faded the non-command comments and more directly inserted command statements, all the while reinforcing compliance without tiquing. We deem it important to note that, as we reintroduced commands more directly, we increased the strength of the reinforcers by doubling the number of points earned each day for no tiquing and decreasing the number of points required to earn most items on the reinforcement menu.

Social Attention

If social attention is maintaining the habit or tic, the primary intervention is to withhold attention when the tic or habit occurs (extinction) and apply social attention contingent upon behavior that is incompatible with the target behavior (differential reinforcement). T.S. Watson and Heindl (1996), in treating a case of habit cough, removed the social reinforcers that were maintaining the cough and made social attention and social activities contingent upon no coughing. In another example, T.S. Watson (1996) found that the repeated cough of a four-year-old occurred only while the child was eating and was maintained by the parent's attention. Therefore, the treatment involved the parent's ignoring the child's cough during times of food consumption and talking to her after gradually longer periods of cough suppression (shaping). Only several days of treatment were required to completely eliminate the coughing.

There are some difficulties involved in extinguishing a habit or tic behavior that is maintained by social attention. First, unless there is a differential reinforcement component added to the treatment regimen, the habit or tic is more likely to increase in frequency or intensity or to change topography (Goh & Iwata, 1994) during the initial stages of treatment. Second, it is extremely difficult for parents and teachers to ignore behavior they consider either embarrassing, annoying, or willful, particularly if the behavior gets worse before getting better. And third, unless all sources of social attention can be controlled, the treatment program may be less than maximally effective.

Negative Reinforcement

If the analysis reveals that the tic or habit is being maintained by escape or avoidance of aversive stimuli, the clinician must design an intervention in which the child cannot escape the aversive stimulus by performing the behavior (escape extinction) and instead allow escape contingent on the display of a more appropriate response. Using the example cited in the "Problem Analysis" section of the child who tiqued to escape academic assignments, we made escape contingent upon completing increasing percentages of work (shaping) and disallowing escape when he tiqued. Although this program proved to be extremely effective, a number of considerations must be taken into account when designing such a program.

The first question the clinician must answer is, "Can the escape response be blocked without harm to the child and without too much stress for the parent or teacher?" If the answer is no, then the best strategy may be to differentially reinforce other behaviors on a thicker schedule or with higher-quality reinforcers than those that are available for the habit or tic. Another question the clinician must address is, "Will tangible reinforcers help accelerate progress?" Even though negative reinforcement is the primary function of the behavior, adding a tangible reinforcer for a nontiquing or nonhabit response may strengthen the desirable alternative of the concurrent schedule (i.e., reinforcement available for tiquing vs. reinforcement available for not tiquing).

Automatic Reinforcement

Many habit and tic behaviors are presumed to be maintained by automatic reinforcement. That is, they often occur when the child is alone and in the absence of any observable socially mediated contingencies. In such cases, the clinician must often devise a treatment strategy that either prevents the behavior from resulting in reinforcement or punishes the behavior. As an example of preventing automatic reinforcement that occurred as a consequence of thumb sucking, T.S. Watson and Allen (1993) attached a post (Allen, Flegle, & Watson, 1992) to a child's thumb to disrupt the tactile/kinesthetic stimulation provided by the thumb contacting the palate. The post was not painful either on the thumb or in the mouth, but prevented the thumb's contact with the palate that was hypothesized to be reinforcing. As a result, the child discontinued thumb sucking and also ceased the hair pulling that covaried with thumb sucking.

The function of some habits and tics may be automatic negative reinforcement. That is, the behavior may result in the attenuation or removal of unpleasant physiological sensations. For example, a child who has a chronic vocal tic may get a tightness in the chest immediately before vocalizing; the tightness is temporarily removed by the vocalization. Children with chronic motor tics often report a tingling or tension in their muscles that is removed by the tic. Considering that the tension is a discriminative stimulus for tiquing and the tiquing results in removal of the tension, muscle relaxation would appear to be the treatment of choice, especially in a functional sense. However, research indicates that the use of relaxation training reduces habit and tic behaviors only by about one-third and is insufficient, by itself, for reducing habit and tic behaviors (Azrin & Peterson, 1989; Peterson et al., 1994). Other strategies that may be applied to augment the effects of relaxation training include differential reinforcement and punishment.

As noted earlier, some habits or tics that appear to be automatically reinforcing may be conditioned reinforcers because they have, in the past, resulted in delays in the onset of other reinforcers (delay reduction). When a habit or tic behavior becomes a conditioned reinforcer, one of the ways to treat the behavior is through punishment and differential reinforcement. For example, one of the most effective treatments for thumb sucking involves placing an unpleasant-tasting substance on the thumb (e.g., Stopzit, Thumbz) and reinforcing behaviors other than thumb sucking (DRO) (see Friman & Leibowitz, 1990, for a full description of the procedure). Many of the earlier studies on aversive taste treatments (ATT) concluded that ATTs were ineffective for reducing thumb sucking and nail biting. Those earlier studies, however, did not include any type of reinforcement-based procedure. It is extremely important to emphasize that punishment, by itself, is not recommended as a treatment for habits or tics. If some type of punishment procedure is to be used, then a concurrent reinforcement program should be implemented in which more appropriate responses are reinforced to teach the child a more appropriate or new behavior.

General Treatment Procedures

Habit Reversal

Some treatment approaches merit special attention because of their demonstrated effectiveness for both habits and tics. Habit reversal (Azrin & Nunn, 1973) is one such treatment. Habit reversal has been used effectively for problems as diverse as temporomandibular pain associated with bruxism (Peterson, Dixon, Talcott, & Kelleher, 1993), tics (Azrin & Peterson, 1990; Miltenberger, Fuqua, & McKinley, 1985), trichotillomania (Rothbaum, 1992), bruxism (Peterson et al., 1993; Rosenbaum & Ayllon, 1981), stuttering (Wagaman, Miltenberger, & Andorfer, 1993), and nail biting (Silber & Haynes, 1991), to name just a few.

We call habit reversal a nonspecific treatment because it appears to be effective regardless of the function of the behavior. Azrin and Nunn (1973) identified thirteen steps in the original habit reversal program. Recent research has questioned whether all thirteen components of habit reversal are necessary to effectively treat habit and tic disorders. Based on a comparative analysis, Miltenberger and Fuqua (1985) suggested that only five components of the habit reversal package are necessary for effectiveness: (a) self-monitoring, (b) competing response, (c) relaxation training, (d) social support, and (e) habit inconvenience review. Silber and Haynes (1991) examined the efficacy of competing response with self-monitoring, punishment (i.e., bitter substance painted on nails) with self-monitoring, and self-monitoring alone in treating severe nail biting in adults. Both the competing response and punishment conditions were superior to self-monitoring, but subjects in the competing response condition had more treatment gains and maintained treatment outcomes better than did subjects in the punishment condition.

Azrin and Peterson (1989) used a soft blink (competing response) procedure to treat an eye tic in a child. Relaxation training, competing response, and a combination of relaxation and competing response were compared to determine which treatment resulted in the greatest reduction of eye tics. Results indicated that competing response alone resulted in the greatest reduction (over 90%) of tics in the subject. Thus, it appears that the competing response is the active component of habit reversal and functions as a punisher because of its effects on the target response.

Despite the effectiveness of habit reversal, there may be situations where either parents or children or both do not comply with the required treatment procedures. Habit reversal requires effort on the part of the child during each display of the target behavior and also requires parental monitoring. If the parents and/or child cannot or will not complete the necessary procedures, the procedure will not be effective. Thus, it may be necessary to reinforce compliance with the treatment program. That is, the child earns reinforcers for completing the treatment procedures. One way to do this is for the clinician to model the parent's role in monitoring and prompting the procedure and socially reinforcing compliant child behavior. Monetary rewards for habit-free periods have proven to be effective in reducing target behaviors (Wagaman et al., 1995) and can easily be applied to treatment compliance. Grab-bags filled with small toys, coins, or notes that can be traded for small outings and edibles have been effective in our clinic for maintaining interest and promoting child compliance with treatment.

Massed Negative Practice

Massed negative practice is one of the most often cited treatments for tics (Peterson et al., 1994). In this procedure, the child is required to repeatedly practice the exact topography of the target behavior as quickly and with as much effort as possible for a specified period of time. Despite its widespread use, massed practice has been shown to reduce tics by an average of only 50% (Peterson et al., 1994). Although massed practice has also been used in the treatment of bruxing, mixed results have been found using this approach. Some studies have found moderate to high success rates using massed practice (Azrin, Nunn, & Frantz-Renshaw, 1992), whereas others have met with little to no success (Pierce & Gale, 1988).

Biofeedback

Nocturnal bruxism provides a case for special consideration. Because the child is asleep, he or she is not aware of the behavior. Thus, procedures that require awareness of the habit will not be effective in treating nocturnal bruxism. Biofeedback has shown promise in treating some habit behaviors, es- pecially bruxism (Cassisi & McGlynn, 1988). Biofeedback instruments measure muscular activity in a specified area and sound an alarm when a threshold level is reached for that muscle area, thus making biofeedback machines function much like the bell-and-pad devices used in the treatment of bed-wetting. In the case of nocturnal bruxism, the individual is aroused once the alarm sounds. Although biofeedback devices have potential in treating habit disorders like bruxism, Peterson and colleagues (1994) found reports that bruxing rates return to baseline levels once use of the device is discontinued. In addition, biofeedback machines are expensive to purchase and require specialized knowledge of how to use them appropriately.

Perhaps the ineffectiveness of the biofeedback technology was due to simple arousal being insufficient for reducing bruxism, as T.S. Watson (1993) found that arousal with overcorrection was superior to simple arousal in reducing nocturnal bruxism. It may also be that nonbruxing came under the stimulus control of the electrodes on the skin so that when they were removed, the bruxing returned.

Planning for Generalization

Regarding the treatment of tics and habits, the most salient form of generalization is stimulus generalization. That is, one of the goals of treatment is to ameliorate the habit or tic behavior not only during one specific set of stimulus conditions (e.g., home) but under many different stimulus conditions. The best ways we have found for promoting stimulus generalization are to conduct treatment in several target situations (e.g., at home with parents, at school, with friends, at church, at a restaurant, at the clinic) and to frequently reinforce the absence of tics or habits randomly throughout the day (Stokes & Baer, 1977).

Plan Evaluation

The primary goal of plan evaluation is to compare treatment data with baseline data to determine whether the treatment is having the desired effect on the target behavior (see Chapter 2). Generally, the data recording procedure that was used during problem identification is continued so that accurate comparisons may be made pre- and posttreatment.

Because data evaluation is a continuous process, many questions must be answered as treatment progresses. For example, How long should the clinician wait for changes to occur in the target response? What should be done when treatment is deemed ineffective. How can the formal program be faded so that the results are maintained over time? and How often should follow-ups be conducted?

There are no hard and fast rules about how much time should elapse before the intervention has an effect on the target behavior. In those cases where the intervention is not working as rapidly as we would like or is not working at all, we generally ask the following questions, in order: (a) Was the problem correctly identified or is the appropriate behavior being targeted? (b) Was the function correctly identified, or did the function of the behavior change since problem analysis? (c) Is the plan consistent with the data from the functional assessment/analysis? (d) Is the intervention being implemented with a high degree of integrity? and (e) Has the treatment been implemented long enough that we would reasonably expect some change in the target behavior? Obviously there are other variables that might influence treatment, but these questions address the most likely sources of problems hindering treatment success.

A common concern among parents and teachers is that they will have to implement the treatment indefinitely. As behaviorists, we know that formal treatments are not required to maintain gains, but clients are less certain. Therefore, we tell them during the plan implementation stage that our ultimate goal is to remove the treatment without the habit or tic returning. A number of strategies are available to gradually fade the treatment program, including behavioral trapping (using reinforcers in the natural environment to maintain the behavior as opposed to relying reinforcers in the treatment program; Kohler & Greenwood, 1986), moving to increasingly thinner schedules of reinforcement, or incorporating some form of self-management into the treatment program.

Social Validity

Wolf (1978) identified three levels of social validation: (a) importance of target behaviors for the client and society; (b) consideration of the acceptability of the procedures used to change the behavior; and (c) satisfaction of clients (child, parents, and/or teacher) with the results. With regard to the importance of target behaviors, it is relatively clear that the habit or tic itself is a socially important behavior. As mentioned previously, habits or tics may cause physical damage to the individual as well as hinder social functioning by evoking negative interactions with peers and important adults.

When considering acceptability of treatment procedures, we are less concerned with pretreatment acceptability because caregivers often do not have enough a priori information to make an accurate estimate of acceptability and, more important, there is no empirical evidence to indicate that acceptability is in any way related to treatment integrity (Sterling, Watson, Wildmon, Watkins, & Little, 1996). Although we do not intentionally make treatments aversive to the user, our research indicates that treatments with aversive components will be implemented with integrity given the proper training. Consequently, if the treatment is implemented with high integrity, there is an increased likelihood of positive results, which in turn renders the treatment more acceptable to the user and leads to greater satisfaction with the treatment process.

Treatment Integrity

One of the most important issues in behavior therapy is treatment integrity, which is defined as the degree to which the treatment procedure was carried out as intended. Regardless of the potential effectiveness of the intervention, if it is not carried out with a high degree of integrity then the plan is unlikely to be effective and the relationship between the intervention and any changes in behavior are unclear. Therefore, we always assess treatment integrity during our interventions by having the clients (parents/child) demonstrate the procedures in the clinic, keep track of the number of times they implement each component of treatment (e.g., escape extinction, reinforcement, competing response), and ask others in the environment if the plan is being carried out.

Summary and Directions for Further Research

Despite the relatively benign nature of habits and tics, they can cause marked disturbances in social and interpersonal functioning. In some instances, habits and tics can result in physical damage to specific parts of the body (e.g., bruxism). From a behavioral perspective, both habits and tics are learned behavior (either through operant or respondent conditioning) that can be successfully treated through techniques like habit reversal or by assessing function and linking treatment to function. It is in linking function to treatment that the largest gap exists in the professional literature on tics and habits. A preponderance of the research on tics and habits has focused on identifying effective treatments rather than on identifying function, either descriptively or experimentally, and then linking treatment to the results of the functional assessment/analysis. Although two recent studies have attempted to investigate, experimentally, the function of habits (Woods & Miltenberger, 1996; T.S. Watson, 1996), they are only preliminary attempts at using functional methodology with habits. The lack of functional studies may be due, in part, to the success of treatments like habit reversal that seem to work regardless of the function of the behavior. The question that remains, however, is, "Can a functional approach yield more effective and efficient treatments than those currently available to the behavioral practitioner?" The answer lies in empirical investigation, which has yet to be conducted.

References

Achenbach, T.M. (1991). *Manual for the Child Behavior Checklist/4-18 and 1991 profile.* Burlington: University of Vermont, Department of Psychiatry.

Allen, K.D., Flegle, J.H., & Watson, T.S. (1992). A thermoplastic thumb post for the treatment of thumb-sucking. *American Journal of Occupational Therapy, 46,* 552–554.

American Psychiatric Association. (1994). *Diagnostic and statistical manual of mental disorders* (4th ed.). Washington, DC: Author.

Anthony, W.Z. (1978). Brief intervention in a case of childhood trichotillomania by self-monitoring. *Journal of Behavior Therapy and Experimental Psychiatry, 9,* 173–175.

Azrin, N.H., & Nunn, R.G. (1973). Habit reversal: A method of eliminating nervous habits and tics. *Behavior Research and Therapy, 11,* 619–628.

Azrin, N.H., & Nunn, R.G. (1978). *Habit control in a day.* New York: Simon and Schuster.

Azrin, N.H., & Peterson, A.L. (1989). Reduction of an eye tic by controlled blinking. *Behavior Therapy, 20,* 467–473.

Azrin, N.H., & Peterson, A.L. (1990). Treatment of Tourette syndrome by habit reversal: A waiting-list control group comparison. *Behavior Therapy, 21,* 305–318.

Azrin, N.H., Nunn, R.G., & Frantz-Renshaw, S.E. (1992). Habit reversal vs. negative practice treatment of self-destructive oral habits (biting, chewing, or licking of the lips, cheeks, tongue, or palate). *Journal of Behavior Therapy and Experimental Psychiatry, 13,* 49–54.

Balsam, P.D., & Bondy, A.S. (1985). Reward induced response covariation: Negative side effects revisited. *Journal of Applied Behavior Analysis, 18,* 79–80.

Barabas, G., Matthews, W., & Ferrari, M. (1984a). Somnambulism in children with Tourette syndrome. *Developmental Medicine and Child Neurology, 26,* 457–460.

Barabas, G., Matthews, W., & Ferrari, M. (1984b). Tourette's syndrome and migraine. *Archives of Neurology, 41,* 871–872.

Bruun, R.D. (1984). Gilles de la Tourette syndrome: An overview of clinical experience. *Journal of the American Academy of Child Psychiatry, 23,* 126–133.

Cash, R.C. (1988). Bruxism in children: Review of the literature. *Journal of Periodontics, 12,* 107–127.

Cassisi, J.E., & McGlynn, F.D. (1988). Effects of EMG-activated alarms on nocturnal bruxism. *Behavior Therapy, 19,* 133–142.

Christenson, G.A., Mackenzie, T.B., & Mitchell, J.E. (1991). Characteristics of 60 adult hair pullers. *American Journal of Psychiatry, 148,* 365–370.

Comings, D.E., & Comings, B.G. (1985). Tourette syndrome: Clinical and psychological aspects of 250 cases. *American Journal of Human Genetics, 37,* 435–450.

Fantino, E. (1969). Choice and rate of reinforcement. *Journal of the Experimental Analysis of Behavior, 12,* 723–730.

Fisher, W.W., Ninness, H.A., Piazza, C.C., & Owen-DeSchryver, J.S. (1996). On the reinforcing effects of the content of verbal attention. *Journal of Applied Behavior Analysis, 29,* 235–238.

Frank, M.S., Sieg, K.G., & Gaffney, G.R. (1991). Somatic complaints in childhood tic disorders. *Psychosomatics, 32,* 396–399.

Freud, A. (1965). *Normality and pathology in childhood.* New York: International Universities Press.

Friman, P.C., & Leibowitz, J.M. (1990). An effective and acceptable treatment alternative for chronic thumb- and finger-sucking. *Journal of Pediatric Psychology, 15,* 57–65.

Friman, P.C., Larzelere, R., & Finney, J.W. (1994). Exploring the relationship between thumb-sucking and psychopathology. *Journal of Pediatric Psychology, 19,* 431–441.

Glaros, A.G., & Melamed, B.G., (1992). Bruxism in children: Etiology and treatment. *Applied and Preventive Psychology, 1,* 191–199.

Goh, H.L., & Iwata, B.A. (1994). Behavioral persistence and variability during extinction of self-injury maintained by escape. *Journal of Applied Behavior Analysis, 27,* 173–174.

Hansen, D.J., Tishelman, A.C., Hawkins, R.P., & Doepke, K.J. (1990). Habits with potential as disorders: Prevalence, severity, and other characteristics among college students. *Behavior Modification, 14,* 66–80.

Houlihan, D., Hofschulte, L., & Patten, C. (1993). Behavioral conceptualizations and treatments of Tourette's syndrome: A review and overview. *Behavioral Residential Treatment, 8,* 111–131.

Hunt, W.A., Matarazzo, J., Weiss, J., & Gentry, W.D. (1979). Associative learning, habit, and health behavior. *Journal of Behavioral Medicine, 2,* 111–124.

King, A.C., & Ollendick, T.H. (1984). Gilles de la Tourette disorder: A review. *Journal of Clinical Child Psychology, 13,* 2–9.

Kohler, F.W., & Greenwood, C.R. (1986). Toward a technology of generalization: The identification of natural contingencies of reinforcement. *Behavior Analyst, 11,* 115–129.

LaPouse, R., & Monk, M.A. (1964). Behavior deviations in a representative sample of children: Variation by sex, age, race, social class, and family size. *American Journal of Orthopsychiatry, 34,* 436–446..

Lauterbach, W. (1990). Situation-response (S-R) questions for identifying the function of problem behaviour: The example of thumbsucking. *Brititsh Journal of Clinical Psychology, 29,* 51–57.

Leckman, J.F., & Cohen, D.J. (1988). Descriptive and diagnostic classification of tic disorders. In D.J. Cohen, R.D. Brown, & J.F. Leckman (Eds.), *Tourette's syndrome and tic disorders: Clinical understanding and treatment* (pp. 4–19). New York: Wiley.

Leckman, J.F., Riddle, M.A., Hardin, M.T., Ort, S.I., Swartz, K.L., Stevenson, J., & Cohen, D.J. (1989). The Yale Global Tic Severity Scale: Initial testing of a clinician-rated scale of tic severity. *Journal of the American Academy of Child and Adolescent Psychiatry, 28,* 566–573.

Leonard, H.L., Lenane, M.C., Swedo, S.E., Rettew, D.C., & Rapoport, J.L. (1991). A double-blind comparison of clomipramine and desipramine treatment of severe onychophagia (nailbiting). *Archives of General Psychiatry, 48,* 821–827.

Lichstein, K.L., & Kachmarik, G. (1980). A non-aversive intervention for thumbsucking: Analysis across settings and time in the natural environment. *Journal of Pediatric Psychology, 5,* 405–414.

Matthews, L.H., Leibowitz, J.M., & Matthews, J.R. (1992). Tics, habits, and mannerisms. In C.E. Walker & M.C. Roberts (Eds.), *Handbook of clinical child psychology* (2nd ed., pp. 283–302). New York: Wiley.

Messiha, F.S., & Carlson, J.C. (1983). Behavioral and clinical profiles of Tourette's disease: A comprehensive overview. *Brain Research Bulletin, 11,* 195–204.

Miltenberger, R.G., & Fuqua, R.W. (1985). A comparison of contingent vs. non-contingent competing response practice in the treatment of nervous habits. *Journal of Behavior Therapy and Experimental Psychiatry, 16,* 195–200.

Miltenberger, R.G., Fuqua, R.W., & McKinley, T. (1985). Habit reversal with muscle tics: Replication and component analysis. *Behavior Therapy, 16,* 39–50.

Nolan, E.E., Gadow, K.D., & Sverd, J. (1994). Observations and ratings of tics in school settings. *Journal of Abnormal Child Psychology, 22,* 579–593.

Peterson, A.L., & Azrin, N.H. (1993). Behavioral and pharmacological treatments for Tourette's Syndrome: A review. *Applied and Preventive Psychology, 2,* 231–242.

Peterson, A.L., Dixon, D.L., Talcott, G.W., & Kelleher, W.J. (1993). Habit reversal treatment of temporomandibular disorders: A pilot investigation. *Journal of Behavior Therapy and Experimental Psychiatry, 24,* 49–55.

Peterson, A.L., Campose, R.L., & Azrin, N.H. (1994). Behavioral and pharmacological treatments for tic and habit disorders: A review. *Journal of Developmental and Behavioral Pediatrics, 15,* 430–441.

Pierce, C.J., & Gale, E.N. (1988). A comparison of different treatments for nocturnal bruxism. *Journal of Dental Research, 67,* 597–601.

Pray, B., Kramer, J.J., & Lindskog, R. (1986). Assessment and treatment of tic behavior: A review and case study. *School Psychology Review, 15,* 418–429.

Redig, G.R., Rubright, W.C., & Zimmerman, S.O. (1966). Incidence of bruxism. *Journal of Dental Research, 45,* 1198–1204.

Robertson, M.M. (1989). The Gilles de la Tourette syndrome: The current status. *British Journal of Psychiatry, 154,* 147–169.

Robertson, M.M., Trimble, M.R., & Lees, A.J. (1988). The psychopathology of the Gilles de la Tourette syndrome: A phenomenological analysis. *British Journal of Psychiatry, 152,* 383–390.

Rosenbaum, M.S., & Ayllon, T. (1981). Treating bruxism with the habit-reversal technique. *Behavior Research and Therapy, 19,* 87–96.

Rothbaum, B.O. (1992). The behavioral treatment of trichotillomania. *Behavioural Psychotherapy, 20,* 85–90.

Shapiro, A.K., & Shapiro, E. (1981). Do stimulants provoke, cause, or exacerbate tics and Tourette syndrome? *Comprehensive Psychiatry, 22,* 265–273.

Shapiro, A.K., & Shapiro, E. (1982). An update on Tourette syndrome. *American Journal of Psychotherapy, 36,* 379–390.

Shapiro, A.K., & Shapiro, E. (1984). Controlled study of pimozide vs. placebo in Tourette's syndrome. *Journal of the American Academy of Child Psychiatry, 23,* 161–173.

Shapiro, S., & Shannon, J. (1966). Bruxism as an emotional reactive disturbance. *Psychosomatics, 6,* 427–430.

Silber, K.P., & Haynes, C.E. (1991). Treating nailbiting: A comparative analysis of mild aversion and competing response therapies. *Behavior Research and Therapy, 30,* 15–22.

Steingard, R.J., Goldberg, M., Lee, D., & DeMaso, D.R. (1994). Adjunctive clonazepam treatment of tic symptoms in children with comorbid tic disorders and ADHD. *Journal of the American Academy of Child and Adolescent Psychiatry, 33,* 394–399.

Sterling, H.E., Watson, T.S., Wildmon, M., Watkins, C., & Little, E. (1996). Treatment acceptability, direct training, and treatment integrity: Applications to consultation. Manuscript submitted for publication.

Stokes, T.F., & Baer, D.M. (1977). An implicit technology of generalization. *Journal of Applied Behavior Analysis, 10,* 349–367.

Stroud, J.D. (1983). Hair loss in children. *Pediatric Clinics of North America, 30,* 641–657.

Torup, E. (1972). A follow-up study of children with tics. *Acta Paediatrica, 51,* 261–268.

Wagaman, J.R., Miltenberger, R.G., & Andorfer, R.E. (1993). Analysis of a simplified treatment for stuttering in children. *Journal of Applied Behavior Analysis, 26,* 53–62.

Wagaman, J.R., Miltenberger, R.G., & Williams, D.E. (1995). Treatment of a vocal tic by differential reinforcement. *Journal of Behavior Therapy and Experimental Psychiatry, 26,* 35–39.

Walkup, J.T., Rosenberg, L.A., Brown, J., & Singer, H.S. (1992). The validity of instruments measuring tic severity in Tourette's Syndrome. *Journal of the American Academy of Child and Adolescent Psychiatry, 31,* 472–477.

Watson, J.B., & Rayner, R. (1920). Conditioned emotional reactions. *Journal of Experimental Psychology, 3,* 1–14.

Watson, T.S. (1993). Effectiveness of arousal and arousal plus overcorrection to reduce nocturnal bruxism. *Journal of Behavior Therapy and Experimental Psychiatry, 24,* 181–186.

Watson, T.S. (1996). Functional assessment and analysis of habit cough. Manuscript submitted for publication.

Watson, T.S., & Allen, K.D. (1993). Elimination of thumb-sucking as a treatment for severe trichotillomania. *Journal of the American Academy of Child and Adolescent Psychiatry, 32,* 830–834.

Watson, T.S., & Heindl, B. (1996). Behavioral case consultation: An example using differential reinforcement to treat psychogenic cough. *Journal of School Psychology, 34,* 365–378.

Werry, J.S. (1986). Physical illness, symptoms, and allied disorders. In H.C. Quay & J.S. Werry (Eds.), *Psychopathological disorders of childhood* (3rd ed., pp. 232–293). New York: Wiley.

Westling, L. (1988). Fingernail biting: A literature review and case reports. *Journal of Craniomandibular Process, 6*(2), 182–187.

Winchel, R.M., Jones, J.S., Molcho, A., Parsons, B., Stanley, B., & Stanley, M. (1992). The Psychiatric Institute Trichotillomania Scale (PITS). *Psychopharmacology Bulletin, 28,* 463–476.

Wolf, M.M. (1978). Social validity: The case for subjective measurement or how applied behavior analysis is finding its heart. *Journal of Applied Behavior Analysis, 11,* 203–214.

Woods, D.W., & Miltenberger, R.G. (1996). Are persons with nervous habits nervous? A preliminary examination of habit function in a nonreferred population. *Journal of Applied Behavior Analysis, 29,* 259–261.

Yates, A.J. (1970). *Behavior therapy.* New York: Wiley.

Bibliography

Azrin, N.H., & Nunn, R.G. (1973). Habit reversal: A method of eliminating nervous habits and tics. *Behavior Research and Therapy, 11,* 619–628. Probably the most influential article on behavioral treatment of habits and tics. The article describes the complete habit reversal procedure, which has led to many developments and refinements in the treatment of habits and tics.

Friman, P.C., & Leibowitz, M.J. (1990). An effective and acceptable treatment alternative for chronic thumb and finger sucking. *Journal of Pediatric Psychology, 15,* 57–65. This article describes a widely used clinical treatment protocol for thumb and finger sucking. It is the only empirical study with a large sample that shows aversive taste treatment with a reinforcement procedure to be effective.

Miltenberger, R.G., Fuqua, R.W., & McKinley, T. (1985). Habit reversal: Replications and component analysis. *Behavior Therapy, 16,* 39–50. This article illustrates the effectiveness of using a brief habit-reversal procedure consisting of awareness training and competing response for reducing muscle tics. One of several original articles that examined modified, brief versions of habit reversal.

Peterson, A.L., Campose, R.L., & Azrin, N.H. (1994). Behavioral and pharmacological treatments for tic and habit disorders: A review. *Journal of Developmental and Behavioral Pediatrics, 15,* 430–441. One of the most recent and comprehensive reviews of habit and tic disorders. This article does a nice job of providing prevalence data and describing the most effective treatment procedures for tics and habits.

Antisocial Behavior in Schools

JEFFREY SPRAGUE, GEORGE SUGAI, AND HILL WALKER

Introduction

Acts of aggression, property vandalism and destruction, and harassment and intimidation by children and youth are increasing in intensity, prevalence, and incidence. In response, more communities are establishing zero-tolerance policies, building more segregated facilities, and increasing security in schools, businesses, and neighborhoods. Unfortunately, these "get-tough" responses have not curtailed the growth of antisocial behavior in our schools and communities. In fact, the pressures and social effects resulting from these behavioral manifestations and failed interventions are threatening to overwhelm the process of schooling for *all* of our students (Walker, Colvin, & Ramsey, 1995). For staff and students alike, school safety has risen to a level of great importance and excruciating national concern. Making schools safe and violence-free is currently one of the most pressing issues before the U.S. Congress. The focus of this chapter is on antisocial behavior in the context of schooling. The nature and characteristics of antisocial behavior, a schoolwide systems response, and behavior support planning for individual students are discussed.

We acknowledge that an interdisciplinary approach represents the most logical response for addressing the complex and persistent challenge presented by students with antisocial behavior. Interdisciplinary models (e.g., systems-of-care,

wraparound) are being implemented and evaluated across the United States. However, economic, political, and social roadblocks and hurdles make it difficult to delineate the critical features of an effective interdisciplinary approach. Thus, in this chapter we have elected to focus on the school as the context for building behavioral support for students with antisocial behavior for two main reasons. First, schools provide a consistent and predictable daily experience for students. A large number of adults are present, appropriate peer models are available, a regular schedule of activities occurs on a daily and weekly basis, and opportunities for academic and social success can be orchestrated. In fact, the scheduled routine of the school day may represent the most consistent and proactive experience in the daily lives of many children and youth. Second, we have a clearly defined and validated knowledge base of strategies that can be applied in school settings. These strategies include academic interventions designed to remediate deficits and prevent academic failure, social skills interventions designed to improve competence with peers and adults, and behavioral interventions used to encourage desirable responding and to discourage inappropriate behavior patterns.

The accelerating number of children and youth who come to school with well-developed patterns of antisocial, aggressive behavior is alarming. Generally, school personnel are not trained to cope effectively with severe levels of antisocial behavior occurring among student populations. Even more egregious criminal acts are being committed on school grounds, including assault, rape, and mur-

JEFFREY SPRAGUE, GEORGE SUGAI, AND HILL WALKER • College of Education, University of Oregon, Eugene, Oregon 97403.

Handbook of Child Behavior Therapy, edited by Watson and Gresham. Plenum Press, New York, 1998.

der. These acts destroy the sense of safety and community that has traditionally characterized school settings. Metal detectors, time locks on doors, video cameras and scanners, and police officers patrolling hallways and school grounds are just a sample of the measures that school administrators are taking in order to secure the safety of the school building. Even more stringent measures than these will be required if present trends continue.

Although schools are vulnerable to the predatory behavior of nonstudents committing criminal acts on school grounds, much of the deterioration in the ecology and sense of safety of schools can be attributed to changes in the student population. More children and youth are entering our schools less prepared to learn, having English as a second language, being culturally diverse, having greater learning and behavioral challenges, and being more different from than similar to their peers (Knitzer, 1993; Knitzer, Steinberg, & Fleisch, 1990; Stevens & Price, 1992). At-risk youth enter our schools having a profile that includes dysfunctional families, poverty, negative peer pressure, popularity "with what's happening," and school failure and leaving.

Coie (1994) argues persuasively that we are experiencing a significant change in the nature of antisocial behavior patterns among today's children and youth. He makes the following observations to buttress his argument:

1. Youth are increasingly carrying high levels of agitation due to such factors as abuse, neglect, drug and alcohol involvement, a sense of hopelessness, and exposure to the widespread social fragmentation of our society.
2. Under the influence of this agitation, such youth are very likely to misperceive social situations and to make serious errors in the interpretation of social cues, body language, and behavioral intentions of others.
3. This agitation often finds expression in *reactive* forms of aggression wherein a youth perceives a hostile act from someone else or interprets their intentions as violent and reacts aggressively in order to get even or to strike first.
4. In far too many cases, this act of reactive aggression ends in tragedy due to the increasing tendency for such youth to use weapons in settling disputes.

As a result, the number of student-to-student conflicts having tragic consequences and the num-

ber of assaults on teacher and school staff have increased dramatically in the last decade. Juvenile crime arrests have increased 68% from 1984 to 1993 (FBI Annual Reports, 1994). In 1993, 3,284 juveniles were arrested for murder, and 116,000 were arrested for other violent crimes (FBI Annual Reports, 1994). Even more troubling than the statistics on violent perpetrators are the victimization data patterns. In 1992, 1.55 million violent crimes were committed *against* juveniles aged 12 to 17 years, a 23.4% increase since 1987 (FBI Annual Reports, 1994). In fact, teenagers are 2.5 times more likely to be victims of violent crimes (APA Commission on Youth Violence, 1993).

In order to combat this phenomenon, schools are placed in the unenviable position of having to socialize students to normative standards that eschew violent and aggressive solutions to problems. Because this challenge is relatively new to the process of schooling, school personnel understand little about the origins and developmental course of antisocial behavior patterns. However, in the past two decades, enormous strides have been made in understanding and treating this disorder (Kazdin, 1987; Reid, 1993; Walker, Colvin, & Ramsey, 1995). Many of these approaches are adaptable to and usable in the school setting.

Antisocial Behavior Defined

Antisocial behavior is defined as "recurrent violations of socially prescribed patterns of behavior" (Simcha-Fagan, Langner, Gersten, & Eisenberg, 1975, p. 7). Antisocial behavior is expressed through such behavioral forms as uncontrolled anger, a general mood of hostility toward others, proactive and reactive aggression, failure to abide by rule-governed forms of behavior, defiance of adult authority, peer conflicts, and a tendency to blame others and to avoid acceptance of responsibility for one's actions. Antisocial behavior is one of the most common forms of psychopathology among children and youth and is *the* most frequently cited reason for referral to mental health services (see Achenbach, 1985; Quay, 1986; Reid, 1993; Walker, Colvin, & Ramsey, 1995). In addition, exclusion or removal to segregated settings is the most common response for conduct disordered, juvenile delinquent, and behavior disordered youth.

Displays of problem behavior are also the number one reason children and youth with disabilities are removed from school, work, and home settings (Reichle, 1990).

In many cases, students who display antisocial behavior in school settings are evaluated and determined to be eligible for special education services. Designations of learning disabilities, attention deficit disorders, or emotional and behavioral disorders often are assigned to these students. In instances where serious emotional and behavioral disorders are indicated, students tend to display "an inability to build or maintain satisfactory interpersonal relationships with peers and teachers," "inappropriate types of behavior or feelings under normal circumstances," "a general, pervasive mood of unhappiness or depression," and/or "a tendency to develop physical symptoms or ears associated with personal or school problems" (Individuals with Disabilities Education Act Regulations, 45 CFR 121a.5[b][1978]). In addition, these students have a history of academic failure and a failure to perform at grade level.

Prevalence of Antisocial Behavior and Conduct Disorder

The prevalence of antisocial behavior patterns among today's children and youth is substantial and increasing. Estimates vary considerably but a large number of experts suggest that up to 9% of the population under age 18 is at serious risk for antisocial behavior disorders (Kazdin, 1993). A preponderance of these youth are male. Half will maintain the disorder into adulthood; the remainder will suffer significant adjustment problems throughout their adult lives (Kazdin, 1993; Robins, 1978).

Although not all students determined to be eligible for special education because of an emotional or behavioral disorder display antisocial behavior or conduct disorders, many students who are considered antisocial or conduct disordered are found to be eligible for special education services. The number of students who have been identified as having emotional or behavioral disorders has been estimated conservatively to be 0.89% of students enrolled in school, or about 414,279 students. Kauffman (1993) indicates that the number of students with emotional and behavioral disorders is grossly underestimated, and that 3%–8% represents a more accurate estimate.

Types of Antisocial Behavior Patterns

Moffitt (1994) makes an important distinction in the population of antisocial children and youth who are at elevated risk for becoming juvenile offenders. Moffitt argues that the construct of delinquency conceals two distinct forms of antisocial behavior (i.e., "adolescent limited" versus "life course persistent"). Most antisocial youth show a temporary pattern of increased offending during adolescence and then return to prior behavior patterns; these youth display an adolescent limited form of antisocial behavior. In contrast, youth with life course persistent antisocial behavior engage in antisocial behavior at every life stage, culminating in serious, persistent criminal behavior and a pathological personality. Life course persistent patterns are characteristics of a minority of juvenile offenders. This taxonomy has great utility for schools and other agencies in developing practices for accommodating the needs and problems of this student population.

Patterson and his colleagues (Patterson, Reid, & Dishion, 1992) have studied the family etiologies, longitudinal paths, and correlates of antisocial behavior patterns for the past three decades. They note that the long-term stability of antisocial behavior is associated with patterns that begin early, are displayed across multiple settings, are severe and expressed in diverse forms. Children and youth who fit this profile are very likely to display life course persistent antisocial behavior patterns throughout their school careers.

Antisocial Behavior and Comorbidity

Comorbidity is a commonly observed occurrence among antisocial students. For example, it is estimated that approximately 50% of hyperactive children and youth either have or will develop conduct disorder during their school careers (Fowler, 1992). Learning disabilities and lower-than-expected achievement levels are also characteristic of antisocial students in many cases (Walker, Colvin, & Ramsey, 1995; Walker et al., 1997).

Dodge and his colleagues have conducted extensive research that documents the attributional biases and social processing deficits of aggressive, antisocial children and youth (Dodge & Frame, 1982). The peer status of these students is also controversial and often reflects rejected social status (Hollinger, 1987).

The above profile of the antisocial student paints a picture of elevated risk for a host of negative developmental outcomes, including school failure. The longitudinal and cross-sectional literatures on antisocial behavior patterns show that children and youth displaying them are at elevated risk of a host of negative developmental outcomes (Kazdin, 1987, 1993; Reid, 1993). These outcomes include school failure and dropping out, delinquency, drug and alcohol involvement, low self-esteem, bad conduct discharges from the military, adult criminality, lifelong dependence on social services, and higher hospitalization and mortality rates.

Antisocial behavior also has been found to be associated with specific family, community, and school features. For example, students with antisocial behavior tend to come from family situations in which behavior management practices are inconsistent, aversive punishment strategies are used, and monitoring of student activities and whereabouts is lacking (e.g., Biglan, 1995; Dumas, 1989; Patterson et al., 1992). These students tend to be associated with communities in which peer networks tend to be antisocial in nature and social engagements tend to be highly negative (e.g., Biglan, 1995). Finally, students with antisocial behavior are often found in schools in which rules and expectations are unclear, consequences for both appropriate and inappropriate behaviors are inconsistently applied, little accommodation is provided for individual student differences, academic failure is high, and rates of reactive management are high (e.g., G. Mayer, 1995).

The economic and social costs of this disorder are potentially enormous. Our society must find cost-effective solutions to this problem and prevention, achieved through socially valid early interventions, offers a realistic goal. We believe strongly that schools must create a context for effective intervention that begins at the level of the whole school and works in concert with families and community service providers (e.g., police and social service agencies).

The remainder of this chapter deals with issues and procedures associated with the effective accommodation of antisocial behavior within the context of schooling. First, we focus on the features of a schoolwide response designed to address the behavior support needs of all students in schools. We then describe the specific features of problem identification and analysis regarding individual students who display antisocial behavior, and the process steps of developing and implementing behavior support plans for these students.

Creating a Schoolwide Context for Effective Intervention

We reiterate that a comprehensive, interdisciplinary approach is recommended; however, because schools represent a closed and predictable system, we emphasize what school personnel can do to address the challenges presented by students with antisocial behavior. To respond effectively and efficiently to the challenge of educating individual students with antisocial behavior, schools first must provide a solid schoolwide foundation from which to develop, implement, and maintain individualized and specialized programs for these students. Features of a proactive schoolwide response to antisocial behavior have been discussed in the literature (e.g., Biglan, 1995; Colvin, Kameenui, & Sugai, 1993; G. Mayer, 1995; G. Sugai & Horner, 1994, in press).

We use the term "proactive" to refer to practices that are positive and preventative in nature. These practices are designed to be preventative by focusing on decreasing the development of new cases of antisocial behavior (i.e., incidence) and reducing and/or controlling the existing cases of antisocial behavior (i.e., prevalence). These practices are designed to be positive in that the use of punitive disciplinary strategies is minimized and the application of constructive and effective interventions (i.e., social skills instruction, academic remediation and curricular modification, behavioral interventions) is emphasized (Biglan, 1995; Lipsey, 1991; G. Mayer, 1995; Tolan & Guerra, 1994). Recent research indicates that the use of punishment-based interventions in schools with students who display antisocial behavior actually results in an increase in the behaviors that were targeted from reduction. In their work with schools, G.R. Mayer and Sulzer-Azaroff (1990) observed that when a proactive system of behavioral support was not provided, episodes of aggression, vandalism, truancy, dropping out, and tardiness actually increased. In this section we address the strategy and process components of schoolwide responses to antisocial behavior.

Schoolwide Strategies

In general, most schools have a disciplinary handbook that delineates the policies and procedures for maintaining a safe school where learning and teaching can occur. Unfortunately, the emphasis is frequently focused on delineating what behaviors represent district and state rule violations and the associated graduated sanctions that accompany each violation. Little information is provided about the expectations for acceptable behavior and the strategies that students, teachers, and parents might employ to encourage these expectations. All students, but especially students with antisocial behavior, must be exposed to clearly specified and consistently implemented discipline systems that both encourage prosocial behaviors and discourage rule violations.

Six main strategy components comprise comprehensive proactive schoolwide behavioral support systems (Colvin, Kameenui, & Sugai, 1993). The first is a simple, clear, and positive purpose statement that serves as the foundation for the learning and teaching process in a school. The following statement from an elementary school exemplifies these characteristics:

> We the staff, students, and parents of Pleasant Hill Elementary School are committed to helping all students acquire the academic, social, and behavioral skills necessary to become productive citizens now and in the future. All students have the right to learn these skills in a safe, caring, and respectful environment. (CARS Project, 1996)

The second component is a set of proactive expectations or rules that serve as the basis for creating and maintaining safe and productive learning and teaching environments. These expectations are always positively stated and small in number. For example, students and staff at Shasta Middle School are guided by five schoolwide expectations:

(a) *Be Responsible,* (b) *Cooperate with Others,* (c) *Treat Others with Respect,* (d) *Keep Hands and Feet to Self,* and (e) *Follow Directions Immediately.* Pleasant Hill Elementary School uses four schoolwide rules: (a) *Cooperate in Work and Play,* (b) *Academic Excellence through Effort and Hard Work,* (c) *Respect Self, Others, and the Environment,* and (d) *Safe Conduct at all Times.* Rule violations (e.g., fighting, defiance, disruptions, harassment) are defined in the back third of discipline manuals.

The third component consists of a set of strategies for teaching the schoolwide expectations. Although most students have learning histories that include mastery and use of typical schoolwide expectations, teaching these expectations to all students ensures that students and staff have been exposed to a common language and meaning for each expectation. Teaching the expectations schoolwide also stresses the importance of these rules to the functioning of the school, and focuses on building a positive schoolwide climate. Expectations are taught using positive and negative examples, across multiple contexts, and with many opportunities to practice the skills.

A planned continuum for encouraging the proactive schoolwide expectations is the fourth component. After all students and staff have been exposed to and practiced the schoolwide expectations, students must have regular and frequent opportunities to receive contingent positive feedback when they display behaviors that represent a given schoolwide expectation. Most commonly, this feedback takes the form of verbal praise and other social acknowledgments. However, to ensure that all staff and all students are involved over time, a continuum of acknowledgments is needed to facilitate the feedback process. For example, Shasta Middle School staff developed a feedback system that consisted of verbal praise, social acknowledgments (e.g., public announcements, popcorn and soda parties), positive office referrals, and large group rewards (e.g., dances, assemblies).

The fifth component is a continuum of strategies for responding to rule infractions. This component usually is specified in great detail in most schools. Sanctions for minor offenses (e.g., tardiness, talking out) are typically handled by individual teachers, whereas major offenses (e.g., fighting, defiance, property destruction, weapons) involve the office and the student's parents. Clear definitions of what is to be handled by teachers and what is to be sent to the office must be provided, and consistent implementation of consequences must occur.

The last component of a proactive schoolwide system is a process for monitoring the implementation of the system and for collecting data to evaluate its effectiveness. Typically, archival information, such as office referrals, behavior incidents, use of positive referrals or acknowledgments, and attendance rates, are used; however, samples of actual student behavior also should be collected to determine the extent to which prosocial and rule violation behaviors are occurring. This information is used to maintain or modify strategies of the schoolwide system.

Schoolwide Process Components

The strategy components of a schoolwide system of behavioral support are relatively straightforward to identify and develop. The more challenging task is implementing the process that establishes and maintains these strategies. Two important considerations serve as the foundation for the process of schoolwide behavior support (G. Sugai & Horner, 1994, in press). First, a systems approach must be taken. This approach organizes the larger schoolwide system into four subsystems. The schoolwide subsystem consists of the strategies and processes that involve all students, all staff members, and all school settings. The classroom subsystem includes the procedures and policies that are implemented in individual classrooms to support the larger schoolwide purpose and expectations. The specific setting subsystem consists of the procedures and strategies that are associated with nonclassroom settings (e.g., cafeteria, hallways, buses, restrooms). The individual student subsystem is comprised of the forms, procedures, and strategies that have been designed to address the needs of the individual student who presents significant behavioral challenges in the school setting. In particular, the first three subsystems must be operating efficiently and effectively to support intensive programming required for individual students who are served in the individual student system.

Second, the process of implementing and maintaining a schoolwide support system requires that the match between problem type and school response is accurate. For example, schools err when schoolwide system changes are made to accommodate the demands and needs of the individual student support system. Schoolwide systems, by definition, consist of universal interventions that are intended for general implementation for all students, by all staff, across all school settings. They are not intended for the individual student who presents significant and chronic behavioral challenges and requires specially designed, individualized programs that require intensive effort and resources.

To increase the efficiency and effectiveness with which schoolwide systems of behavior support are implemented, ten structural and process factors should be considered (G. Sugai & Horner, in press): (a) team, (b) need, (c) priority, (d) commitment, (e) systems approach, (f) administrative participation, (g) proactivity, (h) integration, (I) resources, (j) policy, and (k) competence. Definitions are provided for each of these requirements in Table 1.

Individual Student Behavior Support Planning

Thus far, we have indicated that students with antisocial behavior represent a significant challenge to schools, families, and communities and that schools represent an excellent frontline to address the learning and behavioral needs of these students. A proactive schoolwide effort, consisting of effective procedures and efficient processes, is required to provide the context for effective intervention. However, a schoolwide, universal system will fail to deliver the intensity of support needed by antisocial children and youth. To address the needs of students with significant histories and displays of antisocial behavior, an intensive and individualized response is required. In this section, we describe the features of a behavior support planning process designed to provide specially designed, individualized programming for these students. Problem identification, problem analysis, intervention planning and implementation, and implementation evaluation are discussed.

TABLE 1. Process Components of a Schoolwide Behavior Support System

Priority:	Enhancement of behavior support top three school improvement goals.
Collaboration:	Team-based approach emphasized.
Leadership:	Administrator actively involved.
Need:	Necessity for enhancement of behavior support is defined.
Agreement:	All staff agreement that need exists, and commit to active and long-term participation.
Policy:	Written documents provide direction and significance.
Systems:	All staff, students, and settings included in systemic approach.
Integration:	Behavioral support incorporated into academic programming.
Competence:	Behavioral skills available in building.
Proactivity:	Positive, preventative behavior support emphasized.
Resources:	Time, materials, equipment, FTE, and technical assistance are committed.

Problem Identification

Two major goals must be addressed in dealing with the identification of, and behavior support planning for, students who display antisocial behavior patterns: (a) screening and identification to facilitate early detection and (b) conducting a functional assessment of their behavioral status to guide and inform detailed problem analysis (i.e., functional analysis) and plan implementation. In this chapter, we describe functional *assessment* as part of the problem identification process and juxtapose experimental functional *analysis* as a more rigorous and precise set of methods encompassing problem analysis (J.S. Sprague & Horner, 1995).

Screening and Identification

Because of the aversiveness of their behavioral characteristics, the impact and visibility of students who display antisocial behavior are significant within school environments. Students with more involved antisocial behaviors are relatively easy to identify due to their behavioral salience and the negative impressions experienced by teachers and peers (Hollinger, 1987). However, those students who manifest the "soft" early signs of this disorder (e.g., noncompliance, oppositional behavior, nattering, whining, verbal aggression) are often not re-ferred until their problem behaviors escalate into more serious forms that exceed the tolerance levels of key social agents.

The proactive, universal screening of all students for the signs of antisocial behavior development should be conducted on a regular basis by school personnel. These assessments should be accomplished as early as possible in students' school careers (e.g., preschool and kindergarten). They should be universal in that all students are given an equal chance to be identified through multiagent and multimethod strategies. Excellent multiple gating models for achieving this task have been contributed by Loeber, Dishion, and Patterson (1984); Charlebois, Leblanc, Gagnon, and Larivee (1994); and Walker and his colleagues (Walker & Severson, 1990; Walker, Severson, & Feil, 1995). In addition, comprehensive social skills assessments should be conducted of those students who are identified by the multiple gating assessment procedure as being at risk. An excellent assessment battery for this purpose has been contributed by Gresham and Elliott (1990).

In later grades (e.g., grades 6, 7, 8), office referrals can be used to identify students with behavioral patterns that are likely to lead to failure in later school years. Tobin, Sugai, and Colvin (1996) examined the office referral patterns of students in the first term of sixth grade and observed that as few as one office referral for harassment or fighting in sixth grade was a reliable predictor for significant problem behaviors in grade 8. A later study supported this observation and indicated that males who had been referred for violent, fighting type behavior more than twice in grade 6 and females who were referred even once for violent, harassing type behaviors as sixth graders were not likely to be on track for a standard high school graduation; that is, they were likely to drop out or leave school (Tobin & Sugai, 1996). Although office referrals in general are influenced by teacher tolerance, clarity of discipline rules and procedures, and actual student behaviors, they represent a good means of identifying students with significant antisocial behaviors.

Conducting a Functional Assessment

Although teacher ratings, perceptions, and office referrals are useful screening mechanisms, they do not provide the level of detail required to identify the specific behaviors presented by individual students and the context variables that are associated with the occurrences of these behaviors. In preparation for conducting functional analyses, functional assessments are conducted. In these assessments, information regarding potential influencing factors is collected. Specifically, antecedent triggers or occasioning stimuli, setting events or establishing operations, and maintaining consequences are identified (Horner, 1994; O'Neill et al., 1997). This information can be collected in a variety of ways and from a variety of sources. Archival sources (e.g., previous assessments and intervention attempts) can be reviewed (Tobin & Sugai, 1996). Individuals (e.g., teachers, parents, administrators) who have direct experience with the student can be interviewed (Carr, Levin et al., 1994; Lewis, Scott, & Sugai, 1994; O'Neill et al.,1997). The student can be interviewed (Kern, Childs, Dunlap, Clarke, & Falk, 1994; Reed, Thomas, Sprague & Horner, submitted for publication). Table 2 lists the major outcomes of a functional assessment process (O'Neill et al., 1997; J.S. Sprague & Horner, 1995).

Functional assessment is helpful in intervention design once the information allows prediction of the conditions under which problem behavior is likely to occur and when maintaining consequences have been identified. Recently, researchers have advocated that the intensity of functional assessment procedures should match the complexity of the problem behavior (J.S. Sprague & Horner, 1995). That is, if less rigorous and easier to implement assessment procedures produce an acceptable description of the events that occasion and maintain a problem behavior, then more rigorous procedures may not be required. However, if interviews, rating scales, or archival reviews do not generate clear patterns, then more precise observations and analyses are needed.

Archival reviews and interviews provide indirect information about the nature of the problem behavior and the context in which it is observed. A preferred method of conducting functional assessment focuses on direct observation strategies in which the behaviors of interest and related antecedent and consequence events are recorded (Bijou, Peterson, & Ault, 1968; O'Neill et al., in press; Wolery, Bailey, & Sugai, 1988). When direct observation functional assessments are conducted, recurring antecedent-behavior-consequence patterns are noted as indications of possible testable explanations or hypotheses. A sim-

---

TABLE 2. Five Outcomes of Functional Assessment Process

1. A description of the problem behaviors, including classes of behaviors that occur together;

2. Identification of the events, times and situations that predict when the problem behaviors *will* and *will not* occur (e.g., antecedent stimuli);

3. Identification of the consequences that maintain the problem behaviors (i.e., what function[s] the behaviors appear to serve);

4. Development of one or more hypothesis statements that describe the behaviors, the situation(s) in which they occur, and the consequences maintaining them; and,

5. Direct observation data that support the hypothesis statements.

---

ple model of this relationship is illustrated in Table 3. Determining the validity of these explanations or hypotheses occurs at the next stage, problem analysis.

Problem Analysis

After the features of the problem behavior and context variables have been identified, the validity of testable explanations is examined. The primary purpose of this stage is to analyze the extent to which hypotheses developed during problem identification describe the problem situation and predict future occurrences of the problem behavior. If a testable explanation provides an accurate description of the problem, it is used to develop interventions or behav-

ior support plans. In this section, we discuss (a) the nature of hypothesized functions of behavior, (b) methods of confirming the hypothesized function, and (c) features of the competing behavior model.

Hypothesized Function of Behavior

An important aspect of statements that describe the behavior–environment relationship concerns the outcomes that are associated with the student's display of the problem behavior. Behaviors that are observed consistently and predictably under specified conditions are maintained by consequence events that have reinforcing characteristics (i.e., positive or negative reinforcement). When a relationship between a problem behavior and a

TABLE 3. Simple Direct Observation A-B-C Functional Assessment and Resulting Testable Explanations

Triggering antecedent	Problem behavior	Maintaining consequences
Teacher: Why haven't you completed your worksheet?	Cleo: *It's stupid work, and besides, I already know how to do it.*	Teacher: *You know my policy, "no work, no grade." You have 10 minutes to get it. . . .*
√	Cleo interrupts: *If I don't, what are you gonna do about it?*	Teacher: *You've just earned yourself a trip to the office. Put your stuff away.*
Teacher approaches Cleo.	Cleo: *Yeah, right. You and your school suck. I'm outta here. Any of you wimps going with me?* Points at other students.	Teacher: *If any of you want to join Cleo in the office, go right ahead.*
Two other students get up and follow Cleo out the door.	Cleo: *See . . . they think this class is a joke, too.* Heads for the door.	Teacher: *Get back here . . . all of you. I haven't given you permission to leave.*
The three students smile, and continue out the door.	Cleo slams the door, and leaves the building.	Teacher: *Okay class, now that the disrupters are gone, let's look at how civil disobedience was expressed when the Boston Tea Party. . .*

Testable Explanations:

#1. Cleo fails to complete her in class assignments when
   a.   the task requirements are too easy and she can avoid doing the work, or
   b.   she can get teacher attention

#2. Cleo argues with teachers when
   a.   she receives peer attention for her actions, or
   b.   she can be removed from the classroom.

hypothesized consequence is validated, a *function* is described.

Two major types of functions (i.e., two major consequence classes) can be described. In the first type, a problem behavior occasions the presentation of a reinforcing consequence. In less technical terms, the student *obtains* something "desirable" when the problem behavior is displayed. In the second type of function, a problem behavior occasions the avoidance or removal of an aversive consequence. The student *avoids* or *escapes* something "undesirable" when the problem behavior is emitted. Behaviors maintained by obtaining desirable consequences are described as positive reinforcement, whereas behaviors maintained by escaping or avoiding undesirable consequences are described as negative reinforcement. Figure 1 expands this framework for organizing the possible functions of problem behaviors into six categories (three under "Obtain" and three under "Escape/Avoid") (O'Neill et al., in press).

Under both the Obtain and Escape/Avoid categories, consequences can be further classified in two ways. Some behaviors occasion internal events (e.g., self-stimulation, daydreaming), whereas others are associated with external, socially mediated events (e.g., attention from peers or escape from instruction). Figure 1 provides examples of the types of consequences that might fit into each category, and a descriptive label for each category.

The examples in Figure 1 show that consequences important in the Obtain category for the behaviors of some students also may be important in the Escape/Avoid category for behaviors of other

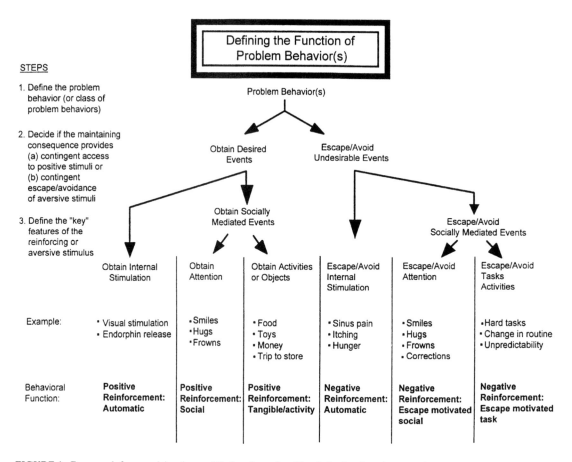

FIGURE 1. Framework for organizing the possible functions of problem behaviors into six categories. *Note.* From *Functional Assessment of Problem Behavior: A Practical Assessment Guide* (2nd ed.), by R.E. O'Neill et al., 1997, Pacific Grove, CA: Brooks/Cole. Copyright 1997 by Wadsworth Publishing Company. Adapted with permission.

students. In other words, a maintaining consequence event that is determined to be a positive reinforcer for one student may be a negative reinforcer for another student. Similarly, a particular behavior or class of behaviors may serve multiple functions for people in different situations (Day, Horner, & O'Neill, 1994). For example, acting out in class may be used sometimes to occasion attention from peers, and at other times to occasion escape or avoidance of completing a work assignment.

Confirming the Function of Behavior

A testable explanation provides a "best guess" that describes the problem behavior, triggering antecedents, maintaining consequence, and functions. However, to be useful in building effective and efficient behavior support plans, the accuracy of testable explanations must be examined. Although functional assessment interviews provide an adequate basis for problem identification, we recommend more rigorous methods for confirming the function(s) of problem behavior. In this section, we describe three methods of checking the function of behavior: (a) descriptive functional assessment, (b) experimental functional analysis, and (c) student-assisted functional assessments.

Descriptive Functional Assessment

One of the simplest and most direct methods of confirming the function of problem behavior is *descriptive functional assessment*. In general, the student with problem behavior is observed systematically and directly in a variety of settings. Systematic, direct observation has long been a foundation of applied behavior analysis procedures (Bijou et al., 1968), and can be conducted by consultants, school psychologists, teachers, direct support staff, and/or family members. The observer records when a problem behavior (or behaviors) occurs, what was happening just before the behavior, what happened after the behavior, and the observer's perception of the function of the behavior in that instance. An example of a simple descriptive functional assessment was illustrated in Figure 3. When such information is recorded across several instances of the problem behavior, across time, and across settings, data patterns are established that confirm (a) problem behaviors that occur together (response classes); (b)

when, where, and with whom problem behaviors are most likely to be observed (setting conditions and triggering antecedents); and (c) events that appear to maintain occurrence of the problem behavior (maintaining consequences and functions).

Testable explanations or hypotheses are confirmed by observing and documenting repeated occurrences of the problem behavior under similar antecedent and consequence conditions. The more often the relationship is observed under specific conditions and not observed under other conditions, the greater our confidence that the explanation accurately describes the functional relationship between the problem behavior and specific environmental conditions.

Experimental Functional Analysis

The most rigorous strategy for gathering functional assessment information involves the systematic manipulation of variables that will and will not result in the occurrence of the problem behaviors, that is, *experimental functional analysis*. The central feature of functional analysis is the conducting of a formal test of the relationship between environmental variables (antecedent and consequent stimuli) and the occurrence of problem behavior (behavioral hypothesis). Functional analysis is the only approach that allows an unambiguous demonstration of a functional relationship between environmental events and problem behaviors.

A variety of experimental functional analyses have been recommended. One frequently used method of functional analysis involves the manipulation of consequences contingent on the occurrence of targeted behaviors (Wacker et al., 1990; Kern, Childs, Dunlap, et al., 1994). Another method involves manipulating structural variables, such as task difficulty, task length, level or type of attention provided during an activity, or the presence or absence of choice in an activity (Axelrod, 1987). A common feature of the various methods is the systematic and controlled manipulation of antecedent and/or consequence events and direct monitoring of student behavior within and across these manipulations. Single case research designs are used to monitor and evaluate the effects of the manipulations on the occurrence of the problem behavior (see Chapter 2).

Two basic types of single case research designs have been used in conducting functional analyses:

(a) reversal or ABAB design and (b) multielement or alternating treatments design (Barlow & Hayes, 1979; Wolery et al., 1988). A reversal design (ABAB) involves (a) gathering data during a baseline (A) phase, where the variable of interest (e.g. antecedent or consequence) is not present; (b) conducting a second treatment (B) phase, in which the variable of interest is present; and (c) repeating the alternation of these baseline and treatment conditions. For example, alternating sessions that present difficult tasks with those that include only easy or preferred tasks should indicate whether the person was performing problem behaviors to avoid having to complete difficult tasks.

A multielement or alternating treatment design involves systematically and sequentially presenting several different conditions within a relatively short period of time. For example, the design might include sessions of difficult instruction with escape contingent on problem behavior performance, sessions in which attention is provided only for problem behaviors, sessions in which the person is ignored for a period of time, and a "control" condition which is unlikely to result in problem behaviors (e.g., sessions of nondemanding social play or interaction with the person) (Iwata, Dorsey, Slifer, & Richman, 1982). By alternating and interspersing the different conditions over a period of time, those variables that have a consistent and differentiated effect can be identified and confirmed. Each condition is repeated to see if any differences become apparent between them.

Iwata and colleagues (1982) pioneered a powerful method for functional analysis of severe self-injury, and this approach has been adapted by many other researchers (Neef & Iwata, 1994). Recent applications to antisocial and typical students provide promising support for the generality of the procedures (Kern et al., 1994; Lewis, Scott, & Sugai, 1994; T. Lewis & Sugai, 1996a, T.J. Lewis & Sugai, 1996b). Functional analysis can be expensive in time and effort, but in some cases, it may be the only way to ensure accurate assessment of problem behaviors. Because the procedure requires presenting conditions that will provoke the problem behavior, functional analyses always should be conducted under supervision of a person trained in conducting behavior analytic research (O'Neill et al., 1997).

Student-Assisted Functional Assessment

The third problem analysis method for confirming the function of problem behavior is *student-assisted functional assessment*. Functional assessment procedures have been most often used with persons with moderate to severe intellectual disabilities. Recently, however, Dunlap and his colleagues (Dunlap et al., 1993, 1994) and others (Lewis, Scott, & Sugai, 1994; T. Lewis & Sugai, 1996a; T.J. Lewis & Sugai, 1996b) have demonstrated interventions based on functional assessments with children who have emotional and behavioral disorders, conduct disorders, mild intellectual disabilities, brain injury, and developmentally typical children.

The success of linking functional assessment and intervention for students with adequate verbal skills raises the possibility of collecting information directly from students. We believe that important functional assessment information can be obtained this way. Our clinical experiences, and those of others (Broussard & Northup, 1995; Dunlap et al., 1993), suggest that many students can (a) state preferences for activities, items, or people; (b) describe complaints about school work; (c) request different activities; and (d) describe conflicts with peers and adults. To the extent that these statements are accurate and consistent, they can supplement information obtained from teacher interviews, direct observations, and functional analysis.

Student-assisted functional assessment interview methods represent promising approaches to including students directly in the functional assessment process and obtaining information that describes testable explanations and behavior function. This methodology is especially encouraging in our work to educate students with antisocial behavior who (a) can be very competent verbally, (b) frequently engage in problem behavior that is hidden (covert) from adults, and (c) interact in complex social networks. To date, development and field-testing has been done in elementary and middle schools (Kern, Dunlap, Clarke, & Childs, 1994; Reed et al., submitted for publication). Preliminary findings indicate moderate agreement between teacher- versus student-provided information on antecedents, behaviors of concern, consequences, and support plan recommendations. Further research is needed regarding the link between student reports, direct observation, and functional analysis results.

Competing Behaviors Model

Teachers may conduct a functional assessment and move directly into writing the behavior support plan. We recommend that an additional step be added once the functional assessment is completed. This step involves using a "competing behavior model" to define the features and strategies of a behavior support plan for a student. The competing behavior model is useful because (a) the link between intervention procedures and functional assessment results is strengthened; (b) the match between the values, skills, and capacity of the people who will carry out the plan is maximized; (c) the fidelity of plan implementation is improved; and (d) the logical consistency among the different procedures used in a comprehensive plan of support is increased.

A competing behavior model is a graphic representation of the variables associated with problem behavior (Horner, O'Neill, & Flannery, 1993). The process of constructing a competing behavior model involves three steps. First, a functional assessment hypothesis statement is diagramed. Second, behaviors are identified that should compete with the problem behaviors. Third, intervention options are identified in four areas (setting events, antecedents, behaviors, consequences). These steps are described below.

Step 1: Diagram the functional assessment hypothesis statement(s). To diagram a hypothesis statement, use information identified during the functional assessment process to list the (a) setting event(s) (b) antecedent stimuli, (c) problem behavior(s), and (d) maintaining consequences. For example, Kiyoshi is a student who displays noncompliance (e.g., pushing papers on the floor,

throwing pencils) and yelling profanities when asked to complete math worksheets. The noncompliance and yelling appear to be maintained by opportunities to escape from math worksheet tasks. The hypothesis is stated as, "When Kiyoshi is presented with math tasks, he displays noncompliance behaviors and yells profanities to escape from the tasks." Figure 2 provides a visual display of the hypothesis statement for Kiyoshi's problem behavior.

Step 2: Define alternative or desired behaviors, and the consequences associated with those behaviors. A fundamental rule of behaviorally based intervention planning is that you should not attempt to reduce a problem behavior without identifying the alternative, desired behaviors the student should perform instead of the problem behavior (White & Haring, 1980; Wolery et al., 1988). Therefore, the behaviors or behavior paths that will compete with the problem behavior must be identified. Two questions should be asked: (a) "When the setting and antecedent events occur, what is the behavior you would like the person to perform instead of the problem behavior?" and (b) "When the setting and antecedent events have occurred, what would be an appropriate behavior that could result in the same consequence as the problem behavior?" The responses to these questions are added to the competing behavior model presented in Figure 3.

The competing behavior model indicates that (a) desired behavior (math worksheets) is not associated with reinforcing consequences and (b) the student does not display appropriate behavior (e.g., asking for a break or assistance) that might result in escape from difficult tasks. The model also suggests that the math worksheets tasks are aversive.

Step 3: Select intervention procedures. We recommend assembling a comprehensive collection

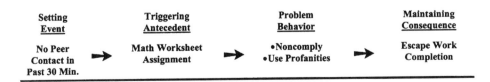

Setting Event	Triggering Antecedent	Problem Behavior	Maintaining Consequence
No Peer Contact in Past 30 Min.	Math Worksheet Assignment	•Noncomply •Use Profanities	Escape Work Completion

FIGURE 2. Diagram of testable explanation or hypothesis based on functional assessment information on Kiyoshi's problem behavior.

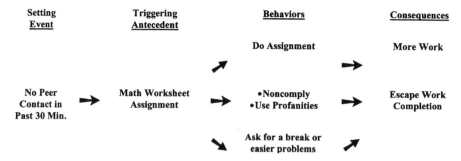

FIGURE 3. Competing behavior model: Diagram summary statement and competing behavior paths. *Note.* From *Functional Assessment of Problem Behavior: A Practical Assessment Guide* (2nd ed.), by R.E. O'Neill et al., in press, Pacific Grove, CA: Brooks/Cole. Copyright 1997 by Brookes/Cole. Adapted with permission by Wadsworth Publishing Company.

of intervention strategies that can be carried out to reduce the likelihood of the problem behavior and increase the likelihood of the alternative appropriate behavior. The selection of intervention procedures should be guided by the outcomes of the problem analysis stage. We now discuss behavior support plan development and implementation.

Plan Implementation

A "behavior support plan" is a plan for teaching and promoting desired behaviors or behaviors that will function as alternatives to the problem behaviors. The development and implementation of behavior support plans must be linked to, and based on, information obtained from functional assessments and functional analysis. In addition, (a) effective interventions must be selected, (b) intervention planning should be comprehensive, (c) behavior support plans should be implemented with high fidelity, and (d) follow-up strategies should be planned and implemented.

Features of Effective Interventions

To be effective for students and those individuals who implement them, behavior support plans should (a) fit the natural routines of the setting; (b) be consistent with the values of the people in the setting; (c) be efficient in terms of time and resources; (d) be matched to the skills of the people who will carry out the procedures; and (e) produce encouraging (reinforcing) short-term results (O'Neill et al., 1997).

Preference should be given to interventions for which research exists to document the conditions (e.g., subjects, settings, behaviors) under which positive intervention effects have been obtained. Other promising methods which have logical or theoretical appeal, but for which validating research has not been conducted, can be considered. Innovative or untested methods should be implemented with caution and safeguards should be put into effect to ensure that negative side effects are avoided and that benefits are maximized. Regardless of whether preferred or promising practices are adopted, formative monitoring and evaluation procedures should be in place.

Comprehensive Intervention Planning

When developing behavior support plans, an array of strategies should be organized to accomplish multiple outcomes: (a) reduction in the problem behavior, (b) increase in the occurrence of alternative or desired behaviors, and (c) acceptable ratings of intervention procedures and effectiveness from the people who carry them out.

A common approach to building behavior support plans is to focus only on the consequences for the problem or desired behavior, for example, only using time-out as a consequence for problem behavior. Adding only single-consequence events (e.g., rewards or punishments) can lead to an excessive focus on problem behavior, overuse of punishment, and increases in the problem behavior (Axelrod, 1987). Thus, the use of a single technique (e.g., time-out) to eliminate or reduce the problem behavior is not recommended. Instead, behavior support plans should be comprehensive and multielement, and focused on the variables highlighted in the competing behavior model. Basic intervention design steps are outlined below (O'Neill et al., in press).

1. *Diagram the competing behavior model, and review the logic and structure of the model.* As mentioned previously, a clear understanding of the contextual variables (setting events, triggering antecedents, and maintaining consequences) that are associated with the problem and desired behaviors must be obtained before intervention development occurs. All individuals who have direct contact with the students should indicate their understanding and agreement with the hypothesis statements created by the competing behavior model.

2. *Identify any changes in setting events that could be made to make them less likely or less influential.* Setting events influence the occurrence of problem behavior by affecting previously existing stimulus–reinforcer relationships. For example, consequence events that once served as powerful positively reinforcing events become less influential because of a setting event (e.g., illness, hunger, peer conflict). Making changes in setting events as part of a comprehensive behavior support plan can make problem behaviors irrelevant by altering the stimulus–reinforcer relationships maintaining problem behavior (Horner, Vaughn, Day, & Ard, 1996).

3. *Change antecedent events.* Several changes can be made in triggering antecedents to make problem behaviors irrelevant or unlikely. These include (a) altering the schedule of activities, (b) adapting the curriculum or features of a task (Dunlap, Kern, Clarke, & Robbins, 1991), (c) changing the size or composition of instructional groups, (d) providing more specific information about when tasks are to be performed and when they will be completed (Flannery & Horner, 1994), shortening task length (Dunlap et al., 1991), (e) interspersing easy tasks with hard tasks (Dunlap et al., 1991; Horner, Day, Sprague, O'Brien, & Heathfield, 1991), and (f) providing precorrections for appropriate behaviors (Colvin, Sugai, & Patching, 1993; J.R. Sprague & Thomas, in press). The goal of each of these antecedent manipulations is to remove or reduce stimuli that occasion the problem behavior, and introduce other antecedent stimulus conditions that occasion the desired or appropriate behavior.

4. *Teach and promote desired and alternative behaviors.* Recent functional analysis research provides strong evidence that many problem behaviors serve as effective means of communication (Carr et al., 1994); that is, these behaviors result in specific outcomes or consequences that serve as reinforcers (positive or negative) for problem behavior. In a comprehensive behavior support planning process, the goal is to identify and teach new behaviors that will be more efficient and effective than are the problem behaviors (Horner et al., 1993). However, to achieve this, three tactics must be applied. First, students must be taught how and when to perform a skill. Teaching content may be chosen directly from the competing behavior path analysis, and also may be augmented with specially designed curricula aimed at preventing antisocial behavior patterns. Two such examples include the Second Step Curriculum (Committee for Children, 1988, 1989, 1990, 1992), which teaches 30 discrete skills related to problem solving, impulse control, and empathy, and First Steps (Walker et al., in press), which provides school and home training for prosocial behaviors such as cooperation, listening, problem solving, and making friends.

Teaching competing behaviors is among the most powerful strategies available. Preferred methods include (a) selecting and sequencing appropriate teaching examples (Engelmann & Carnine, 1982; Horner, Sprague, & Wilcox 1982; Kameenui & Simmons, 1990), (b) presenting teaching trials so they convey unambiguous information (Engelmann & Carnine, 1982), (c) praising correct responses, and (d) ignoring or correcting errors.

Second, effective and powerful reinforcing consequences must be provided whenever the desired replacement behavior is emitted. These consequences must be at least as powerful as those consequences associated with the maintenance of the problem behavior. Third, precorrections (antecedent prompts, reminders) that occasion the desired replacement behavior early in situations or event chains where the problem behavior is likely (Colvin, Sugai, & Patching, 1993) should be included in the behavior support plan.

5. *Change the manner in which consequences are provided to make the positive competing behavior pathway more likely.* To increase the probability that desired behavior is emitted and problem behavior is not occasioned, consequences must be identified and provided that compete with those consequences associated with the problem behavior. In particular, the magnitude of the reinforcer that is associated with the problem behavior must be considered. For example,

the relative magnitude of the relationship between problem behavior and peer attention must be compared to the magnitude of the relationship between the desired replacement behavior and work completion consequences (J.S. Sprague & Horner, in press) If problem behavior is associated with a more powerful consequence than the desired behavior, the problem behavior would be more likely to occur.

Two general strategies are available for changing consequence events (O'Neill et al., in press). The first is to increase the value of the consequences associated with performing the desired be-

havior. The second is to decrease the value of the consequences for performing the problem behavior (e.g., withhold positive consequences or present aversive consequences). The goal is to reduce the comparative value of consequences maintaining problem behaviors and to increase the relative value of consequences maintaining desired behavior.

The competing behavior model with accompanying behavior support plan strategies for the student whose problem behavior was associated with escape from difficult instruction is illustrated in Figure 4. Strategies for changing setting events, an-

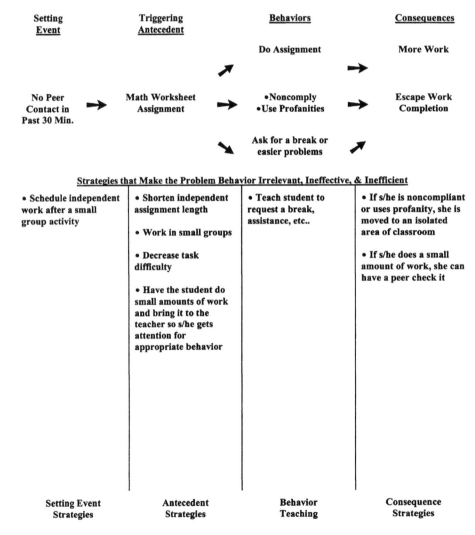

FIGURE 4. Competing behavior model: Diagramed summary statement, competing behavior pathway, and behavior support plan strategies. *Note.* From *Functional Assessment of Problem Behavior: A Practical Assessment Guide* (2nd ed.), by R.E. O'Neill et al., in press, Pacific Grove, CA: Brooks/Cole. Copyright 1997 by Brookes/Cole. Adapted with permission by Wadsworth Publishing Company.

tecedents, behaviors, and consequences are presented. Figure 4 shows how information from the problem analysis stage is used to identify and develop these strategies.

Increasing Implementation Fidelity

A behavior support plan that is well written, carefully developed, and comprehensive is only as good as the accuracy with which it is implemented. However, the behaviors of teachers, parents, counselors, psychologists, and others are vulnerable to the same punishing and reinforcing contingencies that affect and explain student behavior. Thus, ensuring and achieving high intervention fidelity can present major challenges. Resource or capacity limitations; teacher, parent, or student perceptions of intervention acceptability (J.R. Sprague & Horner, 1991); and feedback systems (e.g., lack of objective data collection and review, ineffective reinforcer) delivery can impair the effectiveness of a well-designed behavioral intervention (G.M. Sugai & Tindal, 1993).

We recommend three major strategies for increasing implementation fidelity. First, precise and concise written plans should be used. The competing behavior pathways model and accompanying intervention strategies provide such a concise summary of a behavior support plan. However, because some teachers, parents, and others have limited experience with the strategies and approaches described in these plans, teaching scripts (i.e., lesson plans) may need to be developed to accompany the written plan. These scripts would sequence intervention components and highlight the actual behaviors required to implement the plan.

Second, implementation fidelity can be enhanced by adopting a team-based approach to the provision of behavior support (Colvin, Kameenui, & Sugai, 1993; G. Sugai & Horner, 1994, in press). In this approach, individualized "action teams" are formed around each student for whom behavior support plans are being developed and implemented. These teams are composed of all persons who have daily, direct, and regular contact with the target student; someone with administrative authority to redirect resources, adjust schedules, and so on; and someone with behavioral assessment and intervention competence. This team would conduct functional assessments, develop competing pathway summaries, develop behavior support plan strategies, implement these strategies, and evaluate the effectiveness of their efforts. Most importantly, team members can monitor their behavior and provide any support to ensure high implementation fidelity.

Third, implementation fidelity can be heightened by collecting and using data to evaluate the effectiveness of an intervention. If little, no, or slow change in student performance is observed, two interpretations are possible. First, the intervention strategies that have been selected may be ineffective, and the competing pathways model and behavior support plan may need to be modified or rewritten. Second, the intervention strategies may not have been implemented consistently and/or accurately. In this case, information on who is responsible for the behavior support plan and is actually implementing it would be collected and used to improve the proficiency with which it is implemented.

Follow-up Planning

The final consideration in the development and implementation of behavior support is follow-up planning. The goal of teaching and strengthening behaviors that compete with problem behavior is highly desirable. However, many students with antisocial behavior have had many years to establish and shape their complex behavioral repertoires. Ensuring that behavioral gains endure over time and are applied by students across school, home, and community settings requires solutions that are comprehensive and efforts that are sustained.

Because we lack the technology to produce enduring generalized responding with students who display antisocial behavior, behavior support planning activities should not be based on the assumption that generalized responding will occur automatically. Instead, the following guidelines should be considered. First, interventions must be implemented in contexts where problem behavior must be reduced and desired behavior must be strengthened. Second, students must be taught behavioral self-management strategies (i.e., self-recording, self-delivery of consequences, self-manipulation of antecedents) that can be taken to problem contexts and used to disrupt and prevent the emission of problem behavior. Third, peers should be trained to serve as peer mediators or managers to precorrect for problem behavior and to provide positive reinforcement for avoiding problem behaviors and using desirable behaviors. Fourth, desired behavior should be taught to high levels of mastery and fluency. Fifth, adults should be recruited to respond consistently to behaviors emitted by students in novel, problem, or generalization settings. Finally, teaching efforts should include examples and nonexamples from problem or generalization settings.

Plan Evaluation

Although the outcomes of the problem identification and problem analysis stages improve the development and implementation of behavior support plans, the actual effects of a behavior support plan on the behaviors of a particular student are never certain. As a result, strategies to evaluate the effectiveness of an intervention on the emission of problem behavior are critical. Five questions should be considered: (a) What behaviors and level of performance should be achieved? (b) What data should be collected? (c) How should the data be collected and displayed? (d) How should the effect of a behavior support plan be determined? and (e) What should be done next?

Target Behaviors and Level of Performance

Developing a behavioral objective is an important task in the development of a behavior support plan because the criteria for success and failure are clearly delineated in a well-written and useful behavioral objective. For example, the following behavioral objective states the conditions under which the desired behavior needs to be displayed, focuses on achieving the desired behavior, and specifies the level of performance needed to be able to declare that the behavioral objective has been met: *When working on math word problems and when having no peer interactions for more than 30 minutes, Kiyoshi will ask for assistance by raising his hand in 80% of the opportunities (1 word problem = an opportunity) with no uses of profanity for 5 consecutive days.* The information contained in this behavioral objective serves as evaluation criteria for judging the progress associated with a given behavior support plan.

Selecting the Data to Be Collected

At minimum the frequency at which the problem behavior and the desired behavior are emitted should be recorded. The context (e.g., physical environment, setting events, antecedent events) in which behavioral incidents are observed also should be monitored. This additional information reveals the extent to which generalized reduction of the problem behavior and generalized responding with the desired behavior are achieved. It also helpful to collect information on the extent and accuracy with which the behavior support plan strategies are implemented. This information allows the behavior support team to monitor implementation fidelity.

Collecting and Displaying Data

Data should be collected directly by individuals who have been trained adequately and are facile with behavioral definitions and observation methods. Two general data collection methods are possible. The first method has many variations (i.e., tally, duration, latency, controlled presentation, trials to criterion), all of which have an event based method in common, that is, each emission of the behavior is observed and a feature or dimension (i.e., topography, frequency, latency, duration, force, locus) of that behavioral event is recorded. Depending on the method used, data collected in event based systems are reported as frequency, rate, percent of opportunities, or percent of time, and provide the most direct and accurate estimate of the occurrence of behavioral events.

In the second general method, time is used to provide an estimate of the occurrence or duration of a behavioral event. The presence or absence of behavior at specific times within or at the end of an interval of time is tracked. Three major interval based variations are commonly used: (a) partial interval—the behavior observed at any time within a specified interval length, (b) whole interval—the behavior observed for the entire interval duration, and (c) momentary time-sampling—the behavior observed at the end of the designated interval length. Although relatively easy to use compared to event based data collection procedures, interval based systems can over- or underestimate the occurrence of behavioral incidents depending on the rate at which behaviors are emitted or the amount of variations across behavioral incidents. Regardless of the variation used, interval based data are reported as percent of intervals.

In general, the data collection method should result in information that is equivalent to the information specified in the criteria of the student's behavioral objective. In addition, data should be collected on a formative or regular (e.g., daily) schedule so timely decisions can be made and response patterns (e.g., changes in trend, level, stability) can be assessed. Thus, data should be displayed in a graphic or visual format. An example of a data display showing behavioral performance during baseline (i.e., preintervention) conditions is shown in Figure 5.

Determining Effectiveness

The effectiveness of a behavior support plan is judged by two general methods. The first method examines the extent to which the student's actual behavioral performance has achieved the levels specific in the criteria of the behavioral objective. In this examination the quality or accuracy of the student's performance, the time to achieve this level of performance, and the stability of this performance are scrutinized. In the formative approach advocated in this chapter, the use of visual

guides can enhance the decision-making process. For example, the graphic display in Figure 5 shows an aim line that has been drawn from the last three days of the baseline condition for the desired behavior to an aim star that is based on the criteria specified for the desired behavior in the student's behavioral objective. A trend line (White & Haring, 1980; Wolery et al., 1988; G.M. Sugai & Tindal, 1993) has been drawn through the baseline data to indicate how future behavioral performance is likely to appear if a behavior support plan was not developed and implemented. Finally, a second trend line has been drawn through the intervention condition data. By comparing the intervention trend line to the desired aim line and to the baseline trend line, the effectiveness of the behavior support plan can be examined.

The second method focuses on assessing the degree to which the student and behavior change agents (e.g., teacher, parent, consultant) socially validate the behavior support plan. In general, social validation procedures examine the extent to which individuals consider (a) the goals of the program to be reasonable, (b) the procedures to be used to be appropriate and effective, and (c) the outcomes of the program to be acceptable (Kazdin, 1987; Wolf, 1978). Social validation data are used to corroborate the information obtained through direct observation methods.

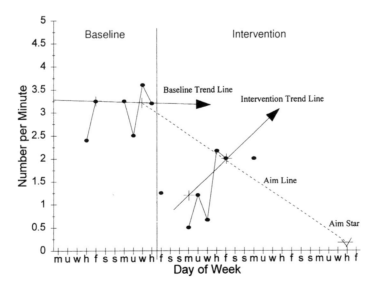

FIGURE 5. Visual display and evaluation of student performance data.

Postintervention Planning

Based on the data that have been collected, displayed, and examined, a number of decisions regarding the behavior support plan are possible. First, if the behavior support plan is effective in achieving the ends specified in the behavioral objective, a new behavioral objective should be developed. Second, if the student is making adequate progress toward meeting his or her behavioral objective, but has not yet achieved the objective, the behavior support plan should be continued. Third, if the criteria specified in the behavioral objective is not likely to be achieved to the level and by the date indicated (i.e., ineffective, inefficient strategy), the procedures of the behavior support plan should be examined. If implementation fidelity is low, efforts should focus on increasing the efficiency with which the plan is being implemented. If implementation is acceptable, modification or termination of the behavior support plan should be considered.

Regardless of the decision, monitoring of performance progress should be continuous and direct. In addition, treatment effectiveness should be judged for its social validity by the student and relevant peers and adults. Finally, progress and treatment effectiveness should be (a) considered against the criteria specified in the intervention or treatment objective and (b) compared with the student's most recent performance (i.e., baseline).

Follow-up

Behavioral intervention often is characterized as a linear process. Problems are identified, assessments are carried out, a plan is developed, staff are trained, the plan is implemented, and the problem behavior shows a dramatic decrease. Unfortunately, in schools, neither the process nor the result typically is this direct. In our experience, the process is much more iterative; we build a plan, evaluate, modify, evaluate, and so on. Some key themes emerge in providing effective follow-up. These are described below.

Long-Term Intervention Support

The task of the teachers and other intervention agents is to provide effective intervention with the aim of reducing problematic behavior and improv-ing the overall development and adjustment of students. The question is not when the intervention will end, but rather what is required now and on an ongoing basis. This perspective is particularly important with students with long histories of chronic and persistent antisocial behavior where simple, one-shot interventions are not likely to have sustained effects. Although the intensity and nature of the intervention might change over time, the removal of behavioral support will be prolonged and systematic.

Measurement and Evaluation Embedded in the Intervention Process

Decisions about whether or how to change the elements of a behavior support plan should be made by the team of people responsible for implementation. These decisions should be based on an analysis of the evaluation data, which can indicate the degree to which the intervention is effective. This approach means that data collection should be an ongoing part of the behavior support process.

Because the environment and the student's behavior may change in unanticipated ways, it may be necessary to periodically collect new functional assessment or analysis data and generate new hypothesis statements. New information should be used to amend existing strategies or to develop new ones.

Summary and Directions for Further Research

The increasing incidence and prevalence of antisocial behavior patterns among youth in our schools and communities is alarming. Multiple community, family, and school factors are correlated with these trends (Hawkins, 1996; Hawkins & Catalano, 1992; Patterson et al., 1992). Antisocial behavior is more likely when children and youth experience the following risk factors: (a) parenting strategies that are punitive, inconsistent, and lacking in careful monitoring and supervision of children's activities and affiliations; (b) communities that tolerate or endorse antisocial attitudes and behavior, and fail to provide prosocial activities; and (c) school environments that have punitive or inconsistent disciplinary approaches, unclear rules and expectations, high rates of academic failure, and poor accommodation of individual differences (G.

Sugai & Horner, 1994; Walker et al., 1996). Persistent and pervasive patterns of antisocial behavior are likely if proactive, early prevention and intervention strategies, and comprehensive intervention approaches are not implemented.

Schools can use preferred and promising practices that can target at-risk children and youth very early in their careers and provide comprehensive interventions with such students and key social agents in (i.e. parents, teachers and peers). These practices have the potential to attenuate risk factors and to enhance protective factors that can redirect children and youth away from antisocial lifestyles and damaging outcomes. Schools need to implement behavioral support systems that are proactive, instructional, sustained, and comprehensive (G. Sugai & Horner, 1994). Unfortunately, efforts to adopt, implement, and sustain these efforts have been reactive, unsystematic, and poorly evaluated (Carnine, 1995).

The interventions we have highlighted in this chapter are designed for adoption and use by schools, particularly at the elementary and middle school level where their impact is likely to be greatest. However, these approaches are not likely to produce meaningful outcomes at any level if they are not implemented with acceptable levels of treatment integrity or implementation fidelity. In particular, schools and school systems must make the following commitments in order to impact this problem (G. Sugai & Horner, 1994; Walker et al., in press):

1. Develop solutions to antisocial behavior from a school and community-wide perspective.

2. Address multiple, coordinated systems (e.g., schoolwide, specific setting, classroom, and individual student).

3. Establish a long-term plan that places the school's commitment to developing solutions as one of the top improvement goals for the building.

4. Obtain commitment from staff, family, and community members to work toward a comprehensive solution to the problem of antisocial behavior.

5. Emphasize a proactive and instruction-based approach.

6. Establish an active leadership role for administrators in the design, implementation, and monitoring of the intervention and evaluation activities.

7. Establish a team-based approach for the development, implementation, management, and evaluation of interventions.

Because they represent the most predictable and supportive environment for many children and youth, schools can serve as primary providers of interventions addressing antisocial behavior patterns. They can screen and identify at-risk students early in their school careers (Walker et al., in press) and provide comprehensive interventions that will reduce the probability of antisocial behavior and long-term adjustment problems.

In this chapter, examples of promising and preferred practices, and effective approaches and practices that are likely to have a significant effect and produce desirable outcomes have been described. Because we have little data on the long-term effects or costs of providing proactive, instruction-based interventions, future research needs to be conducted to document the generality and maintenance of these approaches. The principles and procedures of an instructional and behavior analytic approach hold great potential for positively affecting the prevalence and incidence of children and youth in our schools who display antisocial behavior.

ACKNOWLEDGMENTS

The development of this article was supported, in part, by the Institute on Violence and Destructive Behavior (IVDB) in the College of Education at the University of Oregon. The IVDB is focused on the prevention of violence and destructive behavior at the point of school entry and beyond.

References

Achenbach, T. (1985). *Assessment and taxonomy of child and adolescent psychopathology.* Beverly Hills, CA: Sage.

American Psychological Association, Commission on Youth Violence. (1993). *Violence and youth: Psychology's response.* Washington, DC: American Psychological Association.

Axelrod, S. (1987). Functional and structural analyses of behavior: Approaches leading to reduced use of punishment procedures. *Research in Developmental Disabilities, 8,* 165–178.

Barlow, D.H., & Hayes, S.C. (1979). Alternating treatments design: One strategy for comparing the effects of two treatments in a single subject. *Journal of Applied Behavior Analysis, 12,* 199–210.

Biglan, A. (1995). Translating what we know about the context of antisocial behavior into a lower prevalence of such behavior. *Journal of Applied Behavior Analysis, 28,* 479–492.

Bijou, S.W., Peterson, R.F., & Ault, M.H. (1968). A method to integrate descriptive and experimental field studies at the level of data and empirical concepts. *Journal of Applied Behavior Analysis, 1,* 175–191.

Broussard, C., & Northup, J. (1995). An approach to functional assessment and analysis of disruptive behavior in regular education classrooms. *School Psychology Quarterly, 10,* 151–164.

Carnine, D. (1995). Trustworthiness, useability, and accessibility of educational research. *Journal of Behavioral Education, 5,* 251–258.

Carr, E.G., Levin, L., McConnaichie, G., Carlson, J.L., Kemp, D.C., & Smith, C.E. (1994). *Communication-based intervention for problem behavior: A user's guide for producing positive change.* Baltimore: Brooks.

CARS Project (1996). *Pleasant Hill Elementary School discipline handbook.* Pleasant Hill, OR: Pleasant Hill School District.

Charlebois, P., Leblanc, M., Gagnon, C., & Larivee, S. (1994). Methodological issues in multiple-gating screening procedures for antisocial behaviors in elementary students. *Remedial and Special Education, 15*(1), 44–54.

Coie, J. (1994, July 21). *Antisocial behavior among children and youth.* Keynote address presented at the OSEP National Research Director's Conference. Washington, DC: U.S. Office of Special Education Programs.

Colvin, G., Kameenui, E., & Sugai, G. (1993). Reconceptualizing behavior management and school-discipline in general education. *Education and Treatment of Children, 16,* 361–381.

Colvin, G., Sugai, G., & Patching, W. (1993). Pre-correction: An instructional strategy for managing predictable behavior problems. *Intervention, 28,* 143–150.

Colvin, G., Martz, G., DeForest, D., & Wilt, J. (1995). Developing a school-wide discipline plan: Addressing all students, all settings, and all staff. *Oregon Conference Monograph, 7.* Eugene: University of Oregon.

Committee for Children. (1988). *Second Step, grades 1–3, pilot project 1987–88, summary report.* Seattle, WA: Author.

Committee for Children. (1989). *Second Step, grades 4–5, pilot project 1988–89, summary report.* Seattle, WA: Author.

Committee for Children. (1990). *Second Step, grades 6–8, pilot project 1989–90, summary report.* Seattle, WA: Author.

Committee for Children. (1992). *Evaluation of Second Step, preschool–kindergarten, a violence-prevention curriculum kit.* Seattle, WA: Author.

Day, M.H., Horner, R.H., & O'Neill, R.E. (1994). Multiple functions of problem behaviors: Assessment and intervention. *Journal of Applied Behavior Analysis, 27,* 279–289.

Dodge, K.A., & Frame, C.L. (1982). Social cognitive biases and deficits in aggressive boys. *Child Development, 51,* 620–635.

Dumas, J.E. (1989). Treating antisocial behavior in children: Child and family approaches. *Clinical Psychology Review, 9,* 197–222.

Dunlap, G., Kern, L., Clarke, S., & Robbins, F.R. (1991). Functional assessment, curricular revision, and severe behavior problems. *Journal of Applied Behavior Analysis, 24,* 387–397.

Dunlap, G., Kern, L., dePerczel, M., Clarke, S., Wilson, D., Childs, K.E., White, R., & Falk, G.D. (1993). Functional analysis of classroom variables for students with emotional and behavioral challenges. *Behavioral Disorders, 18,* 275–291.

Dunlap, G., dePerczel, M., Clarke, S., Wilson, D., Wright, S., White, R., & Gomes, A. (1994). Choice making to promote behavior support for students with emotional and behavioral challenges. *Journal of Applied Behavior Analysis, 27,* 505–518.

Engelmann, S., & Carnine, D. (1982). *Theory of instruction: Principles and applications.* New York: Irvington.

Federal Bureau of Investigation. (1994). *FBI annual crime report.* Washington, DC: U.S. Department of Justice.

Flannery, K.B., & Horner, R.H. (1994). The relationship between predictability and problem behavior for students with severe disabilities. *Journal of Behavioral Education, 4*(2), 157–176.

Fowler, M. (1992). *C.H.A.D.D. educator's manual.* Fairfax, VA: CASET.

Gresham, F.M., & Elliott, S. (1990). *The social skills rating system (SSRS).* Circle Pines, MN: American Guidance Service.

Hawkins, D. (1996, May). *Youth violence: Reducing risk and enhancing protection.* Keynote address to the Pacific Northwest Conference on Youth Violence, Seattle, WA.

Hawkins, D., & Catalano, R. (1992). *Communities that care.* San Francisco: Jossey-Bass.

Hollinger, J. (1987). Social skills for behaviorally disordered children as preparation for mainstreaming: Theory, practice and new directions. *Remedial and Special Education, 8*(4), 17–27.

Horner, R., Day, M., Sprague, J., O'Brien, M., & Heathfield, L. (1991). Interspersed requests: A nonaversive procedure for decreasing aggression and self-injury during instruction. *Journal of Applied Behavior Analysis, 24*(2), 265–278.

Horner, R.H. (1994). Functional assessment: Contributions and future directions. *Journal of Applied Behavioral Analysis, 27,* 401–404.

Horner, R.H., Sprague, J.R., & Wilcox, B. (1982). General case programming for community activities. In B. Wilcox & G.T. Bellamy (Eds.), *Design of high school programs for severely handicapped students* (pp. 61–98). Baltimore: Brookes.

Horner, R.H., O'Neill, R.W., & Flannery, K.B. (1993). Building effective behavior support plans from functional assessment information. In M. Snell (Ed.), *Instruction of persons with severe handicaps* (4th ed., pp. 184–214). Columbus, OH: Merrill.

Horner, R.H., Vaughn, B., Day, H.M., & Ard, B. (1996). The relationship between setting events and problem behavior. In L.K. Koegel, R.L. Kogel, & G. Dunlap (Eds.), *Positive behavioral support: Including people with difficult behavior in the community* (pp. 381–402). Baltimore: Paul Brookes Publishing Co.

Individuals with Disabilities Education Act Regulations 45CFR 121a.5 [b][1978].

Iwata, B.A., Dorsey, M.F., Slifer, K.J., & Richman, G.S. (1982). Toward a functional analysis of self-injury. *Analysis and Intervention in Developmental Disabilities, 3,* 1–20.

Kameenui, E.J., & Simmons, D.C. (1990). *Designing instructional strategies: The prevention of academic learning problems.* Columbus, OH: Merrill.

Kauffman, J.M. (1993). *Characteristics of behavior disorders of children and youth* (5th ed.). New York: Merrill.

Kazdin, A. (1987). *Conduct disorders in childhood and adolescence.* London: Sage.

Kazdin, A. (1993). Treatment of conduct disorder: Progress and directions in psychotherapy research. *Development and Psychotherapy, 5,* 277–310.

Kern, L., & Dunlap, G. (in press). Assessment-based interventions for children with emotional and behavioral disorders. In A.C. Repp & R.H. Horner (Eds.) *Functional analysis of problem behavior: From effective assessment to effective support.* Pacific Grove, CA: Brookes/Cole.

Kern, L., Childs, K.E., Dunlap, G., Clarke, S., & Falk, G.D. (1994). Using assessment-based curricular intervention to improve the classroom behavior of a student with emotional and behavioral challenges. *Journal of Applied Behavior Analysis, 27*(1), 7–19.

Kern, L., Dunlap, G., Clarke, S., & Childs, K.E. (1994). Student-assisted functional assesment interview. *Diagnostique, 19,* 29–39.

Knitzer, J. (1993). Children's mental health policy: Challenging the future. *Emotional and Behavioral Disorders, 1* (1), 8–16.

Knitzer, J., Steinberg, Z., & Fleisch, B. (1990). *At the school house door: An examination of programs and policies for children with behavioral and emotional problems.* New York: Bank Street College of Education.

Lewis, T., Scott, T., & Sugai, G. (1994). The problem behavior questionnaire: A teacher based instrument to develop functional hypotheses of problem behavior in general education classrooms. *Diagnostique, 19*(2–3), 103–115.

Lewis, T., & Sugai, G. (1996a). Descriptive and experimental analysis of teacher and peer attention and the use of assessment-based intervention to improve the pro-social behavior of a student in a general education setting. *Journal of Behavioral Education, 6,* 7–24.

Lewis, T.J., & Sugai, G. (1996b). Functional assessment of problem behavior: A pilot investigation of the comparative and interactive effects of teacher and peer social attention on students in general education settings. *School Psychology Quarterly, 11,* 1–19.

Lipsey, M.W. (1991). The effect of treatment on juvenile delinquents: Results from meta-analysis. In F. Losel, D. Bender, & T. Bliesener (Eds), *Psychology and law.* New York: Walter de Gruyter.

Loeber, R., Dishion, T.J., & Patterson, G.R. (1984). Multiple gating: A multistage assessment procedure for identifying youths at risk for delinquency. *Journal of Research in Crime and Delinquency, 21,* 7–32.

Mayer, G. (1995). Preventing antisocial behavior in the schools. *Journal of Applied Behavior Analysis, 28,* 467–478.

Mayer, G.R., & Sulzer-Azaroff, B. (1990). Interventions for vandalism. In G. Stoner, M.R. Shinn, & H.M. Walker (Eds.), *Interventions for achievement and behavior problems* [Monograph]. Washington, DC: National Association of School Psychologists.

Moffitt, T. (1994). Adolescence-limited and life-course-persistent antisocial behavior: A developmental taxonomy. *Psychological Review, 100*(4), 674–701.

Neef, N.A., & Iwata, B.A. (1994). Current research on functional analysis methodologies: An introduction. *Journal of Applied Behavior Analysis 27,* 211–214.

O'Neill, R.E., Horner, R.H., Albin, R.W., Sprague, J.R., Storey, K., & Newton, J.S. (1997). *Functional assessment of problem behavior: A practical assessment guide* (2nd ed.). Pacific Grove, CA: Brooks/Cole.

Patterson, G.R., Reid, J.B., & Dishion, T.J. (1992). *A social interaction approach: Antisocial boys.* Eugene, OR: Castalia.

Quay, H. (1986). Conduct disorders. In H. Quay & J. Werry (Eds.), *Psychopathological disorders of childhood.* New York: Wiley.

Reed, H., Thomas, E., Sprague, J.R., & Horner, R.H. Student guided functional assessment interview: An analysis of student and teacher agreement. Manuscript submitted for publication.

Reichle, J. (1990). *National Working Conference on Positive Approaches to the Management of Excess Behavior: Final report and recommendations.* Minneapolis, MN: Institute on Community Integration, University of Minnesota.

Reid, J. (1993). Prevention of conduct disorder before and after school entry: Relating interventions to developmental findings. *Development and Psychopathology, 5,* 243–262.

Robins, L.N. (1978). Sturdy childhood predictors of adult antisocial behavior: Replications from longitudinal studies. *Psychological Medicine, 8,* 611–622.

Simcha-Fagan, O., Langner, T., Gersten, J., & Eisenberg, J. (1975). *Violent and antisocial behavior: A longitudinal study of urban youth.* Unpublished report of the Office of Child Development, OCD-CB–480.

Sprague, J.R., & Horner, R.H. (1991). Determining the acceptability of behavior support plans. In M. Wang, H. Walberg, & M. Reynolds (Eds.), *Handbook of special education* (pp. 125–142). Oxford and London: Pergamon.

Sprague, J.R., & Thomas, T. (in press). The effect of a neutralizing routine on problem behavior performance. *Journal of Behavioral Education.*

Sprague, J.S., & Horner, R.H. (1995). Functional assessment and intervention in community settings. *Mental Retardation and Developmental Disabilities Research Reviews, 1,* 89–93.

Sprague, J.S., & Horner, R.H. (in press). Low frequency, high intensity problem behavior: Toward an applied technology of functional assessment and intervention. In A.C. Repp & R.H. Horner (Eds.), *Functional analysis of problem behavior: From effective assessment to effective support.* Pacific Grove, CA: Brooks/Cole.

Stevens, L.J., & Price, M. (1992). Meeting the challenge of educating children at risk. *Kappan, 74*(1), 18–23.

Sugai, G., & Horner, R. (1994). Including students with severe behavior problems in general education settings: Assumptions, challenges, and solutions. *Oregon Conference Monograph, 6,* 109–120.

Sugai, G., & Horner, R. (in press). Antisocial behavior, discipline, and behavior support: A look from the schoolhouse door. *Archives of Pediatric and Adolescent Medicine.*

Sugai, G.M., & Tindal, G. (1993). *Effective school consultation: An interactive approach.* Pacific Grove, CA: Brooks/Cole.

Tobin, T., & Sugai, G. (1996). The relationship of middle school discipline referrals to continuing behavior problems. Unpublished manuscript, Behavioral Research and Teaching, University of Oregon, Eugene.

Tobin, T., Sugai, G., & Colvin, G. (1996). Patterns in middle school discipline records. *Journal of Emotional and Behavioral Disorders, 4*(2), 82–94.

Tolan, P., & Guerra, N. (1994). *What works in reducing adolescent violence: An empirical review of the field.* Boulder: University of Colorado, Center for the Study and Prevention of Violence.

Wacker, D.P., Steege, M.W., Northup, J., Sasso, G., Berg, W., Reimers, T., Cooper, L., Cigrand, K., & Donn, L. (1990). A component analysis of functional communication training across three topographies of severe behavior problems. *Journal of Applied Behavior Analysis, 23,* 417–429.

Walker, H.M., & Severson, H.H. (1990). *Systematic screening for behavior disorders (SSBD): User's guide and technical manual.* Longmont, CO: Sopris West.

Walker, H.M., Colvin, G., & Ramsey, E. (1995). *Antisocial behavior in schools: Strategies and best practices.* Pacific Grove, CA: Brooks/Cole.

Walker, H.M., Severson, H.H., & Feil, E.G. (1995). *The early screening project: A proven child-find process.* Longmont, CO: Sopris West.

Walker, H.M., Horner, R.H., Sugai, G., Bullis, M., Sprague, J.R., Bricker, D., & Kaufman, M.J. (1996). Integrated approaches to preventing antisocial behavior patterns among school-age children and youth. *Journal of Emotional and Behavioral Disorders, 4,* 194–209.

Walker, H.M., Kavanagh, K., Stiller, B., Golly, A., Feil, E., & Severson, H.H. (in press). First steps: An early intervention approach for preventing school antisocial behavior. *Journal of Emotional and Behavior Disorders, 5.*

White, O.R., & Haring, N.G. (1980). *Exceptional teaching* (2nd ed.). Columbus, OH: Merrill.

Wolery, M.R., Bailey, D.B., Jr., & Sugai, G.M. (1988). *Effective teaching: Principles and procedures of applied behavior analysis with exceptional students.* Boston: Allyn & Bacon.

Wolfe, M.M. (1978). Social validity: The case for subjective measurement or how applied behavior analysis is finding its heart. *Journal of Applied Behavior Analysis, 11,* 203–214.

Bibliography

Bijou, S.W., Peterson, R.F., & Ault, M.H. (1968). A method to integrate descriptive and experimental field studies at the level of data and empirical concepts. *Journal of Applied Behavior Analysis, 1,* 175–191. This paper describes the classic "ABC" direct observation assessment procedure.

Colvin, G., Kameenui, E., & Sugai, G. (1993). Reconceptualizing behavior management and school-discipline in general education. *Education and Treatment of Children, 16,* 361–381. The authors describe a school-wide, proactive approach to behavior management and school discipline.

Gresham, F.M., & Elliott, S. (1990). *The social skills rating system (SSRS).* Circle Pines, MN: American Guidance Service. Describes the development and use of the SSRS.

Hawkins, D., & Catalano, R. (1992). *Communities that care.* San Francisco: Jossey-Bass. Outlines the critical community and school risk and protective factors contributing to antisocial behavior in children and youth.

Lipsey, M.W. (1991). The effect of treatment on juvenile delinquents: Results from meta-analysis. In F. Losel, D. Bender, & T. Bliesener (Eds), *Psychology and law* (pp. 129–146). New York: Walter de Gruyter. A comprehensive meta-analysis of treatments for antisocial behavior.

O'Neill, R.E., Horner, R.H., Albin, R.W., Sprague, J.R., Storey, K., & Newton, J.S. (in press). *Functional assessment of problem behavior: A practical assessment guide* (2nd ed.). Pacific Grove, CA: Brooks/Cole. A practitioner's guide to conducting functional assessment and analysis procedures. The relationship between functional assessment and program development is illustrated.

Patterson, G.R., Reid, J.B., & Dishion, T.J. (1992). *A social interaction approach: Antisocial boys.* Eugene, OR: Castalia. A comprehensive review and description of effective interventions for antisocial boys.

Tolan, P., & Guerra, N. (1994). *What works in reducing adolescent violence: An empirical review of the field.* Boulder: University of Colorado, Center for the Study and Prevention of Violence. An excellent meta-analysis of effective violence prevention interventions.

Walker, H.M., Colvin, G., & Ramsey, E. (1995). *Antisocial behavior in schools: Strategies and best practices.* Pacific Grove, CA: Brooks/Cole. A comprehensive textbook outlining system and individual student approaches to preventing and treating violent and antisocial behavior.

24

Social Skills Training with Children

Social Learning and Applied Behavioral Analytic Approaches

FRANK M. GRESHAM

Introduction

The skill and fluency with which children navigate the often difficult and unpredictable world of interpersonal relationships are important hallmarks of adaptive child development. The degree to which children learn to establish, develop, and maintain satisfactory interpersonal relationships and terminate deleterious relationships with peers and adults is the essence of social competence. Moreover, the success or failure children have in these interpersonal relationships predicts adaptive or maladaptive psychological outcomes in adulthood (Kupersmidt, Coie, & Dodge, 1990; Parker & Asher, 1987). Empirical literature dating back to the 1950s has consistently shown that children experiencing difficulty in interpersonal relationships with peers, as young as age 8, were at risk for a variety of negative outcomes such as dropping out of school, juvenile delinquency, psychopathology in adulthood, bad conduct discharges from military service, depression, and suicide (see reviews by Cowen, Pederson, Babigian, Izzo, & Trost, 1973; Kohn & Clausen, 1955; Parker & Asher, 1987; Roff, 1961; Roff, Sells, & Golden, 1972; Stengel, 1971). These studies, using follow-back and prospective methodologies, have consistently shown predictive and postdictive relationships between peer difficulties and long-term adjustment problems.

Social Competence and Psychiatric Diagnoses

Dodge (1989) showed that social incompetence was an explicit part of the diagnostic criteria for 17 disorders of childhood listed in the *Diagnostic and Statistical Manual of Mental Disorders,* 3rd edition, revised (*DSM-III-R;* American Psychiatric Association, 1987) and played a role in the diagnosis of an additional 16 disorders. Given the increase in the number of diagnostic categories for children and adolescents in *DSM-IV* (American Psychiatric Association, 1994), social incompetence plays an even greater role in psychiatric diagnoses. For example, in Asperger's Disorder, one essential feature is severe and sustained impairment in social interaction (e.g., marked impairment in nonverbal behaviors regulating social interactions, failure to establish developmentally appropriate peer relationships, lack of social reciprocity). Oppositional Defiant Disorder is characterized by negativistic and defiant behaviors toward adults and peers characterized by disobedience and unwillingness to compromise or negotiate disagreements in social interactions. Children with Conduct Disorder or an antisocial behavior pattern display a repetitive and persistent pattern of aggressive conduct toward others involving bullying, fighting, threatening, or intimidating others. Social incompetence plays a significant role in many other *DSM-IV* disorders that are too numerous to discuss in this chapter (see Major Depressive

FRANK M. GRESHAM • School of Education, University of California–Riverside, Riverside, California 92521-0102.

Handbook of Child Behavior Therapy, edited by Watson and Gresham. Plenum Press, New York, 1998.

Episode/Disorder, Dysthymic Disorder, Attention-Deficit/Hyperactivity Disorder, Autistic Disorder).

Social competence is essential for psychological adjustment because of the importance of establishing and maintaining satisfactory interpersonal relationships. For example, the development of oppositional, antisocial behavior patterns begins early in life and these behavior patterns persist over time (Kazdin, 1987; Oleweus, 1979). Olweus, for instance, found that aggressive, antisocial behavior in boys was as stable as measures of intelligence over one year ($r = .76$) and five-year intervals ($r = .69$). Patterson, DeBaryshe, and Ramsey (1989) presented a developmental model showing that antisocial behavior begins early in life (ages 2–3 years) and continues throughout the school years. A recent review by Lynam (1996) showed that the occurrence of hyperactivity-impulsivity-inattention with behaviors associated with conduct disorder (e.g., bullies, threatens, intimidates others, truant from school, initiates physical fights) were highly predictive of chronic offending in adulthood, or what he termed the development of a "fledgling psychopath."

School entry represents a particularly critical period for children having early onset difficulties in social behavior. Reid and Patterson (1991) indicated that many children demonstrating antisocial behavior patterns before school entry will continue coercive and aggressive behavior patterns with peers and teachers upon entering school. In the absence of intervention, this behavior pattern will be maintained throughout their school careers and beyond (Kazdin, 1987; Patterson et al., 1989; Reid & Patterson, 1991). When children enter school with social competence deficits, particularly characterized by an oppositional, antisocial interaction style, they fail to acquire and perform appropriate social skills in school settings. Consequently, these children are at early risk for school maladjustment, as well as being prime candidates for early referral to special education services (Gresham & Reschly, 1988; Walker, Irwin, Noell, & Singer, 1992).

Social Competence and Mild Disabilities

Clearly, children experiencing difficulties in social or interpersonal relationships are at risk for psychological difficulties. In school settings, children having so-called mild disabilities (behavior disorders, learning disabilities, and mild mental retardation) experience significant difficulties in interpersonal relationships. The definitional criteria of children as seriously emotionally disturbed (SED) use social competence deficits to identify, classify, and place students in this disability category (Forness & Knitzer, 1992; Skiba & Grizzle, 1991). The modern classification system criteria used in mental retardation has consistently emphasized and equally weighted the importance of cognitive and social competence (adaptive behavior) (MacMillan, Gresham, & Siperstein, 1993). Children with specific learning disabilities, in addition to difficulties in academic competence, also experience social competence deficits and problems in interpersonal relationships (Gresham, 1992; Gresham & Elliott, 1990; LaGreca & Stone, 1990).

Although not considered an eligible disability group under the Individuals With Disabilities Education Act (IDEA), it is well known that children with attention-deficit/hyperactivity disorder (ADHD) experience substantial deficits in social competence and peer relationships (Barkley, 1990; Guevremont, 1990). Pelham and Bender (1982) estimated that more than half of children having ADHD experience substantial difficulties in interpersonal relationships with other children, parents, and teachers. Many of their difficulties in social competence can be attributed to their behavioral characteristics of inattention, impulsivity, and overactivity (Whalen, Henker, & Hinshaw, 1985).

Definition of Social Competence

Social competence has been defined and conceptualized from various perspectives in the literature. Gresham and Reschly (1988) conceptualized social competence as a multidimensional domain that included adaptive behavior, social skills, and peer relationship variables (e.g., peer acceptance, friendship, and peer rejection). McFall (1982) articulated a conceptualization of social competence that distinguished between social competence and social skills. In this view, *social skills* are the specific behaviors that an individual uses to perform competently on social tasks. *Social competence* is an evaluative term or concept based on social agents' judgments, given certain criteria, that a person has performed social tasks adequately. These judgments may be based on opinions of significant others (e.g., teachers, parents, and peers), comparisons to explicit criteria (e.g., number of social tasks adequately performed in relation to some criterion), or comparisons to normative samples. McFall's (1982) view of social competence considers social skills as specific behaviors that result in judgments of social competence. As such, social skills are *behaviors* and social competence represents a *judgment* or *evaluation* about those behaviors.

This conceptualization is similar to Gresham's (1983) *social validity* definition of social skills. According to this definition, social skills are those behaviors that, in certain situations, predict important social outcomes for children and youth. Important social outcomes include: (a) peer acceptance, (b) significant others' positive judgments of social competence, (c) friendships, (d) adequate self-concept, and (e) absence of psychopathology. This definition of social competence specifies behaviors in which children may be adequate or deficient and relates them to important social outcomes. It should be noted that social validity is an important consideration in interventions with children and has been a useful standard against which the success of interventions has been judged (Gresham & Lopez, 1996; Noell & Gresham, 1993; Schwarz & Baer, 1991). Social validation will be discussed more thoroughly later in this chapter under the heading of "Problem Evaluation."

Problem Identification

The most important initial step in designing and implementing social skills interventions for children is an accurate identification and classification of social skills difficulties the child is experiencing. Problem identification must deal with two crucial issues of social competence: (a) domains of social competence to be assessed and (b) classification of social skills deficits. Each of these will be described in the following sections.

Domains of Social Competence

One way of understanding how and why children are considered at risk for social competence difficulties is that they do not meet significant others' (e.g., teachers' and parents') social behavior standards. For example, the standards, expectations, and tolerance levels that teachers hold for children's

social behavior influence teaching behaviors as well as peer interactions in classrooms (Hersh & Walker, 1983). For instance, students perceived as being brighter or more competent receive more teacher attention, are given greater opportunities to respond, are praised more, and are given more verbal cues during teaching interactions than are students perceived by teachers as less competent (Brophy & Good, 1986).

I focus on school settings because schools, by virtue of their accessibility to all children, their parents, and teachers, represent an ideal locale for teaching and refining children's social behavior. As a microcosm of society, the school is a place where children and adults work, play, eat, and live together for 6 hours per day, 5 days per week, and at least 180 days per year. By Grade 5, children will spend a minimum of 5,400 hours in school. During this time, these children will be exposed to literally tens of thousands of social interactions with both peers and adults. Not surprisingly, schools are a major socializing institution in our society.

Upon school entry, children have to negotiate two important social–behavioral adjustments: teacher-related and peer-related (Walker, McConnell, & Clark, 1985). Teacher-related adjustment reflects the extent to which children meet the demands of teachers and accomplish tasks in classroom settings. Most teachers would consider a behavioral repertoire to be indicative of successful adjustment if it: (a) facilitated academic performance and (b) is marked by the absence of disruptive or unusual behaviors that challenge the teacher's authority and disturb the classroom ecology (Gresham & Reschly, 1988; Hersh & Walker, 1983). This pattern of social behavior has been described by Hersh and Walker as the *model behavior profile* expected by most teachers.

Walker and colleagues (see Walker et al., 1992) presented an extremely useful model of interpersonal social–behavioral competence for school settings. Table 1 presents Walker and colleagues' model which describes both adaptive and maladaptive teacher and peer social–behavioral domains and outcomes. Note that the adaptive teacher-related adjustment behaviors operationalize the model behavioral profile described earlier and that results in teacher acceptance and school success. The maladaptive domain is characteristic of behaviors that disrupt the classroom ecology and often re-

TABLE 1. Model of Interpersonal Social–Behavioral Competence within School Settings

Teacher-related adjustment		Peer-related adjustment	
Related-behavioral correlatives		Related-behavioral correlates	
Adaptive	Maladaptive	Adaptive	Maladaptive
• Complies promptly • Follows rules • Listens • Completes classwork • Follows directions • Cooperates	• Steals • Defies teacher • Tantrums • Disturbs others • Cheats • Swears • Aggressive • Ignores teacher	• Cooperates with peers • Supports peers • Defens self in arguments • Leads peers • Affiliates with peers • Assists peers	• Disrupts group • Acts snobbish • Aggresses indirectly • Starts fights • Short temper • Brags • Gets in trouble with teacher • Seeks help constantly
Outcome	Outcome	Outcome	Outcome
• Teacher acceptance • Academic success	• Teacher rejection • Referral to special education • School failure • School dropout • Low performance expectations	• Peer acceptance • Positive peer reactions • Friendships	• Social rejection • Loneliness • Weak social involvement

Note. Adapted from "A Construct Score Approach to the Assessment of Social Competence: Rationale, Technological Considerations, and Antici-pated Outcomes," by H. Walker, L. Irwin, J. Noell, and G. Singer, 1992, *Behavior Modification, 16*, 448–474.

sults in teacher rejection, school failure, and refer-ral to special education.

The social behaviors in the adaptive peer-related adjustment domain are substantially differ-ent from those in the teacher-related adjustment domain. These behaviors are essential in the forma-tion of friendships and peer acceptance, but have little to do with classroom success and teacher ac-ceptance. The maladaptive behaviors in this domain are likely to result in peer rejection or neglect, but share many similarities with the maladaptive behav-iors in the teacher-related adjustment domain.

It is extremely important that behavior ther-apists conducting comprehensive assessments of social competence consider both teacher-related and peer-related adjustment and maladaptive be-havioral domains. Walker and colleagues' (1992) model of social–behavioral functioning serves as a useful heuristic for conceptualizing social skills as-sessment procedures leading to accurate problem identification. Note that both adaptive and mal-adaptive behaviors are part of this social–behav-ioral conceptualization; a point to be considered in classification of specific types of social skills deficits.

Classification of Social Skills Deficits

An important parat of problem identification is an accurate classification of the specific type(s) of social skills deficits a child may have. Gresham (1981a, b) distinguished between *acquisition* or *skills* deficits and *performance* deficits. This dis-tinction is important because it suggests different intervention approaches in remediating social skills deficits and may indicate different venues for carry-ing out social skills training (e.g., pullout groups versus interventions in naturalistic settings). A third type of deficit might be called a *fluency* deficit in which the child knows how to and wants to perform a given social skill, but renders an awkward or "un-polished" performance.

Social skills acquisition deficits refer to the ab-sence of knowledge for executing particular social skills even under optimal conditions. Social perfor-mance deficits represent the presence of social skills in a behavioral repertoire, but the failure to perform them at acceptable levels in given situa-tions. Acquisition deficits might be thought of as "Can't do" deficits whereas performance deficits are "Won't do" deficits. Fluency deficits stem from a lack of exposure to sufficient models, from lack of practice, or from inadequate behavioral rehearsal of newly taught or infrequently utilized social skills.

Gresham and Elliott (1990) extended the social skills classification model to include the notion of *interfering* or *competing* problem behaviors. In this classification scheme, two dimensions of behavior, social skills and interfering problem behaviors, are combined to classify social skills problems. Interfering or competing behaviors can include internalizing or overcontrolled behavior patterns (e.g., anxiety, depression, social withdrawal) or externalizing or undercontrolled behavior patterns (e.g., aggression, disruption, impulsivity). Table 2 presents this social skills classification model.

The social skills deficit classification scheme shown in Table 2 is pivotal in linking assessment results to interventions for social skills deficits. It does not make much sense to teach a social skill to children who already have it in their repertoires (i.e., with a performance deficit). Similarly, intervention procedures to increase the performance of a social skill (e.g., prompting, reinforcement) are not particularly efficient in remediating acquisition deficits. Finally, children having fluency deficits do not require that a skill be retaught or need to increase the frequency of its performance. Instead, these children need to have more practice or rehearsal of the skill for adequate and convincing behavioral performances.

Social Skills Assessment Methods

A variety of methods have been used to assess children's social skills, all of which can provide useful information regarding prosocial and interfering problem behaviors. Like all behavioral assessment methods (see Gresham & Lambros, this volume), social skills assessment methods can be broadly classified as *indirect* and *direct*. Recall that indirect behavioral assessment methods assess behavior that is removed in time and place from its actual occurrence. Examples of these methods include functional assessment interviews, ratings by others (teachers and parents), peer assessment methods, and analogue role-play measures. Direct measures assess behavior at the time and place of its actual occurrence and include naturalistic observations (e.g., classroom, playground) and self-monitoring strategies.

For purposes of this chapter, I focus on social skills assessment methods having the most relevance for identifying target behaviors for social skills interventions. These methods include (a) functional assessment interviews, (b) behavior ratings by others, and (c) naturalistic observations of social behavior.

Functional Assessment Interviews

The functional assessment interview (FAI) during problem identification has four primary goals: (a) to identify and define social skills difficulties,

TABLE 2. Social Skills Classification Model

Competing behavior	Acquisition	Performance	Fluency
Present	Acquisition deficit	Performance deficit	Fluency deficit
Absent	Acquisition deficit	Performance deficit	Fluency deficit

(b) to differentiate social skill acquisition, performance, and fluency deficits, (c) to identify competing problem behaviors that interfere with acquisition, performance, and/or fluency, and (d) to obtain preliminary information regarding a possible functional analysis of behavior. Interviews with teachers, parents, peers, and target children represent important sources of information that can assist in a functional analysis of behavior. The first part of Table 3 presents a format that can be used to guide a semistructured FAI during the problem identification phase of social skills assessment.

Professionals designing social skills interventions often work out of a consultation framework in

TABLE 3. Semistructured Functional Assessment Interview

A. PROBLEM IDENTIFICATION

1. What social skills deficits are of most concern to you?
2. Please provide a clear, specific definition of each of the behaviors that concerns you.
3. Do you see these behaviors as being primarily acquisition deficits (Can't Do), performance deficits (Won't Do), or fluency deficits?
4. Approximately how often does this behavior occur? How frequently would you like to see these behaviors occur?
5. What, if any, interfering problem behaviors compete with the acquisition, performance, or fluency of the desired social skill? Provide a definition of each of these behaviors.
6. About how often do these behaviors occur?
7. Are there activities or times of the day when the desired social skill is more likely? Less likely?
8. Are there activities or times of the day when the interfering problem behaviors are more likely? Less likely?
9. Is the desired social skill more likely to occur with some peers than others? Describe these typical social interactions.
10. How does the child's failure to perform the desired social skill affect other children? You?

B. PROBLEM ANALYSIS

11. When the child performs the social skill(s), what happens? What do you do? What do peers do?
12. When the child performs the competing problem behavior(s), what happens. What do you do? What do peers do?
13. What function do you think the interfering behavior serves for the child (social attention, task avoidance/escape, access to preferred activities)?
14. Does the child engage in undesirable behaviors that achieve the same result as the socially skilled target behavior? Are the undesirable behaviors equally or more functional in obtaining reinforcement?
15. If undesirable behaviors are equally or more functional, are they more *efficient* and *reliable* in achieving that function? Do the undesirable behaviors achieve the same reinforcement *more quickly* and *more consistently* than the socially skilled alternative behavior?
16. Are the competing undesirable behaviors associated with the presence of a specific stimulus (person, place, thing, time of day) or are they associated with the presence of many stimuli and situations?
17. What are some situations or activities in which the desired social skill could be taught using incidental teaching?
18. Describe how you might teach or prompt the social skill in these situations or activities.
19. Are there peers in the classroom who might be recruited to assist in teaching or prompting the desired social skill?
20. Do you think the desired social skill(s) would be best taught in a small group outside of the classroom? Why or why not?
21. What types of strategies could you implement to decrease the interfering or competing behaviors? Describe how you might use these.
22. What aspects of the proposed intervention do you like the most? Why? Which do you like the least? Why?
23. Which aspects of the proposed intervention would be easiest to implement? Why? Which aspects of the proposed intervention would be most difficult to implement? Why?
24. Here are some ways in which we could change the intervention. Do these changes make the intervention easier to implement? What additional changes would you recommend?
25. Do you think this intervention is likely to be effective? Why or why not?

C. PROBLEM EVALUATION

26. Describe how you think the intervention worked.
27. What behavior changes did you observe? Did these changes make a difference in the child's behavior in your classroom? How? In other settings? How?
28. Is the child's behavior now similar to that of average or typical peers? If not, do you think the continued use of the intervention would accomplish this goal? Why or why not? How long do you think this might take if we continued the intervention?
29. How satisfied are you with the outcomes of this intervention? Why?
30. Would you recommend this intervention to others? Why or why not? What aspects of the intervention would you change before recommending this intervention to others?

that they work with third parties (teachers or parents) who will be responsible for implementing the social skills intervention. During problem identification, it is extremely important for interviewers to obtain as precise information as possible from these third parties to assist in functional analysis. For example, a teacher might say, "Joe does not fit into a group very well," or "Jack doesn't get along well with others." Although these statements may be true, they are not particularly informative regarding the exact nature of the social skill deficit, much less for a functional assessment of behavior.

Interviewing behaviors should take the form of questions that elicit specific information before embarking on a social skills intervention program. For instance, an interviewer might ask, "What kinds of things does Joe *do* or *not do* that indicates to you he does not fit into a group?" Another useful line of questioning might be, "Does it appear to you that Jack does not know how to initiate play with his peers or that he just doesn't want to or choose to?" These types of questions are likely to provide important information regarding the precise nature of social skills deficits.

Another important task in problem identification is to obtain information regarding competing behaviors that interfere with the acquisition, performance, or fluency of socially skilled behaviors. In some cases, these competing behaviors can block the acquisition of socially skilled behavior, thereby creating social skill acquisition deficits. In other cases, these behaviors can interfere with the performance of socially skilled behaviors. That is, the competing behaviors may be performed more frequently because they are reinforced more often than is the socially skilled alternative behavior. In still other cases, these competing behaviors can detract from the fluency with which socially skilled behaviors are performed.

Finally, interviewers should obtain a tentative description of the environmental conditions surrounding the socially skilled and competing behaviors. In this preliminary functional analysis, interviewers attempt to identify events that precede, occur concurrently with, and follow competing behaviors. These same environmental events may assist in the explanation of the absence of socially skilled behavior (e.g., absence of salient cues for social behavior or low rates of reinforcement for socially appropriate behavior).

Behavior Ratings

Ratings of behavior by significant others in the child's environment represent a useful and efficient method of deriving preliminary information regarding target behavior selection. Behavior ratings can be used prior to functional assessment interviews during problem identification to guide the direction and topics discussed in the interview. It should be noted that behavior ratings are a measure of the *relative* rather than the actual frequencies of behavior. That is, it is best to think of behavior ratings as representing typical performances across a variety of situations over several times rather than actual performances in specific situations at specific times. Raters may also have their own, idiosyncratic definitions of what constitutes any given social skill or problem behavior (e.g., cooperates, argues, initiates conversations) and their own notion of their frequency (e.g., Sometimes versus Not at all).

One effective use of behavior ratings in social skills assessment to identify potential target behaviors is the use of both *frequency* and *importance* ratings of behavior. Most behavior rating scales measure perceived frequency (e.g., Never; Sometimes, or Very Often), but not the perceived importance of behavior for informants (e.g., teachers or parents). The Social Skills Ratings System (SSRS; Gresham & Elliott, 1990) requires raters to rate both the frequency and importance of particular social skills. Importance ratings are made based on the following instructions: "Please rate the behavior concerning how important this behavior is for success in your classroom (teacher) or your child's development (parent), or to your relationships with others (students).

Besides the SSRS, there are other excellent social skills behavior rating scales available. These scales, however, utilize only teacher informants and thus are more limited in scope. Scales with the best psychometric properties include the Walker McConnell Scale of Social Competence and School Adjustment (Walker & McConnell, 1995), School Social Behavior Scales (Merrell, 1993), and Social Behavior Assessment Inventory (Stephens & Arnold, 1992). An excellent comprehensive review of social skills rating scales has been recently published (see Demaray et al., 1995).

During problem identification, behavior therapists can construct Frequency × Importance matrices from SSRS ratings to assist in identifying socially significant target behaviors from the perspectives of multiple consumers (Gresham & Lopez, 1996; Wolf, 1978). Behaviors rated as having low frequencies but high importance are potential target behaviors for intervention. The importance ratings documents the behavior standards and expectations of teachers, parents, and students and identifies behaviors for intervention programs (Gresham & Elliott, 1990; Hersh & Walker, 1983). Table 4 shows such a Frequency × Importance matrix for several potential target behaviors selected during problem identification.

Naturalistic Observations of Social Behavior

Systematic behavioral observations represent one of the most important social skills assessment methods. Observational data are very sensitive to treatment effects and should be included in all social skills interventions. Although there are a variety of elaborate coding systems available for naturalistic observation of social behavior, I recommend that clinicians keep recording procedures as simple as possible. Readers should consult the chapter on behavioral assessment (see Gresham &

Lambros, this volume) for detailed discussion of the behavioral assessment process. Four factors should be considered in using systematic behavioral observations for social skills assessment: (a) operational definitions of behavior, (b) dimension of behavior being measured, (c) number of behaviors assessed, and (d) number of observation sessions.

The first and most important step in collecting social skills observational data is to have a clear, objective operational definition of the social behavior being measured. Operational definitions should describe the specific verbal, physical, temporal, and/or spatial parameters of behavior or environmental events (Gresham, Gansle, & Noell, 1993). Operational definitions should be clear, objective, and complete (Kazdin, 1984).

Walker and Severson (1992) provide a good example of the social skill of *participation:* "This is coded when the target child is participating in a game or activity (with two or more children) that has a clearly specified and agreed upon set of rules. Examples would be kickball, four-square, dodgeball, soccer, basketball, tetherball, hopscotch, and so forth. Nonexamples include tag, jump rope, follow the leader, and other unstructured games" (pp. 23–24).

TABLE 4. Frequency × Importance Matrix from the Social Skills Rating System

Frequency	Importance		
	Critical	Important	Not important
Very often			Initiates Invites others Introduces self
Sometimes			Volunteers Questions rules Listens to others
Never	Receives criticism Controls temper Complies Compromises	Puts work away Makes transitions Pays attention	

An efficient way of formulating an operational definition of social skills is through the functional assessment interview described in the previous section. Recall that the main purpose of this interview is to get a clear and objective definition of target behaviors. Also remember, from the discussion of behavior rating scales, that teachers and parents may have their own operational definitions of social skills when they rate behaviors such as "Controls temper in conflict situations," "Ignores peer distractions," or "Initiates conversations with peers without prompting."

Behavior rating scales can be used to identify general areas of concern in social skills and competing behavior domains. The functional assessment interview can be used to operationally define behaviors of most concern to teachers and/or parents. Finally, direct observation of these behaviors in naturalistic settings (e.g., playground, classroom) are collected as a *direct measure* of social behavior and to conduct a preliminary descriptive functional analysis.

Social behavior can be described and assessed along the dimensions of frequency, temporality, and quality. Frequency, or how often a social behavior occurs, is often used as an index of social competence. Frequency, however, can sometimes be misleading because how often a person exhibits a social skill may not predict important social outcomes for them such as peer acceptance (Gottman, 1977; Gresham, 1983). Some social skills clearly are defined as problems because they occur at low frequencies. Examples include saying "please," "thank you," and "excuse me" or asking permission to get out of one's seat in class or before leaving the home.

Some social skills may be more appropriately measured using temporal dimensions of behavior such as duration, latency, or interresponse times. Examples of social skills that can be measured by durations are duration of social interactions with others, amount of time engaged in cooperative play, or durational ratio of positive to negative social interactions. One easy way of assessing the duration of social skills is to start a stopwatch whenever the child meets the definition of the behavior and stop it when the child is not engaged in the behavior. The process continues throughout the entire observation session. The duration is calculated by dividing the elapsed time by the total time observed and multiplying by 100, thereby yielding a percent duration.

Walker, Colvin, and Ramsey (1995) strongly recommend the use of duration recording of *alone* and *negative social behavior* on the playground (recess) for students demonstrating antisocial behavior pattern. *Alone* can be defined as when a child is not within 10 feet of another child, is not engaged in any organized activity, and is not exchanging social signals (verbal or nonverbal) with any other children. *Negative social behavior* is defined as displaying hostile behavior or body language toward peers; attempting to tease, bully, or otherwise intimidate others; reacting with anger or rejection to the social bids of peers; or displaying aggressive behavior with the intent to inflict harm or force the submission of peers.

Antisocial children spend more time alone and are more negative in their social interactions than are are non-antisocial students. Based on playground recording, if a target student spends between 12% and 15% of the time in solitary activity ("alone") and engages in negative social behavior 10% or more of the time, he or she is at risk for antisocial behavior (Walker et al., 1995). Approximately 90%–95% of non-antisocial students' behavior is positive and they spend little time alone at recess. This procedure has much to recommend it; however, obviously no more than two behaviors can be assessed during any given observation period. This may not be a serious drawback, because perhaps the best way of measuring social skills is at the *response class* level rather than at the discrete behavioral level.

Other social behaviors may best be measured by latencies of responding. Examples include responding to social bids to play, compliance with teacher instructions, or responding to peer requests. Finally, some social skills might best be measured by interresponse times (IRTs). Examples are elapsed time between peer initiations, time between anger outbursts, or time between offers to share play materials.

A particularly important dimension of social behavior is the *quality* of the behavior. In fact, it could be argued that the most important aspect of what makes a behavior "socially skilled" is its quality and not its frequency or its temporal dimensions. Quality of social behavior, however, must be judged by others. This can be accomplished by exposing judges to videotaped or in vivo samples of social behavior and having them rate its quality. This is similar to what is being measured by behavior rating scales except that the measurement is direct rather than indirect and is based on a more limited sample of behavior.

Some children have social skills deficits and interfering problem behaviors limited to one or two behaviors. Other children exhibit multiple social skills deficits and interfering behavior excesses, thereby presenting an unmanageable number of behaviors to assess. An important decision facing behavior therapists is how many behaviors should be observed. This decision is influenced by the nature and severity of the child's social competence difficulties as well as by the degree of teacher and/or parent concern with each behavioral excess or deficit.

It has been our experience in talking with teachers and parents about social competence problems and interfering problem behaviors that some teachers or parents will list as many as 5 to 10 behaviors that are problematic. Although some children will display 10 or more problem behaviors, not all of these behaviors are independent. Some behaviors are subsets of a larger class or category of behavior. These larger categories, known as *response classes,* describe a class or category of behavior that share similarities (topographical response class) or are controlled by the same environmental events (functional response class).

For example, a topographical response class of *social withdrawal* might include the behaviors of sulking, standing alone on the playground, walking away from peers, and ignoring social bids to join games. All of these behaviors may belong to the same response class and the operational definition of social withdrawal would include each of the behaviors listed above. In this example, social withdrawal could be measured using the duration recording procedure described previously. Practitioners should determine which behaviors are and are not members of specific response classes for observational purposes and in conceptualizing social skills interventions. I discuss the use of functional response classes more fully in the section on problem analysis.

Another consideration in using naturalistic observations is the number of times a child should be observed. The central issue here is the *representativeness* of observations. That is, are the observa-tions representative of the child's typical behavior in classroom, playground, or other settings? Based on observation of actual behavior, the observer infers that the observed behavior is typical of the child in that setting. Depending on the representativeness of the observation, this inference may or may not be justified.

Observers cannot be present in classrooms or playgrounds every minute of every day. As such, observers must sample the behavior(s) of concern to obtain reasonable estimates of the baseline rates or durations of behavior. I recommend that at least five sessions of baseline data be collected in the setting of concern (e.g., classroom or playground). These sessions should reflect the setting(s) of most concern to those referring the target child for social skills assessment and intervention. Some behaviors may occur so infrequently that it would be virtually impossible for an observer to directly assess the behavior. Walker and Severson (1992) call these "critical events" or "behavioral earthquakes" that are problematic because of their intensity rather than their frequency (e.g., sets fires, inappropriate sexual behavior, damages others' property). Clinicians should use their judgment regarding the representativeness and typicality of behavior(s) observed as there are no hard and fast rules for making this determination.

Problem Analysis

Most behavior problems addressed in this book have dealt primarily with *behavioral excesses* and the goals of assessment and intervention are to (a) obtain a functional analysis of behavior and (b) design intervention strategies based on this functional analysis information. Social skills assessment and intervention are different from those for the typical behavior problems discussed in this chapter in that they must focus on both behavioral *deficits* (social skills) and *excesses* (interfering problem behaviors). Recall that social skills acquisition and performance deficits have already been identified during problem identification. These deficits represent skills that must be either taught (acquisition deficits) or increased in frequency (performance deficits) or quality (fluency deficits). Thus, a functional analysis of these deficits is obviously not possible since one cannot determine the function of a behavioral deficit. What does require a functional analysis are the interfering problem behaviors that compete with either the acquisition, performance, or fluency of social skills.

Functional Assessment of Problem Behavior

The primary goal in problem analysis is to conduct a *functional assessment* of interfering problem behavior. Fundamentally, behaviors may serve two functions: (a) to *obtain* something desirable (e.g., social attention, preferred activities, or material objects) or (b) to *avoid, escape,* or *delay* something undesirable or aversive (e.g., difficult tasks, social activities, or interruption of desired activities) (O'Neill, Horner, Albin, Storey, & Sprague, 1990). These two functions describe the processes of positive and negative reinforcement, respectively. Functional assessment uses a full range of strategies to identify the antecedents and consequences controlling behavior using descriptive analyses (e.g., functional assessment interviews and observations) and functional analyses (experimental manipulations of antecedents and consequences; Horner, 1994). Based on functional assessments, treatments can be matched to the operant function of behavior using two strategies: (a) weakening the maintaining response–reinforcer relationship for interfering problem behaviors and (b) establishing or strengthening a response–reinforcer relationship for an adaptive behavior class (e.g., social skills) that replaces the function of the interfering or competing problem behavior (Mace, 1994).

Carr (1994) suggests that functional analysis should follow a hypothesis-driven approach in which direct observations are taken in naturalistic settings and correlations between problem behavior and its antecedents and consequences recorded. These observations form the basis of hypotheses concerning the cause(s) of problem behavior and treatments can be designed and implemented based on these hypotheses.

Strategies for Functional Assessment

There are four goals of a functional assessment: (a) description of social skills deficits and interfering problem behaviors in operational terms, (b) prediction of times and situations when interfering problem behaviors occur and do not occur across daily routines, (c) definition of the function(s) that interfering problem behavior(s) perform for the individual, and (d) formulation of behavioral hypotheses regarding the occurrence of problem behavior and identification of a socially skilled alternative that serves the same function (see O'Neill et al., 1990). Three strategies for conducting a functional assessment are the functional assessment interview, naturalistic observation of behavior, and experimental manipulation of environmental events that produce and do not produce the target behavior. Given the time and expense of experimental manipulation, most practitioners rely on the first two strategies for functional assessments.

Section B of Table 3 provides a guide for conducting a functional assessment interview during the problem analysis stage of intervention. Based on the information provided by interviewees, preliminary hypotheses can be formulated regarding the possible functions of behavior. These hypotheses are then confirmed by using direct observations of behavior in naturalistic settings (via a descriptive functional analysis). O'Neill and colleagues (1990) suggest that behavior therapists should ask questions about a wide range of environmental factors that may be related to the occurrence or nonoccurrence of behavior. These include (a) time of day, (b) physical setting (e.g., certain areas of a classroom, playground, cafeteria), (c) social control (with peers, teachers, other adults), and (d) activity (e.g., math, reading, cooperative learning groups). These environmental factors may help predict the occurrence or nonoccurrence of behavior either singularly or interactively. Information about these ecological factors can serve as one basis for behavioral hypotheses concerning problem behavior.

Reliability and Efficiency of Behavior

An extremely important goal of problem analysis is to determine the *reliability* and *efficiency* of interfering problem behaviors relative to socially skilled alternative behaviors. Competing behaviors often are performed instead of socially skilled behaviors because the competing behavior is more efficient than the socially skilled behavior (Horner, Dunlap, & Koegel, 1988). By efficient I mean it: (a) is easier to perform and (b) produces reinforcement more rapidly. By reliability I mean the competing behavior produces the desired outcome more frequently than does the socially skilled behavior. For example, whining and grabbing for food by young children is more efficient and more reliable in obtaining food than politely asking and waiting for food.

Horner and colleagues (1988) have termed this the *functional equivalence of behavior.* That is, two or more behaviors can be equal in their ability to produce reinforcement. Thus, grabbing toys is more efficient than asking for toys, or pushing a peer out of the way is more efficient than asking them to move. All things being equal, preexisting behaviors are likely to successfully compete with socially skilled behaviors if the preexisting behaviors lead to more powerful or immediate reinforcers or more efficiently produce the same reinforcement as the socially skilled alternative (i.e., they are more cost-beneficial). I will return to the concept of efficiency and reliability of social skills in the discussion of generalization programming.

Plan Implementation

Social skills instruction should emphasize the acquisition, performance, and generalization of prosocial behaviors and/or the reduction or elimination of competing interfering problem behaviors. A large number of intervention procedures have been identified for teaching social skills to children. These procedures are based on 10 paramount principles of social skills training presented in Table 5. These principles were derived from a comprehensive review of the social skills training literature as

well as from the work of Walker and colleagues (1995).

Types of Social Skills Training

As discussed earlier, the school is an ideal setting for teaching social skills because of its accessibility to children, their peers, teachers, and parents. Fundamentally, social skills intervention takes place in schools and home settings both informally and formally using either *universal* or *selected* intervention procedures. *Informal* social skills intervention is based on the notion of incidental learning, which takes advantage of naturally occurring behavioral incidents or events to teach appropriate social behavior. Most social skills instruction in home, school, and community settings can be characterized as informal or incidental. Literally thousands of behavioral incidents occur in home, school, and community settings creating rich opportunities for making each of these behavioral incidents a successful learning experience.

Formal social skills instruction can take place in a classroom setting in which the entire class is exposed to a social skills curriculum or in a small-group setting removed from the classroom. Walker and colleagues (1995) refer to these teaching formats as *universal* and *selected* interventions, respectively. Universal interventions are not unlike vaccinations, schoolwide discipline plans, or school rules in that they are designed to affect all children under the same conditions. Universal interventions are designed to prevent more serious problems from developing later in a child's life (i.e., primary pre-

TABLE 5. 10 Paramount Principles of Social Skills Training

1. Social skills are learned behaviors.
2. Social skills can be either acquisition, performance, or fluency deficits.
3. Social skills are highly contextualistic and relativistic.
4. Social skills are best taught in naturalistic settings and situations.
5. Social skills are governed by the Principle of Social Reciprocity.
6. Social skills should be taught by the same procedures used to teach academic skills.
7. There is a direct, positive relationship between the amount and quality (integrity) of social skills training and the amount of change in social behavior.
8. Social skills training strategies must be accompanied by reductive techniques to decrease or eliminate interfering problem behaviors.
9. Social skills training must be supplemented by behavioral rehearsal opportunities, performance feedback, and contingency systems in naturalistic settings to promote their occurrence, fluency, and mastery.
10. For social skills to be integrated into a behavioral repertoire, they must be as or more efficient and reliable in producing desired outcomes as are competing behaviors.

vention). Selected interventions are typically conducted with children who have been identified as being at risk for behavior problems and are based on an individual assessment of a child's social skills deficits and behavioral excesses. These interventions are undertaken to prevent existing behavior problems from developing into more serious behavior problems (i.e., secondary or tertiary prevention). Obviously, these are the types of social skills interventions described in this chapter.

Universal social skills interventions focus on affecting all children in the same setting using the same procedures (Walker et al., 1995). A classwide social skills intervention program designed to teach conflict resolution and social problem solving is an example of a universal social skills intervention. Other examples of universal social skills intervention programs include the Prepare Curriculum (Goldstein, 1988), the ACCEPTS Program (Walker et al., 1983), and the Social Skills Intervention Guide (Elliott & Gresham, 1992). These universal interventions are likely to be used as a means of primary prevention rather than secondary or tertiary prevention. *Selected* social skills interventions, on the other hand, are designed for a single individual or small subset of children using individually tailored intervention procedures based on specific social skills acquisition and performance deficits and functional assessment of interfering problem behaviors.

Objectives of Social Skills Training

Social skills training (SST) has four primary objectives: (a) promoting skill acquisition, (b) enhancing skill performance, (c) reducing or removing interfering problem behaviors, and (d) facilitating generalization and maintenance of social skills. It was noted earlier in this chapter that children will likely have some combination of acquisition and performance deficits, some of which may be accompanied by interfering problem behaviors and others which are not. Thus, any given child may require some combination of acquisition, performance, and behavior reduction strategies. All children will require procedures to facilitate generalization and maintenance of social skills.

Table 6 lists specific social skills training and behavior reduction strategies for each of the four goals of SST. The behavior therapist must match appropriate intervention strategies with the particular deficits or behavioral excesses the child exhibits. Moreover, a common misconception is that one seeks to facilitate generalization after implementing procedures for acquisition and performance of social skills. The evidence is clear that the best practice is to incorporate generalization from the beginning of any social skills training program (Gresham, 1995, 1997b).

Promoting Skill Acquisition

Procedures designed to promote acquisition are applicable when children do not have a particular social skill in their repertoire, when they do not know a particular step in the performance of a behavioral sequence, or when their execution of the skill is awkward or ineffective (i.e., a fluency deficit). It should be noted that a relatively small percentage of children will need social skills intervention based on acquisition deficits: Far more children have performance deficits in the area of prosocial behavior (Gresham, 1995, 1997b; Gresham & Reschly, 1988).

Three procedures represent pathways to remediation of deficits in social skills acquisition: modeling, coaching, and behavioral rehearsal. Specific guidelines for using each of these procedures are presented in Table 7. Social problem solving is another pathway, but it is not discussed here owing to space limitations and the fact that it incorporates the three procedures discussed in this section. More specific information on social problem-solving interventions can be found in Elias and Clabby (1992) and Elias and Branden (1988).

Modeling is the process of learning a behavior by observing another person performing that behavior. Modeling instruction presents the entire sequence of behaviors involved in a particular social skill and teaches how to integrate specific behaviors in this sequence into a composite behavior pattern. Modeling is one of the most effective and efficient ways of teaching social behavior (Gresham, 1985; Schneider, 1992).

Coaching is the use of verbal instruction to teach social skills. Unlike modeling, which emphasizes visual displays of social skills, coaching utilizes a child's cognitive and language skills. Coaching is accomplished in three fundamental steps: (a) presenting social concepts or rules, (b)

TABLE 6. Social Skills Training Objectives and Strategies

I. Promoting skill acquisition
   A. Modeling
   B. Coaching
   C. Behavioral Rehearsal

II. Enhancing skill performance
   A. Manipulation of antecedents
      1. Peer initiation strategies
      2. Sociodramatic play activities
      3. Proactive classroom management strategies
      4. Peer tutoring
      5. Incidental teaching
   B. Manipulation of consequences
      1. Contingency contracting
      2. Group-oriented contingency systems
      3. School/home notes
      4. Verbal praise
      5. Activity reinforcers
      6. Token/point systems

III. Removing interfering problem behaviors
   A. Differential reinforcement
      1. Differential reinforcement of other behavior (DRO)
      2. Differential reinforcement of low rates of behavior (DRL)
      3. Differential reinforcement of incompatible behavior (DRI)
   B. Overcorrection
      1. Restitution
      2. Positive practice
   C. Response cost
   D. Time-out
      1. Nonexclusionary (contingent observation)
      2. Exclusionary
   E. Systematic desensitization
   F. Flooding/exposure

IV. Facilitating generalization
   A. Topographical generalization
      1. Training diversely
         a. Use sufficient stimulus exemplars
         b. Teach sufficient response exemplars
         c. Make antecedents less discriminable (train "loosely")
         d. Make consequences less discriminable ("thin" reinforcement schedule)
      2. Exploit functional contingencies
         a. Teach relevant behaviors
         b. Modify environments supporting interfering problem behaviors
         c. Recruit natural communities of reinforcement
         d. Reinforce occurrences of generalization
      3. Incorporate functional mediators
         a. Incorporate common salient social stimuli
         b. Incorporate common salient physical stimuli
         c. Incorporate salient self-mediated physical stimuli
         d. Incorporate salient self-mediated verbal or covert stimuli
   B. Functional generalization
      1. Identify strong competing stimuli
      2. Identify strong competing interfering problem behaviors
      3. Identify functionally equivalent socially skilled behaviors
      4. Increase reliability and efficiency of socially skilled behaviors (build fluency)
      5. Decrease reliability and efficiency of competing interfering problem behaviors

TABLE 7. Guidelines for Using Modeling, Coaching, and Behavioral Rehearsal

A. Modeling
1. Point out the benefits of learning the skill.
   a. Ask why the skill might be important.
   b. Identify consequences for using the skill.
   c. Use examples from movies, television, books, and so forth in which characters use the skill.
   d. Identify settings and situations where the skill could and should be used.
2. Task analyze skill components
   a. Select a social skill to be discussed (e.g., joining a group of peers playing).
   b. Brainstorrm behaviors a person would have to perform to join a group of peers playing.
   c. Write children's ideas on flip chart or chalkboard.
   d. Discuss relevance of each idea and decide what behaviors would be important in joining peers playing a game.
   e. Decide with the group which behaviors would be the most important in joining peers playing a game.
   f. Decide with the group the order or sequence in which the behaviors should be performed.
   g. Identify potential problems that might occur when performing the skill (e.g., being ignored or teased).
3. Demonstrate the social skill using modeled instruction
   a. Decide whether you or another child in the group will model the skill.
   b. Point out the necessary behaviors for performing the skill. Write these on the board or chart before modeling the skill.
   c. Tell children to watch and see if each behavioral step is performed in the proper sequence.
   d. Model the skill or have another child model the skill.
   e. After modeling, solicit feedback from children in evaluation of the modeling sequence. Discuss comments offered.
4. Rehearse the skill
   a. Have children practice the skill with each other.
   b. Provide specific performance feedback regarding these behavioral rehearsals.
   c. Offer suggestions for how performances might be improved.
   d. Re-model the skill and require repeated behavioral rehearsals to build fluency.
5. Program for generalization
   a. Teach sufficient stimulus exemplars
      1. Role-play a number of situations in which the skill could be used.
      2. Vary the situations in which the skill could be used (e.g., number of persons present, where it is performed).
   b. Teach sufficient response exemplars
      1. Teach a number of variations in performing the skill in the same situation.
      2. Show children how there are numerous ways of accomplishing the same goal in a social interaction.

B. Coaching
1. Present a social concept. For instance, ask the group what is meant by sharing.
2. Ask for definitions of the social concept.
3. Sharpen the group's definition of the social concept. For example, say, "Sharing could also mean . . . as well as . . .
4. Ask for specific behavioral examples of the social concept. For instance, say, "What are some things kids might do to show they are sharing?"
5. Ask for specific behavioral examples of not sharing such as, "What are some things kids might do to show they were not sharing?"
6. Elicit from the group potential consequences for performing or not performing the skill.
7. Generate situations and settings in which the social skill would be appropriate and inappropriate.
8. Use behavioral rehearsal to practice the skill.
9. Use specific performance feedback about the behavioral rehearsals.
10. Build fluency with repeated rehearsals of the skill.

C. Behavioral rehearsal
1. Covert rehearsal
   a. Have children close their eyes. Present a scene involving a social interaction.
   b. Have children imagine themselves performing a social skill in the scene.
   c. Have children imagine how other people in the scene will respond to their behavior.
   d. Have children imagine alternative behaviors they could perform in the scene and the consequences associated with each.
2. Verbal rehearsal
   a. Present a social situation involving a social interaction.
   b. Have children identify each step involved in performing a social skill.
   c. Have children orally arrange these steps in a proper sequence.
   d. Have children describe situations in which the skill would be appropriate.

(continued)

TABLE 7. (*Continued*)

---

   e. Have children describe potential consequences of performing the social skill.

   f. For each situation, have children describe alternative social behaviors and the consequences associated with each behavior.

  3. Overt rehearsal

   a. Describe a role-play situation, select participants, and assign roles for each participant.

   b. Have participants role-play the social situation. Instruct observers to watch performances of each participant closely.

   c. Discuss and evaluate performances in the role-play and provide suggestions for improved performances.

   d. Ask participants to incorporate feedback suggestions as they replay the scene.

   e. Select new participants to role-play the same social situation.

   f. Build fluency with repeated rehearsals of the skill.

---

providing opportunities for practice or rehearsal of a social skill, and (c) providing specific informational feedback on behavioral performances.

Behavioral rehearsal refers to practicing a newly learned behavior in a structured, protective situation of role-playing. In this way, children can enhance their proficiency in using social skills without experiencing adverse consequences. Social learning theory suggests that behavioral rehearsal is essential to learning social behavior (Bandura, 1977). Three forms of behavioral rehearsal can be used in a number of ways and combinations. For example, behavior therapists can ask children to imagine being teased by another child and then to imagine how they would respond (covert rehearsal). Next, one might combine covert rehearsal with verbal rehearsal by asking children to recite specific behaviors they would exhibit in imagined situations. Finally, one might combine covert and verbal rehearsal with overt rehearsal by asking children to role-play the imagined situation.

Enhancing Skill Performance

Most social skills interventions will involve procedures that increase the frequency of prosocial behaviors because most social skills problems are performance rather than acquisition deficits. This suggests that most social skills interventions for most children will take place in naturalistic environments (e.g., classrooms, playgrounds) rather than in small "pullout" groups. Therefore, most social skills interventions can be facilitated by using a consultative framework for intervention. Failure to perform certain social skills in specific situations results from two fundamental factors: (a) inappropriately arranged antecedents and/or (b) inappropriately arranged consequences. A number of specific procedures can be classified under the broad rubrics of antecedent and consequent strategies.

Interventions based on antecedent control assume that the environment does not set the occasion for the performance of prosocial behavior. That is, cues, prompts, or other stimuli are either not present or the child does not discriminate these stimuli in relation to the performance of prosocial behavior. Antecedent control techniques are based on the principle of discrimination learning.

Two general strategies fall under the category of antecedent strategies: peer-mediated interventions and cueing/prompting. Peer-mediated interventions can include three techniques: (a) peer initiations, (b) peer tutoring, and (c) peer modeling (Kohler & Strain, 1990). With peer initiation strategies, a child's peers are used to initiate and maintain social interactions with socially isolated children. This procedure is effective for children who have performance deficits and who evidence relatively low rates of social interaction, but do not have externalizing interfering problem behaviors. Table 8 presents some specific guidelines for using the peer initiation strategy.

A cueing and prompting procedure uses verbal or nonverbal cues or prompts to facilitate prosocial behaviors. Simple prompts or cues for some children may be all that is needed to signal children to engage in socially appropriate behavior. Cueing and prompting represent one of the easiest and most efficient social skills intervention strategies (Elliott & Gresham, 1992; Walker et al., 1995).

Intervention techniques based on consequent control can be classified into three broad categories: (a) reinforcement-based strategies, (b) behavioral contracts, and (c) school–home notes. Reinforcement-based strategies assume that a child knows

TABLE 8. Guidelines for Using Peer Initiation Strategies

1. Recruit peer confederates to be used in peer initiation training. Criteria for selection should be based on children having good social skills, who are well liked by peers, and who display a high level of self-confidence.
2. Train peer confederates in social initiation strategies. Use modeling, coaching, behavioral rehearsal, and direct reinforcement for competent performances during training. If possible, videotape portions of the training sessions and use as a basis for feedback, improvement, and booster sessions.
3. Use procedures in Step 2 to prepare peer confederates for initial rejection or ignoring of their invitation bids.
4. After peer initiation training, use teacher prompting in the natural setting to cue social initiations.
5. Gradually fade teacher prompts to transfer stimulus control of teacher prompts to peers.
6. Periodically conduct booster sessions with peer confederates and discuss unique problems they may be having with target children in their social initiation bids.

how to perform a social skill, but is not doing so because of little or nonexistent reinforcement for the behavior. Reinforcement strategies include attention, social praise, tokens/points, and activity reinforcers, as well as group-oriented contingency systems.

Behavioral contracts (written agreements between children and intervention agents) specify the relation between behavior and its consequences. Behavioral contracts should have the following five components: (a) specification of mutual gains, (b) ways in which the child will demonstrate observable behavior, (c) provisions for sanctions for not meeting contract terms, (d) a bonus clause for consistent performance of desired behaviors (i.e., social skills), and (e) means of monitoring reinforcers given and received (Stuart, 1971). Behavioral contracts are an effective means of enhancing the performance or quality of prosocial behavior and decreasing the frequency of competing interfering problems behaviors.

School–home notes are written communications sent by intervention agents to parents on a daily or weekly basis. School–home notes can be easily incorporated into behavioral contracts to enlist parental involvement and cooperation in facilitating prosocial behavior. More extensive discussion of school–home notes and their use can be found in Kelley (1990).

Removing Interfering Problem Behaviors

The focus in social skills intervention is clearly upon the development and refinement of prosocial behaviors. However, as mentioned earlier in this chapter, the failure of some children to either acquire or perform certain social skills may be due to the presence of interfering problem behaviors. In the case of acquisition deficits, the interfering problem behaviors may block social skill acquisition. For instance, self-stimulatory behaviors of an autistic child may prevent the development of eye contact and conversation skills. In performance deficits, aggressive behavior may be performed instead of a prosocial behavior because it may be more efficient and reliable in producing desired outcomes.

A number of techniques are effective in reducing interfering or competing behaviors. Because of space considerations, only differential reinforcement techniques are discussed in the following paragraphs.

Differential reinforcement derives from the principles of stimulus control in which a behavior is reinforced in the presence of one stimulus and is not reinforced in the presence of other stimuli. After a number of trials of differential reinforcement, a behavior will come under the control of the stimulus associated with reinforcement and thus is said to be under *stimulus control*. Principles of stimulus control can be used to decrease rates of undesirable behavior and increase rates of prosocial behavior. Three types of differential reinforcement have been used most frequently: differential reinforcement of other behavior (DRO), differential reinforcement of low rates of behavior (DRL), and differential reinforcement of incompatible behavior (DRI).

DRO refers to a delivery of a reinforcer after any behavior except the target behavior. The effects of DRO are to decrease the frequency of a target behavior and to increase frequencies of all other behaviors. Technically speaking, *any* behavior except the target behavior is reinforced (appropriate or inappropriate). Practically, only *appropriate* behaviors are reinforced in DRO.

Two types of DRO are used: interval DRO and momentary DRO. Interval DRO involves the reinforcement of a behavior if the targeted behavior does not occur at any time during a specified time interval. Thus, in an interval DRO-2 minute, the first behavior occurring after a 2-minute interval in which the target behavior (e.g., cursing) did not occur is reinforced. If the cursing occurs at any time during the 2-minute interval, the timer is reset to the beginning of the interval. In momentary DRO, behavior is *sampled* at the end of a specified time interval. If the target behavior is *not* occurring at the end of the interval, the first behavior occurring after the interval is reinforced. In a momentary DRO 2-minute, a behavior is reinforced if the target behavior is not occurring at the 2-minute sampling time.

Either DRO schedule can be used to reduce the frequency of problem behaviors in a variety of settings. The primary problem with DRO schedules is keeping up with time intervals and resetting the timer. Momentary DRO schedules are more user-friendly than interval DROs and should be more reasonable for practical purposes.

DRL involves the reinforcement of reductions in the frequency of target behaviors in a specified time interval. Two variations of DRL schedules are described: classic DRL and full session DRL. In classic DRL, the time elapsing between behaviors or interresponse times (IRTs) are gradually lengthened. For example, if a child interrupts frequently, interruptions could be reduced in frequency by reinforcing the child waiting 5 minutes between instances of interruptions. If the child interrupted before the 5 minutes elapsed (e.g., 2 minutes or 4 minutes), the timer would be reset and the 5-minute waiting requirement would remain in effect. This would be called a classic DRL-5-minute schedule of reinforcement.

In full session DRL, reinforcement is provided when the overall frequency of a target behavior is reduced during a specified time session. The difference between a full session DRL and a classic DRL is that full session DRLs do not require longer and longer intervals between occurrences of target behavior. Instead, the requirement is that overall frequency of a target behavior in a specified time interval be reduced. For example, a teacher might set a criterion of five or fewer occurrences of disruptive behavior during a 25-minute reading lesson. If this criterion is met, the child would receive reinforcement. Full session DRLs are more user-friendly than classic DRLs and are easily adapted within the context of group contingency systems.

In DRI, behaviors that are incompatible with the target behavior are reinforced. Whereas DRO and DRL focus on reducing the frequencies of problem behaviors, DRI emphasizes *increasing* the frequencies of prosocial behaviors. DRI reduces the frequency of interfering behavior because prosocial behaviors that are incompatible with problem behaviors are increased in frequency. Several examples should make this clear: sharing behavior is incompatible with stingy behavior; complimenting others is incompatible with teasing others; asking others to borrow a toy is incompatible with grabbing a toy; compromising with others is incompatible with fighting.

DRIs are not effective because of the incompatibility of behaviors, but rather because of the relative rate of reinforcement for each behavior (McDowell, 1982). For example, a child might "choose" to tease others or the child might "choose" to compliment others. Complimenting is incompatible with teasing; however, the child can "choose" to stop complimenting and start teasing at any time. DRI makes particular use of the Matching Law (Herrnstein, 1970), which states that response rate matches reinforcement rate. Based on principles of matching, a child's behavior should follow the Matching Law and incompatible problem behaviors should decrease and prosocial behaviors should increase using DRI.

Facilitating Generalization

At its most basic level, only two processes are essential to all behavioral interventions: *discrimination* and *generalization* (Stokes, 1992). Discrimination and generalization represent polar opposites on the continuum of behavior change. A major problem confronting social skills trainers is that they have been relatively successful in getting some behaviors to occur in one place for a limited period of time. In other words, SST has been highly effective in teaching *discriminations*. On the other hand, getting social behavior to occur in more than one place for an extended period of time has been more difficult to achieve. That is, *generalization* of SST across participants, settings, behaviors, and times has been less unsuccessful. One reason for this may be the way social skills are taught. Social skills are taught under conditions of discrimination rather than under conditions that would lead to generalization. Therefore, we may be teaching social skills under stimulus conditions that may be too tight; this ultimately impedes any generalization effects that might accrue for our treatment procedures.

Generalization is typically regarded from two perspectives. One emphasizes behavioral *form* or *topography* and the other emphasizes behavioral *function* (Edelstein, 1989; Stokes & Osnes, 1989). The topographical description of generalization refers to the occurrence of relevant behaviors under different, nontraining conditions (Stokes & Osnes, 1989). The so-called relevant behaviors (e.g., social skills) can occur across settings/situations (setting generalization), behaviors (response generalization), and/or time (maintenance). Table 6 presents 12 topographical generalization strategies. The topographical approach to generalization suggests that relevant behaviors occurred in other settings, that they led to increases in collateral behaviors, or were maintained over time, but does not indicate *why* this occurred. Topographical generalization merely describes an observed outcome or correlate of a SST intervention program, but does not provide a *functional* account of this outcome.

The functional approach to generalization consists of two types: (a) stimulus generalization, which is the occurrence of the same behavior under variations of the original stimulus (the greater the difference between the training stimulus and subsequent stimuli, the less generalization) and (b) response generalization, which is the control of multiple behaviors by the same stimulus (a functional response class).

One way of understanding generalization errors, functionally, is within the context of competing behaviors. Horner and colleagues (1988) offered the following scenario: A child has acquired a new, adaptive social skill and demonstrates excellent generalization across new situations. A new situation is presented that contains a strong competing stimulus. This competing stimulus is likely to elicit old, undesirable behavior. The practical effect is that the new adaptive social skill does not generalize to situations containing the strong competing stimulus.

The above situation would create no problems if the child did not have to encounter environments

with the strong competing stimulus. However, it is not always possible to arrange this, such as when the strong competing stimulus is a classmate or teacher. The notion of strong competing stimuli may explain why so many problem drinkers "fall off the wagon" (bars and alcohol represent strong competing stimuli for undesirable drinking behavior). One reason, among many, that social skills fail to generalize is that the newly taught behavior is masked or overpowered by older and stronger competing behaviors. This is an important concept for understanding why some behaviors generalize to some new situations but not to others and why a behavior that has been maintained well for a long time may suddenly deteriorate.

The section on reliability and efficiency of behavior described how competing behaviors might be performed instead of socially skilled behaviors because the competing behavior is more efficient and reliable than socially skilled behaviors in obtaining desired outcomes. To program for functional generalization, behavior therapists should ask the generalization questions in Table 3, which are based on Horner and colleagues' (1988) recommendations. Answers to these questions imply two classes of intervention strategies: (a) Decrease the efficiency and reliability of competing, inappropriate behaviors and (b) increase the efficiency and reliability of socially skilled alternative behaviors. The former can be accomplished by many of the procedures listed in Table 6 under Removing Interfering Problem Behaviors. The latter can be achieved by spending more time and effort in building fluency of trained social skills using combinations of modeling, coaching, and, most importantly, behavioral rehearsal with specific performance feedback.

Generalization should never be considered an afterthought with respect to SST. The most important and functional question is how to get social skills to generalize across settings, situations, persons, and time. Social skills that do not generalize are not functional for individuals. Topographical approaches based on training diversely, exploiting functional contingencies, and incorporating functional mediators sometimes are effective. However, the functional approach based on competing behaviors and functional equivalents has more promise for facilitating generalization of trained social skills.

Plan Evaluation

The extent to which SST is effective in increasing the frequency/duration of prosocial behavior and decreasing the frequency/duration of interfering problem behaviors should be evaluated with single case research methodology (see Gresham, this volume). Not all behavior therapists will utilize "true" experimental designs such as withdrawal, multielement, and multiple baseline designs, given financial, time, and personnel limitations. However, at a minimum, therapists should collect adequate baseline and postintervention data (at least 5 data points in each condition) and maintenance probes (e.g., 2–3 data points). This A-B design with follow-up probes will perhaps be the most frequently used method of evaluating the effects of social skills interventions by practicing behavior therapists.

Estimating Effects of Social Skills Intervention

Based on single case methodology, how do behavior therapists know whether or not their intervention "worked"? Gresham (this volume) discussed several methods of quantifying effects in single case methodology: (a) visual inspection, (b) reliable changes in behavior, (c) time series analysis, and (d) effect sizes. For most practical purposes, I recommend a combination of visual inspection, reliable change, and effect size estimates for plan evaluation purposes. With visual inspection, one can get a gross estimate of how the intervention produced changes in *level* and *trend* from baseline to intervention phases. Visual inspection, however, should not be used alone because of possible erroneous conclusions regarding the presence or absence of treatment effects (i.e., Type I and Type II errors) (Knapp, 1983; Matyas & Greenwood, 1990, 1991; Ottenbacher, 1990).

Reliable changes in behavior can be estimated using the *reliable change index* (RCI) to quantify the effectiveness of a social skills intervention for individuals (see Christensen & Mendoza, 1986; Jacobson, Follette, & Revenstorf, 1984). The RCI is defined as the difference between a posttest score and a pretest score divided by the standard error of the difference between posttest and pretest scores. The standard error of the difference is the variation of change scores that would be expected if no

change had occurred. An RCI of $+1.96$ ($p < .05$) is considered a reliable change in behavior.

RCIs can be computed with single case data by averaging the baseline data (pretest) and intervention data (posttest) and dividing by the standard error of the difference between baseline and intervention phases. The standard error of the difference is based on the autocorrelation and variation of baseline and intervention phases. Remember, however, that the RCI is strongly affected by the reliability (autocorrelation) of the dependent variable between pretest and posttest. Thus, small changes in a behavior having high reliability or autocorrelation over time may be statistically reliable, but not socially important. In contrast, large changes in a behavior showing low autocorrelation over time may not be statistically reliable, but could be socially important.

Another way of quantifying your visual inspection of data is by using effect size estimates. Busk and Serlin (1992) recommend using an effect size estimate similar to that used in meta-analytic research based on baseline and treatment phase means. This effect size subtracts the baseline mean from the intervention mean and divides by the standard deviation of the baseline phase. This effect size differs from the RCI in that it uses the baseline standard deviation as the error term rather than the standard error of the difference, which is based on autocorrelation of data points over time.

An effect size estimate that is perhaps the most user-friendly is the percentage of nonoverlapping data points (PNOL) between baseline and treatment phases (see Mastropieri & Scruggs, 1985–1986). PNOL is computed by indicating the number of treatment data points that exceed the highest baseline data point in an expected direction and dividing by the total number of data points in the treatment phase. For example, if 5 of 10 treatment data points exceed the highest baseline data point, the PNOL is 50%. This method provides a reasonable estimate of treatment effectiveness for most purposes; however, it should not be used with data showing inappropriate baseline trends, nonorthogonal slope changes, and floor/ceiling effects.

Social Validation

Evaluating the *social importance* of the effects produced by social skills interventions is a critical step in plan evaluation. The question to be answered in social validation is, Does the quality and quantity of behavior change make a difference in the child's functioning in his or her natural environments? Establishing the social importance of social skills intervention effects is not merely a question of showing changes from baseline to treatment and documenting these with effect size estimates. The issue in social validation is whether the treatment produced noticeable changes that have *habilitative validity* for children.

One problem in evaluating the outcomes of SST is in how we express the amount or degree of behavior change. What we want to do is to produce a degree of behavior change that will make a difference in how children function across a variety of environments. Typical outcome measures in SST research and practice have been rates of positive social interaction, decreases in negative social interaction rates, changes in behavior ratings over time as judged by teachers or parents, improvements in peer acceptance, and so forth. A legitimate question is, Does a change in a score of 75 to 85 on the Social Skills Rating Scale after SST represent a meaningful change? Does increasing a positive social interaction rate of 1 to 5 per minute represent a meaningful change?

Wolf (1978) described one aspect of social validation as the process of determining the *social importance* of treatment effects. Hawkins (1991) argued that we should really be more interested in *habilitative validity*. In other words, SST should produce changes in a child's functional status as it relates to interpersonal relationships. The question is, How do we know or document changes in functional status?

Recently Lee Sechrest and colleagues (see Sechrest, McKnight, & McKnight, 1996) suggested using the method of *just noticeable differences* (JNDs) to gauge outcomes in psychotherapy outcome research. The question here is simple: How much of a difference in scores or behaviors is required to be noticed by those with opportunity to observe behavior of the individual involved? Thus, social skills interventions should produce changes in positive social behaviors that are noticed by significant others (e.g., teachers, parents, peers). According to Sechrest and colleagues (1996), a very large difference between a person's performance on some outcome measure(s) is probably necessary for

it to be noticeable by others. Although we can demonstrate graphically rather large changes in the frequency, rate, or duration of social behavior, this is no assurance that these changes have *habilitative validity* or will be noticed by others.

Recall that the definition of social skills proposed at the beginning of this chapter was a *social validity definition*. Social skills were defined as specific behaviors exhibited in specific situations that predict important social outcomes for children. Important social outcomes include peer acceptance, significant others' positive judgments of social competence, friendships, adequate self-concept, and absence of psychopathology. All of these social validation criteria reflect in some way the degree to which others "notice" changes in a child's social behavior. Therefore, it seems that the ultimate way of evaluating our SST programs would be to produce changes in behavior that are noticed by others (i.e., JNDs) across settings, situations, and times.

References

American Psychiatric Association. (1987). *Diagnostic and statistical manual of mental disorders* (3rd ed.). Washington, DC: Author.

American Psychiatric Association. (1994). *Diagnostic and statistical manual of mental disorders* (4th ed.). Washington, DC: Author.

Bandura, A. (1977). *Social learning theory.* Englewood Cliffs, NJ: Prentice-Hall.

Barkley, R. (1990). *Attention-deficit hyperactivity disorder: A handbook for diagnosis and treatment.* New York: Guilford.

Brophy, J., & Good, T. (1986). Teacher behavior and student achievement. In M. Wittrock (Ed.), *Handbook of research on teaching* (3rd ed., pp. 328–375). New York: Macmillan.

Busk, P., & Serlin, R. (1992). Meta-analysis for single case research. In T. Kratochwill & J. Levin (Eds.), *Single-case research design and analysis* (pp. 187–212). Hillsdale, NJ: Erlbaum.

Carr, E. (1994). Emerging themes in the functional analysis of problem behavior. *Journal of Applied Behavior Analysis, 27,* 393–399.

Christensen, L., & Mendoza, J. (1986). A method of assessing change in a single subject: An alteration of the RC index. *Behavior Therapy, 17,* 305–308.

Cowen, E., Pederson, A., Babigian, H., Izzo, I., & Trost, M. (1973). Long-term follow-up of early detected vulnerable children. *Journal of Consulting and Clinical Psychology, 41,* 438–446.

Demaray, M., Ruffalo, S., Carlson, J., Busse, R., Olson, A., McManus, S., & Leventhal, A. (1995). Social skills assessment: A comparative evaluation of six published rating scales. *School Psychology Review, 24,* 648–671.

Dodge, K. (1989). Problems in social relationships. In E. Mash & R. Barkley (Eds.), *Treatment of childhood disorders* (pp. 222–244). New York: Guilford.

Edelstein, B. (1989). Generalization: Terminological, methodological, and conceptual issues. *Behavior Therapy, 20,* 311–324.

Elias, M., & Branden, L. (1988). Primary prevention of behavioral and emotional problems in school-age populations. *School Psychology Review, 17,* 581–592.

Elias, M., & Clabby, J. (1992). *Building social problem-solving skills: Guidelines for school-based programs.* San Francisco: Jossey-Bass.

Elliott, S.N., & Gresham, F.M. (1992). *Social Skills Intervention Guide.* Circle Pines, MN: American Guidance Service.

Forness, S., & Knitzer, J. (1992). A new proposed definition and terminology to replace "Serious Emotional Disturbance" in Individuals with Disabilities Education Act. *School Psychology Review, 21,* 12–20.

Goldstein, A. (1988). *The Prepare Curriculum.* Champaign, IL: Research Press.

Gottman, J. (1977). Toward a definition of social isolation in children. *Child Development, 48,* 513–517.

Gresham, F.M. (1981a). Assessment of children's social skills. *Journal of School Psychology, 19,* 120–134.

Gresham, F.M. (1981b). Social skills training with handicapped children: A review. *Review of Educational Research, 51,* 139–176.

Gresham, F.M. (1983). Social validity in the assessment of children's social skills: Establishing standards for social competency. *Journal of Psychoeducational Assessment, 1,* 299–307.

Gresham, F.M. (1985). Utility of cognitive–behavioral procedures for social skills training with children. *Journal of Abnormal Child Psychology, 13,* 411–423.

Gresham, F.M. (1992). Social skills and learning disabilities: Causal, concomitant, or correlational? *School Psychology Review, 21,* 348–360.

Gresham, F.M. (1995). Social skills training. In A. Thomas & J. Grimes (Eds.), *Best practices in school psychology–III* (pp. 1021–1029). Washington, DC: National Association of School Psychologists.

Gresham, F.M. (1997a). Designs for evaluating behavior change: Conceptual principles of single case methodology. In T.S. Watson & F.M. Gresham (Eds.), *Child behavior therapy: Ecological considerations in assessment, treatment, and evaluation.* New York: Plenum.

Gresham, F.M. (1997b). Social skills. In G. Bear, K. Minke, & A. Thomas (Eds.), *Children's needs: Psychological perspectives* (2nd ed., pp. 515–526). Washington, DC: National Association of School Psychologists.

Gresham, F.M., & Elliott, S.N. (1990). *Social Skills Rating System.* Circle Pines, MN: American Guidance Service.

Gresham, F.M., & Lambros, K.M. (1997). Behavioral and functional assessment. In T.S. Watson & F.M. Gresham (Eds.), *Child behavior therapy: Ecological considerations in assessment, treatment, and evaluation.* (pp. 3–22). New York: Plenum.

Gresham, F.M., & Lopez, M.F. (1996). Social validation: A unifying concept for school-based consultation research and practice. *School Psychology Quarterly, 11,* 204–227.

Gresham, F.M., & Reschly, D.J. (1988). Issues in the conceptualization and assessment of social skills in the mildly handicapped. In T. Kratochwill (Ed.), *Advances in school psychology* (Vol. 6, pp. 203–247). Hillsdale, NJ: Erlbaum.

Gresham, F.M., Gansle, K., & Noell, G. (1993). Treatment integrity in applied behavior analysis with children. *Journal of Applied Behavior Analysis, 26,* 257–263.

Guevemont, D. (1990). Social skills and peer relationship training. In R. Barkley, *Attention-deficit hyperactivity disorder: A handbook for diagnosis and treatment* (pp. 540–572). New York: Guilford.

Hawkins, R. (1991). Is social validity what we are interested in? Argument for a functional approach. *Journal of Applied Behavior Analysis, 24,* 205–213.

Herrnstein, R. (1970). On the law of effect. *Journal of the Experimental Analysis of Behavior, 13,* 243–266.

Hersh, R., & Walker, H. (1983). Great expectations: Making schools effective for all students. *Policy Studies Review, 2,* 147–188.

Horner, R. (1994). Functional assessment contributions and future directions. *Journal of Applied Behavior Analysis, 27,* 401–404.

Horner, R., Dunlap, G., & Koegel, R. (Eds.)(1988). *Generalization and maintenance: Lifestyle changes in applied settings.* Baltimore: Brookes.

Jacobson, N., Follette, W., & Revenstorf, D. (1984). Psychotherapy outcome research: Methods for reporting variability and evaluating clinical significance. *Behavior Therapy, 15,* 336–352.

Kazdin, A. (1984). Behavior modification in applied settings (3rd ed.). Homewood, IL: Dorsey Press.

Kazdin, A. (1987). Treatment of antisocial behavior in children: Current status and future directions. *Psychological Bulletin, 102,* 187–203.

Kelley, M.L. (1990). *School–home notes.* New York: Guilford.

Knapp, T. (1983). Behavior analysts' visual appraisal of behavior change in graphic display. *Behavioral Assessment, 5,* 155–164.

Kohler, F., & Strain, P. (1990). Peer-assisted interventions: Early promises, notable achievements, and future aspirations. *Clinical Psychology Review, 10,* 441–452.

Kohn, M., & Clausen, J. (1955). Social isolation and schizophrenia. *American Sociological Review, 20,* 265–273.

Kupersmidt, J., Coie, J., & Dodge, K. (1990). The role of peer relationships in the development of disorder. In S. Asher & J. Coie (Eds.), *Peer rejection in childhood* (pp. 274–308). New York: Cambridge University Press.

LaGreca, A.M., & Stone, W. (1990). Children with learning disabilities: The role of achievement in their social, personal, and behavioral functioning. In H.L. Swanson & B. Keogh (Eds.), *Learning disabilities: Theoretical and research issues* (pp. 333–352). Hillsdale, NJ: Erlbaum.

Lynam, D. (1996). Early identification of chronic offenders: Who is the fledgling psychopath? *Psychological Bulletin, 120,* 209–234.

Mace, F.C. (1994). The significance and future of functional analysis methodologies. *Journal of Applied Behavior Analysis, 27,* 385–392.

MacMillan, D.L., Gresham, F.M., & Siperstein, G.N. (1993). Conceptual and psychometric concerns about the 1992

AAMR definition of mental retardation. *American Journal of Mental Retardation, 98,* 325–335.

Mastropieri, M., & Scruggs, T. (1985–1986). Early intervention for socially withdrawn children. *Journal of Special Education, 19,* 429–441.

Matyas, T., & Greenwood, C. (1990). Visual analysis of single-case time series: Effects of variability, serial dependence, and magnitude of intervention effects. *Journal of Applied Behavior Analysis, 23,* 341–351.

Matyas, T., & Greenwood, C. (1991). Problems in the estimation of autocorrelation in brief time series and some implications for behavioral data. *Behavioral Assessment, 13,* 137–157.

McDowell, J.J. (1982). The importance of Herrnstein's mathematical statement of the Law of Effect for behavior therapy. *American Psychologist, 37,* 771–779.

McFall, R. (1982). A review and reformulation of the concept of social skills. *Behavioral Assessment, 4,* 1-35.

Merrell, K. (1993). *School Social Behavior Scales.* Brandon, VT: Clinical Psychology Publishing.

Noell, G.H., & Gresham, F.M. (1993). Functional outcome analysis: Do the benefits of consultation and prereferral intervention justify the costs? *School Psychology Quarterly, 8,* 200–226.

O'Neill, R., Horner, R., Albin, R., Storey, K., & Sprague, J. (1990). *Functional analysis of problem behavior.* Sycamore, IL: Sycamore.

Oleweus, D. (1979). Stability of aggressive reaction patterns in males: A review. *Psychological Bulletin, 86,* 852–875.

Ottenbacher, K. (1990). When is a picture is worth a thousand *p* values? A comparison of visual and quantitative methods to analyze single case data. *Journal of Special Education, 23,* 436–449.

Parker, J., & Asher, S. (1987). Peer relations and later personal adjustment: Are low-accepted children at-risk? *Psychological Bulletin, 102,* 357–389.

Patterson, G., DeBaryshe, B., & Ramsey, E. (1989). A developmental perspective on antisocial behavior. *American Psychologist, 44,* 329–335.

Pelham, W., & Bender, M. (1982). Peer relationships in hyperactive children: Description and treatment. In K. Gadow & I. Bialer (Eds.), *Advances in learning and behavioral disabilities* (Vol. 1, pp. 365–436). Greenwich, CT: JAI.

Reid, J., & Patterson, G. (1991). Early prevention and intervention with conduct problems: A social interactional model for the integration of research and practice. In G. Stoner, M. Shinn, & H. Walker (Eds.), *Interventions for achievement and behavior problems* (pp. 715–740). Washington, DC: National Association of School Psychologists.

Roff, M. (1961). Childhood social interactions and young adult bad conduct. *Journal of Abnormal and Social Psychology, 63,* 333–337.

Roff, M., Sells, S., & Golden, M. (1972). *Social adjustment and personality development in children.* Minneapolis: University of Minnesota Press.

Schneider, B. (1992). Didactic methods for enhancing children's peer relations: A quantitative review. *Clinical Psychology Review, 12,* 363–382.

Schwartz, I., & Baer, D. (1991). Social validity assessment: Is current practice state of the art? *Journal of Applied Behavior Analysis, 24,* 189–204.

Sechrest, L., McKnight, P., & McKnight, K. (1996). Calibration of measures for psychotherapy outcome studies. *American Psychologist, 51,* 1065–1071.

Skiba, R., & Grizzle, K. (1991). The social maladjustment exclusion: Issues of definition and assessment. *School Psychology Review, 20,* 577–595.

Stengel, E. (1971). *Suicide and attempted suicide.* Harmondsworth, England: Penguin.

Stephens, T., & Arnold, K. (1992). *Social Behavior Assessment Inventory: Professional manual.* Odessa, FL: Psychological Assessment Resources.

Stokes, T. (1992). Discrimination and generalization. *Journal of Applied Behavior Analysis, 25,* 429–432.

Stokes, T., & Osnes, P. (1989). An operant pursuit of generalization. *Behavior Therapy, 20,* 337–355.

Stuart, R. (1971). Behavioral contracting within families of delinquents. *Journal of Behavioral Therapy and Experimental Psychiatry, 2,* 1–11.

Walker, H., & McConnell, S. (1995). *Walker-McConnell Scale of Social Competence and School Adjustment.* San Diego, CA: Singular Press.

Walker, H., & Severson, H. (1992). *Systematic screening for behavior disorders.* Longmont, CO: Sopris West.

Walker, H., McConnell, S., Holmes, D., Todis, B., Walker, J., & Golden, N. (1983). *The Walker Social Skills Curriculum: The ACCEPTS Program (A curriculum for children's effective peer and teacher skills).* Austin, TX: Pro-Ed.

Walker, H., McConnell, S., & Clark, J. (1985). Social skills training in school settings: A model for the social integration of handicapped children into less restrictive settings. In R. McMahon & R. Peters (Eds.), *Childhood disorders: Behavioral developmental approaches* (pp. 140–168). New York: Brunner-Mazel.

Walker, H., Irwin, L., Noell, J., & Singer, G. (1992). A construct score approach to the assessment of social competence: Rationale, technological considerations, and anticipated outcomes. *Behavior Modification, 16,* 448–474.

Walker, H., Colvin, G., & Ramsey, E. (1995). *Antisocial behavior in school: Strategies and best practices.* Pacific Grove, CA: Brooks/Cole.

Whalen, C., Henker, B., & Hinshaw, S. (1985). Cognitive-behavioral therapies for hyperactive children: Premises, problems, and prospects. *Journal of Abnormal Child Psychology, 13,* 391–410.

Wolf, M.M. (1978). Social validity: The case for subjective measurement or how applied behavior analysis is finding its heart. *Journal of Applied Behavior Analysis, 11,* 211–226.

25

Current Issues in Child Behavior Therapy

T. STEUART WATSON AND FRANK M. GRESHAM

There are many issues facing behavior analysts/ therapists that will undoubtedly influence the way the science of behavior change is practiced with children, adolescents, and their families and teachers. Some of these issues arise from advancements in the science itself (e.g., functional assessment/ analysis, methods to improve treatment integrity), whereas others arise from changes driven largely by economically motivated contingencies (e.g., prescription privileges, managed care). Other issues arise from the broader field of psychology and have direct relevance to the professional identity of many behavior analysts/therapists (e.g., professional title ["behavior analyst" versus "school psychologist," "clinical psychologist," "counseling psychologist," or "organizational psychologist"]). We will, in this chapter, address each of these issues and offer what we hope is a representative view shared by most behaviorists who read this book. Clearly, we cannot, and do not wish to, speak for all behaviorists. There is considerable disagreement and sometimes professional complacency regarding these issues and, like divorce, there are two sides to every issue. We will try to be fair in our discussion yet maintain integrity with the science to which this book is devoted.

T. STEUART WATSON • School Psychology Program, Mississippi State University, Mississippi State, Mississippi 39762.   FRANK M. GRESHAM • School of Education, University of California–Riverside, Riverside, California 92521-0102.

The Future of Child Behavior Therapy Practice

The chapters in this book have covered a myriad of problems, including academic problems, social/behavior problems, and medical problems. In describing the treatment process, each chapter author has taken a functional approach for treating a variety of child problems. We earnestly believe that a functional approach is the "wave of the future" in child behavior therapy. Prior to the development of functional analysis methodology (Iwata, Dorsey, Slifer, Bauman & Richman, 1982), treatment for child problems usually involved applying reinforcement or punishment contingencies, sometimes in a haphazard fashion, without particular regard to function. From this nonfunctional approach, many effective treatments were developed (e.g., differential reinforcement, extinction, aversive stimulation, habit reversal) for a host of problems (e.g., feeding, stereotypy, self-injury, rumination, thumb sucking). Despite the relative success of these interventions, when treatment was unsuccessful or lost its effectiveness over time, the therapist was often at a loss to explain why the treatment was ineffective. Without knowing the function of a particular behavior, it was almost impossible to specify with any degree of certainty the reason for treatment failure. Often, the behavior was labeled recalcitrant or the client was labeled resistant. These labels did nothing to improve the effectiveness of therapy.

Handbook of Child Behavior Therapy, edited by Watson and Gresham. Plenum Press, New York, 1998.

Functional analysis remedied many of the problems with the traditional method of choosing interventions, by focusing not on the topography of behavior, but on the function of a behavior in the context in which it occurred. Over the past 14 years, this emphasis on functional assessment and analysis has been apparent in the number of journal articles that have featured using functional assessment/analysis methodology to derive treatment for a wide variety of problems. Despite the many advantages of functional analysis and its direct link to treatment, there are some serious drawbacks that have slowed its acceptance and growth in certain areas (e.g., school-based interventions) and that must be addressed in order to increase the use of functional methodology across settings.

One obvious limitation is that not all behaviors lend themselves to an experimental manipulation to determine function. For example, behaviors that occur during sleep (e.g., bruxism, enuresis), with low frequency (a child who fights at school every couple of weeks), or that are covert (e.g., intraverbal negative statements) are more suited to a descriptive assessment than to an experimental functional analysis. Because these behaviors may be infrequent or covert, there may be a greater tendency to apply treatments in a prescribed fashion without assessing their function. Despite, or because of, the difficulty involved in assessing function, behavior analysts must devise innovative methods for analyzing function for relatively inaccessible behaviors.

Another limitation of functional analysis is that, in many cases, it is a time-consuming and complex procedure. To counter this limitation, researchers have developed brief and hierarchical functional analysis procedures to reduce the time involved to conduct the analysis (e.g., Cooper, Wacker, Sasso, Reimers, & Donn, 1990; Harding, Wacker, Cooper, Millard, & Jensen-Kovalan, 1994; Northup et al., 1991). These brief procedures have particular relevance to the typical clinic or school situation where there are limited time and resources to conduct in-depth analyses. In addition, although we obviously prefer the methodological rigor of the experimental analysis, we acknowledge that most practitioners, because of parsimony and economy, will prefer to use descriptive assessments. There is support for the use of descriptive assessments, as research has found that the results of carefully constructed assessments closely match the results from an experimental analysis (Sasso et al., 1992).

A third limitation involves the very nature of the analysis itself. Most published studies on functional analysis have used highly trained experimenters (i.e., researchers with considerable skill in conducting experimental analyses) to manipulate the differing conditions, often in settings apart, and thus different, from where the behavior occurs. Initially, this analogue arrangement was required to establish proper control to illustrate the functional relationships between stimuli and responses. However, this type of setup may or may not have resembled the setting in which the behavior occurred, thus limiting the generalizability of the findings. For example, a behavior may occur in the presence of one person (e.g., experimenter) and be maintained by social attention, whereas in the presence of a different person (e.g., classroom teacher) the behavior may be maintained by escape from an aversive social interaction. Thus, the topography of the behavior may be roughly the same, but the function varies according to the presence or absence of particular discriminative stimuli. If the problem was classroom based and the function was identified in an analogue setting, the treatment would likely be ineffective because the function of the behavior was related to the presence or absence of a particular stimulus.

Some researchers have taken the position that the most reliable and valid functional analysis arises from teaching direct-care providers the analysis procedures. Watson, Ray, Sterling, and Logan (1996), for example, taught functional analysis procedures to a special education teacher who referred a child for self-injurious behavior. After the experimenters explained the rationale for a functional analysis and described and modeled the procedure, the teacher conducted the analysis while receiving feedback from the experimenters. The training resulted in the teacher conducting the analysis with 82% integrity. That is, the teacher performed the analysis correctly 82% of the time. Treatment was then based on the results of the analysis data collected by the teacher, which increased the likelihood that the function was correctly identified and that the ensuing treatment matched the function of the self-injurious behavior.

The fourth limitation of functional analysis is that it was developed and refined using primarily the developmentally disabled population. Persons with developmental disabilities with coexisting behavior problems tend to exhibit overt, high-frequency behaviors (e.g., stereotypy, self-injurious behavior, rumination, skin picking, rectal digging). Behaviors with these characteristics easily lend themselves to a functional analysis. Identifying and controlling stimuli is also easier when working with inpatient developmentally disabled persons than with those who have access to, or can access, many different stimuli. Functional analysis methodology, for the most part, has not been extended to problems evidenced by the non-developmentally disabled population (e.g., temper tantrums, habits, depression, overeating, negative self-statements, anxiety). There are some notable exceptions, such as Lewis and Sugai's (1993) study that used brief functional analyses in regular education classrooms for children exhibiting withdrawn behavior. Until functional analysis is expanded to address problems experienced by "normal" individuals, however, it will not obtain widespread acceptance as a viable therapeutic tool among those outside the relatively small behavior analytic community.

Despite the many advancements in functional analysis methodology, there remains much to be done. For example, most of the research in functional analysis has concentrated on identifying the maintaining consequences and not on identifying the stimuli that evoke, or do not evoke, a particular behavior. As Carr (1994) correctly noted, specifying only the maintaining stimuli for a behavior neglects the possibility of changing behavior by altering stimulus, or antecedent, control. In addition, behavior analysts have discussed the effects of temporally distant stimuli on behavior (i.e., establishing operations, setting events) but have contributed very little in the way of designing a methodology for identifying these stimulus events and demonstrating functional relationships with specific behaviors. Most behavior analysts will concede that there is a variety of temporally distant events that may affect behavior, but instead have focused on the most temporally proximate stimuli because of convenience and a readily available empirical base for doing so.

Treatment Integrity

An issue closely related to functional analysis is treatment integrity, which is defined as the degree to which a chosen intervention is implemented as it was intended. From our perspective, treatment integrity is second in importance only to functional analysis. Regardless of the accuracy of the functional analysis in identifying the maintaining function of a behavior and the potential effectiveness of a chosen intervention, if the intervention is not implemented at all or is implemented with poor integrity, then the chances of positive outcome are greatly diminished. Gresham, Gansle, and Noell (1993) reviewed studies published in the *Journal of Applied Behavior Analysis* (JABA) and found that only 16% of the studies assessed treatment integrity. Considering that JABA is the most prominent and methodologically rigorous behavior change journal, it is unlikely that a greater percentage of studies published in other journals have seriously considered the issue of treatment integrity. In fact, a similar study by Gresham, Gansle, Noell, Cohen, and Rosenblum (1993) revealed that only 15% of articles published in seven prominent behavioral journals assessed and reported treatment integrity. Quite clearly, researchers publishing intervention studies in the leading behavioral journals are not modeling appropriate behavior in terms of measuring integrity of treatment.

For most behaviorists, designing effective treatments is not a difficult matter. The difficulty lies in prompting or teaching others to implement the treatment. Considerable research has examined some of the variables thought to be related to a person's willingness to implement a particular treatment. One of these highly researched variables is treatment acceptability. The idea behind treatment acceptability is that consumers are more likely to implement treatments that they find acceptable. The notion of acceptability, admittedly, carries a certain degree of face validity. However, there is no empirical evidence showing a functional relationship between ratings of treatment acceptability and integrity. In fact, recent research suggests that direct consumer training, not acceptability, is the functional variable for increasing treatment integrity (Sterling, Watson, Wildmon, Watkins, & Little, 1996). Thus, we suggest that behavior therapists spend less time making treatments acceptable and more time training the consumers of our services to implement the chosen intervention.

Prescription Privileges

A current issues chapter would not be complete without at least a brief discussion of the prescription privilege debate currently raging within all camps of psychology. The motivation for pursuing prescription privileges seems to stem from two primary sources: (1) economic incentives and (2) a desire to increase the prestige of the profession by making psychologists more like physicians and psychiatrists. We recognize that some psychologists are seeking prescription privileges so that they can provide more comprehensive services to their clients, but we believe these psychologists are in the minority.

As behaviorists, we cannot ignore the empirical evidence regarding the effectiveness of some psychotropic medications for changing behavior, if only temporarily. That medication changes behavior, however, is not the issue. One of the issues is whether behaviorists, who have worked diligently to separate their science and practice from the medical model view of behavior, will embrace what is decidedly a medical treatment component. Further, there is ample evidence that many of the behavior problems evidenced by children are not well suited for psychopharmacological treatment, as there are high relapse rates after medication is discontinued (see, for example Chapter 13 on enuresis, this volume) and equivocal evidence regarding the effectiveness of medication above and beyond results achieved with behavior therapy alone (see, for example, Chapters 17 and 20 on eating disorders and affective disturbances, this volume). In addition, as DuPaul and Hoff (this volume, Chapter 6) correctly note, Ritalin© and other stimulant medications may help to control inattentive, impulsive behavior, but it has almost no affect on acquisition of academic skills. In our experience, the majority of children diagnosed with ADHD are receiving only medication as treatment and yet they are frequently referred for academic skill deficits. Regardless of whether the child is on medication, our assessment/analysis procedures will not be affected, nor will the resulting treatment. Thus, the practice of using stimulant medication as "the" treatment for ADHD is highly questionable and of little value for the behavior analyst.

Philosophically, some behaviorists are against acquiring prescription privileges because it contradicts their approach to changing behavior. Others oppose it because this is precisely what separates us from psychiatrists, who are not well trained in non-pharmaceutical behavior change. Conversely, some behaviorists support prescription privileges because there is no arguable reason why only medical doctors can prescribe psychoactive medications and because we are the ones who can best empirically evaluate the effects of medication on behavior.

We see prescription privileges for properly trained psychologists as an inevitability. Many other health care professionals (e.g., nurse practitioners, physician's assistants, optometrists, dentists) have prescription privileges that are limited to their area of expertise. Thus, there is very little valid argument against psychologists acquiring prescription privileges, because the precedent has been adequately established in these and other professions.

Professional Identity

Within the American Psychological Association there is a historical precedent for defining one's professional identity largely as a function of where one practices. For example, those who work primarily in VA hospitals and other clinical type settings refer to themselves as "clinical psychologists." Psychologists who work in schools call themselves "school psychologists," and psychologists who work in business or industry settings refer to themselves as "industrial/organizational psychologists." These titles communicate very little about what the behavioral psychologist working in that setting is capable of doing.

We do not believe that location of practice should determine what we call ourselves. The only differences among behavior analysts working in school settings, clinic settings, outpatient counseling settings, business settings, and so forth, is the location of practice. Essentially, the behavior analyst is carrying the same science of behavior change into a variety of settings. Thus, we recommend that behaviorists refer to themselves as "a behavior analyst working in the schools" or "a behaviorist working in a medical setting." Referring to ourselves in the context of our science of behavior change rather than the location of practice will help to establish the credibility of behavior analysis and will educate others about what we do.

A related concern is the dogmatic interpretation of professional titles by some state licensing boards to determine where one is competent to practice. For example, because psychologists who work in the schools are often called "school psychologists," there is often an attempt to prevent school psychologists from working in settings apart from public schools. This is often viewed as "restriction of trade" and a brazen attempt by some psychologists to protect their economic and professional turf from "outsiders." By calling ourselves "behavior analysts" much of the nonsense about *where* one is competent to practice is avoided and opens the door to a variety of settings for appropriately trained behaviorists.

Essence of Child Behavior Therapy

Stokes (1992) said that we should ultimately be concerned with two things: discrimination and generalization. This is the essence of child behavior therapy and of behavior therapy in general. In order to successfully adapt to the environment, humans must know when and where to exhibit a behavior (discrimination), be able to make responses similar to responses in the past (response generalization), and be able to exhibit a response in the presence of many different stimuli that share functional properties (stimulus generalization). Thus, the job of the behavior analyst is to design interventions that teach children when and when not to exhibit a particular behavior and how to use that and similar behaviors in many different situations. Suffice it to say that effective behavior therapy is more than just changing behavior; it is equipping clients with skills (ability to discriminate and generalize) they can use apart from the training situation that make them more successful, likable, sociable, efficient, and so on.

Managed Care

Managed care has permeated the practice of all types of therapy/treatment, including behavior therapy. The primary motivating contingency behind managed care is *profit*. In a capitalist society there is certainly nothing wrong with making an honest profit, which includes controlling the costs of goods and services. Therapy is a service, albeit in most cases a costly one, that, if left uncontrolled, will seriously hinder an insurance provider from making a profit. The basic demands of managed care, relative to psychological treatment, are that a careful assessment is conducted to identify the problem and the related biological, psychological, and social variables, a focused treatment plan is written, the specified treatment has an empirical basis relative to the identified problem, and that outcome data are collected to show that treatment is working (Donovan, Steinberg, & Sabin, 1994).

The demands of managed care are very consistent with the practice of behavior therapy. Managed care is, in a sense, catching up to what behavior analysts have been preaching for decades regarding treatment services. As has been demonstrated in chapter after chapter in this volume, behaviorists identify the problem, identify the variables that are functionally related to the problem, design treatment based on known functional variables, and collect data to show the relationship between intervention and outcome. Because of the rigor involved in behavior therapy and the reliance on empirical data throughout the therapeutic process, there is no reason to fear managed care as a threat to the provision of data-based psychological services to children and their families.

Conclusion

In this book we have tried to establish a different approach for using behavior analysis and therapy for a variety of problems evidenced in childhood. The tack we have taken differs markedly from other child behavior therapy texts where the emphasis has traditionally focused on building effective treatments regardless of function. Quite obviously, this different approach is using functional assessment and analysis methodology for assessing and treating behavior. We hope that novice behavior analysts will embrace the "functional message" and expand on it throughout their careers and that experienced behavior analysts will refine and extend, in future texts and in practice, what we have tried to accomplish.

References

Carr, E.G. (1994). Emerging themes in the functional analysis of problem behavior. *Journal of Applied Behavior Analysis, 27,* 393–400.

Cooper, L.J., Wacker, D.P., Sasso, G.M., Reimers, T.M., & Donn, L. (1990). Using parents as therapists to evaluate appropriate behavior of their children: Application to a tertiary diagnostic clinic. *Journal of Applied Behavior Analysis, 23,* 285–296.

Donovan, J.M., Steinberg, S.M., & Sabin, J.E. (1994). Managed mental health: An academic seminar. *Psychotherapy, 31,* 201–207.

Gresham, F.M., Gansle, K.A., & Noell, G.H. (1993). Treatment integrity in applied behavior analysis with children. *Journal of Applied Behavior Analysis, 26,* 257–264.

Gresham, F.M., Gansle, K.A., Noell, G.H., Cohen, S., & Rosenblum, S. (1993). Treatment integrity of school-based behavioral intervention studies: 1980–1990. *School Psychology Review, 22,* 254–272.

Harding, J., Wacker, D.P., Cooper, L.J., Millard, T., & Jensen-Kovalan, P. (1994). Brief hierarchical assessment of potential treatment components with children in an outpatient clinic. *Journal of Applied Behavior Analysis, 27,* 291–300.

Iwata, B.A., Dorsey, M.F., Slifer, K.J., Bauman, K.E., & Richman, G.S. (1982). Toward a functional analysis of self-injury. *Analysis and Intervention in Developmental Disabilities, 2,* 3–20.

Lewis, T.J., & Sugai, G. (1993). Teaching communicative alternatives to socially withdrawn behavior: An investigation in maintaining treatment effects. *Journal of Behavioral Education, 3,* 61–76.

Northup, J., Wacker, D.P., Sasso, G., Steege, M., Cigrand, K., Cook, J., & DeRaad, A. (1991). A functional analysis of both aggressive behavior and alternative behavior in an out-clinic setting. *Journal of Applied Behavior Analysis, 24,* 509–522.

Sasso, G.M., Reimers, T.M., Cooper, L.J., Wacker, D.P., Berg, W., Steege, M., Kelly, L., & Allaire, A. (1992). Use of descriptive and experimental analyses to identify the functional properties of aberrant behavior in school settings. *Journal of Applied Behavior Analysis, 25,* 809–822.

Sterling, H.E., Watson, T.S., Wildmon, M., Watkins, C., & Little, E. (1996). *Treatment acceptability, direct training, and treatment integrity: Applications to consultation.* Manuscript submitted for publication.

Stokes, T. (1992). Discrimination and generalization. *Journal of Applied Behavior Analysis, 25,* 429–432.

Watson, T.S., Ray, K.P., Sterling, H.E., & Logan, P. (1996). *Evaluating direct behavioral consultation: Teaching functional analysis procedures to a special education teacher.* Manuscript submitted for publication.

Index

ISBN 0-306-45548-X

90000